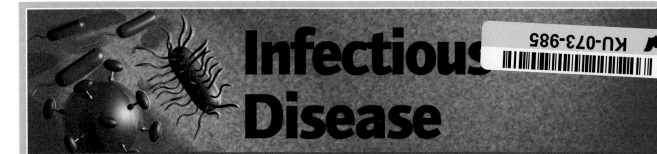

Infectious Disease

Barbara A. Bannister

MSc, FRCP
Consultant in Infectious & Tropical Diseases
Royal Free Department of Infectious & Tropical Diseases
Coppetts Wood Hospital
London

Norman T. Begg

DTM&H, FFPHM
Deputy Director
Public Health Laboratory Service
Communicable Disease Surveillance Centre
London

Stephen H. Gillespie

MD, FRCP (Edin), MRCPath
Senior Lecturer in Medical Microbiology
Royal Free Hospital School of Medicine
London

b

**Blackwell
Science**

International
Edition

© 1996 by
Blackwell Science Ltd
Editorial Offices:
Osney Mead, Oxford OX2 0EL
25 John Street, London WC1N 2BL
23 Ainslie Place, Edinburgh EH3 6AJ
238 Main Street, Cambridge
    Massachusetts 02142, USA
54 University Street, Carlton
    Victoria 3053, Australia

Other Editorial Offices:
Arnette Blackwell SA
    224, Boulevard Saint Germain
    75007 Paris, France

Blackwell Wissenschafts-Verlag GmbH
    Kurfürstendamm 57
    10707 Berlin, Germany

    Zehetnergasse 6, A-1140 Wien
    Austria

First published 1996

Set by Expo Holdings Sdn Bhd, Malaysia
Printed and bound in Italy
by Rotolito Lombarda, Milan

A catalogue record for this title
is available from the British Library

ISBN 0-632-03251-0 (BSL)
    0-86542-619-8 (IE)

Library of Congress
Cataloging-in-Publication Data

Bannister, Barbara A.
    Infectious disease/
    Barbara A. Bannister, Norman T. Begg,
    Stephen H. Gillespie
            p.   cm.
    Includes bibliographical references
and index
    ISBN 0-632-03251-0
    1. Communicable diseases.
I. Begg, Norman T.
II. Gillespie, S.H.
III. Title.
    [DNLM: 1. Communicable Diseases.
WC 100 B219i 1996]
    RC111.B364   1996
    616.9—dc20
    DNLM/DLC
    for Library of Congress   95–42226

DISTRIBUTORS

Marston Book Services Ltd
PO Box 87
Oxford OX2 0DT
(*Orders*: Tel: 01865 791155
            Fax: 01865 791927
            Telex: 837515)

USA
Blackwell Science, Inc.
238 Main Street
Cambridge, MA 02142
(*Orders*: Tel: 800 215-1000
            617 876-7000
            Fax: 617 492-5263)

Canada
Copp Clark, Ltd
2775 Matheson Blvd East
Mississauga, Ontario
Canada, L4W 4P7
(*Orders*: Tel: 800 263–4374
            905 238–6074)

Australia
Blackwell Science Pty Ltd
54 University Street
Carlton, Victoria 3053
(*Orders*: Tel: 03 9347 0300
            Fax: 03 9349-3016)

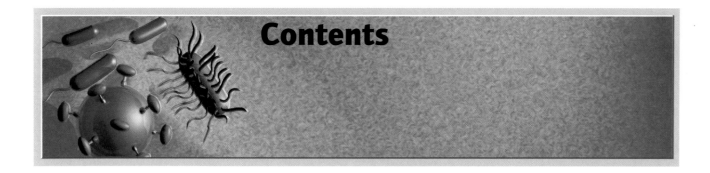

Contents

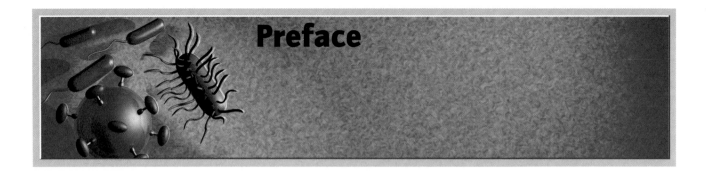

Preface

Infectious Disease encompasses the clinical practice of infectious diseases not in isolation, but as they occur both in hospital and in the community. It has been designed as a problem-solving text which will be equally useful to those preparing for examinations or working in the clinical setting. It is not intended to replace comprehensive textbooks of microbiology or epidemiology.

The introductory chapters set out the important definitions required for the understanding of infectious diseases and describe the nature and presentation of infection, its pathogenesis and scientific investigation. The diagnosis, management and control of individual infectious diseases are described in the systematic chapters. Each chapter introduces the range of diseases affecting the relevant system and a list of pathogens is presented for each disease in the approximate order of importance. For each individual disease there is a discussion of the microbiology and epidemiology of the relevant pathogens, the diagnosis and management of the disease and strategies for their prevention and control.

This textbook is designed to be used either as a basic learning text or as a practical textbook in the clinical setting. It should therefore be most useful for senior medical students and for doctors preparing for the MRCP (UK) and the Primary FRCS. It would also be a useful revision text for those studying for final MRCPath and MFCM and a companion textbook for doctors early in their careers, for physicians, surgeons and public health specialists throughout their training and afterwards. It is intended to provide guidance on the range of conditions which can present in various systems and different situations. It can then be used as a logical guide to diagnosis, management and follow-up. It provides information in the order in which the clinician requires it, based on expert experience in clinical management, microbiology and epidemiology. There are common-sense warnings about avoidable setbacks and complications. It contains much information which will be useful to infection control nurses, community nurses and environmental health officers.

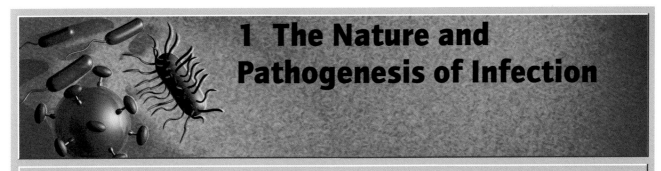

1 The Nature and Pathogenesis of Infection

Introduction

The nature of infection

The terminology used in discussion of infectious diseases is sometimes confusing. Some terms have gone out of use or changed their meaning, often because of recent changes in the knowledge and understanding of infection. We will therefore start by discussing some definitions of terms used in this book.

Pathogen

> **Pathogen**
> An organism which can invade the body and cause disease.

A pathogen is defined as any organism capable of invading the body and causing disease. Such an organism is said to be pathogenic. Koch isolated and identified organisms such as *Mycobacterium tuberculosis* or *Bacillus anthracis*, where the isolation of the organism only occurred in the presence of disease. It is easy to define these bacteria as pathogens. They also fulfil Koch's further definition of a pathogen, that introduction of a pure culture of the organism into a healthy host can cause the disease.

More recently, our understanding of many micro-organisms has improved. For instance, *Escherichia coli* is found in huge numbers in the healthy human bowel, and could therefore be defined as non-pathogenic. However, *E. coli* has now been associated with diarrhoeal diseases, and potent enterotoxins have been found in some strains. Such an organism can behave as a pathogen or a colonizer, depending on various circumstances. A broader definition of a biological agent used in European Union legislation is: 'any microorganism, cell culture or toxin capable of entering the human body and causing harm'.

Changes in medical practice mean that increasing numbers of patients are immunocompromised as the result of immunosuppressive treatments. In these circumstances organisms which are usually non-pathogenic, such as saprophytic fungi, may act as pathogens. Intensive therapy medicine, with insertion of intravascular cannulae, allows *Staphylococcus epidermidis*, a normal part of the skin flora, to enter the cannula and cause significant blood-borne infection, behaving as a pathogen.

Parasites as pathogens

The term parasite is often confusing, as not all 'parasites' cause disease. The real definition of a parasite is an organism that lives on or in another organism, deriving benefit from it but providing nothing in return. Parasitic organisms such as *Entamoeba coli*, a protozoan, live in the human gut without causing human disease and are thus colonizers. The closely related species *E. histolytica* is capable of invading the bowel wall, causing colitis and abscesses in the liver, brain and other tissues. It is thus a pathogen, and this term will be applied to it, and other parasitic pathogens, in this book. Multicellular parasites such as schistosomes may also be pathogens.

Infection

> **Infection**
> A disease caused by a pathogen.

An infection is a disease caused by a pathogen. The human body is colonized on the skin and mucosal surfaces with a large number of microorganisms which form the body's normal flora. These organisms, far from causing disease, often provide benefit to the host, by competing with potential pathogens for attachment sites, by producing antimicrobial substances toxic to pathogens and by competing for nutrients with pathogens. Thus, the mere presence of microorganisms multiplying in the human body does not constitute an infection (Fig. 1.1). It is the presence of the replicating organism *in association with tissue damage* that defines the condition as an infection. *Clostridium tetani* may multiply in a puncture wound, elaborating the neurotoxin tetanospasmin. Because the organism is multiplying in the host's tissues, the resulting disease can be called an infection. In contrast, adult botulism, caused by *C. botulinum*, develops when food is ingested in which this organism has grown and elaborated a neurotoxin; the organism itself does not replicate in the human host. Botulism is therefore an intoxication (poisoning), rather than an infection. *C. difficile* may be isolated from the faeces of 5–20% of normal subjects. However, it is only when conditions within the large bowel are altered by antibiotic therapy that this organism produces its toxin, causing pseudomembranous colitis. In this case colonization, the presence of microorganisms in the human host in the absence of disease, has developed into an infection.

Infections caused by parasites

In the past, diseases caused by metazoan parasites, such as schistosomiasis, were sometimes called infestations. Nowadays all parasitic diseases are called infections.

Communicable disease

> **Communicable disease**
> An infection which is capable of spreading from person to person.

A communicable disease is an infection which is capable of spreading from person to person. Not all infections are communicable diseases. A patient with infective endocarditis caused by *Streptococcus sanguis* is suffering from an infection. This is, however, not a communicable disease as it is unable to spread from this patient to another. Communicable diseases may be transmitted by many routes: direct person-to-person transfer; respiratory transmission; parenteral inoculation; sexual or mucosal contact; and by insect vectors (see p. 5).

Pathogenicity

> **Pathogenicity**
> The ability to cause disease.

Pathogenicity is the ability to cause disease. *Neisseria gonorrhoeae* is the causative organism of gonorrhoea. It is a small Gram-negative diplococcus, some strains of which bear surface projections called pili, while some do not. Those organisms with pili can attach to the urethral epithelium and cause disease. Those which lack this feature cannot and are non-pathogenic. In this example, pili confer pathogenicity. Mechanisms of pathogenicity are numerous, and will later be discussed more fully (see pp. 14–17).

Virulence

> **Virulence**
> The pathogen's power to cause severe disease.

Virulence may be defined as the pathogen's power to cause severe disease. When a pathogen causes infection, the resulting disease may be asymptomatic or mild, but can sometimes be severe. This variation may be due in part to host factors, but may also be dependent on virulence factors possessed by the organism. Influenza virus is constantly able to modify its antigenic structure, on which its virulence depends. The difference in the attack rate and the severity of disease in succeeding epidemics is related to the antigenic structure of the causative virus.

Pathogenicity and virulence are not necessarily related. This is illustrated by *Streptococcus pneumoniae* which depends on its polysaccharide capsule for its pathogenicity. In the absence of the capsule, the lethal infecting dose for a mouse is increased 100 000 times. The biochemical nature of the polysaccharide alters the virulence of the organism. Type 3 and type 30 pneumococci produce copious quantities of capsular material, and both are therefore pathogenic. Infection with type 3 is often associated with severe disease. In contrast, infection with type 30 rarely causes severe disease. For a further discussion of pneumococcal pathogenicity see p. 137.

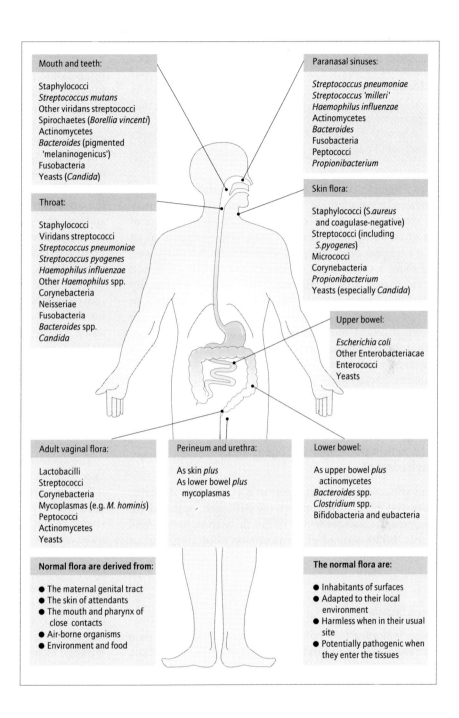

Mouth and teeth:

Staphylococci
Streptococcus mutans
Other viridans streptococci
Spirochaetes (*Borellia vincenti*)
Actinomycetes
Bacteroides (pigmented
 'melaninogenicus')
Fusobacteria
Yeasts (*Candida*)

Throat:

Staphylococci
Viridans streptococci
Streptococcus pneumoniae
Streptococcus pyogenes
Haemophilus influenzae
Other *Haemophilus* spp.
Corynebacteria
Neisseriae
Fusobacteria
Bacteroides spp.
Candida

Paranasal sinuses:

Streptococcus pneumoniae
Streptococcus 'milleri'
Haemophilus influenzae
Actinomycetes
Bacteroides
Fusobacteria
Peptococci
Propionibacterium

Skin flora:

Staphylococci (S.*aureus*
 and coagulase-negative)
Streptococci (including
 S.pyogenes)
Micrococci
Corynebacteria
Propionibacterium
Yeasts (especially *Candida*)

Upper bowel:

Escherichia coli
Other Enterobacteriacae
Enterococci
Yeasts

Adult vaginal flora:

Lactobacilli
Streptococci
Corynebacteria
Mycoplasmas (e.g. *M. hominis*)
Peptococci
Actinomycetes
Yeasts

Perineum and urethra:

As skin *plus*
As lower bowel *plus*
 mycoplasmas

Lower bowel:

As upper bowel *plus*
 actinomycetes
Bacteroides spp.
Clostridium spp.
Bifidobacteria and eubacteria

Normal flora are derived from:

● The maternal genital tract
● The skin of attendants
● The mouth and pharynx of
 close contacts
● Air-borne organisms
● Environment and food

The normal flora are:

● Inhabitants of surfaces
● Adapted to their local
 environment
● Harmless when in their usual
 site
● Potentially pathogenic when
 they enter the tissues

Fig. 1.1 Normal human flora.

Infectiousness

Infectiousness
The ease with which a pathogen can spread in a population.

Infectiousness is the ease with which a pathogen can spread in a population. Some organisms always spread more readily than others. For example, measles is highly infectious and mumps very much less so. A measure of infectiousness is the intrinsic reproduction rate (IRR), which is the average number of secondary cases arising from a single index case in a totally susceptible population. The IRR for measles is 10–18, while for mumps it is 4–7.

Epidemiology of infections

Epidemiology

> Epidemiology
> The study of the distribution and determinants of diseases in populations.

This is the study of the distribution and determinants of diseases in populations. The distribution of diseases may be described in terms of time (day, month or year of onset of symptoms), person (age, sex, occupation) or place (region or country). The determinants of diseases are those factors which are associated with an increased or decreased risk of disease. Their effects are usually identified by analytical studies such as case-control or cohort studies. For example, the epidemiology of meningoccocal meningitis is characterized by its distribution (commonest in winter, peak incidence in young children, worldwide occurrence but especially in sub-Saharan Africa) and its determinants (close contact with a case, passive smoking).

Interaction between host, agent and environment

The behaviour of a pathogen in a population depends upon the interaction between the pathogen, host and environment. Changes in any one of these three factors will affect the likelihood of transmission occurring, and of disease resulting.

Host factors

Host factors affect both the chance of exposure to a pathogen and the individual's response to the infection. Important host factors include travel, sexual behaviour, hygiene, occupation, crowding, previous immunity, nutrition and underlying disease.

Agent factors

Agent factors include infectiousness, pathogenicity and virulence and their ability to survive in human and animal hosts and under different environmental conditions. Other important factors, such as the ability to resist vaccine-induced immune responses, or drugs, also play a large part in the effect of some diseases.

Environmental factors

Environmental factors such as temperature, dust and humidity, and the use of antibiotics and pesticides affect the survival of pathogens outside the host.

The spread of malaria is a good example of the interaction between host, pathogenic agent and environment. The agent, *Plasmodium* sp., is a protozoan parasite transmitted by the bite of an infected female anopheline mosquito. Subsequent asexual and sexual development of the organism takes place within the human hepatocytes and erythrocytes. In some forms of malaria (e.g. *P. vivax*) the organism may remain dormant in hepatocytes to mature months later and produce relapses. This does not occur in infections due to *P. falciparum*.

Many host factors affect the transmission of malaria: individuals who live in endemic areas develop partial immunity as a result of repeated exposure and rarely suffer severe disease. This immunity is lost after 1 or 2 years away from endemic exposure. Newcomers to endemic areas will usually suffer severe disease if infected. Certain genetic factors also affect the outcome of infection. For example, individuals with sickle-cell trait have a relatively low parasitaemia when infected with *P. falciparum*, because this parasite cannot derive effective nutrition from haemoglobin S.

The agent of *P. falciparum* malaria has developed resistance to an increasing range of prophylactic drugs, making it harder for travellers to protect themselves from infection. The very variable antigenic structures of the different stages of the parasite life cycle have made the development of an effective vaccine impossible up to now.

Environmental factors are particularly important in the spread of malaria. Transmission occurs predominantly (although not exclusively) in tropical zones, especially during the rainy season. The anopheline mosquito breeds in stagnant fresh-water environments, and malaria is particularly common in these areas. Drainage of ponds and tanks is an effective means of reducing malaria transmission. Residual insecticides have been used to control adult mosquito vectors; however this measure has had limited success due to the emergence of insecticide-resistant mosquitoes.

Sources and reservoirs of infection

Pathogens are either endogenous, arising from the host's own flora, or exogenous, arising from an external source. The reservoir of infection is the human or animal population, or environment in which the pathogen exists, and from which it can be transmitted. Infection can be transmitted from carriers of an organism as well as from those suffering active infection.

Person-to-person transmission is the most common method of spread. Horizontal spread is between individuals in the same population, as in the case of whooping cough. Vertical spread is also possible, from mother to fetus during gestation or birth, as in the case of congenital rubella or hepatitis B. Many pathogens can cross the placenta, but only a few cause fetal damage. The consequences of vertical transmission are usually, but not always, most serious when infection occurs during early pregnancy (see Chapter 12).

Animal diseases which spread to humans are called zoonoses. The normal infectious cycle between animals is accidentally entered by humans, most frequently where there is close contact between humans and animals, for instance in occupations such as farming or veterinary work or in recreations such as breeding fancy animals or birds.

Zoonosis
An animal disease which can spread to humans.

Many pathogens are environmental organisms, for example *Listeria monocytogenes*, *Legionella pneumophila* and *Clostridium tetani*. Spread from environment to humans can occur by ingestion (*Listeria monocytogenes*), inhalation (*Legionella pneumophila*) or inoculation (*C. tetani*).

Routes of transmission of infection

Fomites

Occasionally, inanimate environmental objects act as intermediaries, transporting pathogens from source to host. Fomites such as towels or bedding may transmit *Staphylococcus aureus* between hospital patients. Make-up applicators, towels and ophthalmic equipment have all been shown to carry bacterial or viral pathogens from eye to eye, when shared without adequate cleaning between uses.

Vectors

Vector
A living creature which can transmit infection from one host to another.

Vectors are living creatures which transmit infection from one host to another. Many arthropod species are able to transmit pathogens (Table 1.1).

Direct contact

Where pathogens are present on the skin or mucosal surfaces, transmission may occur by direct contact. Skin

Arthropod	Diseases
Mosquito	Malaria, dengue fever, filariasis, yellow fever
Sandfly	Leishmaniasis, sandfly fever
Fly	Trypanosomiasis, onchocerciasis
Flea	Plague, rickettsial infection
Tick	Relapsing fever, rickettsial infection
Mite	Rickettsial infection
Louse	Relapsing fever, typhus

Table 1.1 Arthropod vectors of medical importance

infections such as impetigo spread by this means. More fragile organisms cannot survive in a dry, cool environment, but can spread via sexual contact. In children, among whom direct contact is greater than in adults, pathogens in respiratory secretions may also be transmitted by direct contact. A few environmental pathogens can penetrate the skin and mucosae directly. An example of this type of spread is leptospirosis in which organisms excreted in the urine of infected animals penetrate the mucosae or broken skin of a human. Exposure usually occurs via contact with contaminated fresh water, e.g. during swimming, diving and water sports.

Inhalation

Droplets containing pathogens from the respiratory tract are expelled during sneezing, coughing and talking. Droplet nuclei (1–10 μm in diameter) are formed by partial evaporation of these droplets, and they remain suspended in air for long periods of time. Inhalation of droplet nuclei is the principal route of transmission for many human respiratory pathogens, e.g. influenza and measles. Transmission of pathogens by inhalation can also occur from animal to humans, e.g. *Chlamydia psittaci*, which is present in the droppings and secretions of infected birds. Inhalation of the organism usually occurs when infected birds are kept in a confined space.

Environmental pathogens can also be transmitted by inhalation. The most important example is *Legionella pneumophila*, the causative agent of legionnaire's disease, which is present in aerosols generated from air-conditioning cooling towers, cold-water taps, showers and other water systems. Depending upon wind speed, these aerosols can travel up to 500 m and infect large numbers of individuals.

Ingestion

Enteric pathogens are usually transmitted via contaminated food, milk or water. Many foods are produced from animals, thus ingestion commonly results in animal-to-person transmission. The two most important pathogens causing bacterial food poisoning (salmonellae and campylobacters) are both zoonotic pathogens readily transmitted to humans. Food-borne transmission is most likely if food is eaten raw or undercooked, as the pathogens are killed by heat. Many milk-borne infections are also zoonoses acquired by ingestion of unpasteurized milk products from infected cows, sheep or goats.

Spread by ingestion can occur when pathogens discharged in faeces, vomit, urine or respiratory secretions contaminate the hands of an infected individual or fomites such as handkerchiefs, clothes, and cooking and eating utensils. Subsequent spread to food or water is favoured by conditions of poor sanitation. A common form of transmission by ingestion occurs by direct contact between faecally contaminated hands and oral mucosa (faecal–oral transmission). Hepatitis A can spread by all of these means. *Salmonella typhi* may also be transmitted by these routes; a few organisms deposited in food will multiply to achieve an infective dose.

Transmission from environment to humans by ingestion is less common. However, the soil- and sewage-borne bacterium *Listeria monocytogenes* is an example, as it can contaminate food and cause invasive disease following ingestion.

Inoculation

Transmission can occur when a pathogen is inoculated directly into the body via a defect in the skin. Inoculation of contaminated transfusions, blood products or material from unsterile needles and syringes can transmit viruses such as hepatitis B and human immunodeficiency virus (HIV). Malaria may also be transmitted by contaminated blood transfusions.

Animal-to-person transmission occurs when an infected animal bites, scratches or licks an individual. Rabies is usually spread by this route. Alternatively, the skin may be broken by sharp animal bristles, or rough bone meal containing pathogens such as *Bacillus anthracis*.

Environment-to-person spread by inoculation also occurs: *Clostridium tetani* is usually introduced through a puncture wound contaminated with soil, dust or animal faeces.

Definition and types of outbreaks and epidemics

The terms outbreak and epidemic are usually synonymous. The word outbreak is used to describe a localized epidemic. This is the preferred term, as it avoids the sensationalism associated with the word epidemic. An outbreak is defined as an occurrence of a disease clearly in excess of normal expectancy. Outbreaks occurring in animal populations are called epizootic.

> **Outbreak**
> An occurrence of a disease clearly in excess of normal expectancy.

There are three main types of outbreaks — point-source, common-source and person-to-person (Fig. 1.2).

Point-source outbreak

A point-source outbreak occurs when a group of individuals is exposed to a single source of infection at a defined point in time. An example of this is a group of wedding guests who consume a contaminated food item at the reception. All those affected develop symptoms within a few days of each other.

Common-source outbreak

A common-source outbreak occurs when a group of individuals is exposed to a single source, but not necessarily at the same time. An example is an outbreak of hepatitis B associated with a tattoo parlour using contaminated equipment that is inadequately sterilized between customers. Common-source outbreaks may extend over long periods of time.

Person-to-person outbreak

In a person-to-person outbreak there is no common source: the outbreak is maintained by chains of transmission between infected individuals, for example a measles outbreak in a school.

Two other terms which sometimes cause confusion are endemic and pandemic. Endemic refers to a disease that occurs commonly all the year round, for example malaria in West Africa. A pandemic is an epidemic that affects all or most countries in the world at the same time. Only four communicable diseases have caused pandemics: influenza, plague, cholera and acquired immunodeficiency syndrome (AIDS).

Mechanisms of resistance to infection

The defence of the human host to infection can be classified into two parts: the non-specific, or innate immune system, and the specific immune system. Each

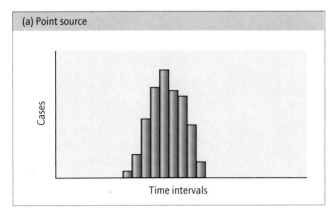

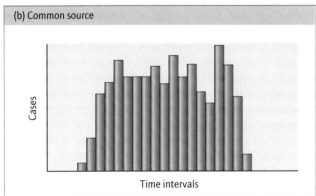

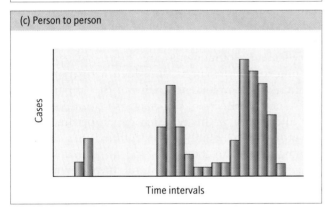

Fig. 1.2 Three types of outbreak: (a) point-source cases occur in a cluster after a single exposure, for example to a contaminated meal.
(b) Common-source cases occur over a period of time after continuing exposure, for example to a commercial distributed food.
(c) Person-to-person cases occur in clusters, separated by an incubation period.

is vital for survival against the continuous pressure of microorganisms.

Non-specific immunity

Many components of this function are normal mechanical and physiological properties of the host. They include the skin, the mechanical flushing activity of urine and intestinal contents, ciliary removal of mucus and debris, the enzymatic action of lysozyme in tears, the phagocytes and the normal flora.

The skin

Natural defences of the skin
1 Keratinous surface.
2 Antibacterial effects of sebum.
3 Effect of normal flora.

The skin forms a mechanical barrier to invasion. As well as this, sebum secreted by the skin inhibits the multiplication of microorganisms. The skin's resident bacterial flora competes with any potential invaders, and may produce metabolic products inhibitory to other species. This combination of effects is called colonization resistance and is also important in the pharynx and the bowel. Scratches, ulcers and other defects in the skin surface can penetrate its protective mechanisms and permit the entry of skin pathogens such as staphylococci or herpes simplex viruses, as well as more invasive organisms such as *Leptospira* spp.

Parasites such as hookworm larvae and schistosome cercariae are capable of invading through intact skin. Cercariae, which hatch from infected water snails, swim towards potential hosts. The head part of the cercaria secretes proteolytic enzymes which break down the skin (and, incidentally, cause a local dermatitis or 'swimmer's itch').

The physical barrier of the skin can also be breached by biting arthropods. Many types of pathogen are transmitted by this route. Intravenous access devices enable coagulase-negative staphylococci and corynebacteria from the skin to enter the blood stream and cause septicaemia and endocarditis. HIV and hepatitis B virus infection are transmitted by this route, through the use of contaminated needles.

Mucosal defences against infection

Natural defences of mucosae
1 Mechanical washing by tears or urine.
2 Lysozyme or antibody in surface fluid.
3 Surface phagocytes.
4 Ciliary action moving mucus and debris.

Many bacteria and viruses can invade through intact mucosal surfaces, which are not keratinized, and are often only one cell thick. Nevertheless, mucosal surfaces also have natural defences. They are usually moistened by tissue fluids, which contain lysozymes capable of destroying microbial peptidoglycan. If previous immunization has occurred, secretory immunoglobulin A (IgA) may also be present at the mucosal surface. Phagocytic neutrophils are often expelled at mucosal surfaces, and can ingest foreign material, including pathogens. The mucosae of the gut and the urinary tract are 'washed' by the constant throughput of liquid contents. The respiratory tract can move material upwards towards the pharynx by the action of mucosal cilia. These defence mechanisms are so effective that the urinary tract and respiratory tract are bacteriologically sterile, except for areas near the exterior, such as the mouth and the lower urethra. Sites which possess a colonizing flora, such as the bowel, also benefit from the additional colonization resistance that this confers.

Obstruction of a bronchus, ureter or bile duct, will overcome many of these defences, permitting pathogens to accumulate at sites of stagnation, thus predisposing to infection. Similarly, inserting a urinary catheter or an endotracheal tube will alter clearance mechanisms, encourage stagnation of mucus secretions around the tube and provide an inanimate substrate, encouraging the entry and establishment of a bacterial flora.

Defences against infection via the gut

Natural defences of the gut
1 Gastric acid.
2 Chemical environment produced by normal flora.
3 Bacteriocins.

The gut provides an important route for the acquisition of microbes. The first barrier to infection is gastric acid which inhibits the survival of many intestinal pathogens. Patients with achlorhydria are more susceptible to infections which are transmitted by the faecal–oral route. The normal flora also provides defence against invaders by competing for nutrients and attachment sites. Facultative and obligate anaerobes produce potent inhibitors of bacterial growth called bacteriocins. These protein antibiotics act to inhibit the growth of competing organisms. In addition the metabolic pathways of many obligate anaerobes produce free fatty acids and alter the local redox potential, making the environment less supportive to other microorganisms. This delicate competitive balance can be upset by disease or by antimicrobial therapy. The most dramatic example of this is pseudomembranous colitis, when patients treated with antibiotics have an overgrowth of *Clostridium difficile* in the intestine. This organism produces a toxin which causes severe ulcerative disease of the large bowel.

Classical and alternative complement systems

The complement system is a complex of serum enzymes which, when they act together, are capable of lysing bacterial cell walls and infected cells (Fig. 1.3). Activation of the classical pathway depends heavily on a specific immune response: C1q binds to the Fc component of immunoglobulin attached to the cell wall. This pathway can also be initiated by binding to C-reactive protein, an acute-phase protein which is non-specifically elevated during acute inflammation.

The alternative complement pathway depends on the breakdown of C3 at bacterial cell surfaces. In both pathways the generation of active C3b initiates the formation of the 'attack complex' of C6–C9, which perforates and disrupts cell membranes. The alternative pathway is initially slower-acting than the classical, but it can act in the absence of a specific antibody and it provides early, non-specific defence against such severe infections as meningococcal septicaemia. Complement can act to enhance resistance to bacterial and parasitic infection by the action of breakdown products such as C3a and C5a which promote capillary permeability and are chemotactic to neutrophils and macrophages. C3b deposited on the surface of bacteria will opsonize them for phagocytosis.

Patients with congenital deficiencies of the early complement components are more susceptible to pneumococcal infections, in which activation of the alternative complement pathway is important in resistance to infection. Deficiencies in components of the alternative pathway, such as properdin, render the individual highly susceptible to invasive meningococcal infection.

Sialic acid inhibits the natural breakdown of C3. Successful pathogens, such as meningococci, have significant amounts of sialic acid on their surface, which probably reduces the effectiveness of the alternative complement pathway.

Phagocytosis

Phagocytosis of invading organisms is an important non-specific defence mechanism (Fig. 1.4). Neutrophils and macrophages are attracted to the site of inflammation by mediators such as complement components. The efficiency of phagocytosis is enhanced when organisms are 'opsonized' by attached complement or specific antibody, which provide receptors for the attachment of phagocytes. Organisms are taken up into phagosomes

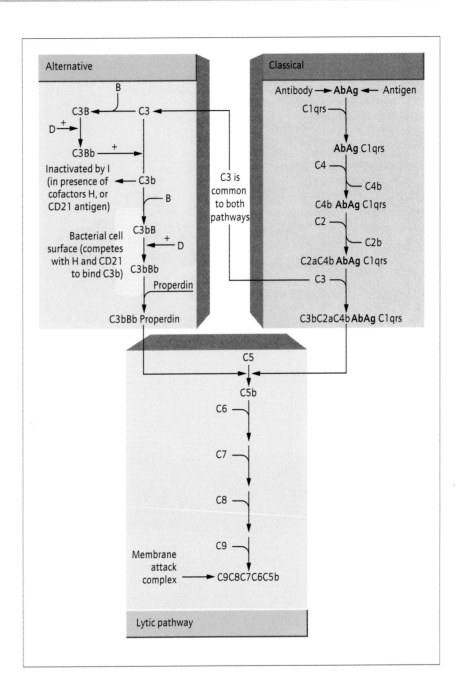

Fig. 1.3 The alternative and classical complement pathways (see also Figs 15.3 and 15.4).

which fuse with the lysosomes containing free radicals and lytic enzymes, resulting in killing.

Patients with deficiencies in phagocyte function suffer repeated pyogenic infections, and develop chronic suppurative granulomata (see pp. 404 and 405).

Specific immune responses

The specific immune response is a series of adaptive changes whereby the host develops defensive responses to individual microorganisms. This is based on recognition of, and response to, specific antigens which the pathogen posesses. Antigens are made up of individual amino acid or sugar residues linked together to form short sequences. The sequences are displayed in an array on the pathogen's surface because of the way they are integrated into the tertiary structure of the surface chemicals. These short sequences are called epitopes. Immunogenic epitopes may also be parts of toxin molecules, or the abnormal surface proteins displayed on

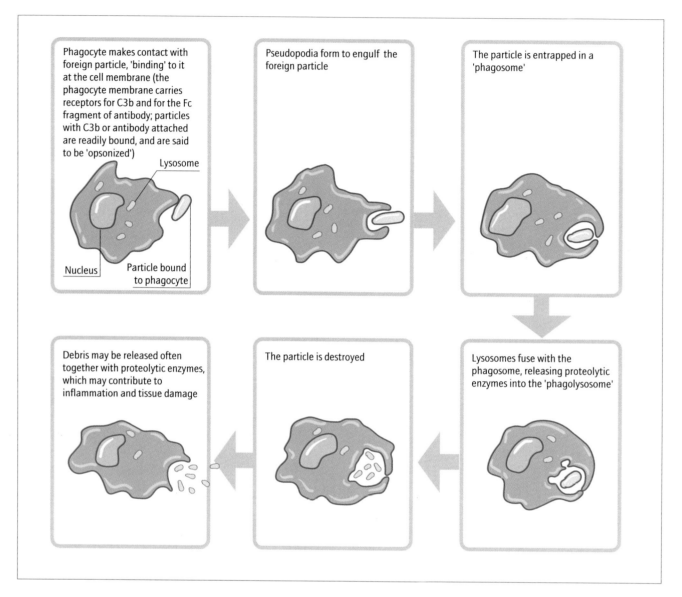

Phagocyte makes contact with foreign particle, 'binding' to it at the cell membrane (the phagocyte membrane carries receptors for C3b and for the Fc fragment of antibody; particles with C3b or antibody attached are readily bound, and are said to be 'opsonized')

Lysosome

Nucleus   Particle bound to phagocyte

Pseudopodia form to engulf the foreign particle

The particle is entrapped in a 'phagosome'

Debris may be released often together with proteolytic enzymes, which may contribute to inflammation and tissue damage

The particle is destroyed

Lysosomes fuse with the phagosome, releasing proteolytic enzymes into the 'phagolysosome'

Fig. 1.4 Phagocytosis.

virus-infected host cells. Different epitopes stimulate T- and B-cell immunity. Organisms each contain many antigens, within which are many different epitopes.

Antigen presentation by macrophages

As well as acting simply as phagocytes, macrophages have an essential role in the development of specific immunity to individual pathogens. Like other phagocytes, the macrophage takes up foreign material into phagosomes and fuses these with lysosomes to form phagolysosomes.

Substances secreted during the resulting burst of metabolic activity include cytokines (chemicals which modulate the activity of other reticuloendothelial cells). These include interleukin-1 (IL-1) and IL-6, which modulate the activity of lymphocytes and of other macrophages. They also act on the hypothalamus, causing an increase in body temperature. Tumour necrosis factor (TNF) is also released, and acts as an important mediator in the action of endotoxin.

Some of the ingested antigen is altered (processed), and processed antigen is expressed at the cell surface, bound in close association with the cell's own class II antigens (the class II human leukocyte antigens (HLAs) of the major histocompatibility complex). The double structure of microbial antigen and class II antigen is recognized by helper T lymphocytes with the same class II antigens, which become activated and capable of displaying chemicals with helper function. Helper T cells also display CD4 lymphocyte antigens.

Activation of the immune response also sets in motion a mechanism which causes the gradual degeneration and death of activated cells. This process is called apoptosis. It is important in limiting the duration and extent of an immune reaction, avoiding the progressive tissue damage which might result from an uncontrolled response.

B lymphocytes express immunoglobulin molecules at their surface, and can recognize the combination of antigen and helper function, which in turn activates them to proliferate. Many enlarge and mature into plasma cells, which secrete immunoglobulin. This leads to the formation of clones of cells which will recognize the antigen in future, and respond by secreting immunoglobulin. This is the basis of immunological memory.

Helper cells are important to both cell-mediated and humoral immune responses (see below). Patients who lack helper-cell function suffer severe cell-mediated immunodeficiency, and mount a poor humoral immune response to new antigens.

Cell-mediated immune responses

This is a system of lymphocyte-mediated attack, which is not based on major production of antibody. It depends on a system of antigen recognition and cytokine production among macrophages and T cells (Fig. 1.5).

When a macrophage ingests and presents antigen, it can interact with a T4 cell of the same HLA class II tissue type and a receptor specific for the antigen. These processes stimulate the macrophage to produce IL-1 which has several actions, including a hypothalamic action leading to fever, and a lymphocyte-stimulating action increasing the density of IL-2 receptors. The T4 cell is also stimulated, and produces IL-2. When a stimulated T cell encounters free antigen, it, too, will produce IL-2. The system not only causes IL-2 production, but also increases the sensitivity of T cells to its effects. The effects of IL-2 are to cause proliferation of T cells which recognize the antigen, and to mediate interactions between T4 (helper) cells and other lymphocytes (including the stimulation of B cells: see below).

Among T-cell populations are cytotoxic cells (with T8 antigens). These recognize antigen on cells bearing HLA class I tissue-type antigens, and kill the cells, lysing them by an unknown mechanism. There is also a population of T8 suppressor cells, which have an inhibitory or modulating role in lymphocyte interactions.

Patients who lack effective cell-mediated immunity are unable to combat viral infections, particularly those caused by enveloped viruses, such as the herpesvirus family, and infections with intracellular bacteria such as mycobacteria. They may also suffer from yeast infections, such as candidiasis and cryptococcosis (see Chapter 21).

Humoral immune responses

This is the system by which clones of antibody-secreting plasma cells are produced by B lymphocyte clones responding to 'their' specific antigen (Fig. 1.6). B cells possess large amounts of surface-bound antibody. This allows them to recognize and bind to antigen. In the presence of helper cells activated by the same antigen, the B cells proliferate, and many of them are transformed into antigen-secreting plasma cells.

Early in the humoral immune response, IgM is produced, but later, in the so-called mature immune response, large amounts of IgG are released. The early IgM response is called the primary response; the prompt and large IgG response to continued or subsequent exposure is called the secondary response. It represents the activation and proliferation of memory cells to form IgG-secreting plasma cells. IgM may also be produced on second or subsequent exposure to a pathogen, but a large memory response of IgM does not occur. Inactivated vaccines are often administered in carefully timed multiple doses to obtain an optimal and long-lasting secondary response.

Antibody can enhance cell-mediated cytotoxicity in the antibody-dependent cell-mediated cytotoxicity (ADCC) response. In this case, killer lymphocytes (K cells) recognize the antibody of bound antigen–antibody complexes on cell surfaces, and kill the antigen-bearing cells.

T-cell-independent antigens

Some antigens can induce a humoral immune response without the involvement of T-helper cells. They are usually rather large polymeric molecules, composed of multiply repeated subunits. It is thought that they bind to many adjacent antigen receptors on the B-cell surface, accidentally influencing intervening receptors concerned with recognizing helper function.

The primary immunoglobulin response to T-cell-independent antigens is usually a rather small and short-lived IgM response. The secondary response is similarly

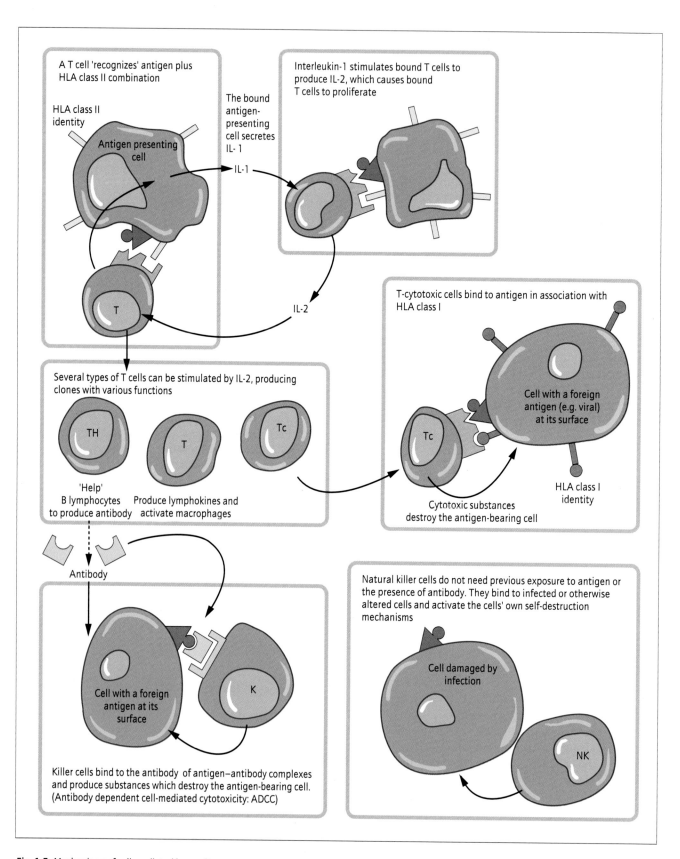

A T cell 'recognizes' antigen plus HLA class II combination

HLA class II identity

Antigen presenting cell

The bound antigen-presenting cell secretes IL-1

IL-1

T

Interleukin-1 stimulates bound T cells to produce IL-2, which causes bound T cells to proliferate

IL-2

Several types of T cells can be stimulated by IL-2, producing clones with various functions

TH   T   Tc

'Help' B lymphocytes to produce antibody   Produce lymphokines and activate macrophages

T-cytotoxic cells bind to antigen in association with HLA class I

Tc

Cell with a foreign antigen (e.g. viral) at its surface

HLA class I identity

Cytotoxic substances destroy the antigen-bearing cell

Antibody

Cell with a foreign antigen at its surface   K

Killer cells bind to the antibody of antigen–antibody complexes and produce substances which destroy the antigen-bearing cell. (Antibody dependent cell-mediated cytotoxicity: ADCC)

Natural killer cells do not need previous exposure to antigen or the presence of antibody. They bind to infected or otherwise altered cells and activate the cells' own self-destruction mechanisms

Cell damaged by infection

NK

Fig. 1.5 Mechanisms of cell-mediated immunity.

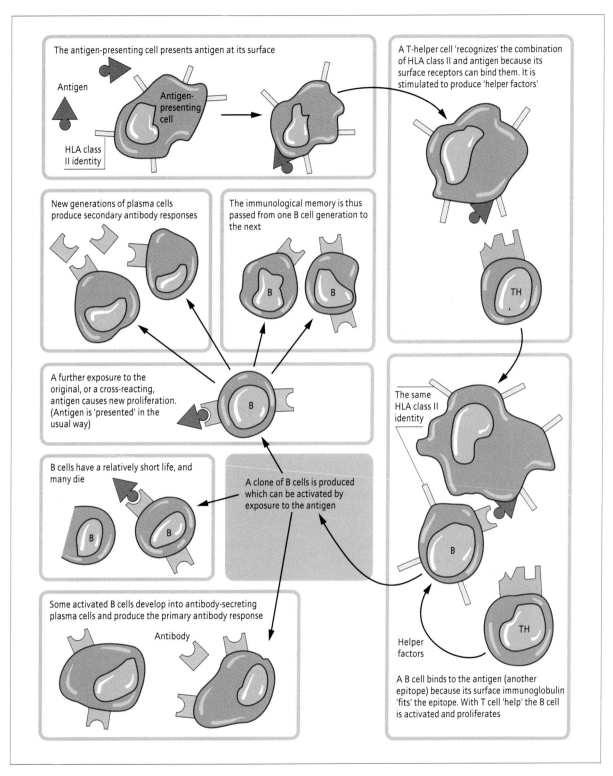

The antigen-presenting cell presents antigen at its surface

Antigen

Antigen-presenting cell

HLA class II identity

A T-helper cell 'recognizes' the combination of HLA class II and antigen because its surface receptors can bind them. It is stimulated to produce 'helper factors'

TH

New generations of plasma cells produce secondary antibody responses

The immunological memory is thus passed from one B cell generation to the next

B

B

A further exposure to the original, or a cross-reacting, antigen causes new proliferation. (Antigen is 'presented' in the usual way)

B

The same HLA class II identity

B cells have a relatively short life, and many die

B

B

A clone of B cells is produced which can be activated by exposure to the antigen

B

Some activated B cells develop into antibody-secreting plasma cells and produce the primary antibody response

Antibody

Helper factors

TH

A B cell binds to the antigen (another epitope) because its surface immunoglobulin 'fits' the epitope. With T cell 'help' the B cell is activated and proliferates

Fig. 1.6 Humoral immune responses.

small, and is usually a further IgM response, without significant IgG production. The absence of a mature IgG response is associated with rather poor and short-lasting immunological memory. This is important as many polysaccharide antigens, such as pneumococcal capsular antigens, act as T-independent antigens, especially in young children.

Superantigens

These antigens do not require processing before they are presented to lymphocytes. Lymphocyte activation is mediated by a different pathway than that of standard antigen-mediated activation, using V-beta receptors, which are possessed by up to 30% of all lymphocytes. This pathway does not require the association of HLA class II antigens. Superantigen presentation does not activate the process of apoptosis. Superantigens therefore cause a very intense immune reaction which is not limited or terminated in the usual way. Staphylococcal enterotoxins, toxic shock syndrome toxins (TSST) and some viral antigens act as superantigens.

Pathogenesis of infection

While the spread of a disease is influenced by characteristics of the host, the agent and the environment, the effects of disease in the host depend on a number of factors particular to the agent or pathogen. The presence and effect of agent factors are important determinants of pathogenicity. They are termed the pathogenicity factors of the organism.

The pathogen exploits its host to best advantage if it achieves optimum levels of survival and multiplication. The death of the host is not an advantage unless this contributes to the transmission of microbial genes. Pathogenicity factors are genetically maintained, by natural selection, because they facilitate survival or transmission via the host.

Characteristics of successful pathogens

Features of a successful pathogen
1 Survival and transmission in the environment.
2 Attachment to the surface of the host.
3 Overcoming the body defences against infection.
4 Ability to damage the host, e.g. by toxin production.

Survival in the environment

Many microorganisms are killed by drying, ultraviolet light and variation from their optimum temperature for growth. To overcome these difficulties, organisms have developed many strategies. Organisms which are predominantly environmental have developed tough survival mechanisms. The bacterial endospore is an example of this. It is a structure which contains a single copy of the bacterial DNA in a keratinous protective 'shell', which has little retained water and a very low metabolic rate. Adverse environmental conditions are the stimulus for sporulation, for example the rise in pH in the duodenum for *Clostridium perfringens*. Bacterial spores are capable of survival for many years, 'germinating' to form vegetative cells when conditions are more favourable. The Scottish island of Gruinard was contaminated with anthrax spores early in the Second World War, and was only declared free of infection 50 years later.

Other organisms have found protected ecological niches in the environment: *Legionella pneumophila* inhabits fresh water and can survive in the protected environment within the cytoplasm of free-living amoebae.

Some have evolved a close relationship with an animal host where they can exist reversibly, either as pathogen or commensal. To increase the chances of survival, some organisms will infect a wide range of species, for example rabies virus, which is able to infect all mammals. This diversity provides a large and adaptable reservoir of infection which will ensure survival of the pathogen if one host group is eliminated.

Transmission

The problem of transmission between hosts is related to survival; organisms which have developed a close relationship with a host are often readily killed by exposure to the external environment. Some organisms with moderate survival potential are transmitted by spreading in the air on droplet nuclei (see p. 5).

Bacteria such as *Neisseria gonorrhoeae* are extremely delicate and are unable to survive outside the host. Sexual transmission overcomes this difficulty by depositing the pathogen directly on to the genital mucosa of the new host, and in addition ties the organism's life cycle into an essential part of the host's life cycle, ensuring the survival of the pathogen.

Attachment of organisms to body surfaces

For organisms to gain access to the body via the mucosal surfaces they must first attach themselves. They have to overcome the natural defence mechanisms which are present in each area.

Organisms may gain attachment by specialized organelles of attachment, or more simply with attachment molecules. Uropathic *Escherichia coli*, which has to overcome the flushing action of urine, uses fimbriae to attach to the urinary epithelium. These fimbriae are pathogenicity determinants. Influenza virus adheres to the host's respiratory mucosal cells via its haemagglutinin molecule.

Microbial defence against immunological attack

From the moment the pathogen enters a new host, it must defend itself against immunological attack. Against organisms which invade via the mucosal surfaces, host secretory IgA is an important defence mechanism. Many respiratory tract pathogens, including *Streptococcus pneumoniae*, *Haemophilus influenzae* and *N. meningitidis*, elaborate a protease which selectively destroys IgA.

Bacterial capsules are an important defence against phagocytosis by neutrophils or macrophages. Capsulate organisms resist phagocytosis unless opsonized by the attachment of specific antibody. Resistance to phagocytosis probably depends on the negative charge on the capsular polysaccharide molecules.

For organisms such as the pneumococcus which activate the alternative complement pathway at their cell wall, the capsule acts as a physical barrier, preventing attached C3b on the cell wall being recognized by phagocytes. Some organisms are able to exploit phagocytes to enhance their life cycle. Once they have entered the phagocyte they are protected from antibody, and in this site can survive for very long periods. *Mycobacterium tuberculosis* is an intracellular pathogen which can survive inside macrophages and from this site reactivate if the host's immune defences become compromised.

Intraphagocytic survival depends on safe entry into the phagocyte, and subsequent avoidance of enzymic degradation by lysosymes.

Phagocytic ingestion of a particle is usually accompanied by a 'respiratory burst' which produces intensely toxic oxygen radicals. *Leishmania* spp. overcome this by utilizing alternative mannose/fucosyl and C3b receptors which, unlike the Fc receptors, do not trigger a respiratory burst. Once inside the phagocyte, there are three main mechanisms by which pathogens can survive: the organism may prevent phagolysosomal fusion, avoiding contact with lysosyme, and continuing to multiply within the phagosome. *Toxoplasma gondii* and chlamydiae act in this way. *Leishmania* survives inside the phagolysosome by metabolic adaptation to the hostile environment, and by excreting a factor which scavenges oxygen radicals. Mycobacteria escape from the phagolysosome into the cytoplasm where they are partly protected from digestion by their high lipid content. This effect has been demonstrated by coating staphylococci with the phenolic glycolipid of *M. leprae*. Although successfully ingested, these coated staphylococci are not killed, while uncoated control staphylococci are destroyed.

Antigenic variation

For organisms which are obliged to live extracellularly, antibody attack poses a major problem. Some organisms are able to evade the humoral immune system by varying the antigenic make-up of their surface. The major surface antigen of *Trypanosoma brucei* var. *rhodesiense* is the variable surface glycoprotein (VSG). As a result of a complex series of molecular events, the trypanosomes are able to express a different VSG every few days. Thus, as a humoral immune response is produced and parasite numbers are falling, a new clone of trypanosomes emerges with a different VSG and is able to multiply unhindered by the immune system. This process is continued through a preprogrammed set of variations, which are reflected by the episodic nature of symptoms in the early phases of the infection. *Borrelia recurrentis* and *B. duttoni* also undergo antigenic variation, producing a characteristic, relapsing fever.

Influenza virus survives as a pathogen by antigenic variation because its genome can undergo antigenic 'drift' and 'shift'. Drift is the process of gradual changes in the genes coding for viral surface haemagglutinin, enabling the virus partly to escape the effects of population immunization by previous epidemics. Shift is a major change in the antigenic structure of the virus, producing a novel strain to which nobody has any immunity. Antigenic shift often initiates a worldwide epidemic (pandemic).

Immune suppression

Immune suppression can take a number of forms, reducing the effectiveness of the humoral or cellular immune response.

Many parasitic infections cause overstimulation of the humoral immune system. High concentrations of ineffective antibodies are produced at the expense of the response to intercurrent infections. African trypanosomiasis and leishmaniasis are examples of this; not only is the parasitic infection uncontrolled, but many sufferers die of intercurrent bacterial infections such as acute pneumonia.

The cellular immune response can also be depressed: this occurs in severe tuberculosis and in lepromatous leprosy, where the infection induces a specific cell-mediated immune defect limiting T-cell responses to the mycobacteria. Acute viral infections, such as measles and infectious mononucleosis, cause temporary suppression of cell-mediated immune responses.

Immune suppression can be non-specific, when a whole arm of the system is impaired by the action of a pathogen. HIV causes a selective depletion of CD4 cells, resulting in susceptibility to those infections where cell-mediated responses are important, such as herpesvirus infections, tuberculosis, *Pneumocystis* infections and toxoplasmosis. Depletion of T-helper-cell function causes an increased susceptibility to many other pathogens, including pyogenic bacteria.

Ability to damage the host

Toxin production

Toxins are responsible for many of the symptoms, signs and complications of infection. They are also excellent vaccine targets as chemically modified toxin vaccines (toxoids) stimulate strong immune responses and have resulted in the virtual elimination of diseases such as tetanus and diphtheria. Toxins are often essential for the life cycle of the pathogen; their potential for pathogenicity may be coincidental. Diphtheria toxin, for example, is responsible for the pharyngeal, cardiac and neurological features of diphtheria. The gene coding for diphtheria toxin exists in a beta-phage, and only organisms with a lysogenic phage infection are toxin producers. In this symbiosis, the phage requires *Corynebacterium diphtheriae* as a host and *C. diphtheriae* is given a biological advantage in colonization of the human host by possession of the toxin gene.

Bacterial toxins are conventionally classified into exotoxins and endotoxins. Exotoxins are toxic substances which are excreted by organisms. The word endotoxin is usually used to describe the lipopolysaccharide antigen of Gram-negative bacterial cell walls. However, it is now known that many bacterial structural antigens can have toxic effects.

Endotoxin

The lipopolysaccharide of Gram-negative bacteria is an important pathogenicity factor. Lipopolysaccharide is made up of three main parts: (i) the core region, lipid A, which is responsible for the main toxic events; (ii) an oligosaccharide region which contains heptoses and hexoses linked to lipid A via the unusual sugar ketodeoxy-octanoic acid (KDO); and (iii) attached to this is a long polysaccharide chain which is responsible for the anti-genic specificity of the lipopolysaccharide. This polysaccharide partly protects Gram-negative bacteria such as salmonellae against the bactericidal activity of serum (Fig. 1.7).

Lipid A acts by stimulating cells of the macrophage series to produce cytokines, such as IL-1 and TNF. These are important factors in the stimulation of the complement and clotting cascades, in causing endothelial damage and in mediating other metabolic and physiological changes associated with Gram-negative septicaemia.

Toxic activity also resides in the cell wall of some Gram-positive bacteria. The C-polysaccharide and F (Forssman) antigen of *S. pneumoniae* are released into the host's tissues, and activate the alternative complement pathway. The products of the complement cascade are responsible for increased capillary permeability and exudate together with leukocyte chemotaxis to the site of infection.

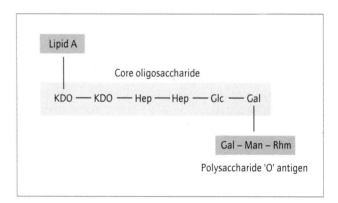

Fig. 1.7 An example of the structure of endotoxin.

Exotoxins

Bacterial exotoxins are diverse in function and clinical effect. They may be classified according to the symptoms produced — enterotoxin, neurotoxin or cytotoxin. Toxins can also be classified according to their mode of action, when this is known (Table 1.2).

Effects of microbial toxins

Some toxins cause important features of a disease, and it is convenient to consider a few examples here.

Streptococci and staphylococci can produce toxins which cause specific rashes. The erythrogenic toxin of *Streptococcus pyogenes* can cause the rash of scarlet fever.

Type	Examples
Extracellular cytotoxins (directly poison cells)	Streptococcal hyaluronidase *Pseudomonas aeruginosa* exotoxin A
Transmembrane cytotoxins (enter cells via implanted receptor/transporting molecule)	*Escherichia coli* verotoxin Shiga toxin Diphtheria toxin
Membrane-damaging toxins (cause haemolysis or cytolysis)	Streptolysin O *Clostridium perfringens* alpha toxin *Staphylococcus aureus* P-V leukocidin
Deregulating toxins (cause overactivity of secretory mechanisms)	*E. coli* heat-labile toxin Cholera toxin
Competitive inhibitors (competitive blockers of natural transmitters)	Botulinum toxin Tetanus toxin

Table 1.2 Actions of bacterial exotoxins

Staphylococcus aureus may produce similar toxins, toxic shock syndrome toxins (TSSTs), causing toxic shock syndrome with a scarlet fever-like rash. TSSTs also behave like the enterotoxins of *S. aureus* and cause diarrhoea. Some organisms produce toxins which can damage blood cells; *Clostridium perfringens* can cause severe haemolysis by this mechanism. Some are directly toxic to tissues.

Microbial synergy

Microbes can act together to establish infection, facilitate tissue invasion, reduce the immune response of the host and enhance the virulence of pathogens. *Streptococcus pneumoniae* is unable to bind to intact respiratory epithelium, but can bind to basal membrane. Influenza virus causes damage to, and shedding of, respiratory epithelium, allowing pathogens such as *S. pneumoniae* to attack the underlying basement membrane.

Many pyogenic infections are polymicrobial, with obligate and facultative pathogens multiplying together and creating the conditions for each other to survive. In synergistic gangrene the metabolic products of facultative organisms reduce the redox potential sufficiently to enable obligate anaerobes to multiply and cause extensive tissue necrosis.

Infection with HIV is an example where one infectious agent reduces the immune response of the host, allowing other organisms to invade. Many parasitic infections (leishmaniasis, trypanosomiasis and malaria) can trigger

polyclonal activation of B cells with the production of large quantities of antibody, and reduce the ability of the host to respond to specific bacterial infections.

Chronic schistosomiasis is associated with recurrent *Salmonella* infection. Salmonellae can bind to schistosome eggs, which provide a niche for salmonellae to cause persisting colonization and recurrent infection.

Manifestations of infection

Fever

This is the most common accompaniment of infection, occurring in all but the most trivial or unusual cases.

The body temperature of a healthy person is set and maintained by the hypothalamus. It follows a circadian cycle in which the temperature is lowest in the early morning and highest at about 10 p.m., varying by 0.5°C or more. Also, in women who ovulate, a monthly variation in temperature can be detected, with an abrupt step at the time of ovulation.

Infection, in common with a number of other events, can cause a resetting of the hypothalamus to a higher body temperature. This change may be initiated in more than one way, but the final common pathway is the release of cytokines, particularly IL-1, TNF and interferon-alpha by activated mononuclear phagocytes.

A raised body temperature is probably useful in combating infection. Many pathogens replicate best at temperatures at or below 37°C. Included among these are many respiratory viruses, pneumococci and other bacteria, and many agents of tropical skin infections. Such pathogens will be adversely affected by higher temperatures. Even if the pathogen is unaffected by temperature change or, like some campylobacters, replicates well at higher temperatures, fever can still help by making immune responses more efficient. Phagocytosis, antibody production and interferon production are all enhanced at raised temperatures.

Adverse effects of fever

Delirium

Delirium is a state of confusion, often with agitation. It can occur at any age but is most common in children and the elderly. The confusion tends to occur when the temperature is at its highest, especially at night, when it may manifest itself as distressing dreams. Although sometimes caused directly by the disease process (toxaemia or cerebral infection), it can often be improved or cured simply by reducing the temperature.

Febrile convulsions

Febrile convulsions are a specific problem in children between the ages of 6 months and 6 years. They are rarely a sign of true epilepsy, and usually cease spontaneously as the child reaches age 4–6. The convulsions most often happen as the temperature is rising.

Treating fever and its complications

> **Treatment of fever**
> 1 Tepid sponging.
> 2 Paracetemol.
> 3 Aspirin.

This is done by sponging the patient with tepid (not cold) water, or by giving antipyretic drugs. Aspirin is an effective antipyretic, but should not be given to children under 12, because of the association of aspirin treatment with Reye's syndrome. Paracetamol is equally effective and is the drug of choice for children.

Convulsions can usually be terminated by lowering the body temperature. If this is unsuccessful it may be necessary to give specific anticonvulsant treatment. Often a once-only dose of diazepam is enough to avert further attacks during a brief illness. On rare occasions a short course of regular anticonvulsant dosage is required; in this case valproate or carbamazepine is the drug of choice, as in true childhood epilepsy.

Pre-existing disorders

Pre-existing disorders may be adversely affected by fever. Epilepsy may become poorly controlled, and is better managed if possible by treating fever than by altering established drug routines. The neurological deficits of multiple sclerosis are reversibly exacerbated by fever.

Inflammation

Inflammation is a complex combination of events, whose pathogenesis is still poorly understood. Several important components can be recognized:
1 Vasodilatation at the affected site.
2 Exudation of tissue fluid from dilated capillaries.
3 Accumulation of neutrophils and macrophages at the site.
4 Release of active chemicals from neutrophils (Fig. 1.8).

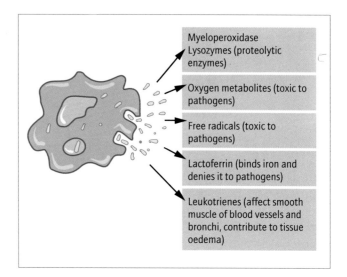

Fig. 1.8 Active substances released by neutrophils.

These events combine to cause local heat and redness, sometimes with the advantage of adversely affecting the responsible pathogen. The tissue exudate contains complement components, which comprise one of the immediate defences against bacteria. Some complement activation products are chemotaxins and attract phagocytes to the site.

The phagocytes ingest bacteria and debris, becoming activated and releasing chemicals which both attack the pathogens and contribute to inflammation. These include enzymes which promote rapid synthesis of prostaglandins, a variety of chemicals which are vasoactive and also affect platelet activation. Prostaglandins are important initiators of inflammation. The effects of non-steroidal anti-inflammatory drugs are due to their strong inhibition of prostaglandin synthesis.

> **Useful anti-inflammatory drugs**
> 1 Ibuprofen (adult and child preparations).
> 2 Aspirin (over-12s only).
> 3 Intramuscular or rectal diclofenac.

Detecting inflammation

The signs and symptoms of inflammation are classically described as pain, heat, redness and swelling. These features are helpful in indicating the site of a localized infection, for instance an abscess or an infected joint. They should always be sought during clinical examination when assessing a patient with suspected infection.

Neutrophils which collect at sites of inflammation may be shed, e.g. in the urine, or discharged from the tissues as pus. Microscopical examination of the appropriate specimen will therefore reveal evidence of infection, even when the patient cannot indicate the affected site.

The swelling of inflammation may be deep in the body and undetectable by surface examination. An X-ray may show the tell-tale soft-tissue shadow, isotope scans may demonstrate the site of hyperaemia, and other imaging procedures such as computed tomography or nuclear magnetic resonance scans are excellent for demonstrating oedema.

Fast-reacting proteins

Several plasma proteins show a large rise in concentration in the presence of inflammation. Notable among these are caeruloplasmin, haptoglobin, alpha$_1$-antitrypsin, alpha$_1$-glycoprotein (orosomucoid) and C-reactive protein (CRP). Levels of transferrin, fibronectin and albumin tend to fall.

The function of these changes, which can be induced by prostaglandins, alpha-interferon or IL-1, is unknown. Caeruloplasmin and haptoglobin will bind to oxygen radicals, perhaps inhibiting their damaging potential in blood. Alpha$_1$-acid glycoprotein can inhibit platelet aggregation, possibly protecting against platelet activation and thrombus formation.

C-reactive protein

CRP is produced in the liver, and synthesis is greatly increased in acute inflammation. It is a disc-shaped pentameric molecule which readily binds a number of substances, including the C fraction of pneumococcal lysates (from which it gets its name). In its bound form it strongly activates the classical complement pathway, possibly acting as a non-specific defence against infection. It is elevated in many acute bacterial infections, but also in severe viral infections and other inflammatory conditions. Because of its rapid response to inflammation it is useful for monitoring responses to treatment in conditions such as endocarditis.

Plasma viscosity and erythrocyte sedimentation rate

The protein changes in inflammation alter the viscosity of the plasma. This can be measured directly, or more often inferred, from changes in the erythrocyte sedimentation rate (ESR: the rate at which red blood cells settle in anticoagulated blood on standing). The normal ESR is not more than about 20 mm/h. This rises to 30–50 mm/h in acute infections, but may reach 70–100 mm/h in some atypical pneumonias and chronic conditions such as abscess formation or immunological disease. It has non-specific diagnostic value, like CRP levels, but responds less rapidly than CRP to changes in the degree of inflammation.

Rashes

Rashes are a particular form of inflammation or tissue damage, affecting the skin. They can be generalized, or localized to a specific site. The rash of an infectious disease often evolves in a predictable way, starting at a particular site, spreading in a particular direction and containing typical types of skin lesions. Some of the skin lesions that occur in rashes are illustrated in Fig. 1.9.

The rashes of infectious diseases, unlike those of hypersensitivity reactions, are rarely painful or even significantly irritating. The lesions of chickenpox may itch quite severely, but this is not so in every patient. However, in rashes caused by severe tissue damage, e.g. the meningococcal rash caused by intravascular coagulation, the more necrotic lesions can be painful.

Harmful effects of immune responses

Immune reactions can be clinically detectable as part of the acute disease, or as a late effect of the disease. This is described as the immunopathology of the disease.

The rashes of some viral infections such as measles are thought to be the manifestation of an immune vasculitis of the skin. The lung damage of respiratory syncytial virus infection is immunopathological, and can be made worse in experimental conditions by immunization against the virus.

Antibodies which accidentally damage human tissues may be manufactured in the course of an infection. Examples include immune thrombocytopenia after rubella and other viral infections, and red-cell agglutination in *Mycoplasma pneumoniae* infections.

Interferon is a lymphokine with many effects, including the inhibition of viruses and reduction of the metabolic activity of virus-infected cells. It also causes the symptoms of fatigue, malaise and myalgia which are typically seen in acute viral infections. High concentrations may contribute to the neutropenia of some viral diseases by a toxic effect on the bone marrow.

The primary function of cell-mediated immunity is to destroy infected cells. Occasionally a very vigorous response can cause severe tissue damage, such as hepatic necrosis in viral hepatitis. It is thought that a similar but slower-onset mechanism is responsible for the encephalitis that can follow acute viral infections.

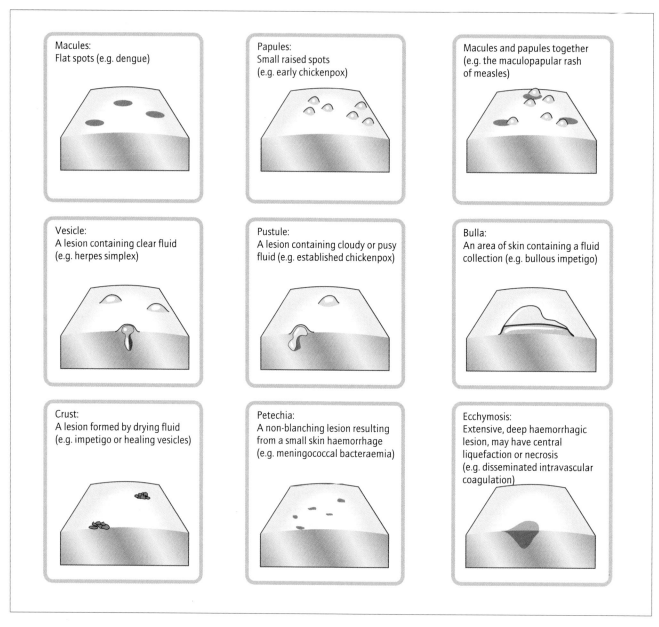

Macules:
Flat spots (e.g. dengue)

Papules:
Small raised spots
(e.g. early chickenpox)

Macules and papules together
(e.g. the maculopapular rash
of measles)

Vesicle:
A lesion containing clear fluid
(e.g. herpes simplex)

Pustule:
A lesion containing cloudy or pusy
fluid (e.g. established chickenpox)

Bulla:
An area of skin containing a fluid
collection (e.g. bullous impetigo)

Crust:
A lesion formed by drying fluid
(e.g. impetigo or healing vesicles)

Petechia:
A non-blanching lesion resulting
from a small skin haemorrhage
(e.g. meningococcal bacteraemia)

Ecchymosis:
Extensive, deep haemorrhagic
lesion, may have central
liquefaction or necrosis
(e.g. disseminated intravascular
coagulation)

Fig. 1.9 The nomenclature and appearance of rashes.

Antibody–antigen complexes often form during immune reactions to infection. Most are harmlessly destroyed or cleared, but some may lodge in tissues such as glomerular capillaries or synovial membranes. If they combine with complement there is a risk that the complement will be activated, causing local inflammation and tissue damage. This takes time to develop, but the late effects can produce autoimmune-like postinfectious disorders. Rheumatic fever after *Streptococcus pyogenes* infections is a classic example of this, but postinfectious arthritis, nephritis and neuritis are nowadays more common (see Chapter 24).

These relatively rare complications of infection probably depend also on genetic factors in the patient. A good example of this is the predisposition of HLA B27-positive individuals to develop Reiter's syndrome. Other recognized factors include secretor status — non-secretors appear to be at greater risk of acquiring disease from organisms which they carry and also of developing some postinfectious disorders.

Of course, an immunodeficient patient may lack the immunopathological features of a disease. Thus, a child with leukaemia may have severe respiratory features of measles or chickenpox with little or no rash, or a patient with AIDS may fail to develop granulomata in organs infected by mycobacteria (see Chapter 11).

Dynamics of colonization and infection

When a microbe encounters a potential host, a sequence of events takes place. On making contact with the host's mucosa or skin, an organism may be able to adhere to and colonize this surface. If successfully established, colonization often continues without ill effect to the host for a variable length of time. During this period the host may develop immunity to the organism (by the development of specific antibody or T-cell responses). This is a common means of development of immunity to a number of pathogens such as *Haemophilus influenzae* and *Neisseria meningitidis*. This process is also important since organisms which have little capacity to cause disease may share some antigenic markers with human pathogens. Antibodies developed to these agents of low pathogenicity may provide immunity to powerful pathogens. This effect of cross-immunity is exploited when bacillus Calmette–Guérin (BCG) vaccine is given to confer protection against tuberculosis or leprosy.

Alteration of the host–microbial interaction may permit the pathogen to extend from colonization to invasion of local tissues or the whole body. For many infectious agents the majority of interactions are restricted to colonization.

For other agents, such as poliomyelitis viruses, invasion of the host may take place as part of the life cycle of the organism. In an unimmunized population, newly exposed to the virus, many individuals will be infected. The great majority suffer only a mild bowel or throat infection and become immune to further attacks. In a few cases this infection is complicated by self-

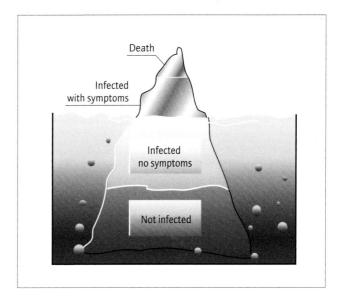

Fig. 1.10 The epidemiological iceberg.

limiting viral meningitis, and a minority of meningitis cases develop anterior horn cell infection and paralysis. Paralysis is most likely to affect older children and adults. In populations where the disease is already common almost all adults are immune, so most infections occur in young children, who rarely develop paralysis. The disease therefore exists in equilibrium with the population, where the combination of host factors and microbial pathogenicity does not favour the occurrence of symptomatic or severe disease. This situation is often described as 'the iceberg of infection' where the majority of host–microbial interactions are colonization–clearance episodes and only a small proportion result in morbidity or mortality (Fig. 1.10).

The manifestation of an infectious disease is a complex balance between the direct effect of the pathogen or its toxins, and the response of the affected patient. The patient's response depends on several factors, including immune competence, previous experience of the same or similar pathogens and his or her own genetic structure.

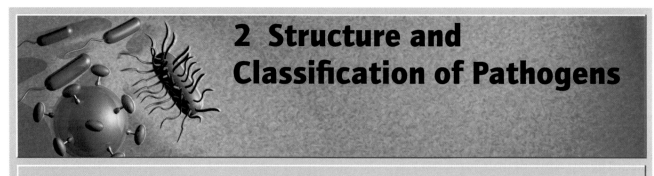

2 Structure and Classification of Pathogens

Introduction

Taxonomy is the process of classifying living organisms into groups (taxa) of related individuals or species. Knowledge of taxonomy is very important for microbiology. However, while taxonomists weigh individual characteristics equally, clinical microbiologists do not, as they consider ability to cause disease more important than, say, the ability to ferment a particular sugar. The microbiologist aims to classify microorganisms into clinically relevant groups. A range of characteristics of organisms is therefore investigated to identify the most reliable and reproducible distinguishing features of each pathogen.

Pathogens can be classified into five main groups: viruses, bacteria, fungi, protozoa and metazoa (usually helminths). Viruses are smaller than bacteria and consist of a piece of either DNA or RNA supported by nucleoprotein, some enzymes for replication and a 'casing' of structural protein. Some viruses possess an envelope which is derived from host cells (Fig. 2.1). Viruses cannot replicate independently but grow inside host cells, taking control of cellular biochemical processes and subverting them for virus production.

Classification of microorganisms
Viruses, bacteria, protozoa, fungi and metazoa.

Bacteria are single-cell organisms with a single circular DNA chromosome, which is not enclosed in a nucleus (such organisms are called prokaryotes). They have a plasma membrane, and a cell wall of characteristic composition. They replicate by binary fission. Specialized surface structures serve special functions: pili and fimbriae are for attachment and flagella for motility (Fig. 2.2), but they have no internal organelles. Some bacteria can form extremely durable spores. The detailed structure of bacteria is discussed below.

Mycoplasmas are small bacteria, lacking peptidoglycan-containing cell walls. They are the smallest organisms able to live and replicate independently.

Rickettsiae and chlamydiae are also small and structurally resemble Gram-negative bacteria. They lack some enzymes needed for independent existence, and must replicate intracellularly, borrowing host enzyme systems.

Protozoa are single cells whose name is derived from the Greek words for first animals. They are diploid, possessing paired chromosomes, and as they also possess a nucleus they are eukaryotes. They have several specialized organelles (see below). Protozoan life cycles may be simple, involving only one species, or require the intervention of intermediate hosts or vectors.

Fungi are also eukaryotes with cell walls containing chitin, cellulose or both. They reproduce by sexual or asexual processes, forming germinative spores.

The final group of organisms which must be considered are the metazoa or multicellular organisms. Virtually all metazoa pathogenic to humans are helminths (worms or flukes).

Structure and classification of viruses

The classification of pathogenic viruses developed later than the classification of other organisms. Original classifications simply described the diseases caused (e.g. rubella), the site of viral shedding (e.g. enteroviruses) or the means of transmission (arthropod-borne; arbo-

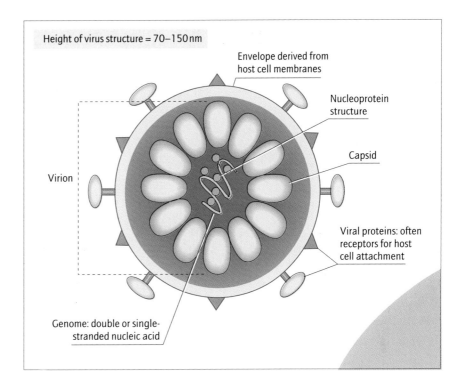

Fig. 2.1 General structure of a virus.

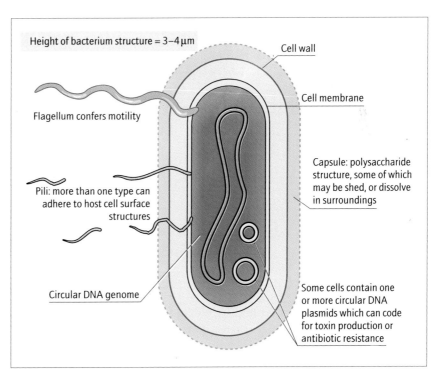

Fig. 2.2 General structure of a bacterium.

Name of family	Type of nucleic acid	Genome size (kB)	Envelope	Examples: genera of medical importance
Poxviridae	ds DNA	130–280	No	Molluscum contagiosum
Herpesviridae	ds DNA	120–220	Yes	Herpes simplex, Epstein–Barr virus, etc.
Adenovirus	ds DNA	36–38	No	Adenovirus
Papovaviridae	Circular ds DNA	8	No	Human wart virus
Parvoviridae	ss DNA	5	No	Parvovirus
Hepadnaviridae	ds DNA with ss portions	3	Yes	Hepatitis B virus
Picornaviridae	ss(+)RNA	7.2–8.4	No	Poliovirus
Togaviridae	ss(+)RNA	12	Yes	Rubella virus
Flaviviridae	ss(+)RNA	10	Yes	Yellow fever virus
Caliciviridae	ss(+)RNA	8	No	Norwalk agent
Rhabdoviridae	ss(−)RNA	13–16	Yes	Rabies virus
Paramyxoviridae	ss(−)RNA	16–20	Yes	Measles virus
Orthomyxoviridae	ss(−)RNA	14	Yes	Influenza virus
Reoviridae	ds segmented RNA	16–22	No	Rotavirus
Arenaviridae	ss(−)RNA	10–14	Yes	Lassa
Retroviridae	ss(+)RNA	3–9	Yes	HIV-1

Table 2.1 Classification of viruses

viruses). Modern classification is based on genetically determined structure (Table 2.1). Three determinants are considered in the classification of viruses: (i) the type of nucleic acid and its means of transcription; (ii) the structure and symmetry of the structural proteins (capsids); and (iii) the presence or absence of an envelope.

Genomic structure in viruses
DNA viruses
Double-stranded DNA.
Single-stranded DNA.

RNA viruses
Positive single-stranded RNA (sense).
Negative single-stranded RNA (antisense).
Double-stranded RNA.
Positive single-stranded RNA (retroviruses; cannot act as messenger).

Nucleic acid

Both the type of nucleic acid and its method of transcription are considered, as there is considerable variation in the mechanisms that viruses employ in their reproductive process.

DNA viruses

The DNA of viruses can be either double- or single-stranded (ds or ss). The double-stranded DNA viruses

include a number of important families which cause human disease. The poxvirus family, the agents with the largest viral genomes, includes the causative agents of smallpox, molluscum contagiosum and also the important vaccinia virus, which was utilized in the smallpox eradication programme, and may in the future be used as a vaccine vector. The herpesvirus family includes herpes simplex, varicella-zoster, cytomegalovirus and Epstein–Barr virus. Adenoviruses also possess double-stranded DNA. Hepatitis B virus is double-stranded with a single-stranded portion. The papovaviruses and polyomaviruses are small viruses containing double-stranded DNA. These viruses are associated with benign tumours (warts) and malignant tumours (cervical, genital and laryngeal cancer).

The only single-stranded DNA virus is parvovirus, responsible for 'fifth disease' or 'slapped cheek syndrome'.

Viral DNA is usually replicated in the nucleus of host cells. It encodes its own DNA polymerase. Newly formed viral DNA is not usually inserted into host chromosomal DNA.

RNA viruses

Single-stranded RNA viruses adopt one of three reproduction strategies, depending on whether the RNA is positive or negative. (Positive and negative are sometimes referred to as sense and antisense.) If it is positive, or sense, it can serve directly as messenger RNA (mRNA) and be translated into protein, which includes structural proteins and an RNA-dependent RNA polymerase which is used to replicate the viral RNA.

If the RNA is negative or antisense, a completely different strategy must be adopted. These viruses encode an RNA polymerase (or transcriptase) which transcribes the viral genome into positive RNA, which can act either as a template for further viral genomic (negative-strand) RNA or as mRNA for translation into proteins (Fig. 2.3).

The reoviruses, which include rotaviruses, possess a segmented, double-stranded RNA genome. Their complex reproductive strategy includes the use of a double-stranded RNA single-stranded RNA polymerase which produces positive (sense) RNA from the double-stranded portion of viral RNA using the antisense strand as a template. The positive (sense) RNA is extruded from

the virus, serving both as mRNA and also as a template to make further antisense RNA, which is then annealed with the complementary strand to form double-stranded RNA.

The third RNA-based strategy is that of the retroviruses. They possess single-stranded positive (sense) RNA which cannot act as mRNA. It is transcribed into DNA by an RNA-dependent DNA polymerase (reverse transcriptase, or RT). The DNA enters the host nucleus and is inserted into host DNA. In the host DNA molecule, it is under the control of host transcriptase enzymes which make mRNA and viral genomic RNA.

Capsid symmetry

Viral nucleic acid is contained within a protein coat made up of repeating units known as capsids arranged in either icosahedral or helical structures. Helical symmetry is found in some RNA viruses in which the capsids are bound around the helical nucleic acid. (Fig. 2.4a). Icosahedral symmetry occurs in both DNA and RNA viruses, the capsids forming an approximately spherical polyhedral structure (Fig. 2.4b). Using simple, repeating capsid structures minimizes the amount of nucleic acid devoted to viral coat production and simplifies the process of viral assembly.

Envelopes

In some viruses the nucleic acid and capsid (the nucleocapsid) are surrounded by a lipid envelope derived from the host cell or nuclear membrane (Fig. 2.5). The host membrane is itself altered by virus-encoded proteins or glycoproteins which may fuse several host cells together, thus facilitating the passage of viruses from cell to cell. Viruses possessing an envelope are sensitive to ether and other substances which dissolve the lipid membrane.

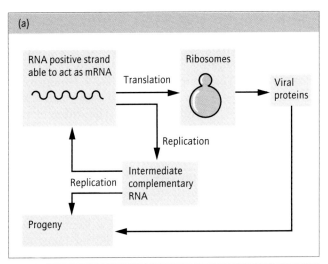

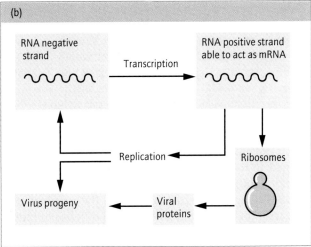

Fig. 2.3 (a) Replication of RNA virus with positive polarity (able to be read as messenger (m)RNA). (b) Replication of RNA virus with negative polarity.

Virus attachment

Virus attachment to host cell membrane is a critical step in the process of infection, and in determining tissue tropism. Viruses have evolved specific antigens which target receptors on the host cells. These are sometimes known as virus attachment proteins or VAPs. The VAP of influenza virus is a haemagglutinin, whereas that of human immunodeficiency virus (HIV) is a glycoprotein which binds to the CD4 antigen of T-cells.

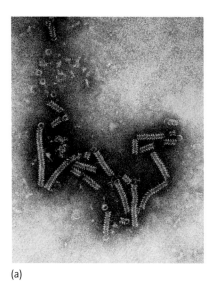

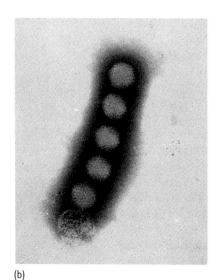

Fig. 2.4 (a) Electron micrograph of a virus with helical symmetry. Parainfluenza type 3 virus × 100 000. (b) Electron micrograph of a virus with icosahedral symmetry. Adenovirus × 100 000.

(a)   (b)

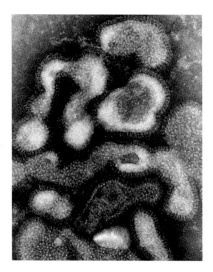

Fig. 2.5 Electron micrograph of an enveloped virus. Influenza virus × 100 000.

Structure and classification of bacteria

For descriptive purposes bacteria are often grouped by four main characteristics: the Gram reaction, shape, atmospheric requirements for respiration and the presence of spores.

Classification of bacteria
Gram reaction, atmospheric requirement, shape, presence of spores.

The Gram reaction or Gram stain uses the ability of stains such as crystal violet to bind to the cell wall teichoic acids found in Gram-positive cells, and resist decoloration by alcohol or acetone. Gram-positive cells stain blue, therefore, but Gram-negative cells are stained pink by the application of a counterstain after the decolorization step. This simple reaction easily demonstrates the marked difference in structure of Gram-positive and Gram-negative cell walls (Fig. 2.6). The different cell-wall structure confers different pathogenic potential and different antibiotic susceptibilities in the two groups of microorganisms.

Bacterial cell walls provide a basis for defined shape which is consistent for individual genera. Cocci are spherical. They include important human pathogens such as streptococci and staphylococci. Bacilli are rod-shaped and may be short (coccobacilli) or long. They may also vary their shape throughout their length, as do *Fusobacterium* spp. Spiral organisms are a diverse group of bacteria, including *Treponema pallidum*, the causative organism of syphilis, which has a very short wavelength, and *Borrelia* spp., which have a longer wavelength, and include the organisms of Lyme disease and relapsing fever. Other spiral organisms, such as the intestinal pathogens *Campylobacter* and *Helicobacter*, have only a few turns.

Bacteria may be classified by their atmospheric requirements into five groups. **Obligate aerobes** are obliged to use oxygen as a terminal electron acceptor. Included in this group is *Bordetella pertussis*. **Micro-aerophilic** organisms use oxygen as the terminal electron acceptor but only grow under conditions of reduced oxygen tension. These include *Campylobacter* spp. Many human pathogens are **facultative anaerobes** capable of growing aerobically or anaerobically. These include staphylococci, streptococci and enteric organisms.

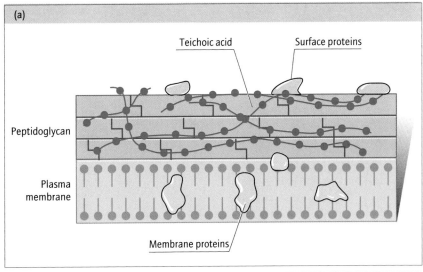

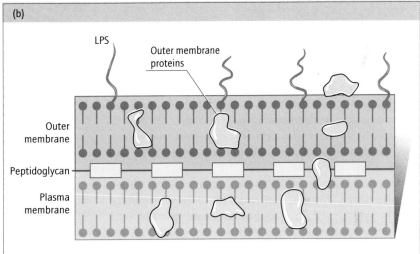

Fig. 2.6 Structures of (a) Gram-positive and (b) Gram-negative bacterial cell walls. LPS, lipopolysaccharide.

Obligate anaerobes only grow in the absence of oxygen. They are divided into aerotolerant and strict anaerobes, depending on their sensitivity to oxygen. This difference has practical importance as strictly anaerobic organisms do not survive long in specimens and are much more difficult to isolate in the laboratory.

Atmospheric requirements of bacteria
Obligate aerobes, microaerophiles, facultative anaerobes, strict and aerotolerant obligate anaerobes.

Two genera of bacteria found in humans possess a bacterial endospore: *Clostridium* and *Bacillus*. The shape, size and position of this spore may be helpful in the determination of species identification, especially in the genus *Clostridium* (Fig. 2.7).

Bacterial structures

The cell wall

The bacterial cell wall is essential for survival, as it must maintain the physical integrity of the organism against the immense osmotic pressure difference between the interior and exterior of the cell. Its strength and rigidity depends on peptidoglycan, a polymer of muramic acid and *N*-acetylglucosamine, cross-linked by peptide bridges.

The Gram-positive cell wall has two layers, consisting of the plasma membrane and a thick peptidoglycan layer. In contrast, the Gram-negative wall has three layers: the plasma membrane, a thinner peptidoglycan layer and an outer membrane (see Fig. 2.6). Cell walls

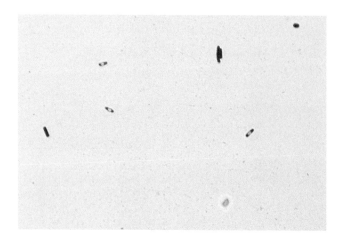

Fig. 2.7 Structure of *Clostridium* sp. showing endospore.

are important targets for beta-lactam and glycopeptide antibiotics (see Chapter 4).

Many bacterial antigens present in the cell wall have an important role in pathogenesis (see Chapter 1). Lipopolysaccharide (endotoxin) is an integral part of the Gram-negative outer membrane. Teichoic acid from *Streptococcus pneumoniae* causes complement activation and is responsible for attraction of neutrophils to the site of infection.

Mycobacteria possess a cell wall of an entirely different structure. This cell wall consists of approximately 40% lipid, including lipoarabinomannan, mycolic acid and phenolic glycolipids. It will not stain satisfactorily with conventional Gram stain. Vigorous staining and decolorizing methods are required to demonstrate it (see Chapter 18). Several of the surface lipids of mycobacteria are implicated in inhibiting macrophage function (e.g. arabinomannan) or phagocytosis (phenolic glycolipid from *Mycobacterium leprae*).

The plasma membrane

The bacterial plasma membrane is like that of other cells: it consists of a trilaminar membrane with two outer hydrophilic layers and an inner lipid core. In the absence of internal membrane-bound structures the plasma membrane is an important site of bacterial metabolism.

Bacterial capsules

These are starchy or gelatinous exterior structures, which surround some of the most important pathogens,

including *S. pneumoniae*, *Haemophilus influenzae*, *Neisseria meningitidis*, *Streptococcus agalactiae*, *Salmonella typhi* and *Bacillus anthracis*. *Klebsiella pneumoniae* and *Pseudomonas aeruginosa* sometimes produce such abundant alginate capsular material that it appears as gelatinous pus at infected sites, or flows over culture plates (Table 2.2).

Capsules protect pathogens from phagocytosis, and from the activation of the alternative complement pathway and humoral immune attack (see Chapter 1).

Species	Associated diseases
Streptococcus pneumoniae	Meningitis, pneumonia, septicaemia
Neisseria meningitidis	Meningitis, septicaemia
Haemophilus influenzae	Meningitis, septicaemia
Streptococcus agalactiae	Neonatal septicaemia and meningitis
Klebsiella pneumoniae	Pneumonia, septicaemia, wound infection
Pseudomonas aeruginosa	Pneumonia in cystic fibrosis patients
Escherichia coli	Meningitis, septicaemia
Bacillus anthracis	Anthrax

Table 2.2 Bacterial pathogens whose capsules are important in pathogenesis, and used to identify pathogenic strains.

Capsulation is not, in itself, a pathogenicity determinant as many organisms which are not usually recognized as human pathogens possess a polysaccharide capsule. The bacterial capsule may have evolved as a mechanism for enabling organisms to survive during conditions of desiccation.

Immune response to polysaccharide capsular antigens

The human host does not respond efficiently to polysaccharide antigens. Such antigens are called T-cell-independent, as T cells are bypassed in the development of antibody to them, and immunological memory is not, therefore, well-established. T cells are, however, involved in the modulation of humoral responses to these antigens. Suppressor and contrasuppressor T cells have been identified in the response to *S. pneumoniae* capsular polysaccharide. Humoral responses are mainly with the immunoglobulin G_2 (IgG_2) isotype.

The spleen has an important role in the control of infection with capsulate organisms, as intrasplenic phagocytes can ingest particles which have not been opsonized.

Protein 'capsules'

The M antigen of *Streptococcus pyogenes* is a fibrillar protein which forms an extracellular capsule-like structure. Its major role appears to be in preventing phagocytosis by polymorphonuclear leukocytes. Strains of *S. pyogenes* cannot be ingested unless opsonized with specific anti-M antibody. There are more than 80 antigenically distinct M-types, and immunity to one M-type does not protect against strains carrying different M antigens. This accounts for the recurrent attacks of streptococcal tonsillitis which occur in the population.

The M antigen is capable of cross-reaction with a number of tissues in the human host, with important pathological consequences. Cross-reaction with myocardial antigens is found in many different M-types and is thought to be responsible for the pancarditis associated with rheumatic fever. Infection with a second type of *S. pyogenes* may cause a recrudescence of rheumatic fever. In contrast, poststreptococcal glomerulonephritis is confined to a narrow group of M-types, including 4, 12 and 49, resulting from cross-reaction with the glomerular basement membrane. Infection with another strain of *S. pyogenes* will not result in a recrudescence unless it too is a 'nephritogenic' strain (Table 2.3).

Glycolipid capsules

Many species export extracellular glycolipid material which appears to be important to the organism as a pathogenicity determinant. *Mycobacterium leprae* can survive inside macrophages. It has been shown that the phenolic glycolipid capsule inhibits the activity of the macrophage myeloperoxide-halide microbicidal system, possibly by scavenging free radicals.

Bacterial extracellular material
1 Polysaccharide capsules.
2 Extracellular slime.
3 M protein.
4 Phenolic glycolipid.

Bacterial adhesins
1 Capsular polysaccharide.
2 Extracellular slime.
3 Fimbriae.
4 Lectins.

Extracellular slime

Many organisms of low virulence such as *Staphylococcus epidermidis* colonize intravascular prosthetic devices. This causes fever or septicaemia in patients with many intravenous cannulae or those with long-term intravascular devices such as Hickman catheters. Slime-producing organisms adhere better to the cannulae and more readily colonize and cause infection.

Pseudomonas aeruginosa is an important pathogen of children with cystic fibrosis. The organisms can convert to a mucoid phenotype in which copious amounts of exopolysaccharide alginate are produced. Alginate is a non-repeating co-polymer of beta-D-mannuronate and its C5 epimer, alpha-D-glucuronate, similar to an alginate produced by brown seaweed. Alginate production assists the organism because it enables the formation of microcolonies protected from humoral and cellular immune responses. Curiously, the alginate-producing strains are often exquisitely sensitive to antimicrobial agents.

Fimbriae or pili

Fimbriae have an important role in adhesion and assist bacteria in allowing access to a new host or locating the organism close to a nutrient supply. Pili are filamentous proteins capable of binding to host antigens by acting as lectins (proteins which bind to carbohydrate residues). An individual bacterial strain may express several different pili and may up- and down-regulate different types as required. For some organisms such as *N. gonorrhoeae*, pili are necessary for pathogenesis. Possession of pili may assist the adhesion of organisms to epithelia. Uropathic *Escherichia coli* express not only type 1 fimbriae, which are common to many Enterobacteriaceae, but P fimbriae, which bind to a digalactoside found in the urinary tract. The role of fimbriae is discussed in more detail on p. 207.

M-type	No. of isolates			
	Scarlet fever	Acute glomerular nephritis	Rheumatic fever	Puerperal infections
1	21	24	5	10
2	10	3	0	2
3	85	6	3	11
4	75	10	2	9
9	0	2	1	20
12	9	20	0	10
R28	8	3	0	48
49	0	8	0	2
75	3	0	0	15

Table 2.3 Number of *Streptococcus pyogenes* isolates from different sites from 1980 to 1990 by M-type. Data courtesy of the Streptococcal Reference Laboratory, Public Health Laboratory Service.

Flagella

The flagellum is the main organ of bacterial motility. It is made up of a globular protein, flagellin, arranged in a multistrand helix. The flagellum is bound to the plasma membrane via the motor unit, where the energy provided by the ion gradient across the membrane is converted into rotary movement.

Flagella are not usually associated with increased virulence or pathogenicity, but may be used in laboratory procedures as an identification feature. Flagellar antigens are frequently used in the classification of organisms such as salmonellae.

Structure of protozoa

Protozoa are unicellular microorganisms. They are found in almost every type of environment, over a wide range of pH (3–9.5), temperature, salinity and redox potential.

Classification

The classification of protozoa can be very complicated but may be simplified by subdivision into four main groups: spore-forming, flagellate, amoeboid and ciliate.

> **Classification of protozoa**
> 1 Sporozoa (e.g. *Microsporidium*, *Plasmodium*, *Toxoplasma*).
> 2 Flagellates (e.g. *Leishmania*, trypanosomes, *Trichomonas*).
> 3 Amoeboid (*Entamoeba histolytica*, *Acanthamoeba* spp.).
> 4 Ciliates (e.g. *Balantidium coli*).

Spore-forming protozoa

These can be divided into two groups:
1 Microspora are organisms which have recently been recognized as human pathogens, particularly in acquired immunodeficiency syndrome (AIDS) patients (see Chapter 11). *Encephalitozoon cuniculi*, *Enterocytozoon beneusii*, *Pleistophora*, *Septata intestinalis*, *Nosema connori* and *N. corneum* are the most important species reported.
2 Sporozoa. This group includes many of the important human protozoan pathogens. The sporozoa possess a complex of organelles known as the apical complex which is important in cell invasion. In the Eimeridia (which include *Toxoplasma gondii*), sexual reproduction occurs in the intestine of the definitive host. In contrast, the sexual stage of haemosporidians, such as *Plasmodium* spp., occurs in arthropods.

Eimeridia:	*Isospora belli*, *T. gondii*, *Cryptosporidium parvum* Sarcocystis
Haemosporidians:	*Plasmodium* spp.
Piroplasms:	*Babesia* spp.

Flagellate protozoa

These may be divided into the intestinal flagellate protozoa and the blood flagellates. The intestinal flagellates include *Giardia intestinalis*. *Trichomonas* spp. should also be included in this group, although it mainly causes disease in the vagina (*T. vaginalis*). Other non-pathogenic members of this genus are found as commensals in the mouth and bowel (e.g. *T. hominis*).

The blood flagellates are also known as the Trypanosomatidae and are characterized by the possession of a kinetoplast (a dense body at the base of the flagellum). They are transmitted to humans by the bite of arthropod vectors: sandflies in the case of *Leishmania*, *Glossina* (or tsetse) flies for African trypanosomiasis and triatomid bugs in the case of South American trypanosomiasis. *Leishmania* spp. exist in a flagellate form in the arthropod vector (Fig. 2.8) but transform after injection into the human host and live intracellularly as non-flagellate amastigotes.

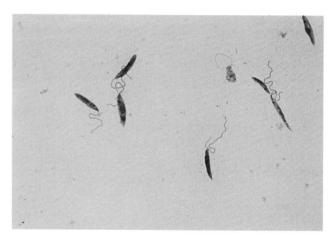

Fig. 2.8 Flagellate appearance of *Leishmania* sp.

Amoeboid protozoa

The most important genus of human amoebae is *Entamoeba*. Recent research has solved one of the classification problems of this group of organisms. The main pathogenic species, *E. histolytica*, could be subdivided by electrophoresis of certain enzymes into pathogenic and non-pathogenic subgroups (or zymodemes).

It is now known that these groups can be separated by monoclonal antibodies, lectin binding and serum sensitivity and these differences now define two different species: *E. histolytica*, which includes the pathogenic organisms, and *E. dispar*, which contains the non-pathogenic strains.

Naegleria fowleri causes a rare but usually fatal form of meningitis. It has an amoeboid form in the tissues, and a cyst and a flagellate form in the environment. It could therefore be classified with either group.

Blastocystis hominis is an organism of uncertain pathogenic potential but has been associated with diarrhoeal disease. Its taxonomic position is also uncertain but it is often classified with the amoebae.

Ciliate protozoa

Balantidium coli is the only ciliate protozoan regularly found in human specimens. It is sometimes identified in faeces, but is rarely implicated in disease.

Nuclear structures

Protozoa are eukaryotes, whose DNA exists as chromosomes within a nucleus. The nucleus is surrounded by a tough nuclear membrane which has multiple channels connecting the nucleoplasm with the endoplasm. Some organisms have a single nucleus, and others may be binucleate (e.g. *Giardia*) or have multinucleate cysts, e.g. *Entamoeba histolytica*. The nucleus may contain single or multiple linear chromosomes. Reproduction is by both sexual and asexual mechanisms.

Cytoplasm

The endoplasm is the inner portion of the cytoplasm immediately surrounding the nucleus. It contains chromatidoid bodies, endoplasmic reticulum, Golgi bodies, mitochondria, food vacuoles and microsomes. The ectoplasm is the metabolically active portion of the cell. It is also involved in locomotion, respiration, osmoregulation and phagocytosis. The cell is limited by the plasma membrane which controls the intake and output of food, secretions and metabolic waste products. It may vary in shape and can often form pseudopodia for locomotion.

Protozoa have a number of structures external to the plasma membrane, and these include an external glycocalyx (as in *Leishmania donovani*), or a tough cyst wall to enable the organism to survive in the external environment (as in *Giardia lamblia*). Encystation is triggered by alteration in food supply, excess of catabolic components, pH changes, desiccation or alteration in oxygen supply. Some protozoa have specialized organelles. *Leishmania* spp. possess flagella which arise from a specialized kinetoplast containing its own DNA, and metabolic processes. Others, such as *B. coli*, express cilia, which beat in formation to propel the organism.

Life cycle

Protozoa have reproductive cycles which may involve a number of different hosts and environments. Vectors may also be included, acting to transmit the infection between hosts and reservoirs of infection. A good example of this is the life cycle of *Plasmodium* sp., the cause of malaria (Fig. 2.9). Vectors can also act as a reservoir of infection by sustaining vertical transmission in the vector, for example certain viral encephalitides in ixodid ticks.

Intermediate hosts

Examples of protozoa that may be transmitted by vectors
1 Mosquitoes (*Plasmodium*).
2 *Glossina* spp. flies (*Trypanosoma brucei*).
3 Sandflies (*Leishmania*).
4 Ticks (*Babesia*).
5 Bugs — triatomid (*Trypanosoma cruzi*).
Protozoa may be transmitted by water, air, vectors, sexual intercourse, food and the faecal–oral route.

Many different species may act as intermediate hosts for human protozoa. These may also be the insect vectors.

Sexual stages

Unlike bacteria which have only limited sexual activity (e.g. fertility factors and transposons), protozoa have well-developed sexual reproduction. In amoebae, simple exchange of DNA is thought to take place, and in ciliates conjugation occurs and microgametocytes are exchanged. Sporozoa have asexual and sexual generations in their life cycle; in coccidia, including *Toxoplasma*, the essential stages of schizogony, gametocyte and zygote formation takes place in one host. In sporozoa, including malarial parasites, schizogony and gametocyte production occur in the vertebrate host and gametogeny is completed in the invertebrate host.

Like other pathogens, protozoa may be transmitted by many different routes (Table 2.4).

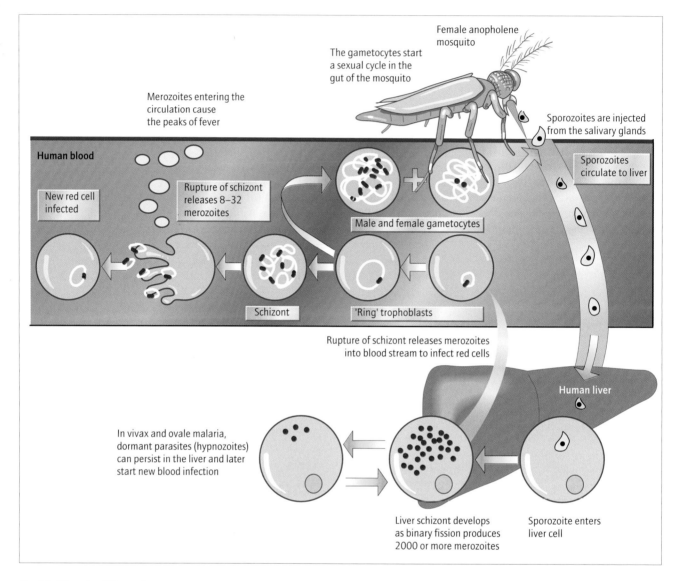

Fig. 2.9 Life cycle of *Plasmodium* sp.

Route	Example
Faecal–oral	*Entamoeba histolytica*
Water	*Cryptosporidium parvum*
Food	*Toxoplasma gondii*
Air	*Pneumocystis carinii*
Sexual	*Trichomonas vaginalis*
Vector	*Plasmodium vivax*

Table 2.4   Transmission of protozoa

Classification of fungi

Clinical classification of fungi of medical importance
Cutaneous, e.g. dermatophytes.
Systemic, e.g. *Coccidioides*, *Histoplasma*.
Fungal infections of immunocompromised hosts, e.g. *Aspergillos*.

The formal classification of fungi is based upon means of reproduction and morphology of sexual and asexual stages (Fig. 2.10). Unfortunately, the schemes derived have little clinical relevance so a simplified clinical classification is described. This divides pathogenic fungal species into three groups: (i) the superficial and subcutaneous; (ii) the systemic fungi; and (iii) the fungi associated with immunocompromised patients.

Superficial fungal infections are common. They include infection with dermatophytes, such as *Microsporon*, and *Trichophyton*. The yeast-like fungus *Malassezia furfur* is the causative organism of pityriasis versicolor. Rarer cutaneous fungal pathogens include *Sporothrix schenckii*, the cause of sporotrichosis, and the agents of piedra.

The systemic fungi include *Histoplasma capsulatum*, *Coccidioides immitis* and *Paracoccidioides braziliensis*.

These are dimorphic fungi, which have yeast-like and filamentous forms. They are environmental organisms which usually gain access to the human body via the respiratory tract. Infection is geographically localized and often clinically mild. Severe disease can occur, however, particularly in immunocompromised subjects.

The main organisms associated with fungal infection of immunocompromised patients are *Candida albicans* and related species such as *C. krusei* and *Torulopsis glabrata*. *Aspergillus* species are important filamentous fungi, usually causing pulmonary or disseminated infection. The commonest species implicated in human infection are *A. niger*, *A. fumigatus* and *A. flavus*. The yeast *Cryptococcus neoformans* was a rare cause of chronic lymphocytic meningitis, usually in patients with deficient cell-mediated immunity. This is now a common infection as a result of the HIV epidemic.

Introduction to helminths

The term helminth is derived from a Greek word which means worm. It was initially applied to roundworms but has been generalized to include all metazoan internal parasites. Helminths are complex multicellular organisms with developed organs. Adult worms may possess an alimentary canal whose morphology can be helpful in identification (e.g. hookworms). Adult females have developed uteri and produce large numbers of eggs daily. Many pathogens possess specialized organs of attachment, especially the hookworms and the tapeworms.

In some helminth diseases (Tables 2.5 and 2.6), humans are the only host and the pathogen produces eggs which are excreted, and survive in the environment. The life cycle is completed when eggs, or free-living larvae from excreted eggs, are ingested by a new host and a new infection develops. Such infections include those by threadworms and roundworms.

The life cycle of some helminths is complex, involving an intermediate host (e.g. the pig or cow in tapeworm diseases) or a vector (e.g. the mosquito in filariasis). The eggs of schistosomes are deposited by humans into water, hatch, invade snails, are released as infectious cercariae and reinfect humans by penetrating intact skin. Humans can be infected as an essential part of the life cycle in the case of filariasis or ascariasis, but hydatid disease is a zoonosis, in which humans replace the sheep in a dog–sheep–dog life cycle.

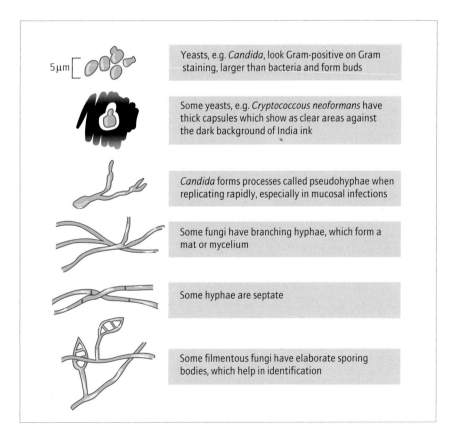

5 µm

Yeasts, e.g. *Candida*, look Gram-positive on Gram staining, larger than bacteria and form buds

Some yeasts, e.g. *Cryptococcous neoformans* have thick capsules which show as clear areas against the dark background of India ink

Candida forms processes called pseudohyphae when replicating rapidly, especially in mucosal infections

Some fungi have branching hyphae, which form a mat or mycelium

Some hyphae are septate

Some filamentous fungi have elaborate sporing bodies, which help in identification

Fig. 2.10 The morphologies of pathogenic fungi.

Family	Species	Disease
Trichuroidea	*Trichinella spiralis*	Trichinosis
	Trichuris trichuria	Trichuriasis
	Capillaria hepatica	
	C. phillipinensis	
Rhabditoidea	*Strongyloides stercoralis*	Strongyloidiasis
	S. fuelleborni	
Ancylostomatoidae	*Ancylostoma duodenale*	Hookworm disease
	A. ceylonicum	Ancylostomiasis
	Necator americanus	
Metastronguloidea	*Angiostrongylus cantonensis*	Eosinophilic meningitis
Oxyurida	*Enterobius vermicularis*	Threadworms
Ascarididae	*Ascaris lumbricoides*	Ascariasis
	Toxocara canis	Visceral larva
	T. cati	migrans and ocular disease
Dracunculoidea	*Dracunculus medinensis*	Guinea worm
Filaroidea	*Wuchereria bancrofti*	Lymphatic filariasis
	Brugia malayi	
	B. timori	
	Onchocerca volvulus	River blindness
	Loa loa	Loiasis

Table 2.5 Nematodes which cause human disease

Family	Species	Disease
Schistosomatoidea	*Schistosoma mansoni*	Bilharzia
	S. haematobium	
	S. japonicum	
Echinostomatoidae	*Fasciola hepatica*	Liver flukes
Taeniidae	*Taenia solium*	Tapeworms and cysticercosis
	T. saginata	
	Echinococcus granulosus	Hydatid disease
	E. multilocularis	

Table 2.6 Most important platyhelminths which cause human infection

Classification

Helminths are classified into the nematodes or round-worms, the cestodes or tapeworms and the flukes.

Helminths are divided into two main groups: round-worms (nematodes) and flatworms (platyhelminths). The flatworms are further divided into the cestodes (tapeworms) and the trematodes (flukes). The flukes are then further subdivided into blood, liver and lung flukes.

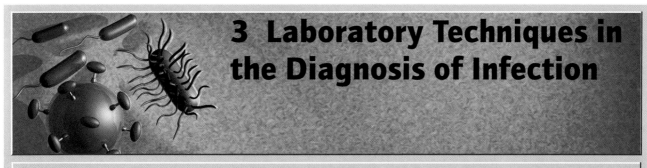

3 Laboratory Techniques in the Diagnosis of Infection

Introduction

The microbiology laboratory plays a crucial role in the diagnosis of all infectious diseases. Although there are many different tests available for the diagnosis of individual patients, there are only three main ways of making a microbiological diagnosis.
1 Microscopical methods.
2 Cultural methods.
3 Serological methods.
In addition, new diagnostic techniques such as DNA probes and the polymerase chain reaction (PCR) are now developing rapidly.

Collection of specimens

A wide diversity of specimens can be examined microbiologically. Many tests must be taken at a particular time, for example malaria parasites are best sought at the peak of fever and a short time afterwards, whereas blood culture should be taken as the fever begins to rise. Special precautions must be taken when some specimens are collected, e.g. careful preparation of the perineum before a midstream specimen of urine is collected. Many organisms are fragile, surviving poorly outside the body, and must be transported to the laboratory with minimal delay. Some anaerobic species die if exposed to atmospheric oxygen and must be transported rapidly or in a dedicated anaerobic transport system. *Neisseria*

gonorrhoeae dies rapidly outside the body and specimens likely to contain this organism should be inoculated on to microbiological medium near to the patient.

Specimens may contain hazardous pathogens and must be handled with care. The concerns about the risk of transmission of blood-borne viruses have led to the introduction of a system of universal precautions which delineates the personal protective measures to be taken in collecting and examining specimens irrespective of their source. The idea is based on handling specimens on the assumption that they may contain a blood-borne virus rather than relying on clinical suspicion or written clinical details which may be faulty or absent.

Direct microscopic examination

Ever since Anthonie van Leeuwenhoek first saw 'animalcules', the light microscope has been a vital tool in the study of microorganisms. It was by seeing the characteristic microscopical morphology of staphylococci in samples of pus that Alexander Ogston discovered their role in pyogenic sepsis.

Microscopy is extremely important in clinical diagnosis. The equipment required is relatively inexpensive, reagent costs are low and early results can be obtained. Microscopy gives such rapid results that the diagnosis of malaria or vaginal trichomoniasis, for instance, can be made while the patient waits at the clinic. The organism being sought need neither multiply nor even be alive.

This aids the detection of microorganisms which may be difficult or even dangerous to grow.

Many different microscopical techniques have been developed and serve different purposes.

> **Types of microscopy for the diagnosis of infections**
> 1 Unstained preparations.
> 2 Simple stains — Gram, Giemsa.
> 3 Special stains — Ziehl–Nielsen, Gomori–Grocott, India ink.
> 4 Immunofluorescence — direct and indirect.
> 5 Electron microscopy.

Microscopy of unstained preparations

> **Direct microscopy of unstained preparations**
> Faecal protozoa and helminths, vaginal discharge, urine for bacteria and pus cells.

Pathogens may be demonstrated by direct microscopical examination of unstained 'wet' preparations. This technique is most suitable for rapid diagnosis in the outpatient setting. The pathogens may have a diagnostic morphological appearance, as does *Entamoeba histolytica*, or may appear in diagnostic circumstances, for instance bacteria, together with white cells, in the urine from a case of acute urinary tract infection. Examination of unstained preparations can, for example, be applied to the diagnosis of trichomoniasis and candidiasis in vaginal secretions or intestinal parasites in saline wet preparations of faeces (Fig. 3.1).

Specimens can be examined directly by electron microscopy, using a negative-staining technique. The viruses are concentrated by vigorous centrifugation and then suspended in a heavy metal solution. As it dries,

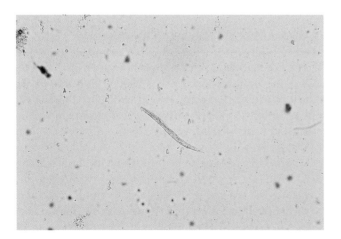

Fig. 3.1 Unstained wet preparation of faeces showing larva of *Strongyloides stercoralis*. × 94 approximately.

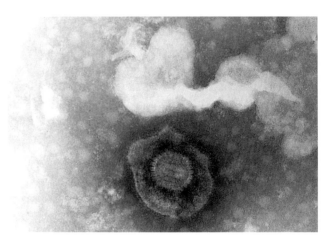

Fig. 3.2 Negatively stained electron micrograph of herpesvirus. Courtesy of Dr David Brown, Central Public Health Laboratory.

the heavy metal salt fills in the spaces between the viruses, providing an electron-dense background against which the virus structures can be demonstrated. This technique is useful for the demonstration of viruses with distinctive morphology, such as poxviruses in scrapings from the lesions of orf and molluscum contagiosum, herpes simplex virus or varicella-zoster virus in vesicle fluid, or one of the many gastrointestinal viruses, such as rotavirus or calicivirus in diarrhoea stools (Fig. 3.2).

Microscopical examination of preparations stained with simple stains

Gram stain

Dried fixed preparations of specimens can be examined using simple stains, such as Gram stain, which dye the bacteria. This technique can demonstrate the shape of the bacteria and their ability, or not, to retain the blue Gram dye (Fig. 3.3). It provides a rapid answer to the clinical question: 'are there any organisms present?' It is therefore most useful when usually sterile fluids such as cerebrospinal fluid (CSF) or pleural fluid are examined. However, the sensitivity of Gram stain is relatively low; more than 100 000 organisms per millilitre must be present for a diagnosis to be made.

> **Gram stain**
> Sterile fluids (cerebrospinal fluid, ascites, pleural fluid), sputum (to exclude poor-quality specimens), pus from any site, urethral discharge.

Gram-staining alone is rarely able to answer the question: 'what organism is present?' because the morphology

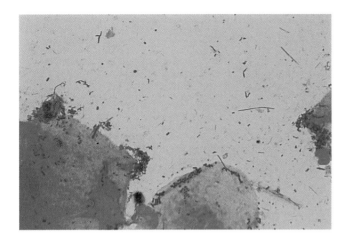

Fig. 3.3 Gram stain of a smear from the mouth, showing a mixture of Gram-positive and Gram-negative cocci and bacilli.

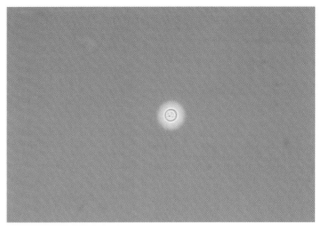

Fig. 3.4 India ink-stained preparation of cerebrospinal fluid, showing *Cryptococcus neoformans* with a thick, clear capsule.

of bacteria is rarely diagnostic. Important exceptions to this include the finding of Gram-positive or -negative diplococci in CSF from a patient with meningitis, or the characteristic appearances of *Borrelia* and *Fusobacterium* in Vincent's angina. Similarly, a Gram-stained preparation of urethral pus showing Gram-negative intracellular diplococci is sufficiently characteristic to allow a presumptive diagnosis of gonorrhoea.

Other simple stains

Other simple stains include acridine orange (which is more sensitive in demonstrating organisms than Gram stain, but more prone to confusing artefactual staining effects), lactophenol blue to demonstrate the morphology of fungi, or India ink, which is used to detect the presence of *Cryptococcus neoformans* in the CSF by negative staining (Fig. 3.4).

Stains such as Ziehl–Nielsen (ZN) are utilized to demonstrate specific features of organisms which are useful for identification. Specimens are stained with carbol fuchsin which is driven into the organism by, for example, heating with phenol. The preparation is destained with an acid–alcohol solution and then counterstained with methylene blue. Mycobacteria possess a lipid-rich cell wall which retains the pink dye against the decoloration of the acid–alcohol solution. The organisms are then seen as pink bacilli against the bright methylene blue counterstain background (Fig. 3.5). The number of species which are acid-fast is limited and this technique is therefore useful in the diagnosis of mycobacterial infection, including tuberculosis and leprosy, and parasitic infections such as cryptosporidiosis.

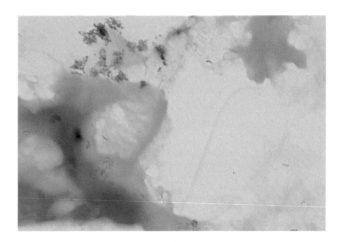

Fig. 3.5 Ziehl–Nielsen-stained smear, showing acid-fast bacilli.

A variation of this technique uses the naturally fluorescent substance auramine to stain the organisms. The specimen is processed in a similar way to the ZN method, and acid-fast organisms fluoresce bright yellow under an ultraviolet light. Auramine microscopy is used for screening large numbers of specimens but, because it lacks the specificity of the ZN stain, all positive specimens must be overstained by the ZN method, and re-examined to confirm the findings.

Romanowsky stains

Romanowsky stains colour cytoplasm and chromatin, and are normally used to demonstrate blood cells. Stains such as Giemsa are used in the diagnosis of blood parasites. Taking malaria or filariasis as examples, Giemsa-stained smears not only demonstrate the presence of the

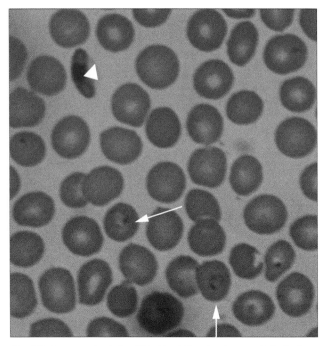

Fig. 3.6 Romanowsky-stained thin blood film, showing morphologically typical trophozoites of *Plasmodium falciparum* (arrows) and a gametocyte (arrow head).

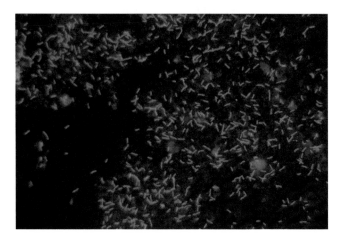

Fig. 3.7 Immunofluorescence-stained preparation of legionellae. Courtesy of Dr Tim Harrison, Central Public Health Laboratory.

organisms, but permit speciation by demonstration of morphological details (Fig. 3.6).

Simple stains used in microbiology	
1 Albert's stain	*Corynebacterium diphtheriae.*
2 Ziehl–Nielsen	*Mycobacterium* spp.
3 Gomori–Grocott	Fungi, *Pneumocystis carinii.*
4 Giemsa	Malaria, *Filaria.*

Immunofluorescence

In direct immunofluorescent techniques, organisms can be revealed by their reaction with fluorescence-labelled antibodies. The patient specimen is dried on a multiwell slide, together with control positive and negative specimens. A specific antibody labelled with fluoroscein is applied to the specimen which is then incubated at 37°C in a humidified chamber for approximately 1 h. The slides are then washed and examined microscopically under ultraviolet light. Where a specific antigen–antibody interaction has taken place, labelled antibody is bound to the pathogen, which will be demonstrated by an apple-green fluorescence (Fig. 3.7).

This technique is both sensitive and specific and provides a rapid, presumptive diagnosis. It can be applied to a wide range of specimens and is used in the diag-

nosis of chlamydial urethritis, influenza, parainfluenza, respiratory syncytial virus, measles and rhabdovirus infections.

Examples of direct immunofluorescence	
1 Viruses	Parainfluenza, respiratory syncytial virus.
2 Bacteria	*Legionella, Treponema pallidum.*
3 Protozoa/fungi	*Giardia intestinalis, Pneumocystis carinii.*

Immunofluorescent techniques are also used for the detection of specific antibody. This will be described in more detail below.

Cultural methods

Microbiological culture consumes much time and resources in the laboratory, but the diagnostic rewards can be modest if the limitations of culture are not appreciated.

Culture can contribute to diagnosis in bacterial, parasitic and viral diseases. In bacteriology, culture allows isolation of bacteria on solid media, aiding recognition by their morphological and biochemical characteristics. It is the main means of obtaining pure cultures for antimicrobial susceptibility testing.

Modern bacterial culture is made possible by the use of agar, a gelatinous substance derived from seaweed, which melts at 90°C but solidifies at 50°C. It is highly stable, rarely affected by organisms in cultures and can be mixed with nutrients such as blood, serum and protein digests to make solid media. Koch introduced agar to microbiology to replace gelatin, which melts at a lower temperature near to that used for incubation. He heard that a woman who lived in Batavia (modern-day Jakarta) used agar to make jellies, as those made with gelatin were prone to melt at tropical temperatures.

Bacteriological culture in solid agar is usually performed on Petri dishes — plastic dishes, 90 mm in diameter, with a vented lid. When prolonged culture is necessary, as in the diagnosis of mycobacterial or fungal infection, it is usually performed in sealed universal containers to prevent the entry of contaminating organisms. Various specimens are usually incubated in a range of atmospheric conditions to allow the growth of organisms which require oxygen (obligate aerobes), reduced oxygen and enhanced carbon dioxide (microaerophilic organisms) or no oxygen (obligate anaerobes) to multiply. Organisms which can multiply with or without oxygen are called facultative.

Media

Three types of bacteriological media are used: enrichment, selective and indicator.

Bacteriological media
1 Enrichment.
2 Selective.
3 Indicator.

Enrichment media

Enrichment media are required when fastidious organisms such as *Streptococcus* spp., *Haemophilus influenzae* or *Bacteroides fragilis* are being sought. Their main purpose is to ensure that small numbers of fragile pathogens will multiply to a sufficient degree to be readily detectable.

Simple base media may be enriched by the addition of blood, yeast extracts, brain and heart infusions, meat, etc. Enrichment media can be solid, for example blood agar, or liquid, as with Robertson's cooked meat broth. Liquid media are especially valuable for investigating body fluids which are normally sterile. Such specimens often contain very small numbers of organisms which, however, rapidly multiply in the rich medium, and can then be subcultured on to solid media for identification and sensitivity testing.

Enrichment medium aims to amplify the organism by more rapid growth, e.g. for *Neisseria* spp., *Streptococcus* spp. or *Vibrio* spp.

Selective media

Selective media are used when a pathogen must be identified in a mixture of organisms. Many body sites,

Medium	Selective agent	Specimen	Organism/s sought
Crystal violet–blood agar	Crystal violet	Throat swab	*Streptococcus pyogenes*
Desoxycholate citrate	Desoxycholate	Faeces	*Salmonella* *Shigella*
New York City medium	Lincomycin, colistin, amphotericin, trimethoprim	Urethral/ cervical smear	*Neisseria gonorrhoeae*
Selenite broth	Selenite F	Faeces	*Salmonella*
Sabouraud's agar	High dextrose content	Many	Fungi

Table 3.1 Examples of selective media for bacteriological culture from sites containing a normal flora

such as the upper respiratory tract or the gut, have a normal resident flora, and pathogens must be isolated from this bacterial competition. Selective media contain compounds which may be chemicals (e.g. selenite F), dyes (crystal violet) or mixtures of antibiotics (such as lincomycin, amphotericin B, colistin and trimethoprim in New York City medium), which selectively inhibit the normal flora, enabling the pathogen to grow through (Table 3.1). It can be seen from Table 3.1 that these media can be complex mixtures requiring careful preparation.

Although the selective agents have their maximum effect on the unwanted organisms, some inhibition of the target organism inevitably occurs. Therefore when selective media are being used, an enrichment medium should be inoculated in parallel so that small numbers of pathogens can be detected.

Selective cultures, e.g. sputum, stool or throat swab specimens, aim to identify, for instance, *Haemophilus* spp., *Salmonella* spp. or *Streptococcus* spp. from among normal flora.
Antibiotics, dyes, antiseptics, chemicals and bile salts are examples of substances used in selective bacteriological media.
Culture of pathogens from sites with normal flora requires selection, and from sterile sites requires enrichment.

Indicator media

Indicator media are used to identify colonies of pathogens among the mixture of organisms able to grow on the selective medium. An example of a selective indi-

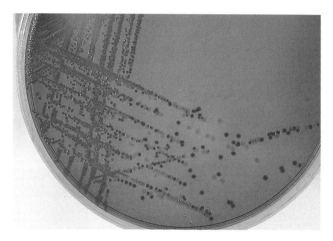

Fig. 3.8 Mixed growth of Enterobacteriacae on MacConkey's agar plate, showing pink, lactose-fermenting colonies of *Escherichia coli* among the colourless non-lactose-fermenters.

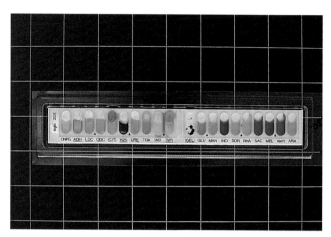

Fig. 3.9 A typical bank of biochemical tests for the identification of species of Enterobacteriacae.

cator medium is MacConkey's agar, which uses bile salts to select for bile-tolerant enteric organisms. It also contains lactose and the indicator neutral red. Colonies of lactose-fermenting organisms produce lactic acid, and are coloured red by the neutral red indicator. Pathogens are usually non-lactose-fermenters, which produce colourless colonies in this system (Fig. 3.8).

> **Indicator media (often combined with selective function)**
> MacConkey
>   Selects with bile salts
>   Indicates lactose fermentation with pH indicator.

Commonly used indicator media are usually selective as well. There are many liquid indicator media, containing different sugars or other substrates such as urea and citrate. They also contain indicator dyes which change colour when bacterial metabolic products alter the pH of the medium. Thus an organism which ferments a particular sugar lowers the pH of the medium, or one which metabolizes urea produces ammonia and raises the pH. These indicator media are usually used in banks of tests which allow identification of an organism by its biochemical profile. Pre-prepared sets of mini-culture vials are commercially available (Fig. 3.9).

Limitations of culture

The main limitation of bacterial culture is the time it takes. It is not often, therefore, the primary means of diagnosis. There are exceptions to this of course, for example, bacterial endocarditis where blood culture is

the only definitive test in most cases. Often, however, infected patients are ill and require immediate treatment. The decision to initiate therapy must be made on the basis of the clinical features of the case, rapid tests like Gram stain of CSF and any helpful haematological or biochemical test results. Culture is useful for confirmation or rebuttal of the diagnosis and for bringing to light unusual or unexpected organisms, or those with unusual susceptibility patterns.

Culture is of particular value when the range of potential pathogens and susceptibilities is wide, as in aspirated pus specimens. The initial therapy in such cases may need modification when the result of culture is available.

Culture has an important epidemiological purpose, not related to the treatment of individual patients. Most cases of acute diarrhoea could be well-managed without microbial culture. The isolation of the same *Salmonella* sp. from several individuals, however, might prompt a search for a common source such as an infected food-handler at a restaurant. Similarly, the isolation of a toxigenic strain of *Corynebacterium diphtheriae* from a throat swab should prompt clinicians to initiate surveillance and control measures in the patient's contracts.

Screening

This particular application of epidemiological investigation can be used to screen patients and staff for colonization with pathogens, such as *Streptococcus pyogenes* in a surgical ward, or strains with multidrug resistance, such as epidemic methicillin-resistant

Staphylococcus aureus (EMRSA). It can allow a prompt response to the presence of dangerous or difficult-to-treat organisms in a hospital setting.

Automation

Bacterial culture is time-consuming and labour-intensive. Fortunately, new techniques for automatic detection of bacterial growth are now becoming available. Conventional methods of blood culture, for example, require manual subculture of each bottle after 12, 24 and 48 h, and later subcultures as necessary. Each laboratory usually has its own protocol. Automated methods detect the microbial production of carbon dioxide, or changes in the electrical impedance of the medium, to indicate the need for subculture. Similar methods can be applied to identification of most bacterial species. These methods have shortened the time taken to detect slow-growing organisms such as brucellae or mycobacteria from weeks to days. Computer analysis of results from multiple test systems can allow rapid identification of bacterial isolates.

> Detection of carbon dioxide produced by bacteria or changes in the electrical impedence of the media have allowed automatic detection of bacterial growth.

Antimicrobial susceptibility testing

Testing antimicrobial susceptibility is an important function of the microbiology laboratory. Apart from confirming the expected behaviour of pathogens, it is of particular value when the infecting organisms have unpredictable antimicrobial susceptibilities. This is especially true of Enterobacteriaceae, among which multidrug resistance may develop and spread in the hospital environment. In some geographic areas salmonellae may be resistant to most commonly used therapeutic agents. Some organisms, such as *Streptococcus pneumoniae*, formerly sensitive to many antimicrobials, have recently developed considerable resistance, making empirical therapy difficult. This emphasizes the need for routine antimicrobial susceptibility testing of common isolates.

Almost all currently available methods of antimicrobial susceptibility testing depend on isolation of the organism by culture, and then on reculture of the pure growth, in controlled conditions, in the presence of antimicrobial agents. This is described in more detail on p. 56.

Typing microorganisms

> Typing is the use of further identification methods to distinguish between strains of organisms within the same species.

For most clinical purposes it is sufficient to identify the genus or species of a pathogen. Occasionally, however, further characterization of organisms is desirable. For example, three cases of *Salmonella typhimurium* infection could be caused by different strains of this common pathogen. The only way to prove that the cases truly represent an outbreak is to show that the strains are identical.

The use of further identification methods to distinguish organisms within a species is known as typing. The principal characteristic of a typing system is that it divides microorganisms into clinically relevant groups; a typing system is of no value if all the clinically relevant strains are in one type. Typing methods should be sufficiently reproducible that results from one laboratory can be compared with those of another. The technique should also be simple to perform, as delay in receiving results hinders early control of an outbreak. And finally it should be inexpensive.

Methods of typing microorganisms

Many methods can be used to type microorganisms, ranging from simple biochemical characteristics to complex genetic characterization. It is quite common for two or more methods to be used, to provide adequately distinct separation of strains; for instance, *Legionella pneumophila* is serotyped into nine groups, and then further biotyped for more accurate identification. *Listeria monocytogenes* is serotyped and phage-typed.

Simple laboratory typing

Simple phenotypic markers are often sufficient to demonstrate the identity of isolates and indicate that an outbreak or episode of cross-infection has occurred. It can also be useful to type successive isolates of the same organism from an individual patient; for instance, in a case of *Staphylococcus epidermidis* bacteraemia the organisms isolated from blood or intravascular devices on different occasions could represent a variety of contaminants from the patient's skin. They could be considered identical, and representative of a true infection, if a range of biochemical characteristics and the antibiogram were identical (Fig. 3.10). This approach

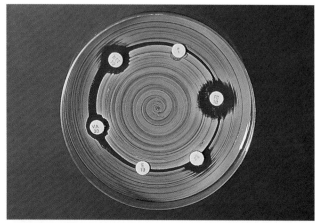

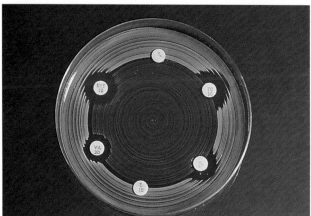

Fig. 3.10 Antibiograms of successive isolates of *Staphylococcus epidermidis* from the blood of a patient in intensive care; although the density of growth is different in the two tests (the centre of the plate) the pattern of inhibition by antibiotic discs is identical, indicating that they may be the true cause of a persisting fever.

could not be adopted for *S. aureus*, however, as many strains can exist which share the same resistance patterns and biochemical phenotypes. For this species phage typing is most appropriate.

Biotyping

Pathogens are often assigned to a species by means of biochemical testing. Biotyping uses the results of additional biochemical tests to assign members of the same species into different groups or biotypes. The tests employed may be sugar fermentation tests, or tests for the action of enzymes such as urease. Strains of *Legionella pneumophila* and *Corynebacterium diphtheriae* are often identified by biotyping (Fig. 3.11).

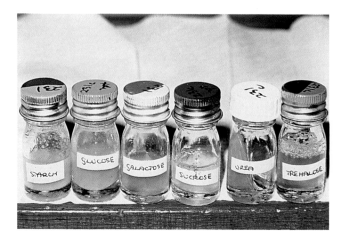

Fig. 3.11 Biotyping of *Corynebacterium diphtheriae*: the sugar tests are typical of the gravis strain.

Auxotyping

This biochemical method tests the ability of an organism to grow on minimal medium and use single chemicals such as arginine as a source of, for example, nitrogen. The profiles detected by the tests, called auxanograms, are most suitable for typing fastidious organisms with complex nutritional requirements, for example *Neisseria gonorrhoeae* or *Haemophilus influenzae*.

Serological typing

Many organisms can be typed by testing a range of serological reactions. Many laboratories use in-house systems for typing enteric pathogens such as *Shigella flexneri* or salmonellas. Antisera are raised in mice or guinea-pigs by immunization with surface protein or polysaccharide extracts of the various strains. Serological typing is performed by suspending a pure growth of the organism in a drop of antiserum on a glass slide and mixing with a rocking movement of the slide. The development of agglutination indicates that the organism carries the antigen specific to the antiserum used.

For organisms where it is difficult to generate sets of typing sera, or the test is rarely required, reference laboratories have been set up to provide a central expert service.

Phage typing

Many bacteriophages lyse the bacteria they infect as part of their life cycle (this is known as a lytic cycle). Different strains of an organism have different sensitivities to the phages which commonly infect the species. This pro-

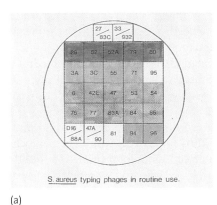
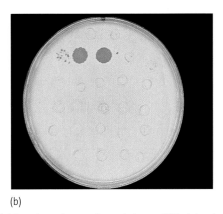
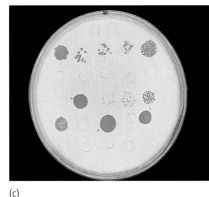

(a)   (b)   (c)

Fig. 3.12 Phage-typing of *Staphylococcus aureus*. (a) Template of currently used phages; (b) lysis by phages 52/52 a; (c) complex type. With permission of Central Public Health Laboratory.

perty is useful in typing staphylococci, *Listeria mono-cytogenes* and some species of *Salmonellae*. A lawn inoculum of the test organism is made, and a battery of suitable phages is inoculated at fixed points. The plates are then incubated overnight and the pattern of lysis indicates the phage type. A *Staphylococcus aureus* may be identified as phage type 88/24 because it was lysed only by the 88 and 24 phages (Fig. 3.12). Some strains are not lysed by any phage, and are called phage-untypable.

Bacteriocin typing

Many microorganisms produce protein antibiotics directed against other bacteria competing for the same ecological niche. These bacteriocins often have different inhibitory effects on different strains within a species, and this characteristic is utilized in bacteriocin typing. A test strain is inoculated as a streak on a suitable agar plate and grown overnight. The growth is then scraped off with a glass slide, and the plate exposed to chloroform to kill any remaining organisms. A battery of indicator strains is then inoculated as a set of streaks at right angles to the test strain, and incubated overnight. The next day some indicator strains will have gaps in their growth where they have been inhibited by the test strain's bacteriocin. The pattern of inhibition is used to assign strains to a bacteriocine type. This method has been used in typing *Shigella sonnei* and *Pseudomonas aeruginosa*.

Molecular methods

Many molecular typing methods have been developed, but they tend to be expensive and at present difficult to standardize between laboratories.

Protein typing

This is a relatively crude method of typing in which the proteins of an organism are simultaneously extracted and suspended in a detergent solution (usually sodium dodecyl sulphate, or SDS). The pattern of proteins is then demonstrated by electrophoresis, often on poly-acrylamide gel (the process called PAGE). SDS-PAGE typing techniques have largely been superseded by nucleic acid profiling.

Nucleic acid typing

Many nucleic methods use the activity of endonuclease enzymes to split the genome into a characteristic range of different-sized fragments. Genomic or plasmid DNA or ribosomal RNA is harvested from the test strains and digested with restriction endonucleases. The resulting fragments are then separated by electrophoresis on an agarose gel, to produce a pattern of bands. Identical organisms have identical bands. The variation in band patterns produced by restriction endonuclease digestion of nucleic acids is called restriction fragment length polymorphism (RFLP; Fig. 3.13).

The main problems with nucleic acid typing arise in gel-to-gel variation, which makes long-term comparisons both within and between laboratories difficult. However, internationally agreed methodology has now been established for *Mycobacterium tuberculosis*, and may soon be available for other organisms.

Meanwhile, less expensive and more reproducible techniques remain the favoured typing methods. Although most typing systems are designed to identify bacterial strains, protozoa and some fungi can also be typed. Protozoa are often typed by the range of enzymes they

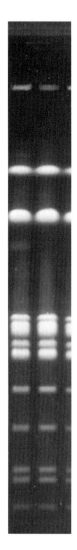

Fig. 3.13 Electrophoresis of DNA restriction fragments of three cytomegalovirus isolates, showing that the infected patients had acquired the same strain.

possess. Enzyme types of protozoa are often called zymodemes.

Methods of typing bacteria
1 Biotyping and auxotyping.
2 Serotyping.
3 Phage typing.
4 Bacteriocin typing.
5 Restriction fragment length polymorphism typing.

Culture of protozoa

Culture of protozoa and helminths is often difficult. In many examples, such as *Cryptosporidium parvum*, culture

of only a single stage in the life cycle may be possible. In others, such as *Strongyloides stercoralis*, the conditions of the natural environment can be reproduced in the laboratory. Using activated charcoal as a culture medium, larvae in faecal specimens will mature and multiply.

In the case of *Plasmodium falciparum* the whole asexual life cycle can readily be maintained by culturing the organism in banked red blood cells. Sensitivity to antimalarial agents can thus be tested. Although this technique is relatively simple it is inappropriate for routine diagnosis, because direct microscopy is sufficiently sensitive to detect even low parasitaemias. In other words, there is no need for the amplification characteristics of culture. Amoebae can also be cultured in solid media if certain bacteria are included, but simple microscopy is an accurate and rapid means of diagnosis, and culture remains a research procedure.

Other protozoan parasites such as *Leishmania* can be cultured in artificial media, but only in the promastigote stage normally found in the insect vector. To achieve a culture of the amastigote, or tissue stage, material must be inoculated into isolated peripheral blood macrophages or macrophage cell lines.

Tissue culture

Viruses are obligatory intracellular pathogens, thus viral culture must be performed in living cells or tissues. Cells are usually prepared as monolayers on to which the specimen is inoculated. The cells may be primary cultures in which cells extracted directly from an organ, e.g. monkey kidney, are cultured in a monolayer. Primary cell lines can be propagated for up to 50 generations, and are essential for isolation of some viruses. Continuous cell lines can be subcultured indefinitely. Cell cultures are maintained at 37°C in an atmosphere of increased humidity and carbon dioxide. Cultured viruses infect the cells and take over their metabolic processes as they do in the human host. The cell monolayer is inspected at intervals for the presence of viral damage to the cells — the cytopathic effect (CPE). Some viruses may be presumptively identified on the basis of a distinctive cytopathic effect (Fig. 3.14). Thus enteroviruses lyse the cells, whereas measles virus produces multinucleated giant cells. For some species there is no visible CPE but growth of the virus is detected by other means, for example adherence of red cells to viral haemagglutinin molecules expressed on the cells (known as haemadsorption). The presence of replicating virus can also be inferred from a change in pH caused by metabolic activity, or viral antigens can be directly demonstrated

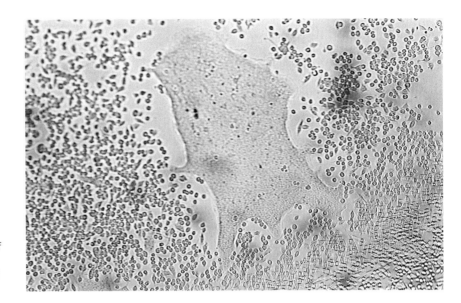

Fig. 3.14 Cytopathic effect of measles virus on lymphoblastoid cells; progressive coalescence of infected cells into a syncytium has formed a giant cell. Such giant cells may contain up to 50 nuclei.

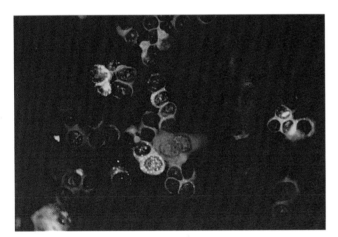

Fig. 3.15 Fluorescence micrograph of Lassa virus-infected vero cells, stained with immunofluorescent-labelled anti-Lassa serum. Courtesy of Dr David Brown, Central Public Health Laboratory.

by fixing the cell monolayer and using immunological techniques such as immunofluorescence (Fig. 3.15).

Evidence of virus growth in cell cultures
1 A cytopathic effect.
2 Haemadsorption.
3 Biochemical change in nutrient medium.
4 Antigen detection.
5 Electron microscopy.

Identification of virus isolates can be achieved by lysing the cells of the monolayer and visualizing the virus under the electron microscope. Alternatively, cultured virus particles can be identified by immunological techniques or virus neutralization (making subcultures of the viruses, and demonstrating inhibition of viral growth by specific antibodies).

Serology in the detection of infection

Serological techniques depend on the interaction between antigen and specific antibody. They are of particular value when the pathogen is difficult or impossible to culture, or is dangerous to handle in hospital laboratories.

The process can be divided into two parts: the antigen–antibody interaction, and the demonstration of this interaction by a testing process. The antigen–antibody reaction depends on the specific binding between epitopes on the pathogen and the antigen-binding sites on the immunoglobulin molecules. The sensitivity of a serological test depends partly on the specificity and strength of the antigen–antibody reaction, but mostly on the ability of the test system to detect the reaction.

In older tests antibody–antigen binding was detected by observing a natural consequence of this interaction: precipitation, agglutination or the ability of the antigen–antibody complex to bind and activate (fix) complement. This approach has stood the test of time and laboratory tests based on these three reactions are still in daily use. Newer tests use modified immunoglobulin molecules to facilitate detection. The main methods employed are labelling with fluorescein, radioiodine or enzymes. Examples of each of these techniques are described in detail below.

Precipitation

The simplest of the serological techniques is precipitation, in which an insoluble complex is formed between antigen and antibody, both of which are in solution. The test can be performed by mixing soluble antigen with serum, and observing any precipitate formation.

More commonly, gel precipitation tests are performed. Wells are cut in an agar gel and antigen and antibody placed in the wells a few millimetres apart. Antibody and antigen diffuse from the wells and at an optimal concentration will form a precipitin line. This can take up to 48 h, but can be speeded up by applying an electrical field to the gel. The charge drives the negatively charged antigen (usually a polysaccharide) towards the anode, while antibody, which is neutral at the pH of the buffer system, is driven towards the cathode in the stream of buffer ions. This means that a precipitin line can be formed in as little as 1 h. This technique, called counter-current immunoelectrophoresis (CIE), has been used in the diagnosis of acute pyogenic meningitis and fungal infections. As the equipment employed is simple and uses only small quantities of reagents, the test is inexpensive. The short time taken to process each sample means that CIE is suitable for rapid diagnosis.

Agglutination

The simplest form is agglutination of bacteria by a specific antibody. This phenomenon can be used to identify the species or serotype of an infecting organism. Slide agglutination tests are particularly useful for identifying faecal pathogens such as salmonellae or shigellae.

Tube agglutination

Tube agglutination is a similar process to precipitation, in which particulate antigens interact with specific antibody, forming a 'lattice' which falls to the bottom of the test vessel in a fine mat. In a positive test, the mat of agglutination is found at the bottom of the reaction vessel, and in a negative test, the particulate antigen falls quickly to the bottom to form a condensed button. This technique has been widely used in the Widal test and the *Brucella* standard agglutination tests. A rapid micro-agglutination test (RMAT) is still the standard test for antibodies to *Legionella pneumophila* (Fig. 3.16).

Specific antibody can be attached to uniform latex particles, or killed protein A-possessing staphylococci. These particles will be agglutinated when they attach in large numbers to antigen molecules. In this way, other-

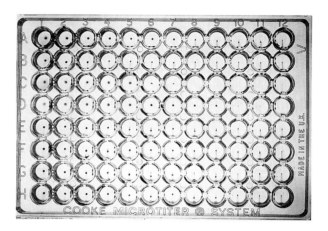

Fig. 3.16 Rapid microagglutination test for the detection of antibodies to *Legionella pneumophila*. Each row is composed of doubling dilutions of an individual patient's serum, mixed with dead organisms. The microtitre plate has conical wells, so that centrifugation 'jams' the agglutinated organism at the bottom of the well. Unagglutinated organisms form a streak when the plate is tipped on its edge: a dot is therefore positive and a streak is negative.

wise soluble antigens may be detected in an agglutination reaction. Such latex and coagglutination techniques are used to detect the presence of the polysaccharide antigens of *Streptococcus pneumoniae*, type b *Haemophilus influenzae*, *Neisseria meningitidis* and *Cryptococcus neoformans* in the CSF or *S. pyogenes* in throat swabs.

Complement fixation

Complement fixation tests are a means of detecting the initial antibody–antigen interaction. Known antigen is added to a patient's serum which has been heat-inactivated (to destroy naturally occurring complement) and supplemented with a measured amount of guinea-pig complement. When specific antibody is present in the serum, it interacts with the antigen, producing immune complexes that bind (or fix) complement. This is the primary reaction. In the secondary reaction, sheep red cells which have been sensitized with rabbit anti-sheep red-cell antibody are added. If complement has been fixed in the primary reaction, none remains to attack the sheep cells and no lysis will occur. In contrast, if no antigen–antibody reaction has taken place in the first reaction, the complement is still available to achieve the second reaction, and lysis of the sheep red cells will occur. Complement fixation tests are a little confusing in that in positive results *no* lysis occurs, whereas in negative tests lysis is found. Positive sera are titrated so that changes in titre can be used to detect a developing immune response. A positive result can be assumed if a serum contains antibody concentrations outside the population norm. More usually, rising or falling titres must be found. A fourfold rise in complement-fixing antibody levels is highly specific but relatively insensitive. The test is technically difficult and requires careful standardization. It is therefore being superseded by those described below.

Indirect fluorescent antibody tests

Specific antigen is fixed on to a multiwell microscope slide. The patient's serum is incubated with this antigen, together with known positive and negative sera in other wells. The slides are then washed and each well is incubated with a fluorescein-labelled antihuman immunoglobulin. After a further wash the slides are examined under ultraviolet illumination, and where a specific antibody interaction has occurred the antihuman globulin is indicated by apple-green fluorescence. Individual positive sera may be titrated. Indirect immunofluorescence is both sensitive and specific. It has found an application in the serological diagnosis of parasitic infections. It is particularly suitable when only a few specimens are received as it is somewhat time-consuming to perform.

Indirect fluorescent antibody tests (IFATs) may be used for the diagnosis of syphilis (FTA) or parasitic disease such as leishmaniasis or amoebiasis.

Radioimmunoassay

Specific antigen is radiolabelled, then mixed and incubated with the patient's serum. The specimen is then centrifuged to separate the bound from the unbound radioactivity. The heavier antibody–antigen complexes collect at the bottom of the tube, where the radioactivity is then counted. The quantity of antibody is determined by reference to a standard curve. Radioimmunoassays are highly sensitive and specific. However, they require expensive radiolabelled reagents which have a short shelf-life and require additional safety measures and disposal arrangements. The processing of each specimen is time-consuming because of the multiple wash stages required to achieve good results. In addition the gamma-counters required for accurate counting are expensive and usually beyond the means of individual microbiology laboratories, but use is usually low, and allows the sharing of equipment by neighbouring laboratories.

Enzyme-linked immunosorbent assay

This technique is in many ways similar to radioimmunoassay, but differs in that either the antigen or antibody in the reaction is allowed to bind to a solid phase, such as the walls of microtitre wells. This eliminates the need for centrifugation. There are many variations of enzyme-linked immunosorbent assay (ELISA) but four will be described here and illustrated in the figures.

Antibody-detection ELISA

In an antibody-detecting ELISA, specific antigen is coated on to the wells of a microtitre ELISA plate. The patient's specimen is added and any specific antibody binds to the antigen. The plates are then washed and an antihuman immunoglobulin which has been labelled with an enzyme is added. Plates are washed again and substrate for the enzyme is added. The enzyme–substrate reaction generates a colour which indicates the specific antibody interaction (Fig. 3.17). The optical density of the wells is measured in a microtitration ELISA reader. A positive result can be determined by reference to control values — a positive result is any serum with an optical density three standard deviations above the mean of a series of control negative specimens. Alternatively, control positive and negative sera can be examined in parallel and a positive result is reported if the optical density is significantly higher than that of the control negative.

As in other serological techniques, sera can be titrated but this is time-consuming and defeats the main advantages of ELISA — simplicity of performance and automation. It is difficult to use an antibody capture assay to answer any question other than: 'is there antibody present?' If a diagnosis is to be made on a single specimen, specific immunoglobulin M (IgM) must be detected. This can be achieved by purifying an IgM fraction from the serum and retesting this in an antibody detection test. A simpler alternative is the antibody-capture ELISA.

Antibody-capture ELISA

By placing antihuman IgM antibody on the solid phase, it is possible to capture all IgM antibody. After washing, labelled antigen is placed in the well so that if the serum contains specific IgM the labelled antigen will bind. A positive result is obtained if specific IgM is detected.

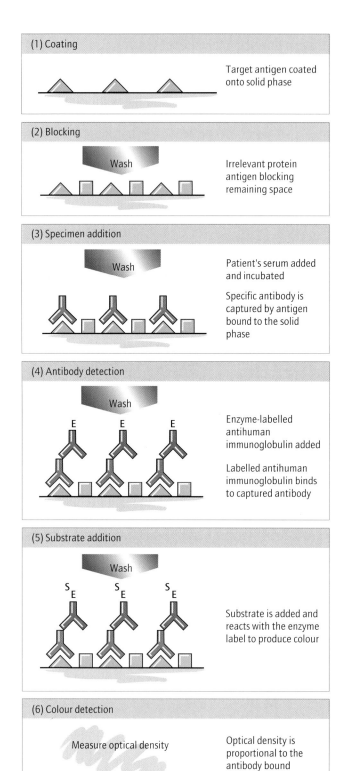

(1) Coating

Target antigen coated onto solid phase

(2) Blocking

Wash

Irrelevant protein antigen blocking remaining space

(3) Specimen addition

Wash

Patient's serum added and incubated

Specific antibody is captured by antigen bound to the solid phase

(4) Antibody detection

Wash

E   E   E

Enzyme-labelled antihuman immunoglobulin added

Labelled antihuman immunoglobulin binds to captured antibody

(5) Substrate addition

Wash

S E   S E   S E

Substrate is added and reacts with the enzyme label to produce colour

(6) Colour detection

Measure optical density

Optical density is proportional to the antibody bound

Fig. 3.17 The principle of antibody-detection enzyme-linked immunosorbent assay.

Antigen-capture ELISA

Antibody directed against a pathogen is placed on the solid phase. If antigen is present in the added serum specimen, it will bind to the antibody. After washing, the bound antigen is then detected by enzyme-labelled specific antibody (Fig. 3.18). The amount of antigen present can be quantified by reference to an antigen standard curve.

Competitive ELISA

Competitive ELISA is a rapid technique which is particularly useful for the measurement of antigen concentrations and is also used to detect antibodies or antibiotic concentrations. Microtitration plates are coated with antibody and the patient serum is added together with labelled antigen. Antigens from the two sources compete for binding sites on the solid phase. The quantity of labelled antigen bound is then determined by the addition of substrate and measurement of the optical density as before. In other words, if antigen is present in the specimen, little labelled antigen will bind and there will be no colour change. Results are computed in comparison with a control antigen curve.

ELISAs have many advantages: they utilize relatively inexpensive reagents and do not require expensive detection systems. These techniques readily lend themselves to automation and in addition the reagents have a long shelf-life. As a result, ELISAs have been widely applied in the diagnosis of bacterial, parasitic and viral infections.

Molecular diagnostics

The development of molecular techniques has opened up a wide diversity of new diagnostic methods. These include the detection of specific sequences of DNA from pathogens by Southern blotting. In this technique the patient's specimen is dried on a nitrocellulose filter, and is then heated in the presence of a specific DNA sequence which has been labelled (this may be a radioactive or a biotin-avidin label). The heating separates the double strands of the DNA. On cooling, some of the labelled DNA will anneal with any corresponding sequence in the specimen. After thorough washing of the nitrocellulose filter to remove left-over single-stranded test DNA, demonstration of the label's fluorescence or colour reaction will confirm the presence of the pathogen's DNA. Southern blotting is not readily applicable to routine diagnosis. It is more useful when

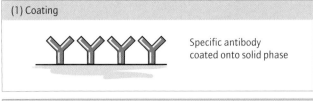

(1) Coating

Specific antibody coated onto solid phase

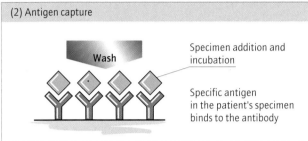

(2) Antigen capture

Wash

Specimen addition and incubation

Specific antigen in the patient's specimen binds to the antibody

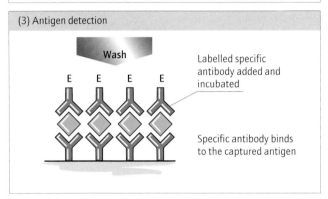

(3) Antigen detection

Wash

E   E   E   E

Labelled specific antibody added and incubated

Specific antibody binds to the captured antigen

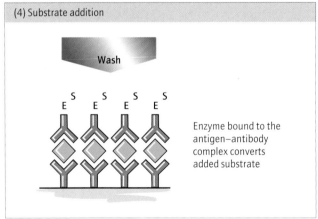

(4) Substrate addition

Wash

S   S   S   S
E   E   E   E

Enzyme bound to the antigen–antibody complex converts added substrate

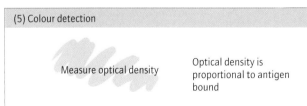

(5) Colour detection

Measure optical density

Optical density is proportional to antigen bound

Fig. 3.18 Antigen-capture enzyme-linked immunosorbent assay, e.g. demonstrating the presence of hepatitis B surface antigen in the test serum.

large numbers of specimens have been collected in epidemiological surveys.

Polymerase chain reaction

The PCR is one of the newest developments in diagnostics. The reaction mixture consists of the specimen together with a pair of primers, which are short sequences of nucleotides specific for the pathogen sought. To this is added nucleotides, and Taq polymerase, an enzyme which catalyses the construction of DNA but is stable at high temperatures. The reaction mixture is heated to separate the two DNA strands. The primers bind to specific sequences in the specimen, the strands are annealed by cooling the mixture, and the Taq polymerase extends the nucleotides to form a complete double-stranded DNA fragment. Each of these stages is performed at a different temperature. At the end of one cycle there are two copies of the specific sequence. The cycle of temperature manipulations is repeated, allowing multiplication to continue exponentially. Positive specimens are detected by performing chromatography of the PCR products on an agarose gel. The presence of the pathogen's DNA sequence can be confirmed by its size relative to DNA markers and the predicted size of the product.

PCR has been applied to the diagnosis of several viral diseases, including human immunodeficiency virus and cytomegalovirus. It is also finding a place in the diagnosis of *Mycobacterium tuberculosis* infection. It can be modified to demonstrate viral RNA in the blood of patients with chronic hepatitis C infection. In many ways PCR is rather like culture as its purpose is to amplify DNA fragments to a degree sufficient for specific detection.

Although it detects organisms, PCR cannot test sensitivities. It is best applied to the diagnosis of conditions for which the choice of treatment is independent of sensitivity testing (as in herpes simplex encephalitis), the antimicrobial susceptibility is predictable (as with *Streptococcus pyogenes*) or normal practice is to treat by a standard multidrug regimen (as in tuberculosis). In the future, however, PCR techniques may contribute to chemotherapeutic decisions by detecting antimicrobial drug resistance genes.

Western blotting (immunoblotting)

Microbial proteins can be separated by SDS-PAGE and transferred electrophoretically to a nitrocellulose membrane. Strips of the membrane are washed in diluted patient serum and antibodies specific to microbial proteins are bound, and can be detected using enzyme-labelled antihuman antibodies. The pattern of antibody recognition can be used in the diagnosis of microbial diseases.

Choice of diagnostic test

The latest molecular techniques can detect very low concentrations of microorganisms. They do not, however, distinguish between living and dead organisms. Those which detect nucleic acid sequences do not even distinguish DNA from a living organism from nucleic acid outside organisms, or inserted into the nucleic acid of a host cell. These facts should be borne in mind when selecting clinical cases to be investigated by various techniques. Also, the oldest, quickest and most economical laboratory methods still hold an important place in modern approaches to diagnosis. A good example is the detection of herpesvirus infections. In herpes simplex encephalitis, the only hope of early microbiological diagnosis may be PCR detection of scanty viral DNA in CSF. In primary herpes simplex stomatitis, electron microscopy of saliva or vesicle scrapings will rapidly demonstrate numerous virus particles. In varicella-zoster pneumonitis, light microscopy of stained cells from bronchial washings can show typical inclusion bodies in infected mucosal cells.

An important skill in clinical infectious diseases and microbiology is the choosing of appropriate diagnostic investigations. While the latest techniques offer new advantages, elegant and timely results are still obtainable using less dramatic methods, as will be seen in the following chapters.

4 Antimicrobial Chemotherapy

Introduction

Most communities have a long tradition of using herbal and other medicines for the treatment of fevers. The underlying religious or scientific theory has varied with time but even very ancient treatments can bear the test of time. The use of cinchona bark originated in the theory that where hazards (marshy land, the bringer of malaria) existed, the natural remedy would be found also. This led to the development of quinine, which is still obtained from its natural source.

Ehrlich thought that the selective staining of micro-organisms by dyes might be used to target and kill organisms. From this he developed salvarsan, the first specific antimicrobial. All modern antimicrobial agents have their effect because of their selective toxicity—interfering with microbial metabolism or function with minimal effect on the host.

> Antimicrobial agents have selective toxicity: they severely damage microorganisms but have much less effect on human metabolism.

Various strategies have been used in the design of antimicrobials. Some interrupt microbial metabolic pathways which are not possessed by host cells. Antimetabolites are often competitive inhibitors of microbial enzymes or false substrates, which participate in the metabolic process but do not result in a useful biological product. The first example of this was the development of sulphonamides by Domagk. These compounds mimic para-amino benzoic acid (PABA) and competitively inhibit the conversion of PABA into dihydropteroic acid, which is an essential precursor of folate. Bacteria rely on this metabolic pathway, as they are unable to take preformed folate from the host, and folate is an essential substrate in the synthesis of DNA. Further down the same pathway, trimethoprim or pyrimethamine inhibits the activity of dihydrofolate reductase, which converts dihydrofolate into tetrahydrofolate (Fig. 4.1).

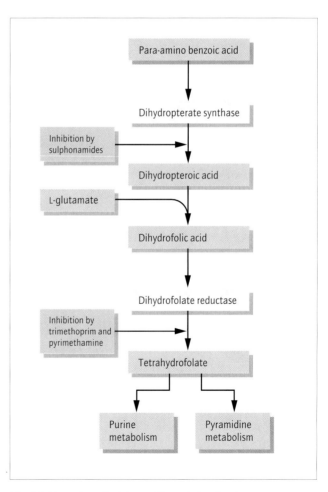

Fig. 4.1 The actions of sulphonamides and trimethoprim.

This also depletes tetrahydrofolate concentrations. These two groups of agents can be used together in the treatment of bacterial infections (trimethoprim–sulphamethoxazole) or parasitic infections such as toxoplasmosis (pyrimethamine and sulphadiazine).

The bacterial cell wall is essential for protecting the organism from lysis caused by the osmotic gradient between the interior and exterior of the cell. The major structural component of the cell wall is peptidoglycan, composed of long polysaccharide chains with alternating *N*-acetylglucosamine and muramic acid molecules. The peptidoglycan chains are cross-linked between short peptide side-chains by an amide linkage (Fig. 4.2). Beta-lactam antibiotics (penicillins, cephalosporins, monobactams and penems) work by inhibiting transpeptidation and preventing cross-linking (Fig. 4.3). Each of these antibiotics possesses a beta-lactam ring which mimics the shape of the amide bond. Inhibition of cross-linking weakens the cell wall and the bacteria are killed by lysis.

Vancomycin and teicoplanin, glycopeptide antibiotics, also affect bacterial cell wall synthesis but the mechanism of action is very different. They act at an earlier stage of peptidoglycan synthesis by blocking prolongation of the peptidoglycan sugar backbone. This activity is limited

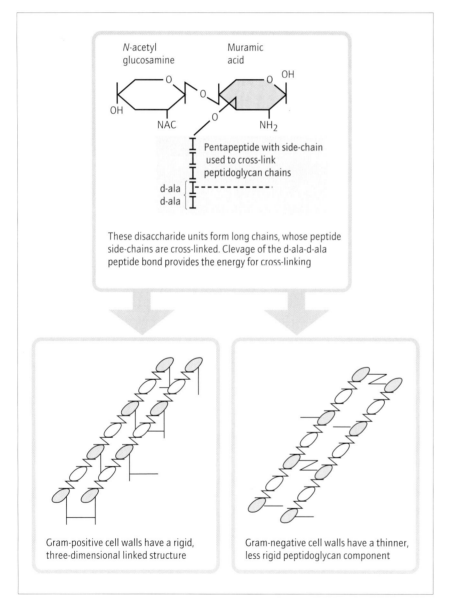

Fig. 4.2 The peptidoglycan cell wall structures in Gram-positive and Gram-negative organisms.

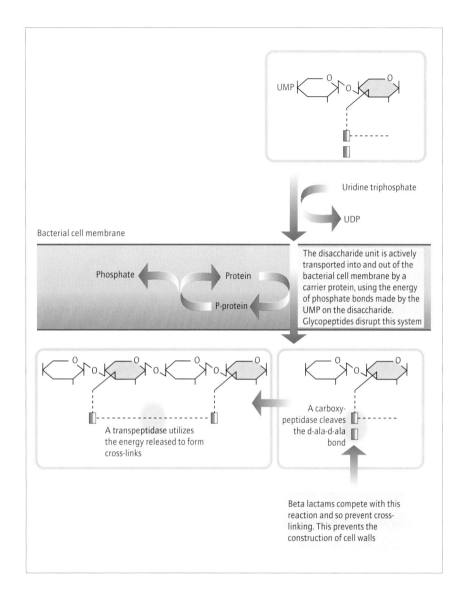

Fig. 4.3 The actions of beta-lactams and glycopeptides. UMP, Uridine monophosphate; UDP, uridine diphosphate.

only to Gram-positive cell walls so these agents have no activity against Gram-negative organisms.

In order to contain the DNA strand in the bacterial cell, the DNA must be supercoiled. It must be uncoiled and recoiled during the processes of replication and transcription. Quinolone antimicrobials, which include nalidixic acid, ofloxacin and ciprofloxacin, work by interfering with the enzyme topoisomerase, or DNA gyrase, which supercoils bacterial DNA (Fig. 4.4).

Rifampicin and rifabutin act by interfering with DNA-dependent RNA polymerase, so preventing transcription of the genetic code.

Bacterial protein synthesis (Fig. 4.5) can be inhibited by a number of different mechanisms. Tetracycline inhibits the binding of transfer RNA (tRNA) to the 30S ribosome, whereas macrolides inhibit RNA-dependent protein synthesis at the 50S ribosome. Chloramphenicol prevents binding of tRNA to the 50S subunit of the ribosome. Aminoglycosides bind to both subunits of the ribosome, interfering with protein synthesis and causing the genetic code to be misread.

Antimicrobial action

1 Antimetabolites interrupt microbial chemical pathways.
2 Cell wall agents prevent the construction of bacterial cell walls.
3 Protein synthesis inhibitors interrupt the transcription and/or translation of microbial genes.
4 DNA gyrase inhibitors damage the tertiary structure of bacterial DNA.

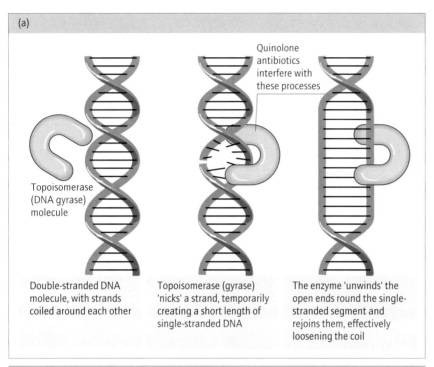

(a)

Quinolone antibiotics interfere with these processes

Topoisomerase (DNA gyrase) molecule

Double-stranded DNA molecule, with strands coiled around each other

Topoisomerase (gyrase) 'nicks' a strand, temporarily creating a short length of single-stranded DNA

The enzyme 'unwinds' the open ends round the single-stranded segment and rejoins them, effectively loosening the coil

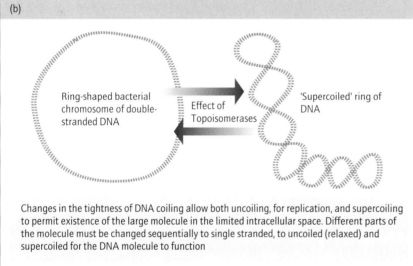

(b)

Ring-shaped bacterial chromosome of double-stranded DNA

Effect of Topoisomerases

'Supercoiled' ring of DNA

Changes in the tightness of DNA coiling allow both uncoiling, for replication, and supercoiling to permit existence of the large molecule in the limited intracellular space. Different parts of the molecule must be changed sequentially to single stranded, to uncoiled (relaxed) and supercoiled for the DNA molecule to function

Fig. 4.4 The actions of quinolone antimicrobials. (a) Topoisomerase tightens (supercoils) or loosens (relaxes) the coiling of the DNA molecule by opening and reclosing small gaps in a DNA strand. DNA must be relaxed for its strands to part during replication or the production of RNA. (b) A bacterial DNA molecule is approximately 1 m long. It must be coiled many times to enable it to fit inside a bacterial cell. It must then be uncoiled, part by part, to allow its code to be read. Quinolone antibiotics prevent these changes in configuration, disrupting the function of the DNA.

Antimicrobial pharmacology

Effective treatment of infection depends on knowledge of the likely infecting organisms and their susceptibility to antimicrobials. It is also affected by the site of infection, the spectrum of action of antimicrobial agents and their absorption and distribution within the body.

Knowledge of the pharmacology of antimicrobial agents is therefore of value in ensuring that an adequate concentration of antibiotic is available at the site of infection (bioavailable). Infection is often localized to special sites such as the meninges, where penetration of antibiotics may be prevented by the blood–brain barrier.

The normal rules of pharmacology apply to the absorption and distribution of antibiotics within the body. Non-polar (lipid-soluble) agents such as chloramphenicol are well-absorbed and cross the blood–brain

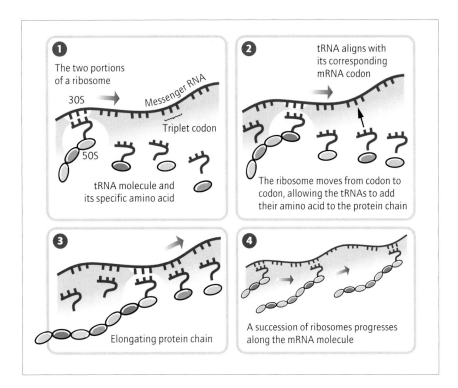

Fig. 4.5 The mechanisms of bacterial protein synthesis. Various aspects of this process are disrupted by tetracyclines, aminoglycosides, macrolides and rifampicin.

barrier easily, whereas the more polar agents, penicillins and cephalosporins are less well-absorbed and are confined to extracellular compartments. Protein binding also has an effect on the duration of action and the bioavailability of antimicrobial agents.

It is important to remember that the conditions at the site of infection may modify the effect of an antimicrobial agent. A concentration gradient of antimicrobial may be set up in an abscess, with lower concentrations at its centre than in the serum. In addition the presence of cellular or bacterial debris and the products of metabolism lower the pH and redox potential, interfering with the action of antimicrobials such as aminoglycosides (gentamicin-like agents) and macrolides (erythromycin-like agents).

The route of excretion also influences the effect of antimicrobial therapy. Agents excreted by the urinary route are likely to be effective in pyelonephritis and cystitis as high concentrations will be found in renal tissue, the bladder and urine. Antibiotics excreted by the kidney are likely to accumulate in cases of renal failure, and the dose must be adjusted to avoid incurring toxic effects. Antibiotics excreted in the bile are likely to be effective in acute cholangitis, as high concentrations are available at the site of infection.

Many antimicrobials are metabolized by the liver, and hepatic disease may interfere with their excretion,

causing an increased risk of side-effects and often necessitating reduction in dosage.

Factors affecting the effect of antimicrobials at the sites of infections
1 The concentration of the antimicrobial (influenced by its ease of access and rate of excretion).
2 Local pH and redox potential.
3 Ability of the pathogen to destroy the antibiotic.
4 Destruction of antimicrobial by host lysozymes and proteases.
5 Renal and/or hepatic damage, which can impair antibiotic excretion.

Antimicrobial sensitivity testing

Concepts of susceptibility testing

Definitions

An organism may be described as sensitive or resistant, depending on whether treatment with the usual recommended dose of the antimicrobial is likely to result in successful therapy. Moderately resistant or susceptible are terms used by some laboratories to describe an organism likely to be susceptible only to doses higher than the standard.

An organism is considered sensitive if treatment with an antibiotic at standard dosage is likely to be successful.

Treatment for a moderately sensitive organism is likely to be successful if an increased dose of antibiotic is used.

An organism which is resistant is unlikely to be successfully treated with a given antibiotic, irrespective of dosage.

These definitions depend on the assumption that the results of laboratory tests reflect what is happening in the patient. Laboratory tests of susceptibility measure the activity of pure drug against bacteria growing exponentially in artificial culture. This is nothing like the situation at the site of an active infection. Antimicrobials, once administered, are absorbed and distributed throughout the body according to their lipid-solubility and protein binding. They may also be metabolized by the liver and other tissues, and excreted or secreted by the kidney. Their breakdown products may or may not have antimicrobial activity. The site of infection may be devascularized, or an abscess with a fibrous cavity may have developed. Many organisms are not 'free' in the tissues but live inside macrophages or other cells. The site of infection may be at a low pH, at which some antimicrobials are relatively inactive. The organisms at the site of infection are not multiplying exponentially, as in the test tube where nutrients are not limited. In infections bacteria may be in a form of stationary phase because of limited nutrients or, in some cases, such as tuberculosis, they may be dormant. In active infection the immune system is a vital contributor to recovery and may enhance the apparent activity of antimicrobials.

In an attempt to overcome these limitations, the laboratory measures directly or indirectly, and under controlled conditions, the inhibitory or killing effect of the antimicrobial agent on the pathogen isolated from the patient. The results of this, together with the known pharmacokinetics of the antibiotic, may predict the likely outcome of treatment with that agent.

Minimal inhibitory concentration and minimal bactericidal concentration

Two concepts are important in this context: the minimal inhibitory concentration (MIC) and the minimal bactericidal concentration (MBC) of the antimicrobial agent for the organism in question. The MIC is defined as the lowest concentration at which growth of the organism is completely inhibited. The MBC is the lowest concentration at which the organism is killed (actually defined as a 99.9% kill). In planning chemotherapy the aim is to ensure that the likely concentration of antimicrobial should exceed the MIC at the site of the infection. In some cases, where the multiplying organisms are inaccessible to the additive effect of phagocytosis and antibody, it is highly desirable that the MBC should be exceeded. This is especially true in endocarditis, in which bacteria are buried in thrombus, and in infections near to artificial material such as implants and prostheses.

The minimum inhibitory concentration (MIC) is the lowest concentration of antibiotic which completely inhibits the growth of an organism.

The minimum bactericidal concentration (MBC) is the lowest concentration of antibiotic which kills an organism.

The MIC can be determined by cultivating organisms in broth cultures or on agar plates which incorporate a range of concentrations of the desired antimicrobial. By subculturing the broth cultures, the death of the organisms can be confirmed, and the MBC can be determined (Fig. 4.6).

Methods of testing antimicrobial susceptibility

MIC determination is too cumbersome to use for all isolates made in a clinical microbiology laboratory. Quicker, indirect methods are therefore used, which allow a large number of isolates to be tested against many antimicrobials. The most popular methods are based on filter-paper discs impregnated with antimicrobials. These are placed on agar plates which have been seeded with bacteria. The antimicrobials diffuse from the disc into the medium, inhibiting bacterial growth. At a certain distance from the edge of the disc, the concentration falls below that which will inhibit the growth of the organism, and a zone of demarcation can be seen. The diameter of this zone is related to the MIC of the organism.

The size of the zone may be altered by a number of factors unrelated to the susceptibility of the organisms tested. These include the composition of the medium, particularly the concentration of divalent cations; the pH of the medium; the molecular size of the antimicrobial; and incubation conditions. These variables must be controlled if reproducible results are to be obtained.

Each of the disc susceptibility methods uses a slightly different way of relating zone size with MIC, and controlling for variation in the conditions of individual tests. These will be discussed in turn.

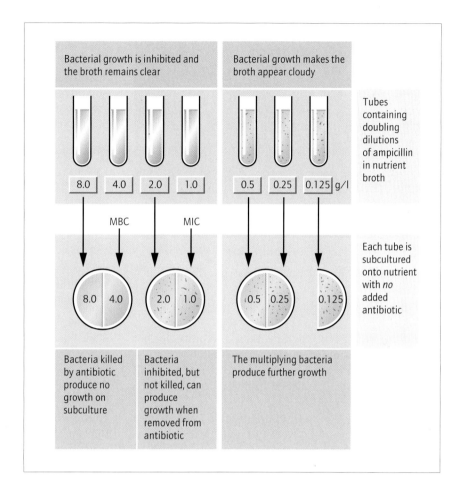

Bacterial growth is inhibited and the broth remains clear

Bacterial growth makes the broth appear cloudy

8.0 | 4.0 | 2.0 | 1.0

0.5 | 0.25 | 0.125 g/l

Tubes containing doubling dilutions of ampicillin in nutrient broth

MBC   MIC

8.0 | 4.0   2.0 | 1.0   0.5 | 0.25   0.125

Each tube is subcultured onto nutrient with *no* added antibiotic

Bacteria killed by antibiotic produce no growth on subculture

Bacteria inhibited, but not killed, can produce growth when removed from antibiotic

The multiplying bacteria produce further growth

Fig. 4.6 The principle of minimum inhibitory concentration (MIC) and minimum bactericidal concentration (MBC) determination.

Stokes method

The Stokes method is popular in British laboratories because of its simplicity and flexibility. In this method the test organism is directly compared with a control organism with known MICs, grown on the same plate. This controls for variation in the composition and characteristics of different media and the conditions pertaining to an individual test. It also relates the result (the zone size) to the zone size for a susceptible organism (Fig. 4.7). Different control organisms are appropriate for different clinical situations and growth characteristics. A sensitive *Staphylococcus* is chosen for most isolates from sterile sites and an *Escherichia coli* for urinary isolates. When organisms have special growth characteristics, controls of the same species are used, for example isolates of *Haemophilus influenzae* or *Pseudomonas aeruginosa*.

Kirby–Bauer method

This is the standard technique used in the USA. The medium and incubation conditions are strictly defined

in this method. The zone sizes are directly related to MIC using a regression line — a graph which plots the known MIC of a series of organisms against zone size. Limits of variation of control results are strictly laid down.

Agar incorporation method

In this method concentrations of antibiotic are incorporated into a solid medium in Petri dishes. The technique has the advantage that many tests can be performed on the same plate, using a multipoint inoculator. It is difficult, however, to obtain an estimate of the MBC in this test.

Breakpoint method

The agar incorporation MIC method can be simplified for routine use by using only two carefully chosen dilutions or breakpoints. Organisms inhibited by the lower concentration of antibiotic would be reported as being sensitive to the antimicrobial at conventional doses. If inhibition occurred only at the higher con-

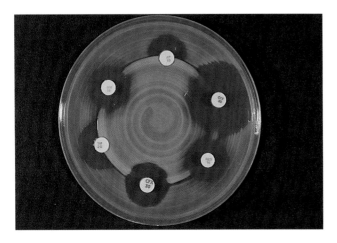

Penicillinase-producing *Neisseria gonorrhoeae* (PPNG) are not inhibited even by high-concentration penicillin discs. Placing the two types of disc on the original selective-medium plate therefore provides an early indication of possible antibiotic sensitivity (Fig. 4.8), but this screening test must be confirmed by formal testing of the purified organism.

Methods of routine sensitivity testing
1 Stokes method.
2 Kirby–Bauer method.
3 Agar incorporation method.
4 Breakpoint method.

Fig. 4.7 Use of the Stokes method for determining antimicrobial sensitivity by disc diffusion. Outer band, susceptible control organism; central band, test organism.

Checking the effectiveness of antimicrobial chemotherapy

centration, successful therapy would require higher doses and this result is reported as moderately sensitive. Organisms not inhibited by either concentration would be reported as fully resistant and therapy would be expected to fail.

High- and low-concentration antibiotic-impregnated discs are sometimes used to test organisms in this way. *Neisseria gonorrhoeae*, for example, is often sensitive to benzyl penicillin, and shows a large zone of inhibition around a low-concentration penicillin disc. Some gonococci have altered penicillin-binding characteristics, and are inhibited only by high-concentration penicillin discs.

In some infections the serum bactericidal concentration is measured while the patient is on antibiotic treatment. In this test, dilutions of the patient's serum are incubated with the patient's infecting organism (the back-titration). The lowest dilution of serum which kills the organism is the bactericidal titre. This is most often used in bacterial endocarditis, when the dosage of antibiotic is chosen so that an eightfold dilution of serum is bactericidal. Of course, more antibiotic will be present in the serum just after dosing (peak concentration) than just before the next dose (trough concentration). It is usually only practicable to perform back-titrations relative to peak levels.

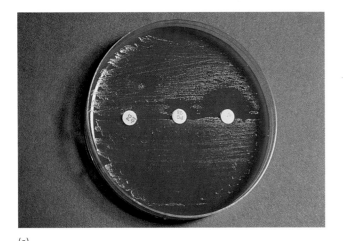

(a)

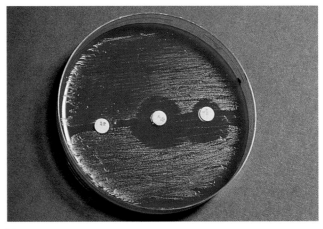

(b)

Fig. 4.8 (a) The organism on the upper half of the plate is a penicillin-sensitive gonococcus with zones to the penicillin 0.25 μg and 1.0 μg disc. Below is a strain resistant to penicillin. (b) The organism on the upper half of the plate is a non-beta-lactamase-producing penicillin-resistant gonococcus as there is only a small zone to co-amoxyclav (right-hand disc). The strain in the lower half is also penicillin resistant: no zone to the ampicillin disc on the left but a wide zone to co-amoxyclav.

A back-titration measures the antimicrobial effect of the antibiotic in the patient's serum against the pathogen isolated from the patient.

Adverse effects of antimicrobials

The basic principle of antimicrobial chemotherapy is selective toxicity, allowing the infecting pathogen's metabolism to be inhibited, with little or no effect on the host. Most antimicrobial agents have very favourable therapeutic indices, meaning that the ratio of toxic level to therapeutic level is high. Adverse effects fall into two major groups: those which are dose-dependent, as in the bone-marrow toxicity of antifolates such as sulphonamides or renal toxicity of aminoglycosides, and idiosyncratic reactions, such as penicillin-induced anaphylaxis or chloramphenicol-induced aplastic anaemia.

Adverse antimicrobial effects
1 Dose-dependent toxicity.
2 Idiosyncratic reactions.

Renal toxicity

There are several ways in which renal damage can occur during antimicrobial chemotherapy. Not all are the direct effects of the antimicrobial drug; for instance, renal failure can follow an anaphylactic reaction, because the accompanying hypotension results in acute tubular necrosis. Obstructive nephropathy can occur if high concentrations of drugs such as long-acting sulphonamides or first-generation cephalosporins form microcrystals in the tubules, or larger crystals in the collecting ducts.

Direct renal cell damage

Direct renal cell damage can be caused by nephrotoxic antimicrobials. Aminoglycosides are toxic to cells of the proximal renal tubules, causing accumulation of membrane structures within the cell. This occurs at serum levels close to those necessary for effective antimicrobial action; the therapeutic index is narrow. There is evidence of mild tubular effects in all patients, and small reductions in the glomerular filtration rate occur in approximately 80% of patients. These mild effects are usually self-limiting.

Elderly patients and those with pre-existing renal compromise, including renal failure induced by sepsis, are predisposed to the toxicity of aminoglycosides. Toxicity is also increased by co-administration of diuretics, of other renal toxic drugs or recent aminoglycoside therapy. A rapid reduction in renal function can occur in patients treated with aminoglycosides for infective endocarditis, because of the additive effects of aminoglycoside toxicity, uncontrolled sepsis and the nephritis which occurs as part of the infective endocarditis syndrome. Aminoglycosides may damage either hair cells of the organ of Corti, resulting in auditory impairment, or the type I hair cells at the summit of the ampullar cristae. In order to prevent the renal and auditory consequences of excess dosage the concentration of these agents must be closely monitored in the serum.

There is a high incidence of renal toxicity in patients treated with amphotericin. The mechanism is not known but may be associated with distal tubular lesions and a decrease in glomerular filtration rate.

Tetracycline can cause renal damage by several different mechanisms. The action of tetracycline is catabolic, producing an increase in nitrogen degradation products, including urea. Some tetracycline degradation products may be directly toxic to the kidneys.

Sulphonamides are a diverse group of agents, some of which can crystallize in the renal tubules, causing obstructive uropathy. Occasionally they cause direct toxicity to the renal tubular cells. Co-trimoxazole, which contains sulphamethoxazole, may accumulate in renal failure, producing a fall in the glomerular filtration rate. Patients with a small urinary volume may develop crystalluria, even with this modern sulphonamide preparation.

Liver toxicity

Damage to the liver may take the form of acute or chronic hepatitis, cholestasis, fatty degeneration or a granulomatous hepatitis.

Hepatocellular damage

Hepatocellular damage is the commonest form of liver damage. It is most frequently associated with the antituberculous agents isoniazid and rifampicin. Among patients given isoniazid prophylaxis, acute hepatitis occurs in approximately 1%. The risk is age-related, becoming more common in patients aged over 35. The mechanism of toxicity is probably formation of a toxic intermediate metabolite, acetylhydrazine. Hepatitis is more likely in patients with previous liver disease, or a history of alcohol abuse.

Rifampicin may also induce hepatitis. A transient 'transaminitis' is common; transaminase concentrations are elevated but return to normal despite continued drug use, and jaundice does not develop. Severe hepatitis associated with jaundice is occasionally seen. Rifampicin may also produce a transient hyperbilirubinaemia due to competition for hepatic excretion. The combination of rifampicin and isoniazid in the treatment of tuberculosis causes hepatitis in about 5% of patients. Hepatitis can complicate the use of erythromycin estolate, parenteral tetracycline, pyrazinamide and ethionamide. Rare cases of hepatitis have been reported following high-dose ampicillin or flucloxacillin treatment.

Cholestatic jaundice

Cholestatic jaundice is a dose-related effect of fusidic acid, occurring at doses above 2 g/day. Tetracycline may induce fatty change in the liver if high doses are given intravenously or if patients are predisposed by pregnancy or renal failure.

Granulomatous hepatitis

Granulomatous hepatitis is a rare complication of prolonged quinine therapy.

Effects on the haemopoietic system

Bone marrow toxicity can be caused by a large number of different agents, and can affect granulocytes alone or the whole haematopoietic system. Bone marrow depression may arise as a result of the normal action of the drug, as an idiosyncratic reaction, or by immune mechanisms.

Aplastic anaemia

Aplastic anaemia can follow chloramphenicol therapy from 10 days after therapy until up to 6 months. This idiosyncratic reaction must be distinguished from a mild, reversible dose-dependent bone marrow depression which occurs in many patients on higher doses. True aplasia has an incidence of 1 in 40 000 to 1 in 100 000, and is often irreversible.

Metabolic bone marrow depression

Metabolic bone marrow depression is a complication of treatment with antimicrobials affecting nucleic acid synthesis, either directly, as with ganciclovir, or by reducing folate availability, as with sulphonamides.

Granulocytopenia

Granulocytopenia is usually idiosyncratic. It is commonest after sulphonamide or sulphone therapy, but rarely follows high-dose benzyl penicillin therapy (> 12 MU/day). Penicillin-associated agranulocytosis is always associated with the same reaction to cephalosporins, and will recur even following small oral doses of these drugs.

Immunologically mediated cytopenias

Immunologically mediated cytopenias are relatively rare. Antibiotics, like other drugs, may act as haptens and induce antibodies to red blood cells or platelets, resulting in a Coombs-positive haemolytic anaemia or immune thrombocytopenia.

Cutaneous adverse reactions

These vary from fixed drug eruptions, urticarial and maculopapular eruptions to erythema multiforme or even life-threatening Stevens–Johnson syndrome. By far the commonest cause of severe skin reactions are sulphonamides, and the risk increases dramatically in the elderly. Mild, itching rashes are common with sulphonamides, penicillins (Fig. 4.9) and cephalosporins. Although not strictly an allergic response, 95% of patients with infectious mononucleosis develop a rash if treated with ampicillin, but this does not recur on re-exposure to the drug after convalescence.

Acute anaphylaxis occurs when an antibiotic generates a type I hypersensitivity reaction, usually as a result of hapten–drug sensitization. This complication is truly uncommon, perhaps affecting 1 : 100 000 treatments. Penicillins are most often responsible. Cephalosporins may cross-react, but in less than 10% of penicillin-sensitive patients. New monobactam agents have even lower cross-sensitivity rates.

Mechanisms of resistance to antimicrobial drugs

Individual antimicrobial agents are effective against only some organisms, usually because the metabolic process with which they interfere does not occur in all species. Vancomycin interferes with chain-lengthening in peptidoglycan in Gram-positive organisms. Thus all Gram-negative organisms are naturally resistant.

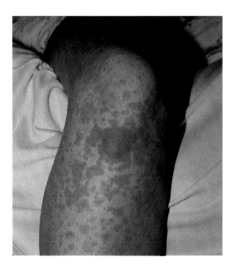

Fig. 4.9 Rash induced by ampicillin; such rashes are usually painful or irritating.

Metronidazole is active at such low redox potentials that only anaerobic bacteria are susceptible. Amphotericin is active against fungi because it inhibits ergosterol synthesis, necessary for cell wall production in fungi, but not in bacteria.

> **Reasons why organisms may be naturally resistant to antimicrobials:**
> 1 They are naturally impermeable to the antimicrobial agent.
> 2 They lack the target binding site.
> 3 They lack the target metabolic pathway.
> 4 They naturally produce antibiotic-destroying enzymes.

Other organisms are resistant to certain antimicrobials because they naturally produce inactivating enzymes. When penicillin was first introduced, 95% of *Staphylococcus aureus* were sensitive, but 5% produced a beta-lactamase which destroyed the beta-lactam ring at the nucleus of the penicillin molecule. As time went on an increasing proportion of strains possessed beta-lactamase. Now almost all *S. aureus* isolated in a hospital are penicillin-resistant. *S. aureus* has acquired resistance due to the selective pressure applied by antibiotics, favouring survival of beta-lactamase-producing strains. In the presence of similar selection pressure, other organisms expressing a beta-lactamase may also be favoured. The genes coding for these enzymes may even be transferred to other organisms, passing on the selective advantage. By this means, antibiotic-destroying enzymes can become widespread. Similar mechanisms exist for other resistance factors (see below).

Bacteria become resistant to aminoglycosides by developing inactivating enzymes which adenylate, hydroxylate or acetylate the aminoglycoside molecule at various sites. Resistance to chloramphenicol depends on possession of an acetyltransferase enzyme.

The action of antibiotics may be inhibited by alteration in binding of the antibiotic to its target. Organisms resistant to macrolides and aminoglycosides have small alterations in binding sites on the ribosomal target. Resistance to streptomycin, for example, may develop in a one-step process in which the ribosomal binding site is methylated, preventing the binding of the antibiotic. Penicillin resistance in *Streptococcus pneumoniae* depends on an alteration in the affinity of penicillin-binding protein (PBP). This has developed in a multiple stepwise fashion under the selective pressure of antibiotics available in the human environment. Recombination has occurred between PBP genes in *S. pneumoniae* and commensal organisms at low frequency (10^{-13}).

Alteration of the permeability of bacterial outer membranes may result in high-level resistance, often affecting all drugs of a class. This form of resistance is common in *Pseudomonas* spp. Some bacteria become resistant to tetracyclines by actively transporting the antibiotic out of the cell (the efflux mechanism). This mechanism results in resistance to all compounds in this class.

The major resistance mechanism for tetracycline among Gram-negative organisms is an alteration of an inner membrane protein which inhibits accumulation of tetracycline within the bacterial cell. Resistance to sulphonamides and trimethoprim occurs due to alterations in the target enzymes — dihydropterate synthetase and dihydrofolate reductase, respectively.

> **Methods by which bacteria can acquire resistance to antimicrobial agents:**
> 1 An alteration in permeability to the antibiotic.
> 2 An alteration in the target binding state.
> 3 Utilizing an alternative metabolic pathway.
> 4 Switching on a gene for an antibiotic-destroying enzyme.
> 5 Acquiring a new gene for an antibiotic-destroying enzyme.

The bacterial genes coding for antibiotic resistance can be transmitted between not only organisms of the same species but also different genera. Transfer of resistance means that organisms which are naturally resistant can transmit this ability to other naturally sensitive organisms. The clinical effect is that resistance to commonly used antibiotics becomes widespread. Bacterial resistance genes, like all other DNA fragments, are transmitted by four main mechanisms: transformation, transduction, conjugation and transposons (Fig. 4.10). Transformation is the process whereby bacteria take up portions of naked DNA and incorporate it into their own genetic make-up. Transduction takes place when fragments of DNA are taken up by a bacteriophage and transmitted when the phage infects a new bacterial cell. Conjugation involves transfer of chromosomal and/or plasmid DNA between bacterial cells. Transposons are movable genetic elements capable of transferring from one bacterial strain to another, between plasmids and between plasmids and the bacterial chromosome.

In the presence of antimicrobial selection pressure, organisms possessing resistance determinants will be favoured. Some strains possess multiple resistance determinants. These organisms can pose significant therapeutic problems to the clinician in the selection of effective chemotherapy. Control of antimicrobial prescribing may be effective in limiting the development of these strains, but must be very strict to eradicate multidrug-resistant strains, as a positive selective pressure exists if any of the antimicrobials to which the organism is resistant are found in the hospital environment.

(a) Transformation

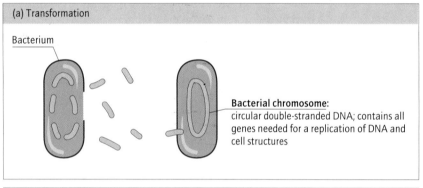

Bacterium

Bacterial chromosome: circular double-stranded DNA; contains all genes needed for a replication of DNA and cell structures

(b) Conjugation

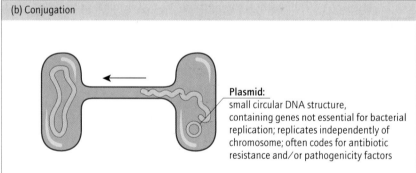

Plasmid: small circular DNA structure, containing genes not essential for bacterial replication; replicates independently of chromosome; often codes for antibiotic resistance and/or pathogenicity factors

(c) Transduction

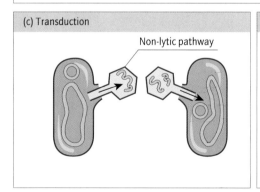

Non-lytic pathway

(d) Transposons

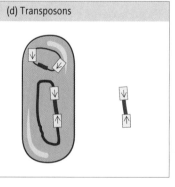

Fig. 4.10 The mechanisms of DNA transfer between bacteria.

Mechanisms for gene transfer between bacteria
1 Transformation (transfer of naked DNA).
2 Transduction (where the gene is acquired with a bacteriophage infection).
3 Conjugation (DNA transfer between conjoined bacteria).
4 Transposons (transposition).

Agents used in treating infection

The main types of anti-infection agents will be reviewed here briefly. Antiviral, antifungal and antiparasitic agents will also be discussed with their main therapeutic targets in the systematic chapters.

Antibacterial agents

Beta-lactam antibiotics

Beta-lactam antibiotics include penicillins and cephalosporins which have similar structures.

Penicillins can be conveniently divided into classes on the basis of their antibacterial activity:
1 Natural penicillins (penicillin G).
2 Penicillinase-resistant penicillins (cloxacillin).
3 The aminopenicillins (ampicillin-like agents).
4 Expanded-spectrum penicillins.
5 Carbapenems.
6 Monobactams.
7 Beta-lactamase inhibitors.

Spectrum of activity

Penicillin G is derived from cultures of *Penicillium chrysogenum*. It is active against Gram-positive bacteria, including streptococci, staphylococci (excluding most *Staphylococcus aureus*), clostridia and corynebacteria, and some Gram-negative cocci, including *Neisseria meningitidis*. *Bacteroides fragilis* is resistant, but *Prevotella* sp., *Porphyromonas* sp. and anaerobic cocci are susceptible.

The beta-lactamase-resistant penicillins, isoxazolyl penicillins such as flucloxacillin, oxacillin and cloxacillin, were developed to deal with the problem of penicillin-resistant *S. aureus*. Their bulky side-chain sterically hinders the binding of penicillinase to these drugs (Fig. 4.11). These agents retain activity against streptococci and *Neisseria*. They are well-absorbed orally.

The aminopenicillins include ampicillin and its esters, and amoxycillin. They are well-absorbed orally, and have an expanded spectrum which includes Gram-negative rods. *Haemophilus influenzae* is susceptible, as are many species of the Enterobacteriaceae, including *Escherichia coli, Salmonella* sp. and *Shigella* sp. Following the introduction of ampicillin, hospitals experienced cross-infection problems with Gram-negative pathogens which were naturally resistant to this agent. These included *Klebsiella* spp. and *Pseudomonas aeruginosa*. Newer penicillins were developed to address this problem and these include the acylureidopenicillins, mezlocillin, azlocillin, piperacillin and the carboxypenicillins: carbenicillin and ticarcillin (Fig. 4.12). All of these agents must be administered parenterally. They are active against some ampicillin-resistant Enterobacteriaceae and *P. aeruginosa* but are susceptible to plasmid-mediated beta-lactamases, which limits their effectiveness.

The carbapenems have a broad spectrum of activity against Gram-positive and -negative bacteria, including beta-lactamase-producing Gram-negative organisms and *B. fragilis*. The monobactams are synthetic compounds which have little activity against Gram-positive organisms but are very active against Gram-negative species, including beta-lactamase-producing strains and *Pseudomonas* sp.

As one of the main reasons for resistance to penicillins is the elaboration of beta-lactamases, co-administration of a beta-lactamase inhibitor is a logical step. These are beta-lactamase stable beta-lactam compounds with minimal antimicrobial activity. It is essential that these compounds have similar pharmacokinetic properties to their companion active agent. Several are available for clinical use, including clavulanic acid and sulbactam. These have been combined with different active agents — clavulanic acid with amoxycillin or ticarcillin, sulbactam with ampicillin or piperacillin.

Pharmacology

Penicillins vary markedly in their oral absorption. Penicillin G is not stable to gastric acid and must be given intravenously. Long-acting derivatives of benzyl penicillin such as procaine and benzathine penicillin are available in some situations for intramuscular administration. Penicillin V, in contrast, is stable to gastric acid and can be given by the oral route. The aminopenicillins and isoxazolylpenicillins such as flucloxacillin are also absorbed orally. The remainder must be administered by the intravenous route.

All the orally active penicillins yield peak levels in the serum at 1–2 h after ingestion and this peak of absorption is delayed by food. Penicillins are excreted and secreted by the kidney. The half-life of penicillins can be

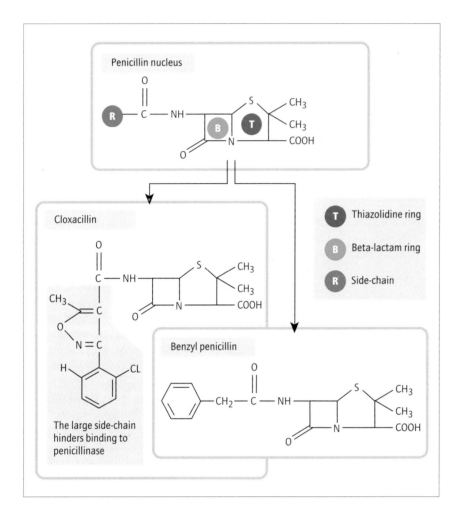

Fig. 4.11 The structure of penicillin G and cloxacillin.

increased by co-administration of probenecid which competes with penicillin for the renal tubular secretory mechanism. The consequence of rapid excretion is a very short half-life, ranging from 30 to 72 min. Protein binding is variable, from 17% for aminopenicillins to 97% for dicloxacillin. Penicillins are distributed in extracellular fluid to most of the body tissues, including lung, liver, kidney, muscle, bone and placenta. They do not cross the blood–brain barrier unless the meninges are inflamed. High concentrations of penicillin are found in the urine. Penicillins are actively secreted into the bile. Imipenem is broken down by renal dihydropeptidase I, so cilastatin, an inhibitor, must be co-administered for this compound to be effective. Meropenem is not broken down, and can be given alone.

Unwanted actions

Penicillins are noted for the infrequency of their adverse effects, and this has contributed to their wide application. The most serious side-effect is acute anaphylaxis which is uncommon but is most likely to develop during treatment with benzyl penicillin. Less severe allergic manifestations include angioneurotic oedema, pruritis and urticaria. In some patients there is a delayed 'serum sickness' reaction with urticaria and arthralgia. Other side-effects include Stevens–Johnson syndrome, dermatitis, morbilliform eruptions and allergic vasculitis. Neutropenia rarely occurs with prolonged high dosage of benzyl penicillin. There is a high salt load associated with the sodium salts and especially the disodium salts of the expanded-spectrum penicillins. High doses in patients with renal failure may result in hypernatraemia, hypokalaemia and convulsions.

Ampicillin can precipitate antibiotic-associated diarrhoea and, occasionally, pseudomembranous colitis due to its activity against obligate anaerobic organisms and the consequent effect on the balance of the intestinal flora.

Mode of action

Penicillins act by interfering with peptidoglycan formation. N-acetylglucosamine and muramic alternate in a

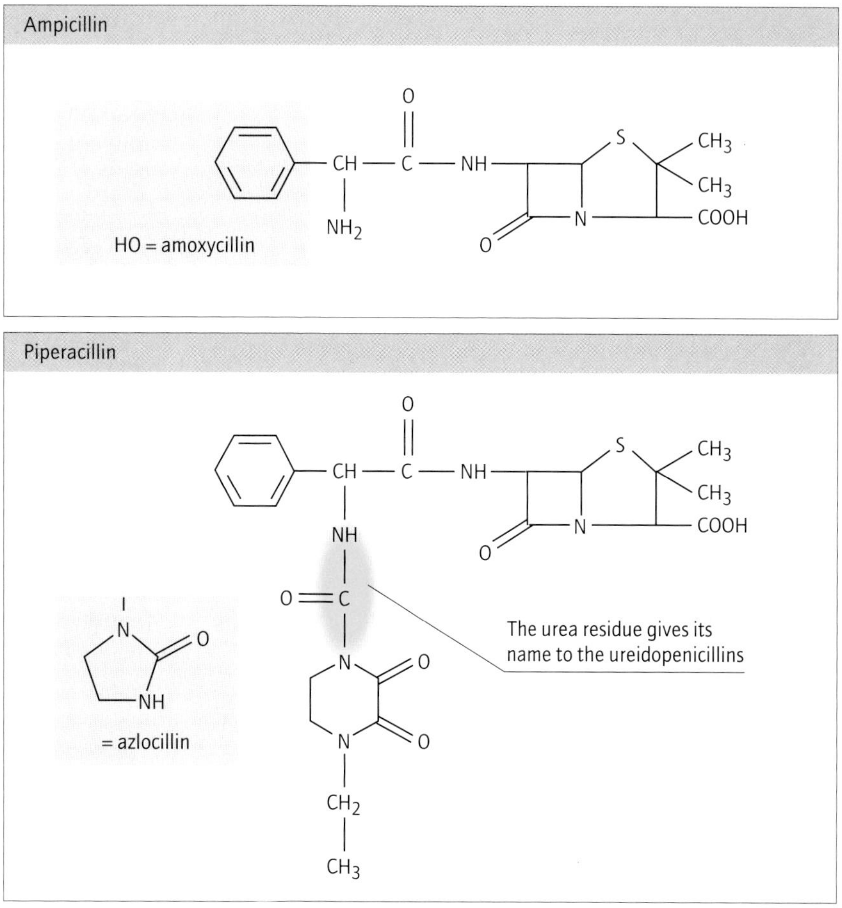

Fig. 4.12 The structure of ampicillin and piperacillin.

linear molecule which is cross-linked through D-alanyl groups. Beta-lactam antibiotics inhibit the transpeptidation part of this process.

> Beta-lactam antibiotics inhibit bacterial cell wall construction by inhibiting cross-linking between peptidoglycan molecules. They are therefore ineffective against bacteria which lack cell walls.

Bacterial resistance

Resistance to beta-lactam antibiotics is mediated by chromosome- or plasmid-encoded mechanisms. Organisms which become resistant may produce a beta-lactamase which destroys the antibiotic. Alternatively, the bacterial outer membrane may become impermeable to penicillin, preventing its access to the site of action. Alterations in the affinity of PBPs may also result in resistance.

Cephalosporins

Cephalosporins are naturally occurring compounds which are closely related to penicillins (Fig. 4.13). They are usually classified according to the route of administration and spectrum of activity.

The first group is the orally active cephalosporins, which all have a strong Gram-positive spectrum. They were initially introduced in response to the spread of penicillinase-producing *Staphylococcus aureus*, but are less effective than either penicillin against susceptible strains or isoxazolylpenicillins against penicillinase-producing *S. aureus*. Some agents such as cefaclor also have useful activity against *Haemophilus influenzae*, making it particularly valuable in the treatment of community-acquired pneumonia.

The second group contains older, injectable agents, such as cefazolin, cefamandole and cefuroxime. These all retain a good spectrum of activity against Gram-positive organisms, but show strong activity against *E. coli* and

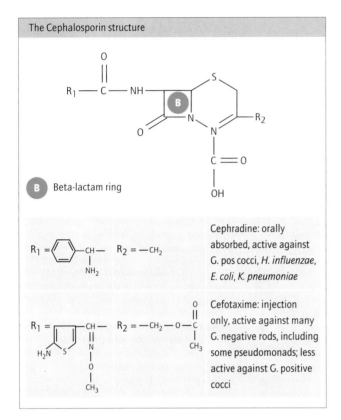

The Cephalosporin structure

B   Beta-lactam ring

R₁ = [phenyl]—CH—   R₂ = —CH₂
        |
        NH₂

Cephradine: orally absorbed, active against G. pos cocci, *H. influenzae*, *E. coli*, *K. pneumoniae*

R₁ = [thiazole, H₂N–S]—CH—   R₂ = —CH₂—O—C=O
                                            |
                                            CH₃

Cefotaxime: injection only, active against many G. negative rods, including some pseudomonads; less active against G. positive cocci

Fig. 4.13 The structure of cephalosporins.

some species of *Proteus*. They have established a role in surgical prophylaxis (e.g. cefazolin and metronidazole before large-bowel surgery). Esters of cefuroxime, such as cefuroxime axetil, are absorbed orally.

Among the newer injectable cephalosporin agents, cefotaxime is active against most Gram-negative organisms, but is less active against *S. aureus*, although it retains good activity against streptococcal species. These agents have gained a place in the management of septicaemia, serious community-acquired pneumonia and neonatal meningitis. Some have only weak activity against *Pseudomonas aeruginosa*. However, cephalosporins such as ceftazidime and cefepime are active against this species. Ceftriaxone has an extended half-life, making single-dose treatment of penicillinase-producing *Neisseria gonorrhoeae* and once-daily therapy of Gram-negative infections possible. More recently, orally active cephalosporins such as cefixime have become available, with a spectrum of activity similar to the newer injectable cephalosporins.

Cephalosporins are mostly rapidly eliminated by the kidney with a half-life of 1–2 h (note the exception of ceftriaxone). They are distributed widely in the extracellular fluid, and penetrate well into tissues. The earlier agents did not cross the blood–brain barrier but the newer injectable cephalosporins such as cefotaxime and ceftriaxone do. Hepatic metabolism is important for some compounds, including cefotaxime.

Cephalosporins have a lower incidence of anaphylaxis, but cross-reactivity occurs in approximately 10% of penicillin-allergic patients. Rashes may also occur, as with the penicillins. The earlier agents cephaloridine and cephalothin are toxic to the kidney but more recent agents have not had this side-effect.

Aminoglycosides

The first aminoglycoside, streptomycin, was isolated from *Streptomyces griseus* in 1943. Since then, a number of different agents have been developed, including kanamycin, gentamicin, tobramicin, netilmicin and amikacin (Fig. 4.14). Aminoglycosides are defined by the presence of amino sugars linked by glycosidic bonds to aminocyclitol. Aminoglycosides inhibit protein synthesis by preventing ribosomes from translating messenger RNA codes into proteins. They are active against aerobic and facultative anaerobic Gram-negative bacilli and *Staphylococcus aureus*. In addition they are active against mycobacteria and *Brucella*.

Aminoglycosides are not absorbed from the gastrointestinal tract and must be administered parenterally. They are polar, and distributed in the extracellular fluid. They are not metabolized by the liver but are excreted unchanged in the urine. Although they have a very low therapeutic index, they are valuable for their activity and effectiveness in treating Gram-negative septicaemia.

The three main adverse events associated with aminoglycoside use are ototoxicity, renal toxicity and neuromuscular paralysis.

Bacteria become resistant to aminoglycosides by three main mechanisms. Methylation of the ribosome prevents the aminoglycoside from binding to its substrate. This mode of resistance is limited to streptomycin. The bacterial cell membrane may become impermeable to aminoglycoside antibiotics. This affects all of the drugs in the aminoglycoside class. Bacteria can also become resistant by developing aminoglycoside-inactivating enzymes. There are three main enzyme groups: *N*-acetyltransferases, *O*-phosphotransferases and *O*-nucleotidyltransferases. Although a wide range of enzyme-mediated resistances can occur, bacterial strains with aminoglycoside resistance are uncommon in hospitals with well-organized infection control and antibiotic policies.

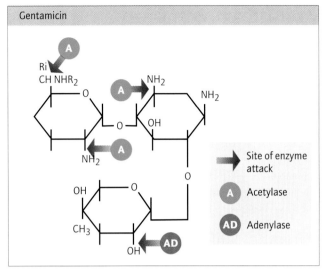

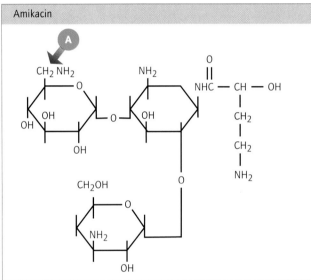

Fig. 4.14 Structure of gentamicin, indicating sites of antimicrobial enzyme attack. Amikacin, by contrast, lacks all but one of these vulnerable sites.

Tetracyclines

Tetracyclines were first isolated from *Streptomyces* species and are based around four fused rings (a hydronaphthacene nucleus). They act by binding to the 30S ribosomal subunit, locking band A of transfer RNA to the septal site on the messenger RNA–ribosomal complex. Although many tetracycline compounds have been described, they have similar spectra of activity but differ in their pharmacokinetics. Tetracyclines are active against *Staphylococcus aureus*, streptococcal species, including *Streptococcus pneumoniae*, *N. gonorrhoeae*, *N. meningitidis*, *H. influenzae* and some species of Enterobacteriaceae. They are active against *Bacillus* species and many other species of anaerobes. They are also effective in the treatment of mycoplasmas, rickettsiae, coxiellae and chlamydiae and spirochaete infections, including those caused by *Treponema pallidum*. Some species of mycobacteria are also susceptible. The activity of tetracyclines is not limited to bacteria but also includes protozoa, such as *Plasmodium* spp. and *Entamoeba histolytica*.

> Tetracyclines act by arresting the sequence of transfer RNA molecules.

Tetracyclines are well-absorbed orally but vary widely in their half-life. Some agents, such as doxycycline, have a long half-life, and adequate therapeutic levels may be obtained by once-daily dosage. Tetracyclines are distributed to many tissues including the lung, liver, kidney, brain and respiratory tract. They are concentrated in the bile but do not cross the blood–brain barrier into the cerebrospinal fluid. They should be used with caution in renal or hepatic sufficiency.

Gastrointestinal intolerance is the commonest adverse event. Skin reactions include photosensitivity and exfoliation. Tetracyclines are concentrated in developing bones and teeth, and are therefore contraindicated in children and pregnant women. Fatty degeneration of the liver, with fatal liver failure, has been reported in pregnant patients. Treatment with tetracycline causes increased protein breakdown and an apparent deterioration in the biochemical status of patients with renal impairment. Irreversible renal failure has developed in some patients treated with tetracyclines.

Because of their wide range of side-effects, tetracyclines are first-line treatment for relatively few infections. They are the treatment of choice for severe rickettsial and chlamydial infections, and for Q-fever.

Chloramphenicol

Chloramphenicol was first isolated from *Streptomyces venezuelae* but is now produced synthetically. It inhibits protein synthesis by reversibly binding to the 50S ribosomal subunit, preventing the attachment of aminoacyl transfer RNA, and subsequent peptide bond formation. It is active against a wide range of agents, including most Gram-positive and Gram-negative aerobic bacteria, and many obligative anaerobes, including *Bacteroides*. It is also active against spirochaetes, rickettsiae, chlamydiae and mycoplasmas. It is bacteriostatic against most microorganisms but is bactericidal against *H. influenzae* and *Neisseria* sp.

> Choramphenicol inhibits protein synthesis by blocking the transfer of amino acids from their respective transfer RNAs to the protein chain.

Chloramphenicol may be given parenterally but is well absorbed orally. It is widely distributed in the tissues and crosses the blood–brain barrier. Chloramphenicol is metabolized in the liver and is excreted by the kidney. A special oily preparation is available and can be given by the intramuscular route. This has proven valuable in developing countries for single-dose treatment of bacterial sepsis.

The principal adverse effect of chloramphenicol is in preterm infants in the neonatal period, when they lack sufficient hepatic enzymes to conjugate chloramphenicol efficiently, and toxic levels build up. The dose must be limited to prevent this. Excessive dosing results in the 'grey baby' syndrome, characterized by circulatory collapse. In adults the principal toxic effect of chloramphenicol is on the bone marrow. There is a reversible dose-dependent bone marrow depression due to the inhibition of mitochondrial protein synthesis. A rare form of idiosyncratic aplastic anaemia occurs in approximately 1 in 40 000 patients. This can occur even after the completion of therapy and is not dose-related. It is unfortunately often fatal.

Despite the wide spectrum of activity of chloramphenicol, fear of toxicity has limited its use for a number of specific indications: alternative therapy of bacterial meningitis, typhoid fever and invasive salmonellosis, brain abscess and rickettsial diseases.

Quinolones

All members of the quinolone group of antimicrobial agents have a similar structure (Fig. 4.15). When DNA is transcribed, the supercoiled molecule must be unwound for transcription to occur. Quinolones interfere with the action of DNA topoisomerase A, the bacterial enzyme responsible for this process. The first agent in clinical use was nalidixic acid, which is active mainly against Enterobacteriaceae, *Haemophilus* and *Neisseria*. *Pseudomonas* spp. and *Serratia* spp. are resistant, as are staphylococci and streptococci. This narrow-spectrum agent was used for the treatment of Gram-negative urinary tract infections, as sufficiently high concentrations could be reached in the urine.

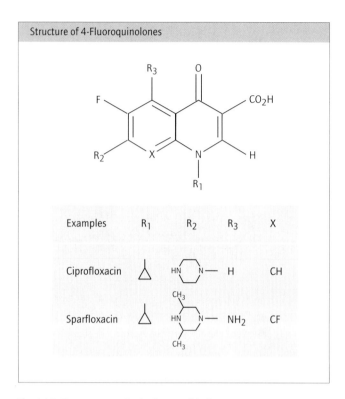

Fig. 4.15 The structure of quinolone antibiotics.

> Quinolones interfere with DNA function by preventing the uncoiling and recoiling of the molecule necessary for polymerization and transcription.

Chemical modification of the basic quinolone nucleus by the introduction of a fluorine at the sixth position produced the fluoroquinolones, resulting in antibacterial activity many times greater than nalidixic acid. Fluoroquinolones such as ciprofloxacin and ofloxacin are highly active against the Enterobacteriaceae, *Pseudomonas* spp., *Haemophilus* spp., *Neisseria* spp., *Chlamydia* spp. and also mycobacteria.

The fluoroquinolones are well absorbed orally, reaching a peak in the serum 90 min after oral administration. Protein binding is low and they are distributed widely in the tissues, including 'difficult' areas such as the prostate. They do not cross the blood–brain barrier. Quinolones penetrate cells, including macrophages and polymorphs. They vary in their degree of metabolism and renal excretion. Ciprofloxacin is partly metabolized and excreted in the urine. The dosage should be reduced in patients with renal insufficiency.

Quinolone antibiotics are well-tolerated but nalidixic acid is associated with nausea, vomiting, diarrhoea, abdominal pain and skin reactions, including photosensitivity. Fluoroquinolones are associated with mild gastrointestinal side-effects, dizziness, tiredness, restlessness and depression. They increase the tendency to seizures in epilepsy, and should be used with caution or not at all in known epileptics. They also have important interactions with some drugs, including aminophylline, increasing their toxic effects.

Fluoroquinolones are useful in the treatment of a wide range of systemic bacterial disease. They are of particular value in the management of hospital Gram-negative septicaemia, especially when *P. aeruginosa* is a likely pathogen, as in neutropenic patients. As they reach high concentrations in bronchial secretions, fluoroquinolones are useful in the treatment of hospital-acquired Gram-negative pneumonia, and in children with cystic fibrosis (who are subject to recurrent *Pseudomonas* infection). They have also gained a place in the management of typhoid, invasive *Salmonella* infections and sexually transmitted diseases, and may be valuable in the management of mycobacterial infections.

Glycopeptides

Vancomycin is a glycopeptide antibiotic first isolated from *Streptomyces orientalis*. It inhibits peptidoglycan synthesis by interfering with chain-lengthening. Glycopeptides are large polar molecules and therefore cannot penetrate the outer membrane of Gram-negative bacteria. All Gram-positive organisms are susceptible, and bacterial resistance to vancomycin is extremely uncommon (but has been reported in some strains of enterococci). Vancomycin and teicoplanin are not absorbed orally and must be administered intravenously, or occasionally locally into the peritoneal cavity. Vancomycin is distributed in the extracellular fluid. It does not cross the blood–brain barrier unless there is meningeal inflammation. More than 80% is excreted unchanged by the kidney.

> Glycopeptides inhibit Gram-positive cell wall construction by blocking the elongation of glycopeptide chains.

Vancomycin causes thrombophlebitis, so administration via a central line is preferred. An idiosyncratic vasodilatation–hypotension ('red man') syndrome develops in up to 15% of patients given bolus doses which is thought to be related to histamine release. To avoid this, the drug is always given by slow infusion. Teicoplanin may be given intramuscularly.

Renal toxicity is important and is more likely to occur in patients receiving concomitant aminoglycosides. Deafness may develop, particularly in elderly patients or those with renal impairment. Toxic manifestations of vancomycin therapy can be minimized by careful attention to dosage schedules and regular monitoring of serum levels.

Vancomycin is indicated for the treatment of patients with severe Gram-positive infections unresponsive to beta-lactam antibiotics, or in patients who are sensitive to beta-lactams. It has an important role in the therapy of invasive methicillin-resistant staphylococcal infection and infections with ampicillin-resistant enterococci. Oral therapy is indicated for the treatment of pseudomembranous colitis, and Gram-positive infections in chronic ambulatory peritoneal dialysis may be treated by the addition of the drug in the dialysis fluid. The dosage of vancomycin should be modified in patients with renal failure, to avoid accumulation and toxicity.

Teicoplanin

Teicoplanin is a new glycopeptide antibiotic isolated from *Actinoplanus teichomyceticus*. It is similar to vancomycin in its spectrum of activity. However, some strains of *Staphylococcus haemolyticus* are naturally resistant. The use of teicoplanin is not associated with the severe adverse reactions reported with vancomycin and serum monitoring is unnecessary. The clinical indications for the use of teicoplanin are similar to those of vancomycin.

Metronidazole

Metronidazole is a nitroimidazole drug active against anaerobic bacteria, *Giardia intestinalis*, *Trichomonas vaginalis* and *Entamoeba histolytica*. The drug acts as an electron-acceptor at low redox potentials, allowing the formation of toxic metabolites which are lethal to the organism.

> Metronidazole acts at low redox potential by generating highly toxic metabolites.

Metronidazole is indicated for the treatment of serious infections in which anaerobic bacteria may play a part — abdominal sepsis, brain abscess, lung abscess, anaerobic lung infections or dental infections. It may also be indicated for parenteral therapy of pseudomembranous colitis. Metronidazole is also used in the therapy of intestinal and vaginal protozoan infections. It is the treatment of choice for giardiasis, intestinal amoebiasis and amoebic liver abscess. It is also valuable for surgical prophylaxis for abdominal and gynaecological surgery (see Chapter 23).

Metronidazole is absorbed orally and rectally, and can also be administered parenterally. It is not strongly protein-bound. It is widely distributed throughout all tissues and fluids. It crosses the blood–brain barrier and achieves high concentrations in brain abscesses. Approximately 30% of the dose is metabolized in the liver and 70% is excreted unchanged in the urine. Initial therapy of serious sepsis and abscesses is via the intravenous route but oral or rectal administration can be commenced as soon as practicable, since adequate concentrations are achieved by these routes.

Metronidazole is usually well-tolerated, but many patients complain of minor side-effects, including fever, dizziness, dry mouth and a metallic taste. More serious side-effects include encephalopathy and peripheral neuropathy, more likely with extended therapy. A disulfiram (Antabuse) reaction can develop in patients who drink alcohol while taking metronidazole.

Metronidazole has mutagenic activity in prokaryotic systems (the Ames test) but there no evidence of carcinogenicity in humans, despite extensive use over a number of years.

Macrolides

The macrolides are a group of related antimicrobials. They have a common macrocyclic lactam ring with 14, 15 or 16 members. The members include erythromycin, clarithromycin, azithromycin and spiramycin. All the agents have a similar antimicrobial spectrum, including Gram-positive organisms, *Neisseria*, *Haemophilus* and *Bordetella*, and some Gram-negative anaerobes. They are also active against *Mycoplasma* sp., *Rickettsia* sp. and *Toxoplasma gondii*. Their mechanism of activity is uncertain but occurs early in the course of RNA-dependent protein synthesis. The macrolides bind to the 50S ribosome. Bacteria become resistant to macrolides by mechanisms which decrease cell permeability and by the alteration of the binding site to the 50S ribosome. Resistance may be inducible or non-inducible (the latter confers resistance to both macrolides and the lincosamide clindamycin).

Macrolides inhibit protein synthesis by an unknown action against ribosomal function.

Erythromycin

Erythromycin is derived from *Streptomyces erthythreus*. Erythromycin base is poorly soluble and inactivated by gastric acid. To improve absorption it may be protected by enteric coating but this may give rise to delayed or incomplete absorption. Esters of erythromycin with stearate, estolate and succinate give improved absorption. A water-soluble preparation is available for intravenous use. Erythromycin is absorbed orally and is distributed throughout the total body water. It is concentrated in alveolar macrophages and polymorphs. It does not cross the blood–brain barrier but does cross the placenta. It is concentrated in the liver and excreted in the bile.

Erythromycin is well-tolerated but some patients complain of nausea and gastric irritation. Thrombophlebitis may follow intravenous use. Jaundice may develop and this is more likely in patients receiving the proprionyl ester. Allergic reactions are reported in a very small proportion of patients. Erythromycin is often indicated as a alternative to penicillin in allergic subjects. It is of benefit in the management of primary atypical pneumonia, including legionellosis. It may shorten the symptomatic period in patients suffering from *Campylobacter* enteritis. It is the treatment of choice in neonatal chlamydial infections. It also used in the treatment of diphtheria and whooping cough, and may be valuable in the management of some mycobacterial infections.

A number of new macrolide antibiotics have been developed, including clarithromycin and azithromycin. These have a similar antimicrobial spectrum to erythromycin, but improved pharmacokinetic properties. Azithromycin may be given in a single daily dose for the treatment of respiratory tract infections and clarithromycin appears to be valuable in the treatment of *Mycobacterium avium intracellulare* infection. Azithromycin reaches very high intracellular concentrations. It may be particularly useful in treating persisting chlamydial infections.

Fusidic acid

Fusidin or fusidic acid is a fermentation product of *Fusidium coccineum*. It is active against Gram-positive bacteria, including the majority of *Staphylococcus aureus* strains and Gram-negative cocci. Streptococci and pneumococci are relatively resistant and Gram-negative bacilli are highly resistant. It has some activity against a variety of protozoa, including *Giardia intestinalis*. Resistance arises naturally and readily develops during therapy, unless a second agent is co-administered to prevent this. It is well-absorbed orally and widely distributed. It does not reach the cerebrospinal fluid but does penetrate into cerebral abscesses and bone. When given orally, sodium fusidate is well-tolerated, although mild gastrointestinal upset and rashes have been reported.

When given intravenously, hepatitis and jaundice can develop but this usually resolves following withdrawal of therapy.

It is indicated for the treatment of severe staphylococcal infection, especially infections of bones and joints. It is also used for the treatment of recurrent furunculosis and for topical therapy of some superficial staphylococcal infections.

Antiviral therapy

The scope of antiviral therapy is still limited despite the understanding of viral replication at the molecular level.

Amantadine

Amantadine is a symmetrical 10-carbon tricyclic amine. It interferes with the replication of influenza type A virus, probably by an effect on cell penetration and viral uncoating. It is used for the prophylaxis and treatment of influenza A during outbreaks. Prophylaxis is usually given to patients with underlying chronic conditions who are at increased risk from severe disease. Resistant influenza A strains do occur and are particularly likely to arise if the drug is given as postexposure prophylaxis.

Amantadine is well-absorbed orally and concentrations in respiratory secretions are equivalent to those in plasma. Side-effects include insomnia, poor concentration, nervousness, dizziness and headaches. In overdose convulsions and psychoses may result. Cardiac failure and arrhythmias can also develop. It is contraindicated in pregnancy, as teratogenicity has been observed in animals.

Aciclovir

Aciclovir is one of a group of nucleoside analogues which are purines or pyrimidines. It is synthetic acyclic purine nucleoside (Fig. 4.16) which has activity against herpes simplex virus (HSV) types I and II and varicella-zoster virus. Aciclovir is activated by virally encoded thymidine kinases which phosphorylate the drug. Cellular thymidine kinases add a further two phosphate molecules to form aciclovir triphosphate (Fig. 4.17). The need for viral thymidine kinase to perform the first phosphorylation means that the drug only becomes active in virally infected cells. The activated drug inhibits HSV DNA polymerase and is a DNA chain terminator. Resistant virus mutants arise naturally and are readily induced in the laboratory but they tend to be of low pathogenicity and rarely cause clinical problems. Aciclovir is absorbed orally and it can be administered parenterally. It is widely distributed and adequate con-

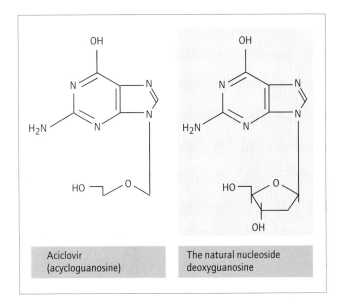

Fig. 4.16 The structure of aciclovir.

centrations are found in the cerebrospinal fluid. The drug is well-tolerated, although renal abnormalities are found if the drug is given in a rapid bolus or in overdosage. Aciclovir is excreted by the kidneys, so the dose must be reduced in patients with renal impairment.

Topical preparations are available for the treatment of herpes simplex infections of the skin and mucous membranes but these have only a weak, local action. Aciclovir is used parenterally for the treatment of severe HSV and herpes zoster infections in immunocompromised or normal subjects.

Other similar nucleoside analogues have recently become available. Esterification of drugs such as penciclovir (producing famciclovir) confers improved oral absorption. This drug is active against herpes zoster but is not effective against all herpes simplex strains.

Ganciclovir

Ganciclovir (Fig. 4.18) is more active than aciclovir against cytomegalovirus (which does not contain the same viral thymidine kinase as herpes simplex and varicella-zoster). It is not well absorbed orally and must usually be given intravenously. It is used in the treatment of life- or sight-threatening cytomegalovirus infections in immunocompromised patients.

Tribavirin

Tribavirin is a synthetic nucleoside derivative (Fig. 4.19). It is active against DNA viruses such as the herpes

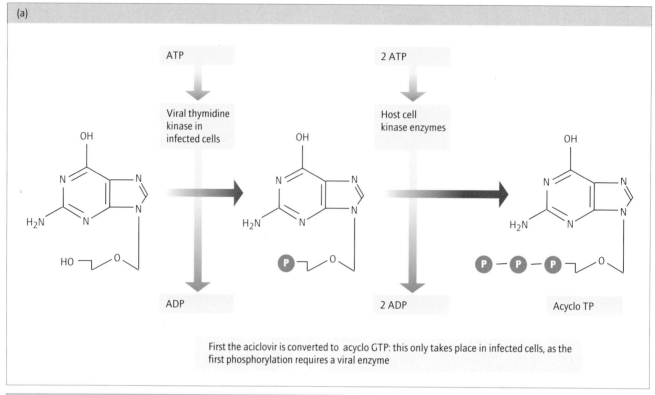

First the aciclovir is converted to acyclo GTP: this only takes place in infected cells, as the first phosphorylation requires a viral enzyme

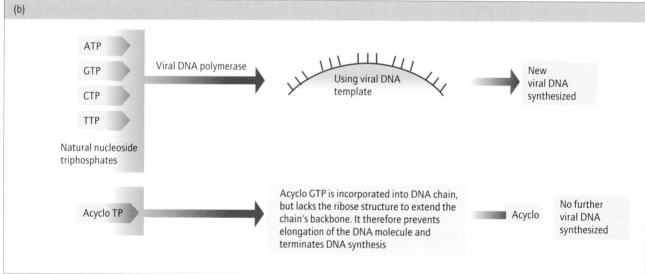

Fig. 4.17 The mechanism of action of aciclovir. (a) Stages in the phosphorylation of aciclovir to a 'false' nucleoside triphosphate. (b) Incorporation of aciclovir into the DNA molecule prevents further chain extension.

viruses and some human RNA viruses such as the orthomyxoviruses, paromyxoviruses, arenaviruses including Lassa virus, Bunyaviridae including Rift Valley virus, and Hantaviruses. It is absorbed orally and can be administered by aerosol for the treatment of respiratory syncytial virus (RSV) infections. The drug is well-tolerated, although elevations in unconjugated bilirubin and a drop in haemoglobin have been described. It is used for the treatment of RSV infections in infants and is effective in the treatment of Lassa fever and Hanta virus infections if given early in the course of infection.

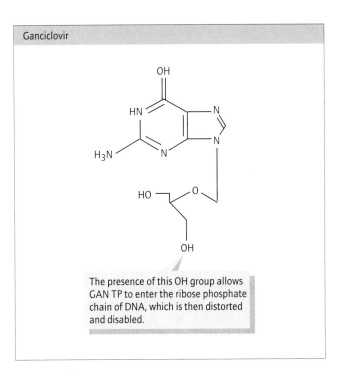

The presence of this OH group allows GAN TP to enter the ribose phosphate chain of DNA, which is then distorted and disabled.

Fig. 4.18 The structure of ganciclovir.

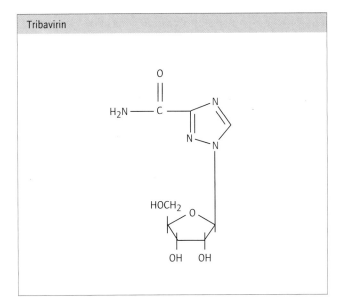

Fig. 4.19 The structure of tribavirin.

Zidovudine

Zidovudine (azidodeoxythymidine or AZT) is a dideoxynucleoside analogue originally developed as an anticancer agent (Fig. 4.20). It is an important inhibitor of

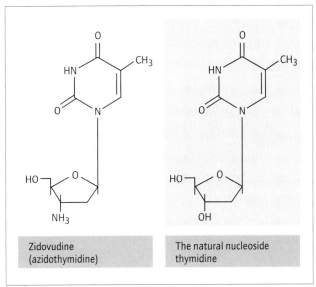

Zidovudine (azidothymidine)

The natural nucleoside thymidine

Fig. 4.20 The structure of zidovudine.

human immunodeficiency virus replication *in vitro* and is therefore used in the treatment of patients with the acquired immunodeficiency syndrome (AIDS).

The drug is phosphorylated to AZT monophosphate by a cellular thymidine kinase and is subsequently converted to diphosphate and triphosphate by cellular thymidylate kinase. It inhibits retroviral reverse transcriptase to which it binds preferentially.

It is well-absorbed orally and is metabolized in the liver. The main side-effects are anaemia and neutropenia which usually occur after about 6 weeks of therapy, particularly in patients with pre-existing neutropenia or anaemia. The drug should be discontinued if the haemoglobin falls below 7.5 g/l or the neutrophil count below $0.7 \times 10^9/l$. These effects are reversible. Other adverse events reported include nausea, headache, rash, abdominal pain, fever and myalgia.

Newer dideoxynucleoside drugs have since been developed. Dideoxyinosine (DDI) and dideoxycytosine (DDC) are finding a place as additional or alternative drugs in managing the emergence of resistance to zidovudine in AIDS patients.

Antifungal therapy

Azoles

The azoles are a large group of synthetic agents which have an imidazole or triazole ring with an N-carbon substitution. These agents act by blocking the 14 alpha-D-methylation step in the biosynthesis of ergosterol. This leads to ergosterol depletion and interference with fungal membrane function. As a group they have a wide spectrum of activity against *Candida* and dermatophytes, and some are active against *Aspergillus* sp. There are two main groups — the systemic agents such as fluconazole and ketoconazole and topical preparations such as clotrimazole and miconazole, which are used for the treatment of dermatophytosis and superficial candidosis.

Systemic azoles

Fluconazole has activity against yeast-like fungi, including *Candida*, *Histoplasma* and *Cryptococcus* spp. It is active in dermatophytosis but ineffective against aspergillosis. It is well-absorbed orally and is well-tolerated. There is a mild induction of transaminases, and warfarin concentrations may be affected. It has proved useful in the oral treatment of vaginal candidosis and the treatment of systemic candidosis in immuno-compromised patients. A closely related agent, *itra-conazole*, is also active against *Aspergillus* spp. It is orally absorbed and achieves high concentrations in the stratum corneum and hair. It has been used in the treatment of superficial mycosis including dermato-phytosis, pityriasis versicolor, and oral and vaginal candidosis. It may also be useful in the treatment of as-pergillosis, histoplasmosis and cryptococcosis as an alternative to amphotericin.

Ketoconazole has a similar spectrum of activity to fluconazole. It is given orally. Side-effects include hepatitis, which occurs in 1 per 15 000 patients. Topical formulations are used in the treatment of fungal infections of the skin and in seborrhoeic dermatitis.

Flucytosine (5-fluorocytosine)

This is a synthetic fluorinated pyrimidine with activity limited to *Candida* spp., *Cryptococcus neoformans* and some fungi causing chromomycosis. It acts by being incorporated into RNA in the place of uracil, resulting in abnormalities of protein synthesis. It also blocks thymidylate synthetase causing interruption of DNA synthesis. Resistance is quite common and may arise during treatment. It is given either orally or parenterally and excreted in the kidney. Dosage must be reduced when the creatinine clearance falls. The main side-effects are marrow aplasia, enteritis and hepatotoxicity. It is used in the treatment of systemic candidosis and crypto-

coccal infections in combination with amphotericin. The advantage of this combination is that the dosage of amphotericin may be reduced, thereby reducing side-effects.

Griseofulvin

This is an antibiotic derived from various species of penicillium such as *Penicillium griseofulvum*. Its mechanism of action is unknown but it does interfere with nucleic acid synthesis. Its activity is restricted to the dermatophytes. The drug is absorbed orally and it appears in keratinized tissues at concentrations which are able to prevent further invasion by the fungus. It is useful for treating nail infections, but must be given for extended periods until the infected keratinized structures are all shed and replaced. Serious adverse events are uncommon but patients complaining of headache and rashes do occasionally occur. Griseofulvin reduces the anticoagulant effect of warfarin.

Polyenes

The polyenes consist of a closed macrolide ring with a variable number of hydroxyl groups along the hydrophilic side. On the hydrophobic side there are a variable number of repeating double bonds. They bind to sterols and eukaryotic cell membranes, causing leakage of the cellular components and consequently cell death. Some polyenes are selectively toxic for fungal membranes but some are equally toxic to fungal and mammalian cells. The most important member of this group is amphotericin, a heptaene with seven conjugated double bonds, which is used as parenteral treatment for systematic mycoses. It is active against most of the fungi which cause disease in humans. As well as this it has activity against *Leishmania* spp. and can be used in the treatment of kala-azar and cutaneous leishmaniasis. Acquired resistance is rare but resistant variants of some *Candida* species, notably *C. tropicalis*, *C. parapsilosis*, *C. lusitaniae* and *C. krusei* have been described. It is administered parentally and is highly protein-bound, thus it does not penetrate well into the cerebrospinal fluid. Treatment causes fever, rigors, headache, vomiting and throm-bophlebitis. Hyperkalaemia and anaemia are also common. The incidence of serious side-effects has been reduced by incorporating amphotericin into liposomes or other lipid carriers. This allows much higher doses to be administered with fewer toxic reactions.

Allylamines

Terbinafine is a recently introduced allylamine drug which is useful for the oral treatment of dermatophyte infections of the nails and of ringworm.

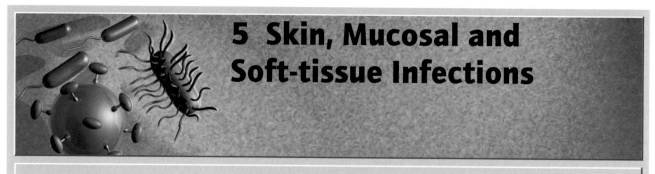

5 Skin, Mucosal and Soft-tissue Infections

Introduction

Structural considerations

The skin consists of a superficial structure, called the epidermis, and the deeper dermis (Fig. 5.1). The epidermis is durable and waterproof, composed of layers of squamous cells, which are increasingly keratinized and flattened as they approach the surface. The keratinous surface is further protected by a film of sebaceous secretion which resists penetration by fluids and microorganisms.

Beneath the deepest, basal cell layer from which the epidermis is generated lies the dermis. This is a sensitive and vascular structure containing a great deal of loose connective tissue, which is well-hydrated and supple. This allows free movement of the skin surface over deeper structures.

The epidermis is penetrated by hair follicles and the ducts of sweat glands arising in the dermis. These can provide a niche for colonizing organisms and, if occluded by keratinous debris or inspissated secretions, they can become sites of loculated or spreading infection. The hair and nails are modified epidermal structures, consisting mainly of keratin.

The epidermis, hair and nails can be locally invaded by organisms which digest keratin or sebum. These are usually fungi. They cause damage and flaking, some-times with a minimal inflammatory reaction. Bacterial infection of the epidermis is more invasive and inflammatory. Some infections spread along the surface of the skin, producing a macerated, weeping lesion, which advances to adjacent areas, or may spread by contact to other skin sites. Such open lesions are often very infectious. Intraepidermal infections are less common. They behave like an expanding intradermal injection, advancing by separating the epidermal cell layers. Erysipelas is an example of this. It has a well-defined advancing edge, and may form vesicles or bullae with roofs of detached epidermal layers.

Infections of the dermis spread widely in the loose connective tissue, and the advancing inflammation has an indistinct edge which gradually merges into normal tissue. This is the typical appearance of cellulitis, an infection of the dermis. The dermis can be greatly expanded by the oedema and cellular infiltrate which accompany infection. Scarring or fibrosis afterwards can tether the skin to the underlying structures such as fascia or muscle. In severe cases the underlying tissue can become infected (for instance, when deep skin ulcer is complicated by osteomyelitis of underlying bone; see Chapter 17).

Skin changes in systemic disease

Being highly vascular and easily visible, the skin displays abnormalities in many systemic diseases, as well

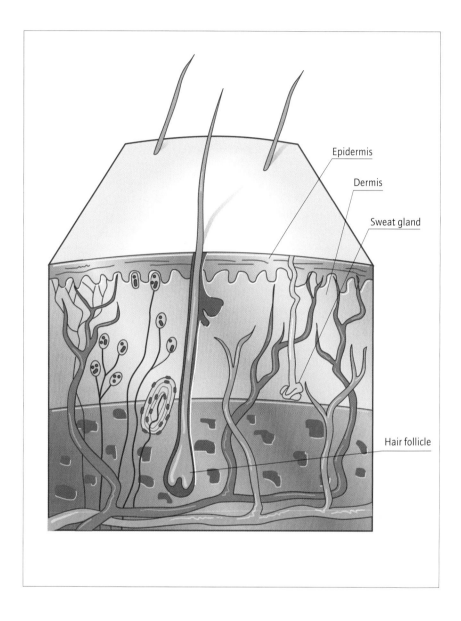

Fig. 5.1 Structure of the skin.

as localized skin disorders. Rashes, jaundice, and vasculitic, embolic and haemorrhagic lesions are valuable physical signs of systemic disease, and may be so typical as to be diagnostic. They may be due to infectious lesions as in the chickenpox rash, to a vasculitic reaction as in the measles rash, or to damage by toxins as in scarlet fever. Vasculitis or intravascular coagulation may produce petechial or haemorrhagic lesions, seen in rickettsiosis or meningococcal disease. Chemical infiltration with bilirubin or methaemalbumin may cause typical discoloration.

Natural defences of the skin

The surface structure and acidic sebaceous secretions are hostile to many pathogens. There is a dense population of normal flora inhabiting the surface, ducts and follicles. These organisms are adapted to the skin environment, which they may further modify by adjusting the pH, redox potential or local concentration of bacteriostatic substances. The rich blood and lymphatic supply of the dermis ensure that both specific and non-specific immune responses can quickly be recruited when pathogens enter the skin.

Important normal skin flora
1 Coagulase-negative staphylococci.
2 *Staphylococcus aureus*.
3 *Streptococcus pyogenes*.
4 Many species of *Corynebacterium*.
5 *Propionobacterium* spp.
6 *Candida* spp.

Skin defences are compromised if the surface is penetrated by injury or thinned and excoriated by inflammatory processes. Sustained wetness of the skin causes maceration of the keratinous epidermis, which can then be invaded by pathogens. Patients who suffer from eczema are highly susceptible to skin infections caused by *Staphylococcus aureus* or herpes simplex.

Natural defences of the skin
1 Keratinous surface.
2 Antibacterial effects of sebum.
3 Effect of normal flora.

Mucosal structure and defences

Mucosae do not have a keratinized surface; they are always moist and some are only one cell thick. They are much more susceptible than skin to invasion by surface pathogens. For defence they rely on the washing action of secretions, which may contain lysozymes or specific secretory immunoglobulin A (IgA). Mucosae adjacent to skin, as in the nose and mouth, are colonized and protected by their own normal flora, which merges into that of the skin at the mucocutaneous margin.

Natural defences of mucosae
1 Mechanical washing by tears or urine.
2 Lysozyme or antibody in surface fluid.
3 Surface phagocytes.
4 Ciliary action moving mucus and debris.

Viral infections of the skin and mucosae

ORGANISM LIST

Papillomaviruses
Herpes simplex virus type 1
Herpes simplex virus type 2
Varicella Zoster virus
Coxsackie A viruses
Molluscum contagiosum
Cowpox
Orf/paravaccinia
Vaccinia.

Papillomavirus infections (warts)

Introduction

There are many types of human papillomaviruses (HPVs), of which the commonest are those associated with common warts, plantar warts (verrucae) and genital warts. Unlike some genital papillomaviruses, particularly HPV16 and HPV18, HPV infections of the skin are rarely associated with malignancy. Exceptions include rare squamous cell transformation of condylomata acuminata, and the uncommon Bowenoid papulosis and epidermodysplasia verruciformis.

Common (plane) warts

These are usually seen in children, as immunity to the viruses is gained by adulthood. They are infectious by contact, the viruses entering tiny fissures, and infecting the epidermal keratinocytes of the prickle-cell layer. The infected cells hypertrophy and multiply, producing a keratinized, nodular papilloma. Curetting the lesion confirms its identity by revealing a group of tiny bleeding points which are dermal capillaries supplying the hypertrophic lesion (in involuting lesions, thrombosed capillaries appear as black dots). While solitary on the palms, plane warts may be multiple in the looser skin on the wrists or dorsa of the hands.

Plantar warts may become large, a centimetre or more in diameter. They are pressed into the foot by the body weight and often develop an eroded central area. Local pressure can cause severe pain on weight-bearing. They can be distinguished from corns by the bleeding points of dermal capillaries revealed on paring the lesion; corns are composed of homogeneous, semitranslucent keratin, with no capillaries.

Treatment of warts is rarely required in children, as immunity gradually develops and the lesions involute. Plantar warts may be reduced in size by paring. Salicylate and lactic acid ointment, painted on to the lesion, allowed to dry and covered with an adhesive dressing, softens the keratin and inhibits the viruses. Warts in adults can be curetted, or preferably ablated by freezing with a cryoprobe or with a small swab dipped in liquid nitrogen.

Plantar warts are highly infectious, especially during swimming, when the uncovered skin is softened by immersion. If the lesions are temporarily covered with a waterproof plaster or latex sock, however, swimming need not be forbidden.

Herpes simplex infections

Introduction and epidemiology

Herpes simplex viruses are colonists and invaders of mucosae. They can also infect skin if entry is available via small punctures, fissures or macerated areas. Typically, infections of the mouth and upper body have been caused by herpes simplex type 1, while infections related to the genital tract have been due to the genetically distinct type 2 virus. In recent years it has been recognized that the epidemiology of the two viruses is less distinct, and either virus may be found in either site.

Like other herpesviruses, herpes simplex has the property of latency; after causing a primary infection it persists in the immune host as a dormant form. It can be reactivated from time to time and may either be shed asymptomatically or cause a lesion, usually less severe than that in the non-immune host.

Herpes simplex infection is spread by direct contact with mucosa or skin from which virus is being shed. In infancy primary infection is often buccal (Fig. 5.2), acquired by oral contact or shared eating utensils. Nailfold or finger pulp infections may follow contamination of the finger with the saliva, and often occur in infants who suck their thumb or nurses who provide mouth care for debilitated patients (Fig. 5.3). Inoculation into the eye may cause infection of the conjunctiva (Fig. 5.4) or the cornea.

Reactivation lesions may be precipitated by acute feverish illness and are therefore called cold sores (Fig. 5.5). Severe herpetic lesions often accompany pneumococcal or meningococcal infections. Overexposure to sunlight is also a common precipitating event.

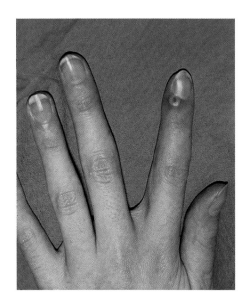

Fig. 5.3 Herpetic whitlow affecting an intensive care nurse.

Sites of skin and mucosal herpes simplex infection
1 Primary gingivostomatitis.
2 Lip margin (cold sore).
3 Nailbed (felon or whitlow).
4 Finger pulp.
5 Facial skin.
6 Eczema affected skin (eczema herpeticum).
7 Cornea (dendritic ulcer).
8 Conjunctiva.
9 Genitalia (see Chapter 11).
10 Central nervous system infections (see Chapter 16).

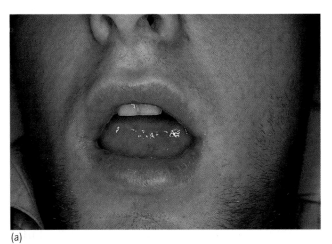
(a)

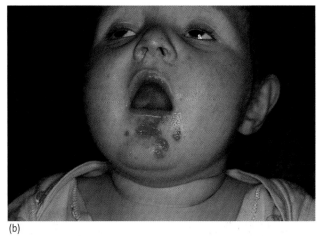
(b)

Fig. 5.2 Primary herpetic gingivostomatitis showing (a) lesions on the tongue (unusually in an adult); (b) in an infant, herpetic lesions on skin macerated by infected saliva.

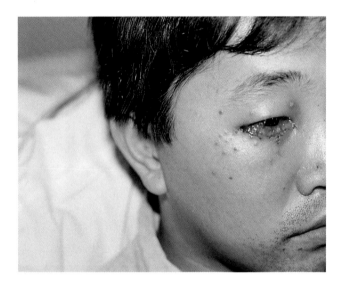

Fig. 5.4 Herpes simplex conjunctivitis.

Effective cell-mediated immunity is essential for the control of herpes simplex infection. Patients treated with cytotoxic drugs, who are undergoing bone marrow grafting, or those with human immunodeficiency virus (HIV) infection are at risk of severe infection.

Pathology

Important structural components of herpes simplex virus (HSV)

1 Core: central protein structure around which DNA winds.
2 Genome: double-stranded linear DNA, coding for approximately 70 proteins.
3 Capsid: icosadeltahedral, with 162 protein capsomeres.
4 Envelope: bilaminar lipid membrane bearing 'spikes' of glycoprotein molecules.
5 Glycoproteins: several, identified by letters:
  (a) gA/B (different forms of same protein) and gD are common to HSV-1 and HSV-2;
  (b) gC, gE and gF are probably important in immune response to HSV;
  (c) gE and gI form a complex which binds IgG Fc, and gC binds to C3b, possibly contributing to pathogenesis of HSV.
6 Tegument: protein found between capsid and envelope.

Herpes simplex is a cytolytic virus that causes acantholysis in the parabasal region of the dermis, leading to vesicle formation. The roof of the vesicle is formed by the keratinized squamous epithelium, but in the mouth and at other mucous membranes the roof is unstable and sloughed away. The vesicle contains cellular debris with Tzanck cells (polykaryocytes; fused keratinocytes), and the base contains cells undergoing ballooning degeneration (Fig. 5.6). Virus spreads from cell to cell.

The virus probably spreads up the sensory neurons via the axon, reaching the sensory ganglion and establishing latent infection. Herpes simplex virus can be isolated from the trigeminal ganglia of approximately 50% of patients tested. If the virus spreads to the brain, encephalitis may develop.

Latency is a dynamic equilibrium with a low-grade viral infection which does not bring about lysis of the cell. Intermittently, the virus reactivates and travels down the sensory neuron to cause a secondary infection. The mechanisms of latency and reactivation are not clearly understood, but specific antisense DNA

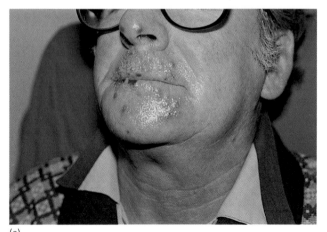
(a)

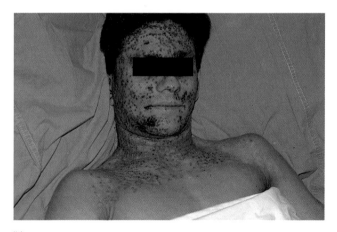
(b)

Fig. 5.5 (a) Herpes simplex reactivation lesion (cold sore); (b) eczema herpeticum originating from a cold sore.

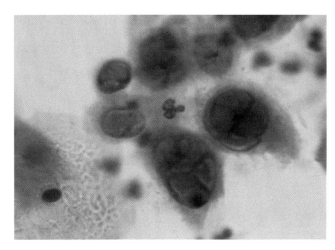

Fig. 5.6 Microscopical appearance of cells from a herpetic vesicle.

sequences from the herpes simplex virus are detectable in latently infected cells.

Clinical features

Primary herpetic gingivostomatitis

Primary herpetic gingivostomatitis is usually seen in infants, though some people escape infection until their teens or early 20s. The illness begins with a day or two of fever and tender enlargement of cervical lymph nodes. Painful, oval, whitish vesicles then appear in the mouth. They may cover the tongue and are common on the soft palate, the gums and inside the lips. Soreness often prevents suckling or taking solid food. Excessive salivation causes dribbling of infectious saliva, often causing secondary lesions on the fingers, the chin or chest.

The natural course of the disease is short. Few new lesions appear after 2 or 3 days of eruption, and most have deroofed and healed within 5–7 days. There is risk of spread to affected skin or, rarely, generalized skin infection in individuals with eczema, even if the disease is currently inactive. This condition is called eczema herpeticum.

Diagnosis

The diagnosis is usually clinically obvious. Oral blisters are seen in hand, foot and mouth disease, but these are accompanied by a typical cutaneous rash. Oval plaques of oral candidiasis sometimes occur in infants, but without associated fever and lymphadenopathy.

Laboratory diagnosis

Direct microscopic examination of scrapings from the base of lesions may reveal cells with intranuclear inclusions typically surrounded by a clear halo and, in skin specimens, fused cells (polykaryocytes). These features are common to other herpesvirus infections. Electron microscopy readily demonstrates virus particles in fresh vesicle fluid and is the investigation of choice in early cases. Older fluid is likely to give false-negative results. Herpes simplex antigen can be detected by immunofluorescence staining of cells from herpetic lesions.

Herpes simplex virus is readily cultivated but, since many individuals have latent infection, recovery of virus is not always indicative of herpetic infection. Fresh vesicle fluid, saliva or scrapings should be inoculated as soon as possible. A cytopathic effect can be seen after only 24 h but may be delayed for up to 7 days. It is characterized by grape-like clusters of refractile cells, usually more pronounced with herpes simplex virus type 2.

> **Techniques for diagnosing herpes simplex infections of skin and mucosae**
> 1 Light microscopy (cytology).
> 2 Electron microscopy.
> 3 Cell culture.
> 4 Serology.

Serology

Herpes virus-specific IgG and IgM are detectable by immunofluorescence, radioimmunoassay (RIA) or enzyme-linked immunosorbent assay (ELISA). Specific IgM antibodies in serum indicate active infection but do not reliably differentiate between primary infection and reactivation. Seroconversion in primary infection can be detected by complement fixation test (CFT), indirect haemagglutination test (IHAT), RIA or ELISA (see Chapter 3). A fourfold rise in antibody titres demonstrated by these methods often indicates reactivation–infection.

Management

Antiviral drugs are rarely indicated in primary infection, as they cannot further shorten the evolution of the oral lesions. Maintenance of hydration is the most important concern. Mild analgesia with paracetamol may help. In severe cases an analgesic gel can be applied sparingly to the gums and anterior tongue. Older children and adults usually cope by taking frequent cool or tepid drinks.

Severe or persisting secondary infections and eczema herpeticum can be treated with oral aciclovir 200 mg five times daily for 5 days. The dose can be doubled in immunosuppressed patients. Intravenous treatment may be given in a dose of 5 mg/kg 8-hourly (doubled in immunosuppressed patients).

Prevention and control

Transmission of herpes simplex infections may be reduced by avoiding direct contact with herpetic lesions, although asymptomatic infections and reactivations, with transient viral shedding, are probably common. To avoid herpetic whitlow those attending dental and tracheostomy patients should always wear gloves. Patients with herpetic lesions should be kept away from immunosuppressed patients, newborns and patients with severe eczema or burns.

Herpes zoster

Introduction

Herpes zoster is the condition caused by reactivation of latent varicella-zoster virus (VZV) whose genomes reside in the sensory root ganglia of the brainstem and spinal cord. Reactivation may be spontaneous or may follow a physical or emotional insult, such as a fever, injury or bereavement. It produces pain and rash in the dermatome corresponding to the affected ganglion.

Most patients are affected in middle or old age, but children and teenagers can develop zoster if they had chickenpox as babies, and neonatal zoster occasionally occurs after intrauterine varicella infection.

The disease begins with inflammation in the affected dorsal root ganglion and the appearance of virus particles in the neurons. There is inflammation in the surrounding meninges and affecting the courses and connections of the neurons in the central nervous system. On reaching the skin the disease causes blistering lesions with the same pathological appearance as those of chickenpox (see Chapter 13).

Clinical features

Illness begins with pain and hyperaesthesia in the affected dermatome, as virus particles migrate down the nerve fibres towards the skin. Virus also spreads centrally, causing intramedullary and meningeal inflammation. A few patients have clinically apparent meningism, and children in particular may present with

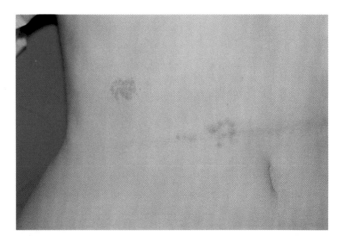

Fig. 5.7 Herpes zoster lesions appearing 2 days after this 8-year-old presented with lymphocytic meningitis; the rash did not extend further.

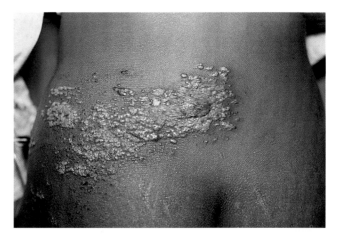

Fig. 5.8 A close-up view of herpes zoster lesions, showing their tendency to coalesce.

viral meningitis and cerebrospinal fluid pleiocytosis before they develop a rash (Fig. 5.7).

The rash begins as small, pink patches at the site of penetrating cutaneous nerves. Vesicles quickly develop in these areas, and the lesions spread until the dermatome is filled. The rash is painful, with a disturbing burning, stabbing quality. Unlike chickenpox vesicles, those of zoster may coalesce to form bullae which become flaccid and lose their roofs, forming ulcerated areas (Fig. 5.8). The vesicles heal by drying and scabbing, rarely leaving a scar.

Multidermatomal and bilateral zoster are rare, occurring when more than one ganglion is affected. Severe zoster in a young person may be an early sign of HIV infection or another immunodeficiency. Blood-borne dissemination of

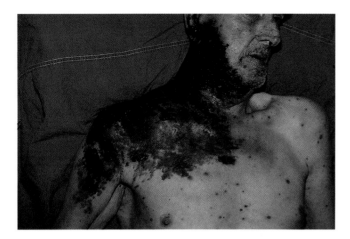

Fig. 5.9 A severe and haemorrhagic herpes zoster rash, with disseminated chickenpox lesions in a patient with chronic lymphocytic leukaemia (the patient recovered fully on treatment).

virus, with the development of a chickenpox-like rash, also indicates immunodeficiency (Fig. 5.9).

Signs of immunodeficiency in herpes zoster
1 Bilateral or multidermatomal dermal rashes.
2 Unusually severe lesions.
3 Recurring herpes zoster.
4 Association with chickenpox-like rash.
5 Association with progressive central nervous system features.

The time course of the illness depends on the patient's age. In children the rash may be minimal; in adults the average duration of rash is 5–8 days. In elderly people there can be weeks of illness, with bullous rash and severe central nervous system disruption causing confusion and debility.

Diagnosis

The diagnosis is usually clinically obvious. If necessary, herpesvirus particles can be demonstrated by electron microscopy of vesicle fluid or scrapings. The virus grows with a typical cytopathic effect in cell culture. Serological testing usually shows a large rise in IgG antibodies (secondary response; see Chapter 1).

Laboratory diagnosis of herpes zoster
1 Light microscopy (cytology).
2 Electron microscopy.
3 Cell culture.
4 Serology.

Management

This may be symptomatic in children and younger adults, who require only rest and analgesia for a few days. The illness can be shortened in older people by early treatment with aciclovir, valaciclovir or famciclovir. Oral aciclovir has poor bioavailability and may not be effective; severe cases benefit from intravenous treatment for 4 or 5 days, or longer in the immunosuppressed. Valaciclovir (an ester of aciclovir) or famciclovir, an ester of penciclovir, are well-absorbed before being hydrolysed to the parent drug in the circulation. They can be given in lower and less frequent dosage than aciclovir.

Treatment of herpes zoster
1 Oral aciclovir 800 mg five times daily for 7 days.
2 Aciclovir infusion 10 mg/kg 8-hourly for 4–7 days.
3 Oral valaciclovir 1 g three times daily for 7 days.
4 Oral famciclovir 250 mg three times daily for 7 days.

Postherpetic neuralgia

Postherpetic neuralgia is persisting severe pain, commonest in the elderly, which can cause misery for months. It responds poorly to analgesics, including opiates. Phenytoin, carbamazepine and vitamin B_{12} injections are ineffective. Tricyclic antidepressants often give some relief, probably by blocking the reuptake of 5-hydroxytryptamine in the presynaptic nerve endings of central pain pathways. They can be given together with standard analgesics. Postherpetic neuralgia is less prolonged in those treated early (within 48 h of rash development) with antiviral agents.

Secondary bacterial infection

Secondary bacterial infection with *Staphylococcus aureus* can affect severe or denuded rashes, especially in the elderly. Oral treatment with cloxacillin, flucloxacillin or trimethoprim is usually effective.

Ascending myeloencephalitis

Ascending myeloencephalitis is an exceptionally rare complication which should be treated with intravenous aciclovir. Immunosuppressed patients are at higher risk, and respond less well to treatment.

Hand, foot and mouth disease

This is a highly infectious disease of toddlers caused by coxsackie A viruses, most often A16. Family outbreaks

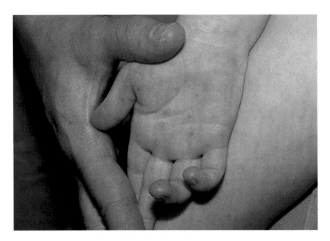
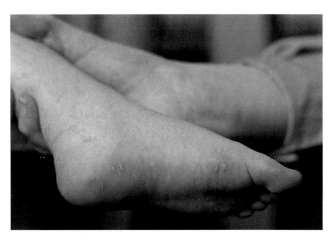

Fig. 5.10 Hand, foot and mouth disease: the typical blisters.

are common, occasionally affecting adults as well as children, though adults are usually immune. A brief feverish prodrome is followed by the simultaneous eruption of several blisters on the hands and feet and in the pharynx. The palms and soles are most affected (Fig. 5.10). There is also a papular rash on the buttocks. There is mild discomfort and soreness of the throat, but the illness is short and self-limiting, requiring no specific treatment.

If microbial diagnosis is needed, the viruses can be identified in cell cultures of vesicle fluid, throat swab or faeces. The laboratory diagnosis of enterovirus infections is discussed in Chapter 6.

Cutaneous poxvirus infections

The poxviruses which infect the skin are molluscum contagiosum, cowpox, orf and vaccinia. Monkeypox and tanapox cause systemic infections with a rash of pocks.

Poxviruses are divided into three groups: (i) orthopoxviruses which include monkeypox and cowpox; (ii) parapoxviruses which include orf; and (iii) the unclassified viruses which include molluscum contagiosum and tanapox. The viruses are large with a double-stranded DNA genome coding for more than 100 viral proteins. They have complex symmetry with a brick-like shape 200–250 × 250–300 nm. Virus uncoating is initiated by host enzymes but completed by viral enzymes. Viral replication takes place in the cytoplasm producing inclusion bodies. Orthopoxviruses are readily cultured on the chorioallantoic membrane of fertilized chicken eggs, producing characteristic pocks. Tanapox grows in cell culture but not on chorioallantoic membrane, and molluscum contagiosum does not grow in cell culture.

Molluscum contagiosum

This is a wart-like condition caused by a poxvirus infection of the prickle-cell layer of the epidermis. The infected cells proliferate, vacuolate and enlarge, protruding above the surface of the skin as typical, pearly lesions up to 3 mm in diameter. They are always umbilicated, with a small central cavity containing

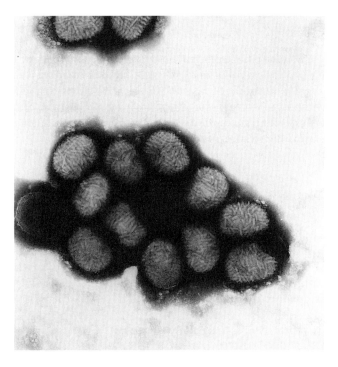

Fig. 5.11 Virion of molluscum contagiosum virus. Courtesy of Professor P. D. Griffiths and Ms G. Clewley, Department of Virology, Royal Free Hospital School of Medicine.

whitish, pulpy material. The vacuolated cells are shed into the lesion, which is highly infectious. Infection is transmitted by skin contact, clothing and towels, and autoinoculation to other skin sites is common.

The lesions are typically in groups, often on the face or arms. HIV-positive patients may have numerous lesions, particularly on the face. Their appearance is diagnostic but, if necessary, poxviruses can be demonstrated by the presence of characteristic molluscum bodies in a scraping stained with, for example, Giemsa or iodine, or by electron microscopy of expressed material (Fig. 5.11).

Spontaneous resolution is uncommon, but adequate treatment is curative. The lesions can be removed by curetting, or 'killed' by inserting the point of an orange-stick dipped in 80% phenol solution into the umbilicated centre.

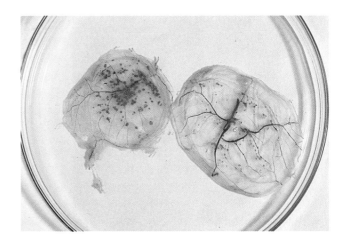

Fig. 5.13 Pocks produced by cowpoxvirus on the chorioallantoic membrane of a hen's egg.

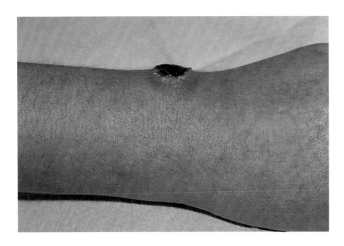

Fig. 5.12 Lesion of cowpox on the wrist of a stable-girl (possibly contracted from the farm cat).

Cowpox and orf

These are zoonoses caused by poxviruses. The natural hosts of cowpox are cattle, in whom lesions occur on the udder. This virus can also affect the skin of cats, and human cases have occurred after contact with both domestic cats and big cats. Transmission occurs by direct contact, and causes large, volcano-shaped pocks with vesicular or necrotic centres, usually on the hand (Fig. 5.12). A large central crater may contain blackened tissue, and a history of animal contact may lead to suspicion of anthrax. Cowpox lesions have no halo of vesicles, however, and the surrounding oedema is rarely as severe or extensive as in anthrax.

Orf is a parapoxvirus whose natural host is sheep. Human infections follow the handling of sheep or their carcasses. The hand or wrist is usually affected by one or more indurated papules 1–2 cm in diameter. There may be a central vesicle or crater, or simply a depression.

Viruses can be identified by electron microscopy or culture of material from the edge or base of the lesions. This can be obtained by biopsy or curettage. Culture of cowpox on the chorioallantoic membrane of hens' eggs produces characteristic lesions (Fig. 5.13).

No specific treatment is required, as the conditions are self-limiting, with a natural history of up to 3 or 4 weeks. Aciclovir and penciclovir are not effective against poxviruses.

Vaccinia

Introduction

Vaccinia exists in many strains whose origins are uncertain. They may have derived from subcultures of cowpox or of variola (the agent of smallpox) (Figs 5.14–5.16). It was used for three centuries as an effective vaccine against smallpox (which was declared extinct from nature in 1979). Vaccinia is now an uncommon laboratory organism, used for manufacturing experimental hybrid vaccines, though canarypox and other animal poxviruses are now more favoured. It is rarely given as a vaccine as the indication no longer exists. Researchers should however be aware that vaccinia is a pathogenic virus. It can cause severe necrotizing or spreading infection in patients with altered immunity. It has a predilection for eczematous skin. It is readily transmitted by the transplacental route. A postinfectious

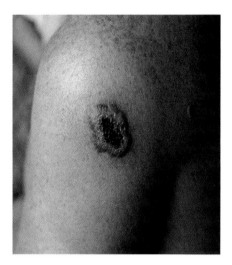

Fig. 5.14 Large vaccinia lesion following smallpox vaccination.

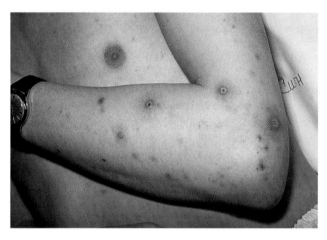

Fig. 5.15 Autoinoculation lesions of vaccinia on the skin.

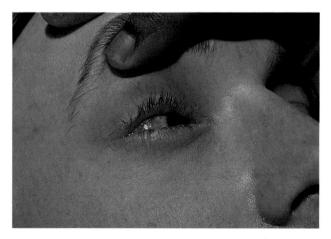

Fig. 5.16 Autoinoculation lesions of vaccinia on the conjunctiva.

encephalitis can follow primary vaccinia infection. Aciclovir is not effective, but vidarabine or methisazone may have some antiviral action.

Monkeypox

Monkeypox is an orthopoxvirus infection which can produce smallpox-like disease in humans. It occurs in Central and West Africa. The diagnosis of monkeypox may be suspected clinically because of the resemblance to smallpox and the presence of significant lymphadenopathy. Specimens of vesicle fluid are suitable for investigation. The virus is stable and survives well while being transported. In recent cases in Zaire the diagnosis was made by a combination of electron microscopy, virus isolation and serology. Distinctive pocks are produced on chorioallantoic membrane culture. Antibody to specific monkeypox antigen can be detected in serum absorbed with smallpox and vaccinia antigens.

Tana

Tana is a milder, systemic poxvirus infection probably spread by insect bites, and usually acquired in Africa. It is unusual to see cases with more than a single skin lesion. The diagnosis is usually suggested by the travel history. The virus can be demonstrated by electron microscopy or cultivated in cell culture. Neutralizing antibodies are produced in convalescence.

Surveillance of systemic poxvirus infections is maintained because of the remote possibility of an increase in virulence.

Bacterial infections of the skin and mucosae

ORGANISM LIST

Staphylococcus aureus
Streptococcus pyogenes
Corynebacterium spp., including *C. minutissimum* and
    C. diphtheriae
Pasteurella spp.
Rochalimaea henselae
Erysipelothrix rhusiopathiae
Mycobacteria, including *Mycobacterium tuberculosis* and
    environmental mycobacteria
Actinomyces spp.

Impetigo and furunculosis

Introduction

Impetigo is a pyogenic infection of the epidermis. Furunculosis is infection of sebaceous glands or sweat glands. Both are usually caused by *Staphylococcus aureus*, and are characterized by an intense local inflammatory response and the production of pus.

S. aureus is distinguishable by phage-typing into many groups, some of which produce powerful toxins. Some toxins act locally, contributing to the pathogenesis of lesions. Others are systemically active, causing severe systemic disease as a consequence of relatively limited local infection. The most important example of this is toxic shock syndrome (see below).

Epidemiology

Pus from skin lesions is highly infectious. Staphylococcal skin infections therefore spread easily, contiguously to adjacent skin sites, by autoinoculation to distant sites or by contact to the skin of other individuals.

Microbiology

Staphylococci are Gram-positive, catalase-producing organisms in the family Micrococcaceae. *Staphylococcus* spp. are facultative, but *Micrococcus* spp. (which rarely cause human disease) are obligate aerobes. The organisms are non-motile and rarely produce capsules.

There are at least 16 *Staphylococcus* species of varying pathogenicity to humans. They can be divided into the pathogenic coagulase-positive *S. aureus*, and the non-pathogenic coagulase-negative staphylococci, on the basis of the coagulase test. *S. aureus* colonies on modern media are not always gold-coloured, and are therefore not morphologically distinguishable from some coagulase-negative staphylococci.

Pathogenesis

The enzyme coagulase catalyses the conversion of fibrinogen to fibrin without the presence of thrombin. It has conventionally been associated with pathogenicity, but not all strains of *S. aureus* are highly pathogenic. Capsules are rarely found in *S. aureus* but are associated with enhanced virulence. Some organisms produce a pseudocapsule in host tissues. Many strains of *S. aureus* express a fibronectin receptor at their surface. This may facilitate adhesion to host tissues, where fibronectin is present, and may be produced in increased quantities during the reaction to acute infection.

The organism also produces extracellular enzymes, such as hyaluronidase, collagenase and lipase, which break down host tissues and may facilitate invasion. Cytolytic toxins, conventionally named haemolysins, are also produced. The way in which these enzymes contribute to the pathology of the disease is not known.

S. aureus may produce extracellular toxins. These include enterotoxins, which are important in food-borne disease (see Chapter 8), and toxic shock syndrome toxins 1 and 2, which, among other effects, act on the skin and destroy the desmosomes. Pyrogenic exotoxins are also produced. These are closely homologous with toxins produced by *Streptococcus pyogenes* and are associated with severe and exfoliative skin rashes.

Factors affecting pathogenicity of staphylococci
1 Coagulase.
2 Capsules (rare).
3 Fibronectin receptor.
4 Extracellular enzymes.
5 Haemolysins.
6 Pyrogenic exotoxins.
7 Enterotoxins A–E.
8 Toxic shock syndrome toxins 1 and 2.

Clinical features

Impetigo

Impetigo often occurs around the mouth or nose, where skin is easily damaged, or in superficial skin lesions such as scratches, insect bites or broken chickenpox vesicles. It is common in children, but adults can also be affected, particularly by secondary 'impetiginization' of skin lesions. Beginning as a small spot, impetigo extends to form a plaque-like inflamed lesion on which a yellowish

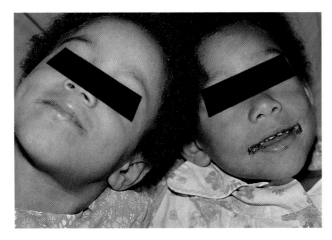
Fig. 5.17 Impetigo in a typical site: both sisters are affected.

exudate forms, and dries into thick scabs. The lesions are irritating and sore; scratching or rubbing contributes to infection of other sites (Fig. 5.17).

Furunculosis

Furunculosis tends to occur in stagnant sebaceous material, and therefore affects children and men more than women. Poor personal hygiene can predispose to furunculosis by allowing blockage of sebaceous ducts. The lesions may be single, when they are often called boils, or multiple. They begin as small papules which increase in size and tenderness to a variable degree. Some will 'point' and discharge yellowish pus before gradually resolving, while others may remain 'blind', gradually healing by becoming less indurated and inflamed.

Concurrent infection of several neighbouring glands causes a composite lesion with several discharging sinuses at the skin surface. These lesions are called carbuncles. They tend to occur in men, often affecting the axilla or the hairline at the back of the neck, and can reach several centimetres in diameter.

Diagnosis

The diagnosis is usually clinically evident. *Staphylococcus aureus* can readily be recovered from cultures of exudate or pus, allowing confirmation of the antibiotic sensitivities of the organism.

A small minority of impetiginous lesions produce *Streptococcus pyogenes* on culture. Such lesions have a tendency to contain bullae, but this is not a reliable distinguishing feature.

Lesions similar to furuncles are occasionally caused by non-staphylococcal infections, especially in secondary infection of pre-existing lesions. Microbiological examination is therefore important in managing lesions which do not readily respond to standard treatment.

Microbiological diagnosis

Staphylococci are not nutritionally demanding and grow readily on simple media. Colonies are readily identified on blood agar because of their opaque, butyrous consistency. Many colonies elaborate a haemolysin, and are surrounded by a zone of complete haemolysis. Colonies of *Staphylococcus aureus* are golden-yellow to creamy-white, whereas coagulase-negative colonies are smaller and white. Strains are identified by confirming the characteristic staphylococcal morphology on Gram staining, catalase production and the presence of coagulase.

The coagulase test detects coagulase, which is either bound to the cell wall (when it is known as clumping factor) or expressed extracellularly. Isolates are usually screened using a slide agglutination technique to detect clumping factor. This identifies more than 89% of strains of *S. aureus*. Negative isolates are then tested using a tube coagulase technique which detects free coagulase. This identifies more than 99% of *S. aureus*.

Other useful tests for the identification of *S. aureus* include the demonstration of deoxyribonuclease. More than 95% of *S. aureus* produce this enzyme (but so do up to 10% of coagulase-negative staphylococci). Once an isolate is identified as a *S. aureus* no further identification is usually necessary. Speciation of the coagulase-negative staphylococci may be indicated when attempting to confirm that several isolated from the same patient are the same, thus indicating an increased likelihood of the isolates being clinically significant. A number of commercial testing kits are available so that identification of these organisms is easily achievable by routine laboratories.

When *S. aureus* must be identified from sites contaminated by other organisms, selective media may be used. Staphylococci can tolerate salt concentrations of 5% or more. Five per cent salt agar will therefore select for these organisms. Mannitol and an indicator are also incorporated, as mannitol is fermented by almost all *S. aureus*, allowing selection of positive colonies for further study. These screening techniques are used to identify carriers of *S. aureus* in outbreaks of infection.

Laboratory tests used to identify *S. aureus*
1 Slide coagulase test.
2 Tube coagulase test.
3 Tests for deoxyribonuclease.

Management

Impetigo is an extremely superficial infection, which responds readily to modest doses of antibiotics. In British practice oral antistaphylococcal agents are usually given, and these are also effective in the minority of impetigo cases caused by *Streptococcus pyogenes*. Cloxacillin or flucloxacillin is usually adequate. In penicillin-allergic individuals oral cephalosporins may be given (unless anaphylaxis was the problem, in which case there is approximately a 10% change of anaphylactic reaction to cephalosporins also). Trimethoprim is also likely to be effective. For methicillin-resistant staphylococci, treatment must be determined by sensitivity testing of the organism.

Topical antimicrobial agents may also be effective. There is a risk of hypersensitivity, especially with topical penicillins and neomycin. Aminoglycosides may be absorbed from the lesions, with risk of toxicity, if used on large areas. Tetracyclines and fusidic acid may be effective, but can encourage the emergence of resistant organisms. The only topical antimicrobials unrelated to commonly used systemic agents (and therefore without risk of devaluing them by encouraging resistance) are mupirocin and silver sulphadiazine. Mupirocin ointment is effective against many bacteria, and promotes healing of superficial infected lesions. It is particularly useful when intolerance or hypersensitivity limits the value of systemic agents. *Staphylococcus aureus* can develop mupirocin resistance, so prolonged or extensive use is not recommended. Silver sulphadiazine also has a wide spectrum and is used for prophylaxis and treatment of infection in burns.

Treatment of staphylococcal skin infections
First choice
Oral flucloxacillin 250 mg or cloxacillin 500 mg 6-hourly for 5–7 days.

Alternatives
1 Oral cephalosporins 250–500 mg 6–8-hourly (see data sheet) for 5–7 days.
2 Trimethoprim 200 mg 12-hourly for 5–7 days.

Mild furunculosis, with small or moderate pustular lesions, will often heal spontaneously if good skin hygiene is maintained. Large lesions and carbuncles are painful and may be accompanied by spreading inflammation and fever. They should be treated with anti-staphylococcal antibiotics, which may need to be given parenterally in severe cases.

Surgical management

Once an abscess has formed, healing is unlikely until the pus is discharged or drained. Continued antibiotic treatment may limit inflammation and abolish systemic features but walled-off pus sometimes remains, with risk of recurrent infection. Large pustules and abscesses should therefore be aspirated or incised. This is usually followed by rapid resolution of the lesion and relief of pain.

Surgical drainage is the most effective treatment for large abscesses and carbuncles.

Complications

Failure to respond to treatment

Skin infections acquired in hot climates may be caused by *Acinetobacter* spp. Vibrios from brackish or marine environments can cause quite severe, sometimes necrotizing, lesions. Both types of organism are resistant to antibiotics commonly used in skin infections. *S. aureus* acquired overseas, even as near as Portugal and Spain, may be resistant to a wide range of agents. Patients whose skin is frequently exposed to disinfectants, for example indoor swimmers, may be colonized with opportunist pathogens such as *Pseudomonas* spp. and develop pseudomonal furunculosis.

Scalded skin syndrome or toxic epidermal necrolysis

This is also called Ritter's or Lyell's syndrome when it affects neonates. It is a special effect of the pyrogenic exotoxins of *S. aureus*. The skin is superficially infected with *S. aureus*, but spreading outwards from each lesion is an area of separation of the superficial layers of the epidermis. Early lesions look pale, and often form flaccid, shallow bullae, which may be very extensive. Affected areas of epidermis are loose and can be rubbed off the underlying layers simply by an examining finger (Nikolsky's sign). In severe cases the lesions become confluent and the whole surface of the skin separates, leaving the typical scalded appearance (Fig. 5.18).

Prompt treatment with antistaphylococcal agents will quickly abort the lesions. The surface epidermal layers separate, leaving regenerating skin areas. Severe cases must be nursed in warm, humid conditions to avoid

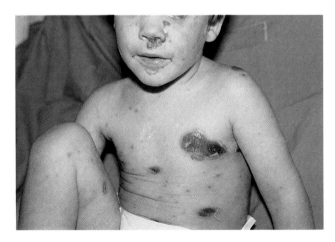

Fig. 5.18 Scalded skin appearance; the child has healing chickenpox, the lesions of which have become infected with *Staphylococcus aureus*.

excessive loss of heat and moisture from denuded areas. This is especially important for small babies, whose surface area is great relative to their body mass.

Toxic epidermal necrolysis is sometimes caused by drug reactions. In such cases there is no evidence of accompanying staphylococcal lesions, but a history of drug ingestion should be obtainable. Commonly implicated drugs include sulphonamides, sulphonylureas, phenytoin, indomethacin and allopurinol. Anti-staphylococcal treatment is not indicated in these cases.

Toxic shock syndrome

This is a systemic disease caused by the toxic shock syndrome toxins (TSSTs) of *S. aureus*. The patient has a staphylococcal infection, commonly a skin abscess or, in women, a vaginal infection associated with the use of highly absorbent tampons during menstruation. This infection is often trivial and forgotten by the patient. Occasionally toxic shock syndrome complicates staphylococcal bacteraemia or endocarditis.

The main features of the illness are fever, diarrhoea, myalgia, rash, hypotension and confusion. The rash is similar to that of scarlet fever, but without the rough, punctate effect. It particularly affects the peripheries, where it may contain petechiae, and is exaggerated in the flexures. Conjunctival reddening or injection is often prominent (Figs 5.19–5.21). Accompanying laboratory findings are raised creatine kinase and other muscle enzymes, low serum calcium, mild thrombocytopenia and a white cell count which may be normal or high but usually with a predominance of neutrophils.

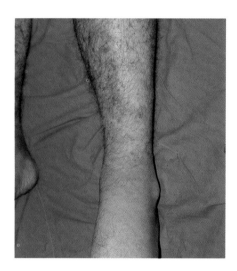

Fig. 5.20 Toxic shock syndrome: petechial component in rash on legs.

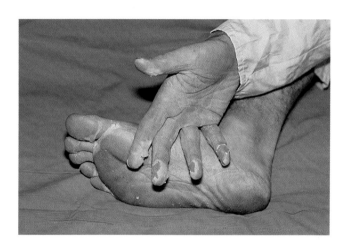

Fig. 5.21 Toxic shock syndrome: typical desquamation of the digits.

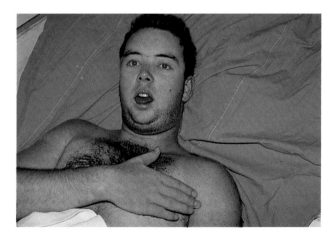

Fig. 5.19 Toxic shock syndrome: erythema and conjunctival injection in a confused and hypotensive patient (the causative infection was a small abscess on the occiput).

Definition of toxic shock syndrome
1 Temperature 39°C or greater.
2 Rash: diffuse macular erythema.
3 Desquamation: 1–2 weeks after onset.
4 Systolic blood pressure 90 mmHg or less;
Plus involvement of three or more of the following organ systems:
1 Gut — vomiting or diarrhoea.
2 Muscles — creatine kinase twice upper limit or more.
3 Mucosae — vagina, mouth, conjunctiva inflamed.
4 Renal — creatinine twice upper limit or more.
5 Hepatic — bilirubin or transaminases twice upper limit or more.
6 Platelets — 100 000/mm³ or less.
7 Central nervous system — altered consciousness without focal signs.

The diagnosis can be made clinically and treatment should be commenced as soon as possible. Anti-staphylococcal antibiotics should be given intravenously. The treatment of choice is cloxacillin or flucloxacillin, to which agents such as rifampicin or fusidic acid may be added, as they readily penetrate into inflamed tissues. Fluid balance and haemodynamic support are important in severe cases. Rare cases of toxic shock syndrome are caused by methicillin-resistant staphylococci. It is therefore important to seek the focus of infection and take pus or swab specimens to identify the organism and check its sensitivity spectrum.

It may take some days for the diarrhoea and hypotension to resolve. The erythema often heals by desquamation, with characteristic shedding of the whole nailfold and skin overlying the finger pulp.

Streptococcal impetigo can be complicated by surgical scarlet fever (see Chapter 6), and, in young children, by poststreptococcal nephritis (see Chapter 24).

Erysipelas

Introduction

Erysipelas is a characteristic intradermal infection caused by *Streptococcus pyogenes*. It is often confused with cellulitis, which is a subcutaneous infection caused by a variety of skin flora and sometimes opportunistic pathogens. The two conditions can often be clinically distinguished from one another, and this is important both in deciding on treatment and in determining which cases may have severe underlying disease, such as bacteraemia.

The origin of the infection is almost always endogenous, from the normal skin flora.

Pathology

The inflammation spreads in the layers of the epidermis, causing an expanding bleb of infection. In severe infection, fluid-filled bullae may form in the epidermal layers. Properties of *S. pyogenes* predisposing to virulence are discussed in Chapter 6.

Clinical features

Erysipelas almost always affects the face or the shin, sites where the skin is easily traumatized or fissured; a small lesion between the toes or at the angle of the nose or mouth may afford entry for the streptococci (Fig. 5.22).

The appearance of the lesion is often heralded by aching, throbbing or tenderness of the skin. This is followed in a few hours by an indurated, hot, tender, erythematous lesion which is clearly demarcated from the normal skin, both visually and by palpation. The patient can easily feel the boundary between normal and infected skin. There is a variable fever, moderate malaise and a neutrophilia with a total white cell count of $11–13 \times 10^6/l$.

If untreated, the lesion spreads rapidly. Tender enlargement of draining lymph nodes is common, and severe cases may have suppurative lymphadenitis (Fig. 5.23) with surrounding erythema and considerable pain. Breakdown of lymph nodes indicates a danger of secondary bacteraemia (Fig. 5.24). Erysipelas other than on the face or shin is extremely uncommon, and is usually a complication of streptococcal bacteraemia.

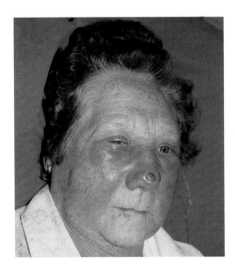

Fig. 5.22 Erysipelas: this rash spread from a tiny fissure in the nose.

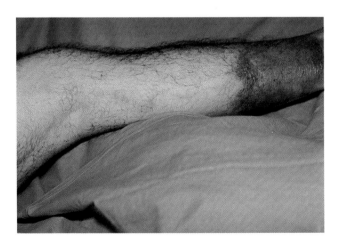

Fig. 5.23 Erysipelas: lymphangitis ascending from the skin lesion (the patient had tender, enlarged inguinal lymph nodes).

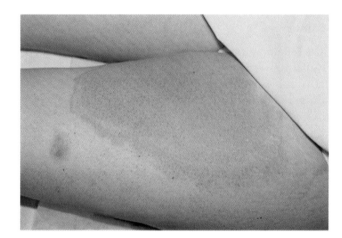

Fig. 5.24 Erysipelas: spreading infection surrounding the draining inguinal lymph node.

Diagnosis

The appearance and site of the lesions are usually diagnostic. As the infection is 'enclosed' in the epidermis, *S. pyogenes* is rarely recovered from swabs. Blood cultures are usually negative. A cultural diagnosis is therefore impossible in the majority of cases. Serological diagnosis is possible, by demonstration of a rising antistreptolysin O titre (ASOT), but the rise in titre is modest. Anti-DNase or antihyaluronidase titres (reference laboratory tests) may show greater rises.

Management

Early treatment is important to limit the extension of the infection. Many cases are successfully treated in general practice with oral antibiotics such as ampicillin and flucloxacillin or with erythromycin. Failure to respond within 36–48 h should prompt admission for intravenous therapy. The treatment of choice in hospital is benzyl penicillin. Cefuroxime and erythromycin are suitable alternatives; however, some streptococci are resistant to erythromycin, which is also irritant and difficult to give intravenously.

> **Treatment of erysipelas**
> **1** Oral treatment in mild cases (7–10 days): amoxycillin 500 mg 8-hourly, ampicillin 500 mg 6-hourly, flucloxacillin 500 mg 6-hourly or erythromycin 500 mg to 1 g 6-hourly.
> **2** Intravenous treatment in severe cases (10–14 days): benzylpenicillin 2.4 g 4–6-hourly, cefuroxime 1.5 g 6–8-hourly or erythromycin 1 g 6–8-hourly.

The skin lesion usually spreads for 12–24 h after treatment is commenced, possibly because of the effect of streptococcal hyaluronidase. Thereafter, the swelling and redness subside and healing is often accompanied by desquamation of the affected skin. Five to 7 days' treatment is usually sufficient, but a few cases prove very difficult to control and may require up to 3 weeks' therapy.

Complications

Complications are generally rare, the only important one being tissue damage with necrosis. This occasionally occurs even after apparently prompt and effective treatment. Full-thickness sloughing of skin may require referral for grafting (Fig. 5.25). Painful suppuration or sloughing of local lymph nodes indicates risk of bacteraemia, and deserves inpatient treatment with parenteral antibiotics.

Recurrence of erysipelas is common, and may occur weeks or months after the first attack. A few patients suffer repeated attacks, usually in the same site. Prophylactic oral penicillin or erythromycin may prevent further attacks, but is not effective in all cases. If no attack occurs after a year of prophylaxis, it may be possible to discontinue the antibiotic.

Cellulitis

Often confused with erysipelas, this is an infection of the loose subcutaneous tissue, with inflammation of the overlying skin. It often results from a penetrating injury or local lesion which allows ingress of pathogenic bacteria. In hospital practice it is a common complication of

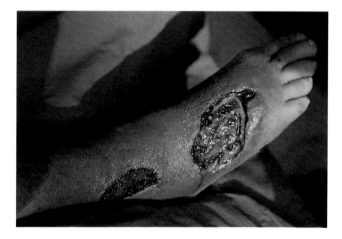

Fig. 5.25 Erysipelas: this patient made a rapid recovery on penicillin treatment, but the affected site sloughed, requiring a full-thickness skin graft.

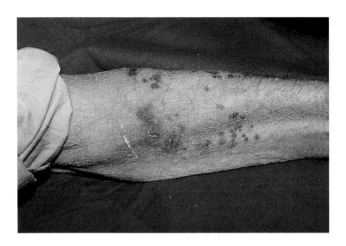

Fig. 5.26 Small area of cellulitis surrounding a venepuncture site (this was caused by a methicillin-resistant *Staphylococcus aureus*).

indwelling cannulation of veins (Fig. 5.26). In rare cases, apparently spontaneous cellulitis is a blood-borne condition complicating bacteraemia. Unlike erysipelas, cellulitis has an indistinct margin; indeed its subdermal or subfascial extent may be much greater than the area of cutaneous erythema. While erysipelas affects the face and lower leg, cellulitis can occur anywhere.

The commonest causes of cellulitis are *Streptococcus pyogenes* and *Staphylococcus aureus*. Other organisms, such as *Pasteurella multocida*, may complicate dog or cat bites. Marine vibrios can enter via scratches or cuts from rocks and coral. Coliforms or enterococci can infect the lower limb in incontinent patients, and pseudomonads may cause hospital-associated cellulitis.

Community-acquired cases often respond well to treatment with oral cloxacillin, flucloxacillin, cephalosporins or trimethoprim. Erythromycin may be effective, but is not a reliable antistaphylococcal drug. Ciprofloxacin is likely to be effective in cases associated with unusual precipitating exposures. In hospital, treatment may need to be guided by culture and sensitivity data. Severe infection, especially in debilitated patients, may require parenteral antibiotics.

Necrotizing infections of skin and soft tissue

Introduction

In general these infections are endogenously acquired but they can also complicate penetrating skin lesions, surgical incisions and wounds and, occasionally, decubitus or diabetic ulcers.

Gas-forming infections of limited extent

These are often polymicrobial infections which arise when devitalized tissue is contaminated by facultative Gram-negative organisms (which often produce gas during carbohydrate metabolism) and various anaerobes. Enterococci or anaerobic cocci may coexist in these infections. The devitalized tissue enables the growth and multiplication of facultative organisms which further lower the redox potential allowing the obligate anaerobes to multiply. There is inflammation and moderate gas formation at the affected site, but significant systemic toxaemia is rare. This type of infection is relatively common in diabetic ulcers and decubitus ulcers, and can complicate diabetic or ischaemic gangrene of the toes or feet.

Clinical examination may reveal slight crepitus in the inflamed area, and X-rays may show streaks of gas in tissue planes. In spite of these appearances, treatment with broad-spectrum antibiotics is often successful. Suitable treatment should include cover for Enterobacteriaceae, enterococci and anaerobes. A broad-spectrum cephalosporin, such as cefotaxime, plus gentamicin or another aminoglycoside should be combined with metronidazole, which penetrates tissues and abscess walls well, and is highly effective in anaerobic environments. Surgery, other than that demanded by the pre-existing condition (such as ray amputation in the diabetic foot or debridement of necrotic ulcers), is rarely necessary.

Gas gangrene

This is a clostridial infection of subcutaneous tissue, particularly of muscle (clostridial myonecrosis). The majority of cases follow the inoculation of *Clostridium perfringens* organisms or spores into a wound or incision. Clostridia, which are spore-bearing, anaerobic Gram-positive rods, are common in faeces and soil, especially manured areas, so that wounds acquired out of doors, in wars or in field sports are at risk. Operations at or near the perineum, or, rarely, gallbladder surgery can also lead to gas gangrene. Rare, apparently spontaneous cases, especially in unusual sites such as the arm or trunk, are often the result of metastatic spread via a malignancy of the colon or genital system. Initiation of infection is also facilitated by the inoculation of foreign material, such as soil or surgical implants.

Several clostridial species are capable of causing gas gangrene. They all produce copious amounts of gas from the metabolism of either saccharides or proteins. Mainly saccharolytic organisms include *Clostridium perfringens*,

C. septicum and *C. tertium*. Mainly proteolytic organisms include *C. oedematiens* and *C. histolyticum*.

C. perfringens, in particular, is a highly toxic organism. It produces an alpha toxin, which is a lecithinase, and strongly haemolytic; a necrotizing beta toxin; a similarly necrotizing epsilon toxin; and a theta toxin, which is strongly haemolytic, producing large clear zones around colonies on blood agar plates. Many other toxins are also produced (including a delta toxin, which causes rare cases of necrotizing jejunitis).

Clinical features

The clinical picture is one of rapidly advancing swelling and devitalization of a limb or other affected tissue. There is gross crepitus of the tissues, and the skin often contains fluid- and gas-filled blisters. The infection may produce a characteristic sickly-sweet smell. The patient is feverish and hypotensive, and may also be severely anaemic.

Diagnosis

The diagnosis is usually clinically evident. The presence of gas in the tissues is easily demonstrated by clinical examination and X-ray. Microscopy of vesicle fluid or wound swabs may show plentiful Gram-positive rods with surprisingly few neutrophils. The white cell count is elevated; serum methaemalbumin is elevated and haptoglobins are often reduced. Fluid and wound cultures readily produce a growth of clostridia on anaerobic culture. Although *C. perfringens* is common, other clostridial and facultative organisms may be present. Blood cultures should be performed, as bacteraemia can coexist.

Treatment

Treatment has three important aspects:
1 Antimicrobial chemotherapy; traditionally this is intravenous benzyl penicillin, but metronidazole penetrates tissues better and is an excellent antianaerobe drug — probably both should be given. A broad-spectrum cephalosporin can be substituted for penicillin if Gram-negative rods may be involved.
2 Surgery is important; extensive debridement or amputation may be necessary to halt the spreading infection.
3 Hyperbaric oxygen therapy has been suggested but has never gained a place in routine therapy. It may save critically devitalized tissue and/or make demarcation between salvageable and necrotic tissue more evident to the surgeon.

4 Anti-gas gangrene serum (AGGS) is available from regional pharmacies. It is directed against *C. perfringens* and its toxins, and may protect tissues from further toxic damage. Its use is unproven.

Prevention

Prevention of gas gangrane is important. Benzyl penicillin or metronidazole is given prophylactically in at-risk operations such as high amputations of the leg, and after contamination of traumatic or military wounds. Adequate cleaning of wounds, removal of debris and devitalized tissue, and avoiding primary closure of severely contaminated wounds all decrease the risk of anaerobic infection.

Necrotizing fasciitis

This is a rapidly spreading infection predominantly affecting subcutaneous and perimuscular fat. Necrotic liquefaction of fatty tissue is the characteristic pathology. It is usually caused by a mixed bacterial infection, which may include pathogens derived from the skin and bowel. Fournier's gangrene is a full-thickness necrosis of the perineal skin which can leave the testicles denuded. It has a similar aetiology. Both are usually treated with broad-spectrum antibiotics plus metronidazole. Surgical management with extensive debridement is almost always essential. Rare cases of necrotizing fasciitis are caused by *Streptococcus pyogenes* infection. The optimum antibiotic treatment in such cases is thought to be penicillin plus metronidazole, or clindamycin alone.

Acute pyomyositis

Acute pyomyositis is a rare infection usually seen in the tropics. It is a pyogenic *Staphylococcus aureus* infection of muscle frequently affecting the leg. It is difficult to treat with antistaphylococcal drugs alone. Surgical drainage and debridement are usually required.

Otitis externa

This is a superficial inflammation of the skin of the external auditory meatus. Eczema is a common precipitating condition. The onset of infection often causes quite severe pain. It can present with erythema and weeping, or may be similar to impetigo or furunculosis. As well as common skin-infecting bacteria, the poorly ventilated auditory canal can be colonized by fungi, including *Aspergillus* spp. Swimmers and divers, whose ears are often wet and exposed to brackish conditions, are prone to pseudomonal otitis externa.

Simple cleaning and drying of the ear canal under direct vision may be sufficient to allow resolution. Short courses of corticosteroid drops may eradicate the eczematous reaction. Mild infection is often treated topically with neomycin, framycetin or clioquinol drops. Such preparations should not be given in courses lasting longer than 7 days. They may predispose to both local sensitization and the establishment of fungi. Topical clotrimazole is useful if fungal infection is present. Staphylococcal infection is best treated with oral cloxacillin or flucloxacillin, as for other skin infections.

Erythema chronicum migrans (cutaneous Lyme disease)

Erythema chronicum migrans (ECM) is the cutaneous manifestation of early Lyme disease (see Chapter 20). It consists of a circular or discoid lesion which begins and expands from the site of an infecting tick bite (Fig. 5.27). It is not known whether different strains of *Borrelia burgdorferi* are more or less likely to produce ECM, but not all infected individuals develop the lesion. Some lesions are large, disappearing when they have traversed a whole limb, while occasional patients have multiple lesions.

Typical ECM is pathognomonic of Lyme disease, which can usually be confirmed by demonstrating IgM antibodies to *B. burgdorferi* in the patient's serum. However, false-positives are relatively common, and false-negatives sometimes occur. A firm diagnosis should rest on a combination of clinical and serological evidence. *B. burgdorferi* can be cultured from blood or

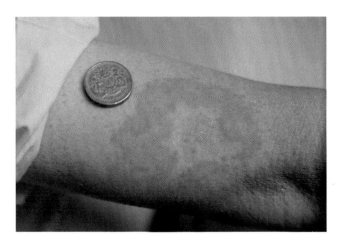

Fig. 5.27 Erythema chronicum migrans expanding from the site of a tick bite on the arm. Courtesy of Dr M.G. Brook.

biopsies of lesions, but this requires experience and is most reliably performed in reference laboratories.

Treatment is important. Although untreated ECM is self-limiting, this leaves the risk of later manifestations of Lyme disease. The treatment of choice is oral tetracycline for 3 weeks. Erythromycin is a second-choice alternative. A small risk of continued infection remains after this treatment. This possibility must be excluded if the patient suffers later, systemic symptoms (see Chapter 20).

Erythrasma

This is a superficial inflammation of the skin, usually of the flexures, caused by *Corynebacterium minutissimum* infection. The advancing flexural erythema can be mistaken for a fungal infection or for erysipelas, but it is not painful, and antifungal treatment is ineffective. When illuminated by ultraviolet light the lesion shows characteristic, salmon-pink fluorescence.

C. minutissimum may be distinguished from *C. jeikeium* and *C. bovis*, which also do not utilize nitrate, hydrolyse urea or digest gelatin, by its lack of dependence on lipid in the culture medium. It produces small colonies which fluoresce red-orange under Wood's light in serum-containing medium.

Erythromycin treatment will cure most cases; the organism is also sensitive to tetracycline. Toe-web infections may fail to respond to oral antibiotics, but can often be eradicated by topical treatment with compound benzoic acid ointment.

Erysipeloid

Erysipelothrix rhusiopathiae is a zoonotic organism which causes erysipeloid in pigs. Human infections result from inoculation injuries, such as puncture wounds from bone splinters. A dull red erythema advances, often spreading from one finger to another via the web. Underlying joints may become sore. Systemic manifestations rarely occur.

Clinical diagnosis is usually possible from the history of exposure (often occupational) to a source of infection, and from the clinical features. The infection responds rapidly to 5–7 days' treatment with oral penicillins or tetracyclines.

E. rhusiopathiae is a facultative, catalase-negative, non-sporing Gram-positive rod, which produces alpha haemolysis on blood agar. Unlike *Listeria*, it is non-motile and it produces hydrogen sulphide in Kligler's triple sugar iron medium. The mechanisms of pathogenesis are uncertain but are thought to be related to neuraminidase production.

Cat-scratch disease

This is a lymphocutaneous disease caused by *Bartonella henselae*. The patient usually has a history of cat-scratch or cat exposure. After 5–10 days' incubation, a nodular or indurated swelling appears at the site of the scratch, and may discharge a little pus. The local-draining lymph nodes enlarge and become tender, occasionally suppurating and discharging.

Diagnosis is usually clinical. The organism does not grow in standard cultures; serological diagnosis is possible, but is not widely available. Small bacteria can be seen in silver-stained sections from lymph-node biopsies.

The disease is self-limiting, but may last for 3 weeks or more. Treatment with oral tetracycline or erythromycin may shorten the course.

R. henselae can cause systemic or bacteraemic infection in the immunosuppressed (see Chapter 21).

Actinomycosis

This is an infection of skin and subcutaneous tissue caused by *Actinomyces israelii* or, rarely, by other *Actinomyces* spp. The organism may invade from underlying mucosa, from the mouth, the pleura or the peritoneum. The commonest lesion is an abscess of the cheek.

The lesion begins as an enlarging, extremely indurated nodule which suppurates and discharges greyish pus containing tiny pale or yellow dots. These 'sulphur granules' are spherical colonies of the branching bacteria; they can be crushed between a slide and a cover slip and stained to demonstrate their variable degree of Gram-positivity (Fig. 5.28). Anaerobic culture allows accurate

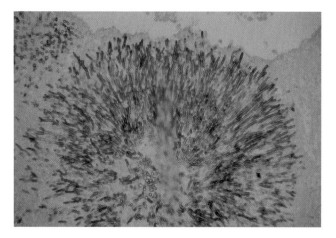

Fig. 5.28 Gram-stained crush preparation of 'sulphur granule', showing a Gram-variable, branching appearance.

speciation and sensitivity testing. Cultures must be maintained for up to 2 weeks to obtain maximum diagnostic yield.

Penicillin or erythromycin are effective in eradicating the infection, but high doses are needed and the course should last for 6 or 8 weeks.

Cutaneous mycobacterial infections

Some 'environmental' mycobacteria can cause skin infections which fail to respond to simple antibiotic treatment and which seem sterile on standard bacterial culture.

Mycobacterium marinum is found in pools and rivers. It may also inhabit aquaria. Infection, probably of small skin defects, produces indolent, nodular lesions, almost always on the hand. These can spread to affect subcutaneous tissue, fascia and tendons. Extensive lesions may ulcerate and/or discharge pus. Mycobacteria can be seen and cultured in curettings or biopsy material (see Chapter 18). Treatment with rifampicin plus ethambutol or clarithromycin will often effect a steady improvement.

M. chelonae and *M. fortuitum* occasionally infect inoculation sites, for instance in diabetics taking insulin. The infection usually causes a 'sterile' subcutaneous abscess. Mycobacteria can readily be recovered by appropriate culture of pus. Treatment with co-trimoxazole or ciprofloxacin will often cure the infection without the need for drainage.

M. tuberculosis can cause skin infection which is traditionally called lupus vulgaris. It is a granulomatous lesion which appears slightly nodular, lichenified and sometimes scaling, often with an atrophic centre. It may have a natural history of years, leading to misdiagnosis as chronic dermatitis. Pressing a glass slide on the lesion to blanch it may reveal the granulomata as translucent granular structures heaped together (called the apple-jelly appearance). Mycobacteria may be demonstrable in, and culturable from, biopsy material.

Many patients also have pulmonary or other foci of tuberculosis. Standard antituberculosis treatment will cure the skin lesion as well as any other focus.

Propionobacterium acnes and acne

Acne is a multifactorial skin disorder, in which excessive sebaceous secretions are produced in response to strong androgenic stimulation. The sebaceous glands become engorged and blocked, causing pustules and comedones. Secondary infection may cause severe inflammation and contribute to later scarring. *P. acnes* can be recovered from the lesions. It is not known what contribution the organism makes to the pathology of acne, or whether other skin flora are also involved, but broad-spectrum antibiotics can control the condition to a large extent. Doxycycline is often given once-daily in courses of several months. Erythromycin is also effective in many cases.

Fungal infections of the skin and its appendages

ORGANISM LIST

Candida albicans

Dermatophytes
  Microsporum spp.
  Trichophyton spp.
  Epidermophyton spp.
Malassezia furfur

Rarities
  Sporothrix schenckii
  Blastomyces
  Histoplasma capsulatum
  Cryptococcus neoformans

Introduction

The fungal infections (mycoses) commonly seen in Europe are superficial mycoses, affecting only the skin and causing superficial inflammation confined to the site of infection. They are usually recognizable by their typical skin lesions, and the organisms are easily identified in swabs or scrapings.

The deep mycoses are rare in temperate countries. Although some are respiratory infections (see Chapter 7), several are infections of subcutaneous tissue, acquired by inoculation through the skin. They tend to produce granulomatous lesions which sometimes invade, either by spread to adjacent tissue or by metastasis to lymph nodes and other body sites. The lesions of deep mycoses must be distinguished from infectious and autoimmune granulomata and from tumours.

Candidiasis

Introduction and epidemiology

Candida albicans is a yeast which is part of the normal flora of the skin, mucosae and bowel. Its balance with other flora and the health of the tissues is important in preventing superficial invasion and infection. Normal skin is rarely affected by candidiasis, but it requires only wetting and slight maceration of the epidermis to allow the establishment of replicating organisms. Antibiotic treatment increases the likelihood of candidiasis. Mild degrees of immunosuppression, including the effects of corticosteroid or cytotoxic therapies, pregnancy, diabetes and other endocrine diseases, can all predispose to candidiasis.

Predisposing conditions to candidiasis
1 Antibiotic treatment.
2 Corticosteroid treatment.
3 Cytotoxic therapy.
4 Diabetes mellitus.
5 Pregnancy.
6 Cell-mediated immune deficiency.

Clinical features

The warm, moist areas of the folds under the breasts, in the natal cleft or under the abdominal 'apron' of the obese are most often affected. Candidiasis is a common infection of the napkin area of infants. The nailfolds can also be infected in individuals who constantly wear rubber gloves for washing-up or other tasks, and whose hands are always sweaty or damp.

Skinfold infection (intertrigo) produces reddening and slight thickening of the skin, causing plaque-like lesions which are clearly demarcated from adjacent, normal skin. Moist lesions are dull and may produce a slight, sticky exudate. Drier lesions often appear shiny or flaky, may have circular satellite lesions nearby, and must be distinguished from psoriasis. This type of lesion is common in napkin rash. Both types of lesion are often irritating or itchy.

Nailfold lesions (paronychia) cause bolster-like swelling, with thickened rolls of skin which may bulge over the nail. A 'cheesy' exudate is sometimes seen in the cleft under the swelling. Inflammation of the nailbed causes ridging of the nail, and in rare cases infection of the nail itself produces an opaque greenish or brownish discoloration.

Diagnosis

The site of the lesions and the cheesy exudate, if present, strongly suggest candidiasis. The differential diagnosis includes erythrasma, dermatophyte infections, contact dermatitis and flexural psoriasis. Swabs from lesions or exudate can be Gram-strained to demonstrate the diagnostic presence of budding yeasts. Inoculation on to

Sabouraud's agar will allow cultural identification of yeasts in cases of doubt. The organism will also grow on blood agar or heated blood agar, but produces tiny colonies which are easily overlooked in mixed cultures of skin organisms.

Management

Removing the predisposition, when possible, will greatly improve the effect of treatment and reduce recurrences. Most candidal infections respond readily to topical treatment. Water-soluble creams are recommended for the skin, as they do not have the occlusive and therefore macerating effect of ointments. The polyenes nystatin and amphotericin are effective and cheap. The imidazoles, miconazole, clotrimazole and econazole are also effective; the last two are available as sprays, solution or lotion for application to large or hairy areas.

In patients with severe or extensive disease, or persisting predisposition, topical treatment may fail. The orally administered triazole itraconazole may be effective in these cases. It is contraindicated in liver disease and should be given with caution during pregnancy and lactation. It has important interactions with astemizole and terfenidine.

Treatment of severe *Candida* infections of skin or mucosae: itraconazole 100 mg daily for 15 days.

Dermatophytoses (tinea infections)

Introduction

Dermatophytes are filamentous fungi which digest keratin. Different species have varying affinities for skin, hair and nails. Although they cannot invade living tissues, their presence in the epidermis can induce an inflammatory reaction in the affected site. Some species are exclusive to humans; others are acquired by contact with infected animals, and these often cause the most severe inflammation.

ORGANISM LIST

Organism	Host	Fluorescence
Scalp infections		
Microsporum canis	Cat, kitten, dog	Positive
M. audouinii	Human	Positive
Trichophyton sulphureum	Human	Negative
T. violaceum	Human	Negative
T. schoenleinii	Human (favus)	Positive
Body infections		
T. mentagrophytes	Animal	Negative
T. verrucosum	Animal	Negative
Groin and foot infections		
T. rubrum	Human	Negative
T. interdigitale	Human	Negative
Epidermophyton floccosum	Human	Negative
Nail infections		
T. rubrum	Human	Negative

Laboratory identification of dermatophytes

Scrapings of infected skin, hair and clippings from nails should be sent dry to the laboratory. These are clarified by gently heating in a solution of potassium hydroxide, and examined under the microscope for the presence of the typical branching hyphal elements.

Dermatophytes grow readily on many microbiological media but a useful selective medium is Sabouraud's dextrose agar. As all are resistant to the action of cyclohexamide, this is incorporated as a selective agent. Chloramphenicol and gentamicin can be added when bacterial contamination is likely. A specialized dermatophyte test medium incorporates all three of these agents together with an indicator which detects the rise in pH which occurs when dermatophytes grow. Cultures are incubated at 30°C for up to 4 weeks.

The identification of dermatophytes is made on the basis of colonial morphology, microscopic appearance of the fungal hyphae and conidia, and on physiological and biochemical testing. Slide preparations of mycelia can be

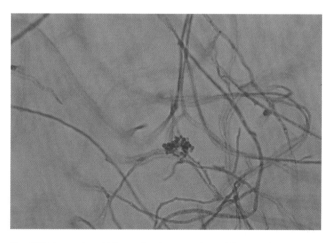

Fig. 5.29 Lactophenol blue-stained preparations of dermatophytes, showing the characteristic morphology of conidia.

stained with lactophenol cotton blue and examined microscopically for the morphology of the conidia and chlamydospores. These structures are often characteristic for different species and some examples are seen in Fig. 5.29. Other tests which may be employed include the ability of the fungal isolate to penetrate an uninfected hair, to hydrolyse urea and to produce characteristic growth on rice grains.

Clinical features

The commonest manifestation of dermatophyte infection is an expanding lesion with a scaly or inflamed advancing edge. This is a typical tinea or ringworm infection. The eruption is usually described by its position on the body, e.g. tinea capitis, tinea corporis or tinea cruris.

Scalp ringworm (tinea capitis)

This is common in children, in whom it is usually caused by a *Microsporum* species. It presents as one or more oval patches of hair loss, which expand steadily and can affect the whole of the scalp. The hairs are damaged, and broken off near to the skin (this distinguishes the condition from alopecia, in which there is no scaling, and hairs are absent in the acute stage).

Infection with *Trichophyton* species can affect both adults and children. Swelling of the scalp is often marked and hairs broken off at the opening of the follicles may appear as black dots. When inflammation is severe there may be a purulent exudate from the follicles, causing hairs to be completely shed. This terminates the infection, but can leave scarring of the scalp and follicles, with permanent hair loss.

Diagnosis can be made presumptively by clinical features. *Microsporum* infections cause a greenish-blue fluorescence of the affected hairs and skin under ultraviolet light (Wood's light). Scales can be gently scraped off and hair stumps removed by plucking, and both examined by microscopy and culture.

Treatment with topical antifungal agents rarely succeeds. The treatment of choice is oral griseofulvin. At least 2 months' treatment is necessary; the need for further treatment may be reduced by applying miconazole or clotrimazole cream.

Reinfection can be prevented by seeking and treating the source of infection. Depending on the species of fungus involved, this may be another child or adult, a family pet or a farm animal.

Ringworm of the body (tinea corporis)

This is usually an obvious round or oval expanding lesion with a scaly, slightly inflamed periphery (Fig. 5.30). It must be distinguished from discoid eczema and isolated lesions of psoriasis. Examination and culture of scrapings will confirm the diagnosis.

Treatment with topical antifungals such as clotrimazole or miconazole cream is adequate for most mild lesions. Very extensive or severely inflamed lesions may be best treated with a 3- or 4-week course of oral griseofulvin. Oral itraconazole is effective in a dose of 100 mg daily for 15 days.

Ringworm of the groin (tinea cruris)

This is an intertriginous infection, often confined to the inguinal folds and adjacent thighs. *T. rubrum* infection, however, can cause extensive lesions spreading down the thighs and posteriorly to the natal cleft and the buttocks. Tinea cruris may be inadvertently treated with topical corticosteroids, which partly inhibits the inflammation. The margin of the lesion may then disappear, but papulopustular lesions often develop. This modified disease is often called tinea incognita. It can also occur on the face in similar circumstances. As in other tinea infections, microscopy and culture of scrapings will make the diagnosis. The important differential diagnoses are intertriginous candidiasis or psoriasis, and erythrasma.

Treatment with topical antifungals should be successful, but the sensitive, inflamed skin may be damaged by the strong agents, or develop contact dermatitis. If this happens, or the skin is intensely inflamed at pre-

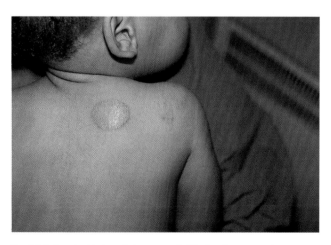

Fig. 5.30 A typical lesion of tinea corporis (the family cat was also affected).

sentation, dilute potassium permanganate soaks can be applied twice a day for 3 or 4 days before commencing a weak corticosteroid cream and topical antifungal. The steroid can be discontinued when the inflammation subsides, and the antifungal continued as required. Itraconazole offers an alternative approach, especially in extensive lesions. The dose is as for tinea corporis.

Ringworm of the hands, feet and nails

Dermatophyte infections of thick keratin often produce extremely scaly lesions which resist treatment with topical antifungals. The interdigital webs may become fissured and macerated, with scaly infection extending on to the digits or the dorsum of the foot (or hand). Nails become opaque, discoloured and brittle, starting at the tip and gradually affecting the lateral margins and then the whole nail plate, which may flake away. The nailfolds do not swell, as they do in candidiasis. The main differential diagnoses are psoriasis and contact dermatitis.

Treatment must be systemic. Oral griseofulvin must usually be given for some months. Six months is the minimum for nail infections; 12 months or more is usual for toenails. As griseofulvin has an Antabuse-like effect and precludes alcohol consumption, many people prefer not to take the necessary course for the toenail infections. Itraconazole may be effective in treating the skin of the hands or feet, but the maximum course of 30 days may not be sufficient for toenail infections. Terbinafine can penetrate thick keratin, and 2–4-week courses of 250 mg daily have proved effective in treating palmar and plantar disease, as well as early nail infections.

> **Treatment for fungal infection of the nail**
> **1** Griseofulvin 500 mg (child 10 mg/kg) daily for several weeks or months until cure is complete. Beware of its Antabuse-like effect.
> **2** Itraconazole 100 mg daily for 30 days.
> **3** Terbinafine 250 mg daily for 6 weeks to 3 months (not recommended for children).

Pityriasis versicolor

This is a very superficial skin infection caused by the filamentous fungus *Malassezia furfur*. Pale brown, fine scaly macules develop on the upper chest or back, forming an irregular pattern which appears slightly brown in a white-skinned person, or slightly pale in a dark skin. There is little or no inflammation, and sensation is normal in the affected areas. When the skin is warm after a bath or during a feverish illness, the plaques may become red or pink (Fig. 5.31).

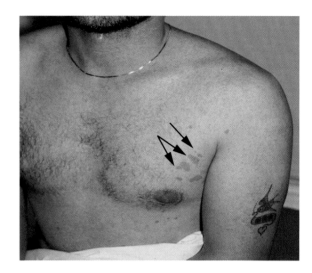

Fig. 5.31 Pityriasis versicolor: this appears red because the patient has a slight fever.

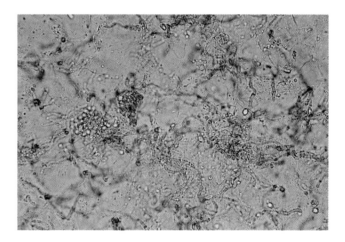

Fig. 5.32 Potassium chloride preparation of scraping from a case of pityriasis versicolor (stained with blue ink (Quink)).

The clinical appearance is characteristic, but the diagnosis can be confirmed by microscopy of skin scrapings. The scrapings are placed on a microscope slide, and mixed with a drop or two of 5% potassium hydroxide. As the keratin softens it is easy to see a mycelium in which are scattered groups of rough, round sporing bodies. This 'meat balls and spaghetti' appearance of the fungus distinguishes it from the dermatophytes, and is diagnostic (Fig. 5.32).

Almost any topical antifungal cream will clear the lesions, but recurrence is common. Washing all clothes and shampooing the hair with selenium sulphide

(Selsun) shampoo may help to remove a reservoir of infection. Oral itraconazole 200 mg daily for a week is also effective.

Sporotrichosis

This is a localized, nodular skin infection caused by *Sporothrix schenckii*, a ray fungus which produces characteristic stellate microcolonies *in vitro*. The fungus exists in wood, soil and vegetation. Infection is usually by inoculation, and leads to nodules, abscesses or ulcers which may expand locally. Satellite lesions may appear along lymphatic pathways, and draining lymph nodes may be affected. Haematogenous spread occasionally occurs in debilitated or immunosuppressed individuals.

The only important differential diagnoses are mycobacterial infections (fishtank granulomata) or rare syphilitic lesions. Histology and culture of biopsy material are diagnostic.

The traditional treatment of sporotrichosis has been oral potassium iodide for courses of several weeks. Amphotericin is also effective, but is reserved for severe spreading or systemic disease because of its toxicity. Results of treatment with itraconazole or ketoconazole have yet to be critically reviewed.

Rarities

Fungal infections of the skin are more common in the tropics than in temperate countries. Several exotic fungi can produce nodular or granulomatous lesions on the skin, typically of the lower legs. Diagnosis is by histology and culture of biopsy material. A positive complement-fixation test is usual in histoplasmosis, which is often a systemic disease with risk of lymph node, buccal mucosa and lung involvement. Expert advice should be sought about management, which may be difficult and is always prolonged.

Pityriasis rosea

This is a disease of unknown aetiology which looks like a fungal infection. The first sign is the 'herald patch', an inflamed, scaly, rather scabby lesion up to 4 cm in diameter on the trunk or upper leg (Fig. 5.33). After anything from 3 to 14 days there follows a symmetrical eruption of oval plaques and smaller macules and papules, which are sometimes itchy. The plaques affect the trunk and proximal limbs ('vest and pants' distribution), and have their long axes aligned with the skin creases, giving the rash a typical 'Christmas tree' appearance (Fig. 5.34).

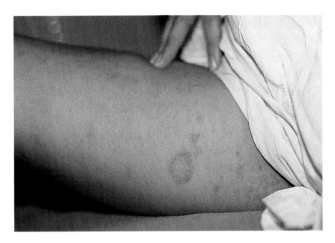

Fig. 5.33 Pityriasis rosea: herald patch on the thigh.

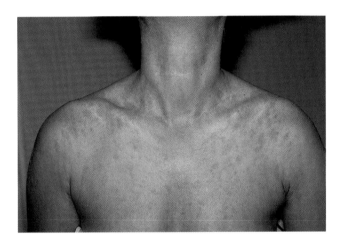

Fig. 5.34 Pityriasis rosea: typical 'vest and pants' rash, with 'Christmas tree' orientation of lesions.

Each plaque, or medallion, has an indistinct, slightly raised margin with central arrays of pointed scales, with the points oriented towards the edge of the lesion. The lesions expand up to 5 cm long in about 2 weeks, and then fade over about 2 months.

The differential diagnosis is of tinea or discoid eczema, or occasionally syphilis. There is no treatment which affects the inevitable evolution of the disorder. The condition is not contagious, and second attacks are extremely rare.

Parasites of the skin

Scabies

Scabies is caused by the mite *Sarcoptes scabiei*, which burrows in the epidermis, the female mites laying eggs along their burrows' tracks. The condition is infectious by direct skin contact; mites attracted by warmth emerge into the area of contact and burrow into the adjacent epidermis. Scabies is easily transmitted between sexual partners, those who share beds or to those who care for infected and bed-ridden individuals.

The infection itself is asymptomatic, but hypersensitivity to the mites, their eggs or surface proteins eventually causes severe itching and leads to scratching and excoriation of affected skin. The soft skin of the flexures, digital webs, perineum and axillae are most affected; the face is spared, except in small children and severe infections. So-called Norwegian scabies is caused by an aggressive strain of mite which causes severe lesions, even affecting the face in adults. Scabies can cause widespread chronic lesions in immunosuppressed HIV patients.

The diagnosis is suggested by the typically distributed, itchy rash. Burrows may be visible, with a tiny, pearly nodule at the advancing end. The nodule may be teased out and shown to be a mite. Often, however, burrows are destroyed by scratching, but scrapings may still contain round, black dots of mite faeces.

Treatment is with topical acaricides. All members of a household should be treated, and the medication should be applied to the whole skin excluding the face. Lindane 1% lotion or cream is inexpensive; malathion 0.5% lotion or liquid may succeed if lindane fails. Permethrin 5% cream is also available, and can be applied to the face if necessary. Monosulphiram solution may be used for treating children. Most cases will respond to one application of acaricide, washed off after 12–24 h. If lindane is used, a second application should be given after 1–3 days. Itching may persist for many days after successful treatment. It is often ameliorated by topical crotamiton cream. Oral albendazole has shown useful additive effects with topical treatment in immunosuppressed patients.

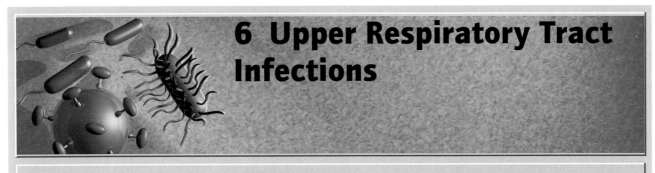

6 Upper Respiratory Tract Infections

Introduction

The upper respiratory tract comprises the conjunctiva, the nose, paranasal sinuses, the middle ear, the nasopharynx, oropharynx and laryngopharynx. It is largely covered with ciliated columnar epithelium. Exceptions are the oropharynx, vocal cords and upper posterior epiglottis which are lined with stratified squamous epithelium. The conjunctiva is also stratified squamous epithelium, continuous with and similar to the epithelium of the cornea. Sqamous epithelium is also found in the mastoid antrum of the middle ear.

The adenoids and tonsils are important structures of the upper respiratory tract. They are lymphoid organs whose surfaces are marked by many deep clefts, both macroscopic and microscopic.

The whole upper respiratory tract is colonized by a variety of normal flora.

Normal upper respiratory tract flora
1 *Streptococcus pneumoniae.*
2 Anaerobic and microaerophilic streptococci.
3 *S. 'milleri'* (found in the sinuses).
4 *Haemophilus influenzae.*
5 Other *Haemophilus* species.
6 Diphtheroids.
7 Coagulase-negative staphylococci.
8 *Staphylococcus aureus.*
9 *Prevotella melaninogenicus* and related species.

Temporary colonization by potential pathogens is also common, and may provide an important reservoir of infection, for instance with *Neisseria meningitidis* or *Corynebacterium diphtheriae*. A variety of viruses are intermittently excreted from the pharynx, including rhinoviruses, paramyxoviruses, enteroviruses, adenoviruses and myxoviruses. These are sometimes associated with symptoms, but often replicate asymptomatically.

Finally, the pharynx is a site of intermittent shedding of latent viruses. Herpes simplex virus and Epstein–Barr virus are the most important of these, but others include cytomegalovirus and possibly other human herpesviruses such as HHV6.

The environment of the upper respiratory tract is varied; different areas are susceptible to infection with different pathogens. While most infections are of surfaces, the middle ear and the paranasal sinuses are hollow structures connected to the surfaces by narrow ducts (the ostia of the sinuses and the eustachian tubes of the middle ears). These cavities can become obstructed, permitting loculated infection and abscess formation. The tissues of the fauces, surrounding the tonsils, are also susceptible to the formation of soft-tissue abscesses when disrupted by intense inflammation.

Conjunctivitis and keratoconjunctivitis

Introduction

The conjunctiva is often mildly affected by infections of the respiratory tract, becoming reddened and injected during infections such as colds, influenza and measles. Being moist and exposed, it is open to attack by many air-borne infections, but is protected to a great extent by the washing action of the tears. Tears contain a number of substances, including lysozymes and immunoglobulins, which also discourage the establishment of infection. Nevertheless, a number of organisms are recognized as causing primary conjunctivitis. Conjunctival infections can also be transmitted directly from eye to eye by fomites such as ophthalmological instruments, shared cosmetic applicators and, in conditions of poor hygiene, by flies. When the cornea is involved, the condition is called keratitis or keratoconjunctivitis.

Occlusion of the conjunctiva by contact lenses increases the likelihood of infection, and poor lens hygiene can lead to severe pseudomonal or even amoebic infections with the risk of corneal damage.

ORGANISM LIST

Adenoviruses
Enteroviruses (especially type 30)
Herpes simplex virus
Moraxella spp.
Streptococcus pneumoniae
Haemophilus influenzae
Neisseria gonorrhoeae
Chlamydia trachomatis
Pseudomonas aeruginosa
Acanthamoeba spp.

Clinical features

These are similar in most types of conjunctivitis. The eye feels sore and itchy, and there is a discharge of watery, mucoid or purulent material, which may dry, especially during sleep, and glue the eyelids together. In severe cases there is swelling of the eyelids which further embarrasses eye-opening and drainage of secretions.

The conjunctiva appears red, often with a thin, clear outline surrounding the iris. Occasionally marked swelling causes it to bulge through the palpebral fissure.

Diagnosis

The clinical diagnosis is usually evident. Important differential diagnoses for a red, painful eye include herpes simplex keratitis (dendritic ulcer — see below) and acute glaucoma. Both of these conditions can be sight-threatening, and should be considered whenever a red eye persists.

In infants the lacrimal sac may drain poorly, causing swelling and a mucus discharge at the inner canthus.

The condition is non-infectious, harmless and self-limiting. Digital lacrimal sac drainage abolishes the 'sticky eye' and can be discontinued after 1 or 2 weeks.

Management

Most viral cases resolve spontaneously in a few days, requiring only gentle washing away of any discharge. Most of the bacterial cases will respond to a short course of chloramphenicol drops. Failure to respond should prompt investigation with swabs for bacterial culture, a search for chlamydial infection and perhaps viral culture. In difficult cases an early ophthalmological examination is advisable.

Childhood conjunctivitis

Childhood conjunctivitis (pink eye) is common and often spreads among small children in families and school communities. It is usually caused by a respiratory adenovirus, begins unilaterally and may spread to the other eye. It is self-limiting and usually mild, with a natural history of a few days.

Shipyard eye

Shipyard eye is a colloquial term applied to a keratoconjunctivis spread by ophthalmological equipment. Often caused by adenovirus type 8, it was common in occupational settings where minor eye trauma and frequent examinations took place. Simple hygiene precautions such as hand-washing by staff and adequate sterilization of equipment prevent continuing spread of infection.

Haemorrhagic conjunctivitis

Haemorrhagic conjunctivitis caused many epidemics worldwide in the early 1980s. The agent was enterovirus type 30. The disease was abrupt in onset, moderate to severe, and associated with intense, haemorrhagic inflammation of the conjunctiva.

Warning
A red eye unresponsive to antibiotic treatment should not be treated with corticosteroids until the possibility of a herpes simplex infection has been ruled out.

Herpes simplex keratitis (dendritic ulcer)

This is an infection of the corneal epithelium which presents as a red, painful eye. Unlike most viral conjunctivitis, it is not self-limiting. It produces a branching ulcer which destroys the corneal epithelium and may damage the underlying tissue, leading to scarring and visual impairment. *It progresses rapidly if treated with topical corticosteroids.*

The diagnosis is suggested by a persistently red eye, unresponsive to topical antibiotic treatment. The branching ulcer can be seen on slit-lamp examination, or by inspection after the instillation of fluorescein drops. Herpes simplex virus can be recovered from corneal scrapings.

The treatment of choice is topical aciclovir, applied as 0.5% ointment. Treatment is continued until healing is complete. Follow-up by an ophthalmologist is important, both to monitor healing and to offer advice if residual scarring remains.

Treatment of herpes simplex keratitis
1 Topical aciclovir 3% eye ointment five times daily (continue for at least 3 days after complete healing).
2 Second choice: idoxuridine 0.5% eye ointment every 4 h (continue for 3–5 days after complete healing).

Bacterial conjunctivitis

Bacterial conjunctivitis is often secondary to upper respiratory infections, and the common causative organisms are *Haemophilus influenzae* and *Streptococcus pneumoniae*, and sometimes *Staphylococcus aureus*. The condition is usually mild and often self-limiting. Unusual bacteria affecting the conjunctiva include *Moraxella lacunata*, which causes indolent or subacute infections (often in outbreaks where spread is by towels, make-up applicators or unwashed hands) and *H. aegyptius*, more common in tropical climates, which causes more acute infection and may also spread by the droplet route.

Pseudomonas aeruginosa can cause keratoconjunctivitis with blurred vision in contact lens wearers. Infection is derived from unsterile cleaning fluids or from inappropriate use of stored tap water. It may require treatment with aminoglycosides, in severe cases by the subconjunctival or parenteral route.

Treatment with chloramphenicol drops speeds healing. Chloramphenicol ointment can be used at night. The course should rarely be longer than a week. Repeated or sustained use of chloramphenicol carries a risk of agranulocytosis and should be avoided. Severe unresponsive or ulcerating eye infections require specialist management which includes subconjunctival injections of antibiotics.

Treatment of bacterial conjunctivitis
1 Chloramphenicol 0.5% eye drops at least 2-hourly, then four times daily when infection is controlled. Continue for 48 h after healing. Chloramphenicol 1% eye ointment may be used instead of drops at night or alone in a dose of three or four times daily.
2 *Pseudomonas* conjunctivitis should be treated with gentamicin 0.3% eye drops in the same regimen as choramphenicol drops; an alternative is tobramycin 0.3% eye drops.

Ophthalmia neonatorum

This severe neonatal conjunctivitis is acquired during birth from the infected maternal genitalia. It is caused by either *Chlamydia trachomatis* or *Neisseria gonorrhoeae* and is clinically apparent in the first 2 or 3 days of life. Gonococcal ophthalmia responds to topical chloramphenicol. Chlamydial infection is nowadays more common. It is treated with tetracycline eye drops and systemic erythromycin. Systemic treatment is needed because respiratory chlamydial infection may follow ophthalmia (see Chapter 12). In both cases the parents should be offered follow-up treatment.

Treatment of ophthalmia neonatorum and chlamydial conjunctivitis
1 Gonococcal: chloramphenicol eye drops and/or ointment (systemic penicillin or other appropriate treatment should be given simultaneously).
2 Chlamydial: tetracycline 1% eye ointment four times daily (systemic erythromycin treatment should be given simultaneously; see Chapter 12).

Chlamydial conjunctivitis and trachoma

Strains of *Chlamydia* which commonly colonize the genital tract can also affect the eye. They are different species from the *Chlamydia* which cause primary respiratory disease, and can be distinguished from one another and from the agent of lymphogranuloma venereum by serotyping. They sometimes cause subacute conjunctivitis which spreads between sexual contacts and from eye to eye. It does not respond to treatment with chloramphenicol. *Chlamydia* can be demonstrated in cells from conjunctival scrapings. Tetracycline eye drops are the treatment of choice for the eye condition and oral treatment, e.g. erythromycin or tetracycline, may also be given. Investigation and treatment of the patient and sexual partner for genital infection are also necessary (see Chapter 11).

Trachoma

Trachoma is a disease of crowding and poor hygiene. It is precipitated by persisting or repeated infection with *C. trachomatis*, spread from eye to eye by unwashed hands, and in warm climates possibly by flies. Untreated infection and repeated superinfections may lead to the formation of a plaque of vascular inflammatory tissue (pannus) which deforms the eyelid. Scarring, leading to entropion and trichiasis, is an important cause of corneal damage and can lead eventually to scarring and blindness. Topical treatment and hygienic measures can control this disease.

Amoebic keratoconjunctivitis

This is a rare condition associated with contact lenses. The lens cleaning fluid becomes colonized by free-living amoebae, usually *Acanthamoeba*, but occasionally *Naegleria*, which are then repeatedly inoculated into the eye. The resulting severe keratitis is very difficult to treat and often damages vision. Control is by the use of only sterile cleaning fluids, which are discarded after use.

Infections of the middle ear

Acute otitis media

ORGANISM LIST

Many respiratory viruses
Streptococcus pneumoniae
Haemophilus influenzae
S. pyogenes
Staphylococcus aureus
Chlamydia pneumoniae and *C. trachomatis*
Mycoplasma pneumoniae.

Introduction

Infection of the cavity of the middle ear causes pain, reddening and opacification of the tympanic membrane and sometimes rupture of the membrane with discharge from the ear. There has been much discussion in the last decade about the pathology and management of the condition. Traditionally it has been thought of as a primary or secondary infection caused by respiratory

tract organisms ascending the eustachian tube to infect the obstructed or virus-inflamed cavity. However, several studies have suggested that antibiotic treatment is rarely more successful than symptomatic treatment, and furthermore that drainage by myringotomy and culture of middle ear contents do not improve the results of treatment.

These findings may be explained by the existence of different types of infection. The eardrum is reddened in many viral respiratory infections, and also in rotavirus gastroenteritis. *C. pneumoniae* has recently been implicated in cases of otitis media, causing mild disease and not responding to treatment with ampicillin or cotrimoxazole. On the other hand, severe infections are sometimes seen, with early rupture of the eardrum and frankly purulent discharge (usually before presentation for treatment). Such severe infections may be spontaneous, but are often seen as complications of catarrhal respiratory infections, including the now rare measles. Implicated organisms include *Streptococcus pneumoniae*, *H. influenzae*, *S. pyogenes* and *Staphylococcus aureus*. It seems reasonable to treat these promptly with antibiotics, and to culture any discharge.

Management

1 Mild pain and reddening of drum, with no fluid level or other features or with general upper respiratory symptoms: offer analgesics, and decongestant if indicated. Review if persistent or worsening.
2 Evidence of *C. pneumoniae* or *M. pneumoniae* infection (see Chapter 7): systemic erythromycin (or tetracycline in an adult) may be beneficial.
3 Severe pain, discharge or important precursor such as measles or influenza: obtain specimen of pus if possible for bacterial culture. Offer antibiotics, which may need to include an antistaphylococcal spectrum. Analgesia is essential.

Complications

Mastoiditis

Mastoiditis is the extension of pyogenic infection into the mastoid antrum. If treated early with antibiotics this may resolve, but obstruction and stagnation of the many cells of the antrum make the infection very difficult to eradicate. There is severe pain behind and within the ear, and often a high fever. There is also a risk that the infection will penetrate the cranial cavity. Treatment must then be surgical, with opening and debridement of the trabeculated cavity of air cells (mastoidectomy).

Attic infection

Attic infection is damage to the high roof of the middle ear cavity, which can involve the facial nerve. This is more common in chronic or neglected infections. A cholesteatoma (tumour of waxy inflammatory tissue) may form, and can erode the cranial bones, predisposing to intracranial infection. The treatment of cholesteatoma is surgical. Rare cases of chronic middle ear infection can be complicated by the presence of anaerobic pathogens.

Paranasal sinusitis

In this condition the paranasal sinuses fill with exudate, and the draining ostia become blocked. Like otitis media, it is often secondary to a catarrhal infection and may be caused by *Streptococcus pneumoniae*, *H. influenza*, *S. 'milleri'*, anaerobes or *Staphylococcus aureus*.

Clinical features are pain and tenderness over the affected sinus, usually maxillary or frontal sinus. There is a loss of transillumination, and X-rays show thickening of the soft-tissue wall of the cavity, often with a fluid level.

Treatment includes elevation of the head and offering decongestants to aid drainage. A broad-spectrum antibiotic such as co-trimoxazole, erythromycin or tetracycline will penetrate the soft tissues and reduce the purulent exudate. In relapsing or chronic cases, surgical treatment can be offered. The ostia of the frontal sinuses can be enlarged, or false ostia can be made to connect the maxillary sinuses to the buccal cavity, allowing improved drainage.

Complications of sinusitis tend to affect the ethmoid and sphenoid sinuses, which are adjacent to the cranial cavity. The thin lateral and superior walls of the ethmoid sinus may rupture. Lateral spread of infection causes orbital cellulitis, while superior spread may lead to meningitis. Inflammation of tissues in the walls of the ethmoid and sphenoid sinuses affects the overlying venous sinus. Cavernous sinus thrombosis is a grave complication of severe, untreated sinusitis. It is best diagnosed by computed tomography or magnetic resonance scan.

Viral infections of the throat and mouth

ORGANISM LIST

Rhinoviruses
Coronaviruses
Enteroviruses
Adenoviruses
Epstein–Barr virus
Herpes simplex virus.

The common cold (coryza)

Introduction

This disorder is most often caused by various types of rhinoviruses and sometimes by coronaviruses, but many mild respiratory virus infections can produce the same symptoms. Colds are extremely infectious by the droplet route. The familiar clinical features are mild fever, swelling of the respiratory mucosa, often affecting the nose and conjunctiva as well as the throat, and finally a copious mucoid exudate. Otitis media in children and sinusitis in adults are common complications.

Pathology

Rhinoviruses are members of the Picornaviridae. They are small RNA viruses 28–34 nm in diameter expressing icosohedral symmetry. The genome consists of a single strand of positive-polarity RNA of approximately 7.2 kb. A single polypeptide is produced and cleaved. There are four capsid proteins, VP1–4. There are more than 100 different serotypes.

Coronavirus is the only genus in the family Coronaviridae. It is a pleiomorphic, non-enveloped RNA virus ranging in size from 60 to 220 nm. The virus has characteristic club-shaped projections 20 nm in length extending from the surface. There are three main structural proteins: the nucleocapsid protein, the surface projection protein and the transmembrane or matrix protein. The nucleocapsid proteins are species-specific whereas strain-specific antigens are found on the surface projections. The surface projections are a high-molecular-weight glycoprotein (180 kDa) and are readily removed by protease activity.

The main mechanism of pathogenesis is probably a direct cytotoxic effect on respiratory epithelial cells.

Laboratory diagnosis

The laboratory diagnosis of rhinovirus infection is rarely attempted due to the frequency and trivial nature of the infection. Nasal washings may be inoculated into humans embryonic lung fibroblasts. A cytopathic effect (CPE) similar to that of enterovirus develops within 8 days, although it may not develop until a second passage has been performed. Rising titres of virus-specific antibody can be detected by the viral neutralizing test, but this is too cumbersome for routine use. An enzyme immunoassay (EIA)-based method is available but has the disadvantage of being serotype-specific.

Coronaviruses are not usually detected in routine practice as they are difficult to isolate, and serological investigations are not readily available. Virus can be isolated from nasal and throat swabs and nasopharyngeal aspirates by inoculation in human embryonic lung fibroblasts. The CPE consists of small granular round cells in the monolayer. Antibodies can be detected by virus neutralization, complement fixation test and HAI.

Management

Treatment is symptomatic and includes antipyretic analgesics, mild decongestants such as pseudoephedrine tablets and bed rest in severe cases. Enthusiasm for intranasal interferon therapy has waned because of local irritation and poor evidence of benefit.

Enteroviral pharyngitis

Epidemiology

Pharyngitis due to enterovirus infection is common. Coxsackie type A10 is frequently responsible, although other coxsackie and echoviruses can cause pharyngitis. Infections predominate during summer and autumn; this distinguishes them from winter viruses whose main target is the respiratory tract (e.g. influenza and adenovirus). Humans are the only known reservoir of infection and transmission occurs by direct contact and through aerosol spread. The disease often occurs as epidemics affecting young children in nurseries, playgroups and schools. Crowding and poor hygiene increase the risk of epidemics.

Virology

More than 70 serotypes of enterovirus have been isolated from human sources. All belong to the family Picornaviridae. The Picornaviridae are divided into four genera, of which two, the rhinoviruses and the enteroviruses, cause disease in humans.

The viruses are 27 nm diameter, symmetrical particles, with icosahedral symmetry. The virion consist of 60 copies of each of four proteins — VP1–4. The genome consists of a single strand of positive-sense RNA. Antiviral antisera neutralize only the homologous virus strain but gentle treatment or denaturation will result in other antigenic determinants being exposed.

Neutralizing antibodies bind to sites on VP1, the complex site involving residues on VP1 and VP2 and to other complex sites involving residues VP1, 2 and 3. Enteroviruses bind to host cells via specific receptor sites and it is thought that differences in these receptors are responsible for different tissue tropisms among enteroviruses.

The enteroviruses can be differentiated into five main groups: (i) polioviruses; (ii) coxsackieviruses group A; (iii) coxsackieviruses group B; (iv) echo (enteric cytopathogenic human orphan) viruses; and (v) five more recently characterized human enteroviruses types 68–72 (type 72 is hepatitis A virus). Each of these has different tissue tropisms (see Chapter 16).

Groups of enteroviruses
1 Polioviruses.
2 Coxsackieviruses group A.
3 Coxsackieviruses group B.
4 Echoviruses.
5 Other recently characterized human enteroviruses.

Pathology

Enteroviruses enter the body through the pharynx and the alimentary tract. The virus multiples locally in the tonsils, Peyer's patches and other bowel-associated lymphoid tissue. A viraemic phase often occurs, and this may be followed by disease in different organs, for example meninges, brain or skin. In poliomyelitis the virus multiplies and causes damage in the anterior horn cells, resulting in a flaccid paralysis (see Chapter 16).

Clinical features

The incubation period is about 1 week, and is followed by abrupt development of a sore throat and fever. The severity and duration of symptoms are very variable. In severe cases headache, stiff neck or frank meningism can accompany the sore throat. Symptoms rarely last more than 5–7 days.

Reddening of the fauces is usual, but varies in severity and is not directly related to the intensity of symptoms. Chains of moderately enlarged lymph nodes are often palpable in the anterior and posterior triangles of the neck. Both echovirus and coxsackievirus infections occasionally produce an accompanying rash of sparse macules or small papules, concentrated on the cheeks and trunk.

Coxsackie A infections may cause a faucial rash of blisters with haloes of inflammation (herpangina; Fig. 6.1). Hand, foot and mouth disease of toddlers

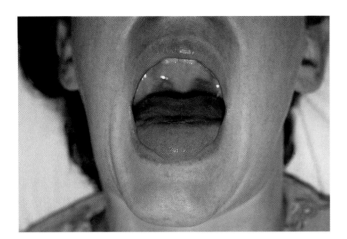

Fig. 6.1 Faucial blisters in a case of herpangina.

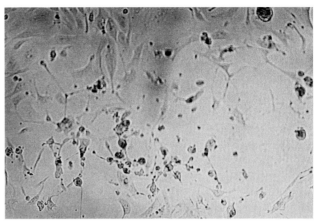

Fig. 6.2 Cytopathic effect of enteroviruses, showing rounding, shrinkage and loss of contiguousness of the cell monolayer. Courtesy of Dr M. Zambon, Central Public Health Laboratory.

causes similar lesions in the mouth, accompanied by blisters on the palmar aspects of the hands and feet, and a papular rash on the buttocks (see Chapter 5).

Coxsackie B infections may be accompanied by pleurodynia (also called Bornholm disease) in which the trunk muscles are severely tender and painful, mimicking pleurisy. There is usually also a high fever and obvious sore throat. Coxsackie B can also cause maculopapular rashes, mild to moderate orchitis and, rarely, myocarditis.

Management

In the absence of specific antiviral treatment, symptomatic treatment is offered. Analgesics, especially non-steroidal anti-inflammatory agents, are helpful. In patients over age 12, soluble aspirin gargles often have a beneficial local effect, and can be swallowed for their systemic effects. Bed rest reduces malaise in severe cases.

Laboratory diagnosis

Enteroviral infections can be diagnosed by a combination of virus isolation and serological tests. For culture, the most useful specimens are faeces, but throat swabs and cerebrospinal fluid should be sent in cases of meningitis. The isolation rate from the latter specimens is poor. However, culture of an enterovirus from a sterile site is diagnostic, whereas isolation from faeces is less certainly so. Enteroviruses grow well in cultures of primary monkey kidney cells and human embryonic lung fibroblasts. A cytopathic effect is produced which is common to all enteroviruses. The infected cells become rounded and refractile before separating from the mono-

layer (Fig. 6.2). Isolates are typed by neutralization using pooled antisera.

Coxsackie group A viruses do not grow well on tissue culture; when virus isolation is essential it can be achieved by intracerebral inoculation of mice. Modern EIA techniques have been applied to the serological diagnosis of enteroviral infections using immunoglobulin M (IgM) antibody capture methods.

Complications

The spectrum of enteroviral infections includes lymphocytic meningitis, pericarditis and acute myocarditis. Patients with significant meningism, precordial pain, dysrhythmias or heart failure require further investigation.

Adenoviral sore throats and pharyngoconjunctival fever

Introduction

The so-called respiratory adenoviruses (particularly types 1–10) are capable of causing severe sore throats. There is usually high fever, intense sore throat, severe faucial inflammation and painful enlargement of lymph nodes in the upper neck. The illness may last as long as 7–10 days and is often followed by debility in the convalescent period.

The same adenoviruses commonly cause conjunctivitis. When conjunctivitis and pharyngitis coexist, the condition is called pharyngoconjunctival fever. It is almost always adenoviral in aetiology.

Human adenoviruses form part of the genus Mastadenovirus which is part of the family Adenoviridae. Adenoviruses are unenveloped viruses with icosohedral symmetry. The virus is made up of 252 identical hexon capsomeres and 12 vertex penton capsomeres with fibre vertex projections. A complement-fixing antigen exists on the hexon and is a group antigen common to all types. Forty-two serotype-specific antigens exist, located on the hexon and the fibre. Antibody to this antigen will neutralize virus of a homologous serotype.

Adenoviruses possess a linear, double-stranded DNA of approximately 35 kDa, located in the viral core in a chromatin-like structure which contains two polypeptides (classified as V and VII). The disease caused varies according to the subgenus and serotype. Subgenus A is highly oncogenic in animals, B and C are associated with respiratory disease, D is associated with keratoconjunctivitis, E with conjunctivitis and respiratory disease, and F with infantile diarrhoea.

Adenoviruses multiply inside the nuclei of epithelial cells. They are cytopathic for human cells, and this is probably responsible for the tissue damage and symptoms associated with infection. Different target specificity of the adenovirus fibres contributes to the different tissue trophisms noted above. A toxin-like activity has been associated with the vertex capsomeres.

Laboratory diagnosis

Adenovirus is most easily isolated from stool but can also be recovered from conjunctival swabs, nasopharyngeal aspirates and cerebrospinal fluid. Human cell lines, e.g. Hep-2, and some monkey kidney cells are suitable for virus isolation. A cytopathic effect is seen in 48 h and is characterized by rounded-up cells with refractile intranuclear inclusion bodies. The identification can be confirmed by electron microscopy. Antibodies to a group-specific antigen can be detected by complement fixation test or EIA.

Infectious mononucleosis

Introduction

Infectious mononucleosis is the clinical disease produced by primary Epstein–Barr virus (EBV) infection. It is a systemic disease, but in 75% of cases its main feature is sore throat (anginose infectious mononucleosis) and so it is discussed in this chapter, especially as the differential diagnosis and main complications fall into this section. However, 15% present as hepatitis with mild jaundice and 10% as fever alone (see Chapters 9 and 22).

> **Clinical presentations of Epstein–Barr virus infection**
> 1 Sore throat 75%.
> 2 Hepatitis 15%.
> 3 Fever alone 10%.
> 4 Rare: viral-type meningitis, mononeuritis or polyneuritis, perisplenic pain.

Although primary disease causes considerable morbidity and convalescence is occasionally slow, the late effects of infection may also be important. Both Burkitt's lymphoma and nasopharyngeal tumours are consequences of EBV infection in early infancy. Cofactors such as early infection with malaria, or ingestion of toxins in certain foods, for example preserved vegetables, may also be important.

Epidemiology

EBV is shed in pharyngeal secretions, and transmission occurs via close oral contact. It may be acquired through kissing, shared eating utensils or in some cultures by a mother chewing food for her infant.

EBV infection is common in young children, when it is usually asymptomatic. Clinical disease occurs mainly in teenagers and young adults; approximately 50% of infections in this age group present as typical glandular fever. The incidence of the disease is not known precisely as many infections are mild and not reported. The estimated annual incidence, based on general practitioner consultations, is 1 per 1000 population.

Virology and pathogenesis

The discovery of EBV arises from the initial observation of Denis Burkitt of a geographically limited lymphoma which he proposed was infectious in origin. The virus was recovered from Burkitt's lymphoma material and later shown to be a herpesvirus.

EBV is morphologically identical to other herpesviruses. It is a DNA virus with isocohedral symmetry consisting of 162 triangular capsomeres of 100 nm diameter. Like other herpesviruses, it is enveloped with a membrane derived from the host plasma membrane. The double-stranded DNA is 172 kb in length — large enough to code for 100–200 proteins. Only a small number of proteins have been studied in detail. These include the Epstein–Barr nuclear antigen (EBNA) complex, the latent membrane protein, the terminal protein, the membrane antigen complex, the early antigen (EA) complex and the viral capsid antigen (VCA). The function of many of these antigens is unknown.

The EBNA complex consists of at least six proteins of unknown function, but which are probably important in maintaining the virus in the infected cell. EBNA 1 antigen is expressed on all infected cells but may be lost as infected cells die. The early antigen (EA) complex is expressed only on cells which have entered a lytic phase. Antibodies to EBNA and EA appear early in the disease and are transient. Antibodies to capsid antigens appear in IgM by the time disease is apparent, and may persist for weeks or months. IgG anticapsid antibodies indicate immunity, and persist throughout life.

Virus invades via the pharynx, from where B lymphocytes become infected and the infection is spread throughout the body. EBV is capable of activation and immortalization of B cells. This is the probable pathogenic mechanism for many of the 'immunological' effects and complications of infection.

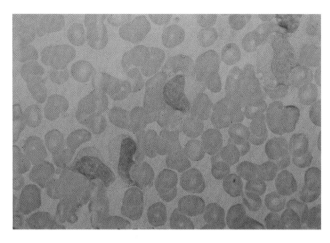

Fig. 6.4 Atypical mononuclear cells in the peripheral blood of a case of infectious mononucleosis.

Clinical features

The incubation period is about 7 weeks. Typical features of fever, sore throat and widespread lymphadenopathy develop more or less simultaneously. The tonsils become covered with a white creamy exudate, which may begin as serpiginous streaks, but becomes confluent within 24–36 h. The exudate is rarely discoloured. It may become bulky, obscuring even grossly enlarged tonsils, but it does not involve the pharyngeal mucosa (Fig. 6.3).

The pharyngeal and nasal mucosae are congested and swollen. Gross pharyngeal swelling may make it impossible to swallow saliva and can even threaten the airway.

The spleen is palpably enlarged in 25–40% of cases; the liver edge is often palpable. A chest X-ray occasionally shows enlarged mediastinal lymph nodes and, sur-

prisingly, as many as 20–25% of patients have a lung opacity suggesting segmental pneumonitis. The X-ray abnormalities resolve spontaneously as the fever abates.

There are important laboratory abnormalities in this condition. Although the infected B cells do not appear in the circulation, there is a vigorous T-cell response which causes activated T cells to spill into the blood stream. These are the 'atypical mononuclear cells' that give the condition its name; they may constitute 40% or more of the total lymphocyte count during the acute infection (Fig. 6.4).

The liver function tests show changes of mild hepatocellular disorder with transaminases usually in the range of 300–500 IU/ml. The alkaline phosphatase may rise during convalescence (in cases with clinical jaundice it

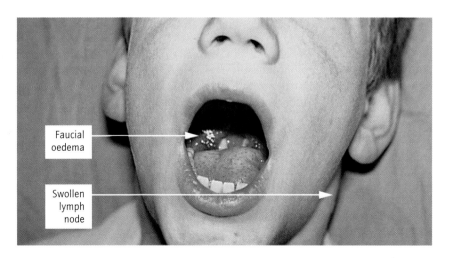

Faucial oedema

Swollen lymph node

Fig. 6.3 Exudative tonsillitis with marked cervical lymphadenopathy in a case of infectious mononucleosis.

can be very high, even approaching 1000 IU/ml, but this rarely causes any clinical consequence and it resolves during convalescence).

The activated B cells produce various antibodies, of which the most common are the heterophile antibodies which agglutinate horse and sheep red blood cells.

Other detectable antibodies include haemolysins, platelet antibodies, antinuclear antibodies, rheumatoid factors and anticardiolipin antibodies. On rare occasions these antibodies are associated with immune cytopenias or with autoimmune-like diseases, but the most common of these effects does not exceed an incidence of 1 in 20 000–30 000 clinical cases.

The duration of fever and exudative pharyngitis varies widely from a few days to as much as 3 weeks. Most patients convalesce steadily after this, but a minority suffer disabling fatigue and lassitude for many weeks. This postinfectious fatigue usually recovers between 3 and 6 months after the end of the feverish illness.

Diagnosis

The clinical picture of exudative pharyngitis, generalized lymphadenopathy and atypical mononucleosis is often sufficient for diagnosis. Exudate is present in many cases of streptococcal pharyngitis, but this is follicular and rarely confluent. The pseudomembrane of diphtheria is sometimes confluent, but it is discoloured, and tends to spread beyond the tonsillar margin. In both bacterial diseases there is a low-grade neutrophilia, quite unlike the atypical lymphocytosis of EBV infection.

In most patients it is not possible to detect rising IgG titres to VCA as concentrations are already high when the patient presents, but the presence of IgM anti-VCA is diagnostic. These antibodies can be detected by immunofluorescence or EIA. A more rapid but less specific test is the heterophile antibody test. Sheep red cell agglutination was the basis of the original Paul–Bunnell test.

A commercial slide test, the Monospot, which measures the presence of this antibody is now available. This utilizes horse red cell agglutination, and is positive in about 95% of patients at presentation. Small children, however, do not produce high levels of heterophile antibodies, so the test is less reliable in patients aged less than 5 years. All patients have IgM anti-EBV capsid antibodies.

Management

There is no specific treatment; most cases recover uneventfully. Analgesia is helpful, and an anti-inflammatory agent may help to limit throat swelling. In older children and adults soluble aspirin in standard doses may be gargled and swallowed. In the under-12s paracetamol may not be sufficient; paediatric formulations of ibuprofen may then be helpful. Stronger analgesics, even mild opiates, may be indicated in some cases.

Complications

Threatened respiratory obstruction

Threatened respiratory obstruction is by far the commonest problem and, apart from pharyngeal pain, is the usual reason for hospital admission. It will often improve overnight with bed rest (preferably with the head elevated to encourage drainage of oedema from the pharyngeal tissues), anti-inflammatory analgesics and reassurance. Danger signs are inability to swallow saliva and a rapidly increasing pulse rate; these may be followed by increasing respiratory rate and cyanosis, requiring emergency intervention. This progression can often be avoided by reducing oedema with an intravenous bolus of corticosteroid. A modest dose of 50–100 mg hydrocortisone is often sufficient, and the patient usually reports improvement within 20–30 min. Fears of adverse effects have been much allayed by controlled trials of similar treatment in croup, showing no significant complications. The corticosteroid has no effect on the general progress of the infection, and dosing can be repeated if non-steroidal anti-inflammatory agents do not maintain the improvement.

Effects of abnormal antibodies

Effects of abnormal antibodies are rarely clinically important. Thrombocytopenia is the least rare, followed by haemolytic anaemia. A handful of cases of systemic lupus erythematosus-like disease are reported; joint pains occur in convalescence and may persist for some months, often improving when anti-DNA antibodies disappear.

Suppurative complications

Rare but well-recognized complications of this type include peritonsillar abscess, pharyngeal abscess, ethmoiditis, infection of other intracranial sinuses and periorbital cellulitis. They probably represent secondary infection of stagnant cavities or damaged tissue resulting from severe mucosal oedema and disruption. They should be investigated and treated as for primary pyogenic infections at these sites.

Rupture of the spleen

Rupture of the spleen, often quoted, is extremely rare. It may be preceded by left upper quadrant and shoulder pain during acute disease (though even this type of pain often subsides spontaneously, perhaps representing distension of the splenic capsule without rupture). In other cases it is precipitated by apparently trivial trauma, such as a blow during play, a sudden movement or a cough. Imaging studies may demonstrate free fluid in the peritoneal cavity, or the disrupted splenic anatomy. Prompt surgical intervention in needed to terminate bleeding. Contact sports or combat sports should therefore be avoided until lymphadenopathy and, by inference, splenomegaly have subsided.

Neurological complications

Neurological complications include lymphocytic meningitis, mononeuritis or brachial plexitis (Fig. 6.5). These are benign and self-limiting. Occasional cases of encephalopathy are reported, of which some are progressive or even fatal.

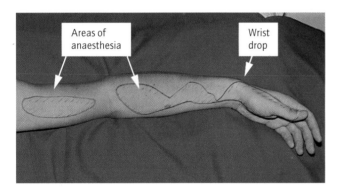

Fig. 6.5 Brachial plexitis complicating infectious mononucleosis: complete recovery occurred within 3 weeks.

Bacterial throat infections

ORGANISM LIST

Streptococcus pyogenes
Haemophilus influenzae
Corynebacterium diphtheriae
Other bacteria, including *Neisseria meningitidis, H. haemolyticum, Chlamydia pneumoniae* and *N. gonorrhoeae.*

Streptococcal tonsillitis

Introduction

This disease is caused by *S. pyogenes*, and is common worldwide, affecting both adults and children. It causes considerable short- and medium-term morbidity, and can be recurrent, as *S. pyogenes* is a tenacious colonist of the throat. It is also important because streptococcal throat infections can be followed by poststreptococcal nephritis or by rheumatic fever (see Chapter 24).

Epidemiology

Streptococcal pharyngitis is common in temperate climates, occurring mainly in the winter. The disease is usually spread by direct contact with respiratory excretions, and less commonly by air-borne droplets or indirect contact by hands. Outbreaks due to contaminated food and milk have been described but are uncommon.

The infection occurs mainly in children, up to 20% of whom may be asymptomatic carriers. Disease is commoner in crowded settings such as children's homes and military camps.

Scarlet fever is a notifiable disease in the UK. The incidence and severity of scarlet fever (and other manifestations of group A streptococcal infection) have declined steadily over the past 50 years. In 1936, when yearly notifications began, there were 104 862 notifications and 440 deaths from scarlet fever in England and Wales — a case fatality ratio of 0.42 per 100. By 1986, this had dropped to 6888 notifications and 3 deaths (0.05 per 100). The incidence (but not the case fatality ratio) increased during 1988 and 1989, but has subsequently declined to around 5000 cases per annum. A similar fall was seen in the USA; however, a reappearance of severe infections complicated by rheumatic fever has been observed since 1986, associated with mucoid strains of *S. pyogenes*.

Pathogenesis

The main pathogenicity determinant is the M protein antigen of which there are many types (see Chapter 2 and Table 2.3). This protein has a fibrillar structure with a similar function to the polysaccharide capsule of other pyogenic organisms, such as *H. influenzae* and *N. meningitidis*. It inhibits bacterial phagocytosis by neutrophils. Bacteria can only be ingested when opsonized by anti-M antibody. This antibody is serotype-specific, providing no protection to infection by

S. pyogenes of other M-protein types. Cross-reactions between M proteins, of *S. pyogenes* and host myocardial muscle are thought to be responsible for the development of rheumatic fever. Cross-reactions between antigens in the glomerular basement membrane and certain 'nephritogenic' M-types of *S. pyogenes* are responsible for poststreptococcal glomerulonephritis.

Pathogenicity factors for *Streptococcus pyogenes*
1 M proteins.
2 Lancefield group antigens.
3 Streptomycin S.
4 Streptomycin O.
5 Hyaluronidase.
6 Collagenase.
7 Deoxyribonuclease.
8 Streptokinase.
9 Pyogenic exotoxins A, (B) and C.

Lancefield group antigens

These are polysaccharide–teichoic acid antigens located in the bacterial cell wall. Lancefield antigens group streptococci into pathologically related groups and species, and constitute the main method of classifying beta-haemolytic streptococci. The Lancefield group antigen has not, however, been directly associated with the pathogenesis of infection.

Lytic enzymes

S. pyogenes elaborates a wide range of lytic toxins, some of which are thought to contribute to the virulence of the organism and some of which are used in diagnosis. The organism produces two haemolysins, one of which is oxygen-stable (streptolysin S) and one which is oxygen- and heat-labile (streptolysin O; anti-streptolysin O (ASO)). The latter is one of a family of cytolytic toxins found in Gram-positive organisms (see p. 17). The antibody response to ASO is used in the serological diagnosis of *S. pyogenes* infections (see p. 116). In addition to this, hyaluronidase and collagenase are produced and these may aid tissue invasion by breaking down collagen and hyaluronic acid in connective tissue. The ability of this organism to disrupt tissue and reduce tissue redox potential is thought to be important in the pathogenesis of synergistic gangrene, where mixed infection with Gram-positive cocci, including *S. pyogenes* and/or *Staphylococcus aureus*, and obligate anaerobes can result in destruction of tissue planes and a rapidly progressive infection.

Streptococcus pyogenes produces streptokinase, which acts as a plasminogen activator, producing clot lysis, which may enhance the spread of the organism. Other lytic enzymes include four serologically different DNAses (A–D). On the surface, the organism expresses C5a- and immunoglobulin-binding proteins which may interfere with host immune responses.

Steptococcal pyrogenic exotoxins (SPEs)

There are three distinct SPEs; A, B and C, of which A and C are structurally similar. These toxins are responsible for the rash of scarlet fever (erythrogenic toxins) and, more importantly, stimulate macrophages to produce tumour necrosis factor, with all the metabolic and immunological consequences. They are superantigens, and have close homology with some *Staphylococcus aureus* exotoxins. They are thought to mediate the shock syndrome in severe group A streptococcal infections.

SPE B has a different structure. It is secreted as a zymogen and is converted to a proteinase which is mitogenic and cardiotoxic.

Clinical features

The usual features are fever, pain in the throat, enlargement of the tonsils and tender swelling of the tonsillar lymph nodes at the angles of the jaw. The severity of the symptoms is variable; some patients with severe pain have only the mildest reddening of the throat, while some with moderate pain have alarming tonsillar inflammation.

The most severe and classical appearance is of follicular tonsillitis, in which the tonsils are enlarged, very red and dotted with patches of soft white exudate (Fig. 6.6). The throat is extremely painful and a large, tender lymph node swells downwards from beneath the angle of the jaw. It is not unusual for one or other tonsil to be predominantly affected, with proportionately greater swelling of the lymph node on that side.

Scarlet fever

Scarlet fever is the response to erythrogenic toxin produced by the infecting *Streptococcus pyogenes*. There is severe malaise, and many children with the condition vomit at the onset of illness.

An erythema appears on the chest and quickly involves all of the skin. It is more marked in the folds and valleys of the skin, e.g. the inguinal and elbow folds (Pastia's sign). The papillae of the skin are swollen, forming tiny conical papules which give the rash a sand-

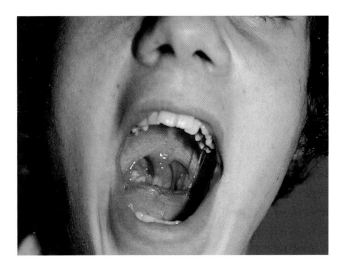

Fig. 6.6 Typical appearance of follicular tonsillitis.

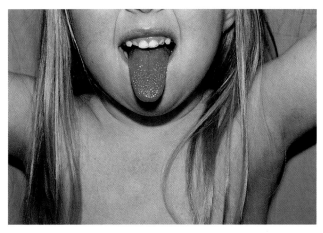

Fig. 6.8 Red strawberry tongue of scarlet fever.

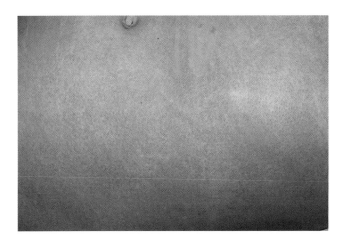

Fig. 6.7 Typical rash of scarlet fever.

paper texture, and a stippled appearance (often called a punctate erythema). There may be a less affected area around the mouth or 'snout' area, but this is neither a constant nor a diagnostic feature (Fig. 6.7).

Initially the tongue is furred and white (white strawberry tongue). Over about 3 days this clears from the tip backwards, leaving a reddened (red strawberry tongue) appearance (Fig. 6.8).

Diagnosis

Mild streptococcal tonsillitis is difficult to distinguish clinically from other causes of sore throat. However, a neutrophilia in the peripheral blood is a strong predictor of bacterial rather than viral aetiology, and allows an early decision for antibiotic treatment to be made.

Follicular tonsillitis with associated tender enlargement of tonsillar lymph nodes is typical of *S. pyogenes* infection, and is clinically diagnostic.

Recovery of *S. pyogenes* from throat swabs strongly suggests the diagnosis, but streptococcal colonization can coexist with viral and other sore throats. Also, *S. pyogenes* does not transfer well from swab to culture, so that there is a 20–30% false-negativity rate in the results of swab cultures.

S. pyogenes is a fastidious organism, growing only on rich nutrient media, usually containing blood. Haemolytic toxins produce the characteristic zone of complete (beta) haemolysis, enabling selection of suspect colonies for identification. The growth of the organism and the haemolysis it produces are enhanced by incubation in an anaerobic atmosphere. When large numbers of specimens are to be screened, a selective medium incorporating antibiotics such as ofloxacin or nalidixic acid, or dyes such as crystal violet, can be used to inhibit Gram-negative and Gram-positive commensal organisms respectively.

For most routine laboratories, identification of *S. pyogenes* is achieved on the basis of colonial morphology (large clear colonies surrounded by a zone of beta-haemolysis) and the presence of the group A Lancefield antigen. The antigen is extracted with an enzyme and its presence detected by agglutination of latex particles coated with antibodies to the different Lancefield groups. The groups, different species and pathogenicity are listed in Table 6.1. A rapid diagnosis can be made by latex agglutination of specimens collected on throat swabs. These techniques are of sufficient simplicity that they may be used in a general practitioner surgery. They are highly specific but of variable sensitivity (as low as 55% in some studies).

Group	Species	Diseases caused
A	*Streptococcus pyogenes*	Acute pharyngitis, quinsy, otitis media, erysipelas, synergistic gangrene, rheumatic fever, poststreptococcal glomerulonephritis
	S. milleri (minute colony)	Metastatic suppurative infection
B	*S. agalactiae*	Neonatal septicaemia, meningitis and pneumonia
C	*S. dysgalactiae* *S. equi* *S. equisimilis* *S. zooepidemicus*	Rare cause of skin sepsis and endocarditis. Postinfectious glomerulonephritis has been reported
D	*S. bovis*	Endocarditis and bacteraemia associated with colonic neoplasm
F	*S. milleri* (see p. 291)	Metastatic suppurative disease, dental sepsis

Table 6.1 Species of beta-haemolytic streptococci and their pathogenicity

---

Laboratory identification of *Streptococcus pyogenes*
1 Chains of Gram-positive cocci growing on blood agar, plus beta-haemolysis, plus Lancefield group A antigen.
2 Serodiagnosis: rapid antigen detection in throat swabs; antibody detection — high or rising titres of antistreptolysin O, antihyaluronidase and/or anti DNAse.

Serology

Acute streptococcal infection can be diagnosed by detecting a rise or fall in antibodies to the oxygen-labile streptolysin (ASO), DNAse B or hyaluronidase. ASO titres (ASOT) above 400 U indicate likely recent infection, while a fourfold rise in titre in paired sera is strong evidence of streptococcal disease. Although these techniques are available in many laboratories, they have limited utility as antibody response may be delayed for up to 4 weeks. Their main use is in providing supportive evidence in the diagnosis of complications such as rheumatic fever or glomerulonephritis. Anti-DNAse B responses usually last longer and may be used as a marker of infection in the late convalescent phase.

Management

The treatment of choice is penicillin. Early and mild cases may respond to oral therapy with ampicillin, but established and severe infections can require inpatient treatment with intravenous benzylpenicillin. Suitable alternative drugs are narrow-spectrum cephalosporins and erythromycin. However, a small proportion of highly virulent strains are resistant to erythromycin, so failure to respond to this drug should prompt an early change of treatment.

It is not easy to eradicate *S. pyogenes* from the throat. Research shows that 2 weeks of vigorous (often parenteral) penicillin therapy is needed. This is important in dormitory or barracks-associated outbreaks of streptococcal sore throat, especially those associated with rheumatic fever. In a domiciliary setting a course of a least 10 days' treatment is probably advisable.

Treatment of streptococcal sore throat
1 Early and mild cases: oral ampicillin 250–500 mg 6-hourly for 10 days, or erythromycin in the same dosage and schedule.
2 Severe cases: benzylpenicillin 1.2–2.4 g 4–6-hourly.

Complications

Peritonsillar abscess

Peritonsillar abscess (quinsy) is the commonest complication of tonsillar sepsis. The tissue of the fauces and soft palate on the affected side becomes boggy and pendulous. The throat is intensely painful and tender, often with severe tenderness and swelling of the draining lymph node. The tonsil may be invisible in the mass of oedematous tissue. A small proportion of cases have bilateral quinsy, which carries a high risk of airway obstruction (Fig. 6.9).

Prompt and vigorous treatment can avert the need for surgical drainage of the developing abscess. High doses of penicillin (up to 2.4 g 4-hourly) can be given intravenously. Sometimes even this will not reduce swelling, fever and pain; many specialists find the addition of metronidazole can initiate improvement. (Streptococci grow very well anaerobically, and metronidazole penetrates the oedmatous tissue well.) Early abscesses will resolve. Those already containing pus will often rupture into the throat, causing a brief rancid taste followed by relief of pain. A few progress and enlarge, requiring formal drainage by an ear, nose and throat surgeon.

Streptococcal bacteraemia

Streptococcal bacteraemia is a rare complication with a high mortality rate. Warning signs are high fever, extreme pain in the draining lymph nodes (rarely, even

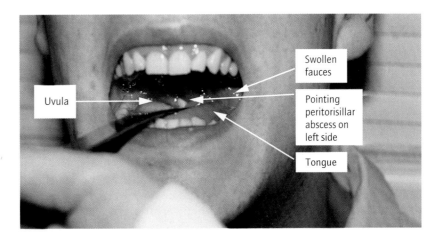

Fig. 6.9 Bilateral quinsies (peritonsillar abscesses).

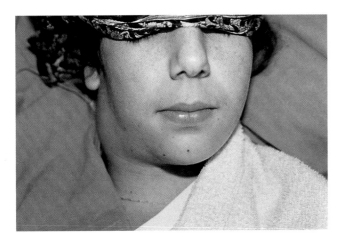

Fig. 6.10 Suppuration of cervical lymph node following tonsillitis (300 ml of pus was drained at surgery).

suppuration or sloughing of the painful nodes; Fig. 6.10) or the appearance of erysipelas-like lesions on the skin. Patients with these features should be treated intravenously while blood culture results are awaited (see Chapter 15).

Poststreptococcal disorders

Poststreptococcal disorders include rheumatic fever, nephritis, erythema multiforme and erythema nodosum. These are discussed in Chapter 24.

Acute epiglottitis

Introduction

This is a severe throat infection which causes massive oedema of the epiglottis and threatens the airway. It is mainly a disease of preschool children, but occasional adult cases are reported. *Haemophilus influenzae* is almost always the cause, although *S. pyogenes* causes a small percentage of cases, mostly among adults. The disease is important for two reasons: first, it must be considered in cases of severe sore throat, as untreated cases may die suddenly of respiratory obstruction; second, it is a bacteraemic disease, and other children in an affected community may suffer from *H. influenzae* bacteraemic diseases such as meningitis or facial cellulitis.

Epidemiology

The peak incidence is at about 3 years of age, and most infections occur during the winter. Boys are affected more commonly than girls. Between 10 and 15% of all invasive *H. influenzae* infections present as epiglottis. The incidence is decreasing since the introduction of routine immunization (see Chapter 16).

Epiglottis due to *S. pyogenes* is uncommon and affects mainly adults.

Clinical features

The illness may begin like a cold and sore throat, with fever and general malaise. It develops rapidly, with swelling and tenderness of the neck and hyoid region, with severe pain in the throat and great difficulty in swallowing. As epiglottic swelling increases the patient drools and then develops stridor.

The temperature is high and sustained. The respiratory rate is often faster than would be expected. There is marked neutrophilia in the peripheral blood, often with a white cell count of 15–$25 \times 10^9/l$. The liver and renal function tests are usually normal.

On examining the throat with the tongue depressed, the red, swollen epiglottis can be seen protruding upwards like a cherry. However, manipulation of the throat can precipitate complete respiratory obstruction and should be avoided if urgent X-ray diagnosis is available. The swollen epiglottis is visible on a lateral X-ray of the soft tissues of the neck, in which it looks like the rounded tip of the thumb, filling the lower oropharynx (Fig. 6.11).

Diagnosis

The diagnosis should be suspected clinically in a feverish child with severe throat pain and drooling or stridor. Adult cases are often missed until a late stage because epiglottitis is not considered.

Clinical confirmation is provided by a lateral X-ray of the soft tissues of the neck, or by direct inspection of the throat if there is no alternative.

Differential diagnoses

Differential diagnoses which can produce similar clinical features include infectious mononucleosis with respiratory obstruction, bilateral peritonsillar abscesses, retropharyngeal abscess and Ludwig's angina. A differential white count and heterophile antibody test will exclude infectious mononucleosis. Cautious examination of the mouth and fauces will exclude the gross sublingual swelling of Ludwig's angina and the faucial swelling of quinsy. The X-ray will show the site of swelling within, rather than behind, the pharynx.

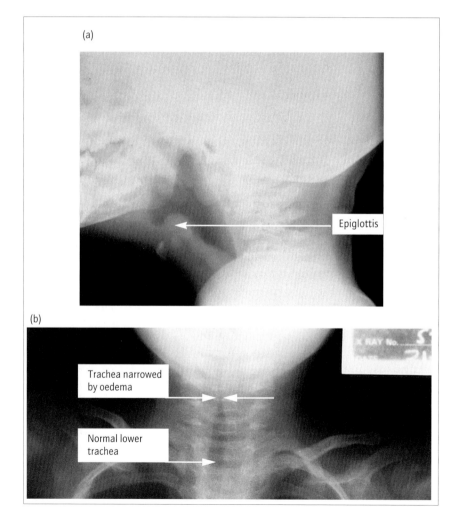

(a)

Epiglottis

(b)

Trachea narrowed by oedema

Normal lower trachea

Fig. 6.11 Acute epiglottitis: (a) enlarged epiglottis demonstrated by lateral X-ray of the soft tissues of the neck; (b) oedema tracking downwards narrows the trachea.

Finally, in patients arriving from rural overseas areas, diphtheria should be considered.

Blood cultures should always be obtained, to provide laboratory confirmation of the diagnosis and to check the sensitivities of the *H. influenzae*. Throat swabs should be deferred until the airway has been made safe.

Management

Acute epiglottitis is a medical emergency. The patient should be allowed to sit up, as this often helps to keep the airway open. An intravenous infusion should be started and high-dose antibiotic treatment begun immediately. The treatment of choice is a broad-spectrum cephalosporin such as cefotaxime. Chloramphenicol is an acceptable alternative with a low risk of resistance. There is approximately a 15% risk of resistance to ampicillin, which is not a drug of first choice. There is a risk of recrudescence if the treatment is stopped too soon. A course of 10 days is adequate for most cases.

Treatment of acute epiglotittis
1 First choice: cefotaxime: child — intravenous 150–250 mg/kg daily in two to four divided doses; adult — 2–4 g 8-hourly. Or ceftriaxone: child — 50 mg/kg as a single daily dose; adult — 2–4 g as a single daily dose.
2 Second choice: child or adult — intravenous chloramphenicol 50–100 mg/kg daily in three or four divided doses; may be continued orally at 50 mg/kg daily.
All above regimens for 10 days.
NB Consider a single bolus dose of corticosteroid to reduce epiglottic oedema.

If the airway is critically obstructed, oxygen should be given by mask while urgent tracheostomy is considered. A bolus dose of corticosteroid may reduce oedema and avoid the need for tracheostomy while antibiotic therapy is taking effect. It will not compromise the response to treatment. Many ear, nose and throat departments keep a supply of heliox (80% helium and 20% oxygen), which has an extremely low viscosity and will pass much better than pure oxygen through a tiny airway or a small cannula in the trachea.

Complications

Once the patient reaches medical care the mortality is low and the complications are mainly those of intubation and ventilation; hypostatic lung infections, pneumothorax in young children, and infected tracheostomy sites. Metastatic complications of the bacteraemia are rare, but a few cases also have pneumonia or skeletal infection, which responds to the treatment for epiglottitis.

Prevention and control

See Chapter 16; *Haemophilus influenzae.*

Diphtheria

Introduction

Diphtheria is an infection of the respiratory mucosa, and sometimes of broken skin, caused by *Corynebacterium diphtheriae*. Although preventable by childhood immunization, it is important because of its severe acute and late effects. Immigrants may suffer from the disease or carry the organism in the nose and throat. Vaccine-induced immunity declines in adult life. Tourists may unwittingly pass through endemic areas, and be unexpectedly infected. Transmission is favoured by crowding; the incubation period is short and many asymptomatic carriers often exist for every case identified. Outbreaks are therefore a severe challenge to public health control measures.

Epidemiology

Humans are the only reservoir of infection. The disease is spread by direct contact with cases or carriers. Patients with cutaneous diphtheria are more infectious than those with pharyngeal and other forms.

Diphtheria was a common disease during the 19th century, with up to 10 000 deaths recorded each year. Most of the deaths were in children under the age of 5. Children living in crowded accommodation were particularly at risk. During the early part of the 20th century, the disease remained common, although the case fatality ratio declined by almost 50%. This decline has been attributed to a number of factors, including a change in virulence of the organism and the availability of antitoxin treatment.

Following the introduction of routine immunization in 1942 in Britain, the incidence declined rapidly and by the 1960s diphtheria had almost been eliminated. Since then a handful of cases have been reported each year. Most of these are in adults and are acquired abroad, although limited indigenous tranmission does occur from time to time. It is noteworthy that the case fatality ratio for diphtheria has increased slightly since 1960 (from 5 to 8 per 100), probably because of failure to recognize the disease now that it is so rare. *C. ulcerans* infection from unpasteurized milk occasionally presents as classical diphtheria.

Immunization also resulted in a decrease in carriers of both toxigenic and non-toxigenic strains of *C. diphtheriae*. This was unexpected, as a toxoid preparation should in theory only protect against the toxic manifestations of disease. The reason for the decline in carriers has not been satisfactorily explained.

In tropical countries where hygiene is poor, diphtheria is still common. Here the usual presentation is the cutaneous form of disease, which is often limited in extent, and confers immunity without a severe, toxic illness. Nasal diphtheria also tends to be mild, but the infected discharge is important in the spread of disease among children.

In recent years there has been a resurgence of disease in the former USSR, due to declining vaccine coverage (Fig. 6.12).

Pathology

The consequences of infection with *C. diphtheriae* are twofold: the effects of the potent exotoxin; and obstruction of the airway by necrotic debris, which forms a tough, pseudomembrane on infected respiratory mucosa (Fig. 6.13).

Diphtheria toxin is the major pathogenicity determinant of *C. diphtheriae*. The genetic sequence encoding the toxin resides on a beta-phage. Bacteria not infected by the phage are non-toxigenic and non-pathogenic. The

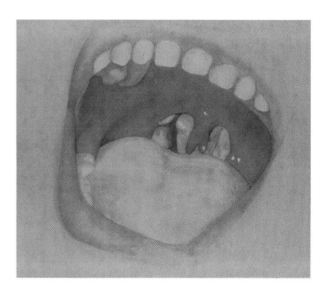

Fig. 6.13 Diphtheria: the off-white, smooth pseudomembrane affects the tonsils and pharynx.

protein toxin posesses three domains. A receptor portion binds to the target cell and the central portion, which is highly hydrophobic, dissolves in the cell membrane, carrying the toxin portion into the cell. The toxin itself is an adenosine diphosphate ribosylase which ribosylates an amino acid diphthamide present in elongation factor 2. Elongation factor 2 is essential for protein synthesis in the host cell, and its inhibition leads to cell death.

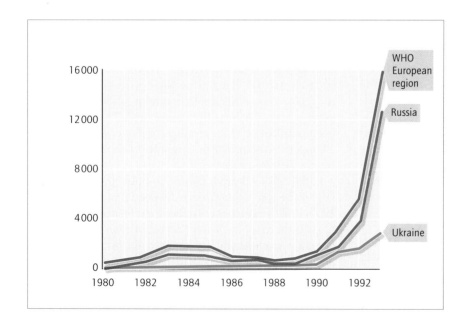

Fig. 6.12 Trends in diphtheria reporting in Europe. Reported cases in the WHO European region, Russia and the Ukraine, 1980–93.

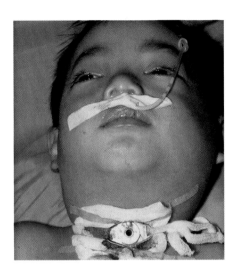

Fig. 6.14 Diphtheria: bull-neck appearance and tracheostomy. Courtesy of the World Health Organization.

Clinical features

After an incubation period of 3–5 days, the infected site becomes inflamed and gradually covered by a spreading, tough, adherent slough (often called the membrane). The resulting symptoms depend on the site affected. The toxic effects of diphtheria are proportional to the extent of the infection, indicated by the area of membrane.

Pharyngeal diphtheria is the commonest respiratory form. This presents with fever, sore throat and marked oedema of the cervical lymph nodes, which may produce a bull-neck (Fig. 6.14). The membrane may affect the tonsils but, unlike the exudate of infectious mononucleosis, also spreads across the pharyngeal mucosa. It is usually greyish and semitransparent, opacified where it contains areas of altered blood, and sometimes blackened and necrotic. It is strongly adherent, and attempts to scrape it away cause pain and bleeding.

The combination of swelling and thickening membrane easily threatens the airway, causing early stridor. Children often assume a characteristic posture, leaning forward with the neck extended, to hold the airway open.

Diphtheria can also affect the larynx and trachea, and then presents as croup. The true diagnosis may be suggested if a membrane is visible in the pharynx, but if it only exists in the lower airways it may be missed. Only a strong index of suspicion will allow prompt diagnosis in such cases.

Other sites which may be affected include the nares, the conjunctiva and small areas of broken skin, such as abrasions or ulcers. These small sites are inflamed, often produce a serosanguineous exudate and may have small adherent patches of membrane. *C. diphtheriae* can colonize sites of other infections and has been found in impetigo, cellulitis and broken chickenpox lesions.

During acute diphtheria there is a modest fever, but disproportionate tiredness or prostration. There is a neutrophilia in the peripheral blood, but minimal disturbance of renal and liver function.

Diphtheria toxin

The diphtheria toxin causes early cardiac damage and late neurological lesions. In the first week there is loss of the fibrillar structure of heart muscle cells and inflammation of the myocardium. Heart failure and conduction defects are likely, and profound heart block is a risk. Attempts to treat failure with digoxin may exacerbate the heart block. The myocardium recovers completely when convalescence is established.

The neurological damage is caused by demyelination. It occurs earliest and most severely near to the site of the membrane. Palatal and ocular palsies are common after throat infections. More severe cases have more extensive defects and after 3 or 4 weeks can develop a generalized weakness or paralysis similar to Guillain–Barré syndrome. Like the myocardial damage, the demyelination is fully reversible.

In rare cases a late nephritis causes impared renal function.

Fatalities are usually due to irreversible heart failure. Intrabronchial or tracheal membrane can cause respiratory failure. Very severe cases occasionally die with a Waterhouse–Friderichsen syndrome of adrenal failure and haemorrhagic features.

Diagnosis

Clinical suspicion is aroused by severe throat or pharyngeal swelling with modest fever, severe prostration and neutrophilia. The presence of a typical, spreading membrane allows clinical diagnosis to be acted upon.

Laboratory diagnosis

Specimens from the throat, larynx, nose or skin may be sent. Swabs are adequate. It is very important to inform the laboratory that diphtheria is suspected, otherwise

Organism	Sucrose hydrolysis	Mannitol hydrolysis	Starch hydrolysis	Glycogen hydrolysis	Urease	Nitrate production	Toxins D	Cp	Both
C. diphtheriae var. gravis	+	+	+	+		+	+		
C. diphtheriae var. intermedius	–	+	–	–		+	+		
C. diphtheriae var. mitis	+	+	–	–		+	+		
C. ulcerans	–		+		+	–	+	+	+

D = diphtheria toxin; Cp = toxin produced only by the animal pathogen C. *pseudotuberculosis* and by C. *ulcerans*.

Table 6.2 *Corynebacterium diphtheriae*: tests to identify and distinguish *gravis, intermedius* and *mitis* biotypes

special media will not be inoculated and the pathogen may be discarded as a diphtheroid. Specimens suspected of harbouring diphtheria should be inoculated on to a slope of Loeffler's medium and a tellurite-containing blood agar such as Hoyle's medium. The Loeffler's slope contains a rich serum medium and the organisms grow rapidly. Sufficient growth is usually available after 6 h to allow staining by Albert's method which demonstrates the volutin granules found in this species. The organism should then be subcultured on to blood agar for biochemical confirmation using sugar tests adapted for corynebacteria (Table 6.2). On tellurite media corynebacteria reduce tellurite to a black substance. The colonies have a black shiny appearance, aiding selection for identification.

Confirmation of toxigenicity is made either serologically by precipitin tests on Elek or Jamieson plates, or biologically by intradermal injection in susceptible guinea-pigs (Fig. 6.15). Polymerase chain amplification allows rapid detection of the toxin gene in C. *diphtheriae* isolates.

It must be emphasized that the laboratory's role is to confirm the presence of toxigenic C. *diphtheriae* and to alert the public health services. The identification of non-toxigenic C. *diphtheriae* requires no public health control measures.

Management

Early intervention greatly reduces the risk both of respiratory obstruction and of severe intoxication.

Antibiotic treatment

Antibiotic treatment consists of intravenous benzyl-penicillin. Parenteral erythromycin or a cephalosporin are reasonable alternatives. The inflammation and fever respond within 24–36 h. As inflammation subsides the membrane loosens. Casts of the upper airway or bronchi may be shed, sometimes needing assisted removal by suction or bronchoscopy.

Antitoxin

Antitoxin is given to neutralize circulating toxin and prevent further damage to myocardium and myelin. Dosage depends on the extent of infection, and ranges from 8000 U for nasal disease to 120 000 U for aggressive nasolaryngeal diphthcria. The average dose is 30 000–40 000 U for tonsillar or pharyngeal disease.

Antitoxin treatment in diphtheria		
Type of diphtheria	*Dose (units)*	*Route*
Nasal	10 000–20 000	Intramuscular
Tonsillar	15 000–25 000	Intramuscular or intravenous
Pharyngeal or laryngeal	20 000–40 000	Intramuscular or intravenous
Combined sites or late diagnosis	40 000–60 000	Intravenous
Cutaneous disease	Not widely recommended: wound toilet and antibiotics preferred	

Precede full dose by subcutaneous test dose of antitoxin, e.g. 50–100 U 30 min before main dose. (From WHO (1994) *Manual for the Management and Control of Diphtheria in the European Region.* World Health Organization.)

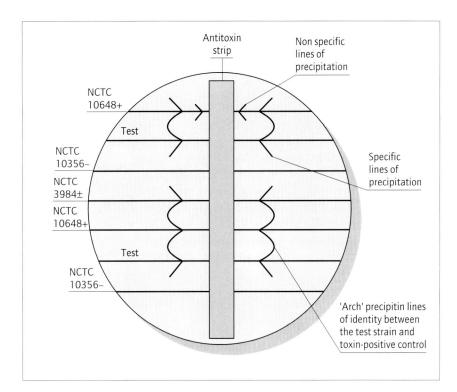

Antitoxin strip

Non specific lines of precipitation

NCTC 10648+

Test

NCTC 10356−

NCTC 3984±

NCTC 10648+

Test

NCTC 10356−

Specific lines of precipitation

'Arch' precipitin lines of identity between the test strain and toxin-positive control

Fig. 6.15 Elek plate showing positive precipitin test for toxin production by *Corynebacterium diphtheriae*. Courtesy of Dr A. Efstratiou, Central Public Health Laboratory. NCTC 10648, toxin-positive control; NCTC 10356, toxin negative; NCTC 3984, weak positive.

Human immunoglobulin is not effective, so diphtheria antitoxin is a horse serum preparation. A small intramuscular test dose is therefore given 30–45 min before the main dose, to detect possible hypersensitivity. In severe cases half of the main dose may be given intravenously and half intramuscularly.

Elective tracheostomy

Elective tracheostomy may be performed soon after admission if membrane and oedema threaten the airway. It avoids possible emergency tracheostomy, which is difficult when the tissues are very oedematous. It also provides airway protection if palatal palsy develops later.

Diphtheria cases require prolonged observation to detect cardiographic changes, rhythm disturbances and late neurological complications, which may require airway protection or other support. When patients have recovered, they are likely to be carriers of *C. diphtheriae*. It is usual to obtain three negative nose and throat swabs to indicate clearance. Carriage is difficult to eliminate, often requiring erythromycin treatment for 10–14 days (penicillin will not eradicate carriage).

Prevention and control

Diphtheria vaccine is a formalin-inactivated toxoid preparation. A standard paediatric dose contains at least 30 IU of antigen. In adults and children over 10 years a low-dose (1.5 IU) vaccine should be used because of the risk of hypersensitivity reactions. Three doses of vaccine given at monthly intervals, starting at 2 months of age, are recommended for primary immunization in the UK, with a booster dose 3 years later and again before leaving school (see Chapter 25). Nowadays over 95% of children in the UK receive a full course of vaccine. Adults born before 1942, when routine immunization was introduced, have only naturally acquired antibody. Up to 25% of people in this age group have no measurable antibody.

Measuring immunity to diphtheria by antitoxin concentration

1 <0.01 IU/ml: no protection.

   0.01–0.10 IU/ml: partial protection.

3 >0.10 IU/ml: reliable protection.

Diphtheria is a notifiable disease. Cases and carriers of toxigenic strains should be isolated until three consecutive throat and nose cultures taken 24–48 h apart (the first at least 5 days after completion of antibiotic therapy) are negative. Close contacts should have cultures taken, and also be kept under surveillance for a minimum of 7 days from the last date of exposure to the case. Contacts should also receive a booster dose of vaccine (or a full primary course if unimmunized) and a course of chemoprophylaxis. The regimen for chemoprophylaxis is erythromycin 250 mg four times a day for 7 days. Bacteriological clearance should be demonstrated in any contacts found to be carriers by taking two consecutive nose and throat swabs, the first at least 5 days after completion of chemoprophylaxis.

Ludwig's angina

This is a suppurative infection of the hypoglossal tissue planes. It may become an ear, nose and throat emergency because the oedema and exudate push the tongue upwards and backwards, deform the pharynx and threaten the airway.

The origins of the infection are probably the mouth and teeth. A range of organisms may be responsible, and most infections are polymicrobial. Typical implicated organisms include *Streptococcus pyogenes*, *Staphylococcus aureus*, viridans streptococci and 'mouth' anaerobes such as *Prevotella melaninogenicus* and *Fusobacterium* spp.

Clinical features develop rapidly. They include pain, fever, difficulty in swallowing and increasing stridor. Examination shows a bull-neck appearance with tenderness of the neck and throat. It is difficult to open the mouth and, when it is open, the tongue is elevated so that its underside is visible above the lower teeth. The fauces may also be swollen.

Treatment should be prompt. Antibiotics should include one active against *S. aureus*. Satisfactory therapy includes penicillin plus cloxacillin or flucloxacillin, or a cephalosporin such as cefuroxime or cefotaxime. Although these agents are effective against mouth anaerobes, metronidazole penetrates oedematous tissues well and may be useful additional treatment. Treatment should usually last for about 10 days.

Oedema may be reduced medically with a bolus dose of corticosteroid, e.g. 200 mg hydrocortisone. If this does not provide significant or sustained relief, drainage of pus from the sublingual space may be effective. This is performed by passing perforated drains through the floor of the mouth and out through the skin anterior to the hyoid bone.

Retropharyngeal abscess

This is a suppurative infection in the tissue spaces behind the pharynx. Normally there is only a narrow space between the posterior pharyngeal wall and the anterior ligaments of the spinal column. If oedema and pus expand this space, the posterior pharyngeal wall is pushed forwards, obstructing the airway.

The abnormal position of the pharyngeal wall is difficult to see on inspection, especially if the abscess is low in the throat. Many patients therefore present as emergencies, with neck or throat pain and difficulty in breathing. The diagnosis can be demonstrated by showing a wide soft-tissue space between the vertebrae and the air-filled pharynx on a lateral X-ray of the neck.

Emergency tracheostomy may be life-saving in urgent cases. Medical treatment is identical to that for Ludwig's angina, as the infection is almost always of mouth origin (and only rarely from a spinal infection). Pus can be released by incising the posterior pharyngeal wall. Spinal infection should be excluded by appropriate imaging of the spinal tissues. Rare cases of retropharyngeal abscess result from cervical infection with tuberculosis or (in endemic areas) brucellosis, so pus should be obtained for culture if the spine is involved.

Vincent's angina

This is a synergistic infection of the mouth which particularly affects the gums. It is associated with poor dental health and poor oral hygiene. The patient presents with extreme soreness of the mouth and gums, accompanied by an offensive halitosis.

The microbial cause is the synergistic action of the mouth spirochaete *Borrelia vincenti* and the anaerobe *Fusiformis*. If laboratory confirmation of the diagnosis is needed, they can be demonstrated in large numbers by making a Gram stain of the material on a mouth swab.

Treatment with metronidazole will quickly eradicate the anaerobic organisms. Penicillin or ampicillin is also effective. Improved mouth care may be needed to avoid recurrence.

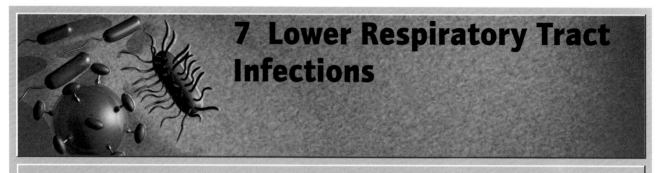

7 Lower Respiratory Tract Infections

Introduction

The lower respiratory tract comprises those structures extending downwards from the vocal cords.

The trachea, bronchi and bronchioles are lined with ciliated columnar respiratory epithelium, within which are distributed mucus-producing goblet cells. The walls of the airways contain smooth-muscle cells, and are also elastic, dilating on inspiration and narrowing during expiration. Any narrowing of the lumen of an air passage therefore becomes more noticeable during expiration.

The smallest bronchioles lose their muscular coating as they approach the alveoli, and their epithelium becomes flat and non-ciliated. The alveoli themselves are lined with two types of cells — smooth, flat cells and slightly thicker cells with a granular cytoplasm. The thicker cells are related to the alveolar macrophages, which are mobile within the alveoli. The alveolar cells are separated from the underlying capillary endothelium by a film of interstitial fluid, which is in hydrodynamic equilibrium with the alveoli (which usually contain no fluid) and the capillary blood.

The normal lower respiratory tract is bacteriologically sterile. Inhaled particles, including bacteria, are trapped in the mucus which lines the airways and is moved constantly towards the pharynx by the beating of the epithelial cilia. The mucus is swallowed when it enters the pharynx, and most of the bacteria and debris it contains are destroyed by gastric acid. Particles which reach the alveoli are phagocytosed by alveolar macrophages, which are also eventually expelled from the respiratory tract by the 'ciliary escalator'.

Common mechanical problems in the respiratory tract include:

1 Paralysis of the cilia by cigarette smoke.
2 Excessive volumes of mucus which cannot be effectively cleared.
3 Mucus too thick to be effectively cleared (in cystic fibrosis).
4 Paroxysmal narrowing of the airways by asthma attacks.
5 Immobilization or damage of alveolar macrophages by particles which they cannot destroy (e.g. silica or asbestos particles).

Each of these adverse factors tends to impair the clearance of bacteria or other particles from the lower respiratory tract. Although the larger airways can be cleared by coughing, this cannot maintain the patency of smaller airways, even when supplemented by vigorous physiotherapy.

The lower respiratory tract is exposed to a variety of inhaled pathogens, which in its healthy state it can often expel before infection becomes established. It must also defend itself against the flora of the pharynx which constantly seek to colonize it. *Streptococcus pneumoniae* and *Haemophilus influenzae* are common colonists, which are also potential pathogens.

Their rich blood supply makes the lungs vulnerable to infection by blood-borne organisms, of which *Staphylococcus aureus* is the most important.

Although the lower respiratory tract has several defence mechanisms, they are interdependent, and many rely ultimately on ciliary clearance and coughing. These can be disrupted by intrinsic lung abnormalities or interrupted by unconciousness, paralysis or intubation.

Non-infectious conditions can mimic lower respiratory infections, by presenting with fever and cough or shortness of breath. These include:

1 Autoimmune disorders such as systemic lupus erythematosus.

2 Granulomatous conditions such as sarcoidosis.

3 Vasculitides, particularly Wegener's granulomatosis or polyarteritis nodosa (both of which can also produce nodular opacities on chest X-ray).

4 Hypersensitivity reactions such as farmer's lung or the more severe Goodpasture's syndrome.

5 Malignancies, such as infiltrating lymphomata.

Laboratory diagnosis

Introduction

A comprehensive diagnosis of lower respiratory tract infections is difficult, due to the diversity of possible causative pathogens. For most patients, therefore, diagnostic efforts are directed at the common important pathogens. For most patients adequate diagnosis can be achieved by a combination of sputum microscopy and culture, and serological tests on blood.

Sputum examination

This is one of the commonest procedures carried out in the microbiological laboratory but one about which there is most controversy, because of the difficulty in obtaining adequate specimens. The help of a physiotherapist is often valuable in obtaining lung secretions, rather than a specimen containing mostly saliva and buccal epithelial cells.

The specimen is examined initially by microscopy of a Gram-stained smear. Specimens containing few polymorphs and more than 25 epithelial cells per low-power field are largely salivary, and are likely to yield only upper respiratory tract flora on culture. Alternatively, a specimen containing neutrophils and ciliated columnar cells is largely of bronchial origin. Some organisms, such as *Klebsiella pneumoniae*, have a characteristic morphology and are seen in high numbers when causing infection.

One of the main problems facing the microbiologist is that the common respiratory pathogens also occur in the normal upper respiratory tract flora. This can be overcome by estimating the numbers of organisms in the specimen, using semiquantitative methods, assuming that organisms acting as pathogens reach higher concentrations than those acting as commensals. Organisms present at more than 10^6 cfu/ml are considered more likely to be acting as pathogens. The results of semiquantitative sputum culture can compare favourably with the culture of specimens obtained directly from the lower respiratory tract (e.g. by cricoid puncture or by bronchial aspiration).

Bronchoalveolar lavage

Bronchoscopy is a valuable aid in the diagnosis of lower respiratory infections with unusual pathogens or in immunocompromised patients (who rarely produce excess sputum because of their reduced inflammatory responses). The bronchoscope is passed into a lower airway and 100–200 ml of sterile saline is injected and aspirated. Although the material has come directly from the alveoli without having to pass through the pharynx, semiquantitative methods are advisable, as contamination can still occur from the advancing end of the bronchoscope. Organisms present at more than 10^3 cfu/ml may be pathogens. Bronchoalveolar lavage is of particular value for the diagnosis of infections such as tuberculosis, legionellosis, fungal infections and *Pneumocystis carinii* infection.

> **Obtaining specimens from the lower respiratory tract**
> 1 Sputum obtained by coughing.
> 2 Cricoid puncture.
> 3 Direct bronchial aspiration.
> 4 Broncheolar lavage.

Viral infections of the lower respiratory tract

Introduction

Viral respiratory infections are among the most common infections of humanity. Many infections of the lower respiratory tract pass unremarked. These are often part of a systemic disease such as measles, varicella or infectious mononucleosis, or mild cases of influenza or respiratory syncytial virus (RSV) infection, and are only recognized if a chest X-ray is carried out. Nevertheless, viral infections can cause severe, and occasionally life-threatening, pulmonary disease.

Laboratory diagnosis

Specimens of nasopharyngeal secretions, which always contain shed respiratory cells, should be obtained from children under the age of 5 years. A fine-bore catheter is passed through the nostril into the nasopharynx and secretions are aspirated using gentle suction either via a 20 or 50 ml syringe or a low-pressure suction apparatus. In order children and adults, specimens may be obtained by gargling normal saline.

Direct immunofluorescence is a useful rapid laboratory test for those viral infections against which strongly binding antibodies are available. RSV can be demonstrated by this method, which is also occasionally used for influenza, parainfluenza or measles. Nasopharyngeal secretions are dried on a Teflon-coated slide, acetone-fixed and incubated with rabbit antibody to the expected virus. If viral antigen is present in the respiratory cells, the rabbit antibody will bind to it, and is demonstrated by staining with fluorescein-labelled antirabbit antibodies.

ORGANISM LIST

Influenza virus
Parainfluenza viruses
RSV
Adenoviruses
Measles, varicella and Epstein–Barr viruses.

Croup

Introduction

Croup is a syndrome of laryngotracheobronchitis, which usually affects children but also occurs occasionally in adults. Its importance is that almost every young child has at least one episode, it is often a child's first severe illness, the physical signs are distressing and there is a risk of respiratory obstruction in the most severe cases. Most of the obstruction is caused by gross oedema of the airway just below the vocal cords; the common syndrome of croup must be distinguished from rarer causes of obstruction such as epiglottitis or diphtheria.

Epidemiology

Croup is common in infants. The principal causal agents are parainfluenza viruses types 1 and 2 which circulate during the late autumn and winter months. They are highly infectious by the air-borne route. Prodromal measles causes a similar cough; influenza can cause croup in both adults and children.

Organisms which may cause croup
1 Parainfluenza virus.
2 Influenza virus.
3 Measles virus.
4 Respiratory syncytial virus.
5 *Haemophilus influenzae*
6 *Corynebacterium diphtheriae*

Pathology

Parainfluenza viruses are classifed in the genus *Paramyxovirus* within the family Paramyxoviridae. Four parainfluenza virus types (types 1–4) are pathogenic to humans. The virus is pleomorphic with a roughly spherical shape, 120–300 nm in diameter, and possesses an envelope. The envelope contains glycoprotein projections of haemagglutinin and a neuraminidase. The virion contains a helical nucleocapsid, with single-stranded negative-sense RNA. Negative-sense RNA is transcribed by virally encoded transcriptase into positive complementary RNA.

The virus invades epithelial cells throughout the tracheobronchial tree. Involvement of the aryepiglottic folds of the larynx causes swelling, obstruction and the characteristic stridor and croup.

The infection falls mainly on the columnar ciliated cells with loss of ciliary function. There is oedema of the mucosa, with an acute neutrophilic infiltrate. In a minority of cases a severe pneumonia develops; in fatal cases the lungs are dark red, with a haemorrhagic bronchiolitis and also loss of ciliated epithelium. Polymorphs and macrophages are found in the alveolar exudate.

Clinical features

The syndrome develops rapidly, with bursts of harsh, barking coughs interspersed with noisy breathing. Many cases are trivial or mild, with no other features. In more severe cases there is fever and increasing stridor, sometimes with recession of the intercostal spaces on inspiration. Initially the patient may lie quietly, but restlessness and tachycardia increase as respiratory obstruction develops. Auscultation of the chest rarely reveals abnormal sounds, unless the bronchi are involved enough to be loaded with mucus. Cyanosis is a late and grave sign. Most cases resolve within a week, but a croupy cough may return if there are further respiratory infections in following weeks.

Diagnosis

In most cases this is clinical, based on the presence of a typical cough. A low or normal white cell count supports a probable viral aetiology. In patients with neutrophilia, other causes of croup or pharyngeal obstruction should be considered. These include epiglottitis and occasionally diphtheria.

A parainfluenza virus may be demonstrable by immunofluorescent staining of nasopharyngeal aspirate, or may be recovered by cell culture of respiratory secretions. Serodiagnosis is rarely undertaken.

Management

The classic management of surrounding the patient with a warm, steamy atmosphere is often effective. It relieves pain, reduces cough, and the heat may inhibit viral replication. Controlled trials have recently confirmed that short courses of corticosteroids also reduce oedema and improve airway function without causing adverse effects. Intravenous doses of 25–50 mg hydrocortisone (100–200 mg in an adult) may be repeated three or four times on the first day. Oral prednisolone 1–2 mg/kg

daily (up to 40 mg daily for an adult) should be continued for a further 2 or 3 days.

In suspected bacterial cases, antibiotic treatment should be commenced while efforts are made to confirm the diagnosis by X-ray and/or culture (see Chapter 3).

Bronchiolitis

Introduction

This is similar in its pathology to croup, but the small bronchioles are affected instead of the upper airways. In this condition respiratory difficulties often develop suddenly in a child with an apparently mild illness. This causes considerable morbidity in infants, but with modern treatment mortality is very low.

Epidemiology

The infection principally affects infants up to the age of 2 years. Epidemics occur during late winter and early spring (Fig. 7.1). These are usually due to RSV, although other viruses may cause epidemics. Epidemics often coincide with increases in the incidence of sudden infant death syndrome, suggesting a possible role of RSV in its aetiology. Preterm infants and those with congenital heart disease are at particular risk of severe infection. Serious outbreaks have been reported among newborn babies on intensive care units.

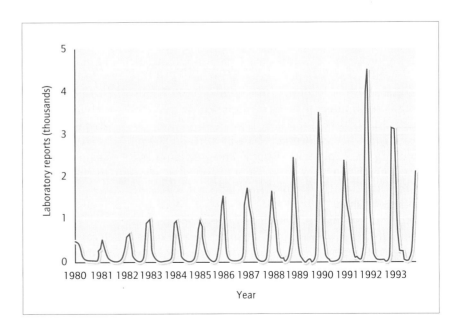

Fig. 7.1 Epidemic curve of respiratory syncytial virus infections, showing regular winter/spring epidemics.

Humans are the only source of infection. The incubation period is 5–8 days and the patient remains infectious for about 7 days after the onset of symptoms.

Pathology

RSV is a member of the genus Pneumovirus in the family Paramyxoviridae. It is an enveloped virus of 120–300 nm diameter, with 12 nm glycoprotein projections lying 10 nm apart. The helical RNA genome codes for at least 10 polypeptides including F and G envelope-associated glycoproteins. The F or fusion protein is associated with penetration of the virus into cells, and spread from cell to cell. The larger G protein is responsible for initial attachment of the virus to host cells. There is antigenic variation among strains of RSV but this is not easy to demonstrate, as human sera produce neutralizing antibody which neutralizes all viruses of this genus.

RSV is acquired through the upper respiratory tract and spreads throughout the respiratory epithelium. Infection is characterized by peribronchial inflammation, associated with oedema of the submucosa and adventitium. There is necrosis of the bronchiolar epithelium and plugging of these airways. This has a particular impact on infants, whose small airways are prone to obstruction. When the bronchiolar lumen is incompletely obstructed a ball-valve effect occurs, which results in air trapping, and the characteristic hyperinflation seen in this condition.

Clinical features

Initially the child seems to have a cold with catarrh and a loose cough. Then after 3 or 4 days the respiratory rate suddenly increases, and intercostal recession appears. Paradoxically, fever usually becomes less severe at this stage. Breathing is laboured and wheezy, and bottle-feeding is often impossible, as crying or feeding causes cyanosis.

Examination of the chest reveals widespread wheeze, particularly in expiration. Patchy areas of dullness, reduced breath sounds or adventitious sounds are common and may change with coughing, which is repetitive and often constant.

Complete bronchiolar obstruction causes atelectasis in parts of the lung, while partial obstruction causes air trapping and hyperinflation elsewhere. The chest X-ray therefore shows areas of both opacity and lucency, which often change from day to day.

Slow improvement begins after 5 or 6 days. It may take a week or two for the child to return to normal, but the capillary oxygen saturation is often subnormal for twice as long.

Diagnosis

Clinical diagnosis is often obvious.

Laboratory diagnosis

Laboratory diagnosis of RSV infection can be made by immunofluorescence or enzyme immunoassay (EIA) performed on nasopharyngeal secretions. Sensitivity between 70 and 100% can be expected. RSV can also be cultured in HEp 2 or HeLa cells. The characteristic cytopathic effect is the formation of syncytia, generally seen between 2 and 7 days after inoculation.

A retrospective diagnosis can also be achieved by detecting rising titres of RSV antibodies, by complement fixation, virus neutralization, EIA and indirect immunofluorescence tests.

> **Laboratory diagnosis of respiratory syncytial virus infection**
> 1 Direct immunofluorescence of respiratory secretions.
> 2 Cell culture.
> 3 Serological: complement fixation, enzyme immunoassay or indirect immunofluorescence.

Management

Oxygenation and adequate hydration are the immediate requirements. Humidified oxygen can be given in a cot-sized oxygen tent. The inspired oxygen concentration is adjusted to maintain as near normal arterial oxygen saturation as possible. Pulse oximetry is a useful means of monitoring saturation.

Bronchospasm plays little part in the bronchiolar narrowing, so bronchodilators are rarely helpful. A trial of nebulized salbutamol is worthwhile however if there is a past or family history of atopy.

Hydration is best maintained by intravenous infusion, as this also gives access for antibiotic or other supportive treatment if needed.

Nebulized tribavirin

Nebulized tribavirin shortens the duration of hypoxia and fever in bronchiolitis, and is licensed for this use. Its effect is small and is of limited benefit in otherwise healthy infants. Morbidity from bronchiolitis is great, however, in those with pre-existing cardiac or lung disorders; tribavirin may be of benefit to these children.

Complications

Secondary bacterial infection is uncommon, but can threaten life. The reappearance of high fever, change from mucoid to purulent sputum, sustained deterioration in oxygen saturation and rising neutrophil count are all warning signs. The chest X-ray may show a segmental opacity or an air bronchogram, suggesting consolidation.

Blood and sputum cultures should be obtained and antibiotic treatment started without delay. A cephalosporin such as cefuroxime or cefotaxime will be effective against *Streptococcus pneumoniae* or *Haemophilus influenzae*, which are the likely pathogens. Treatment must usually be given intravenously.

Influenza

Introduction

Influenza is a moderate to severe illness most often caused by influenza A or B viruses. It is highly infectious to susceptibles, and with its short incubation period it can cause overwhelming epidemics. Sudden loss of staff caused by epidemics adversely affects commerce, industry and public services. Individuals with the disease can be seriously ill, and severe secondary bacterial infections cause as much morbidity and mortality as the influenza itself.

Pathology

Influenza virus infects ciliated respiratory cells, killing many, and causing shedding of the majority. This leaves denuded airways, which are susceptible to colonization and invasion by bacterial pathogens. There is a vigorous immune response to the infection, with much production of interferon and temporary impairment of cell-mediated immunity (the tuberculin reaction cannot be elicited until convalescence is complete). Although influenza viraemia is difficult to demonstrate, viral genome is present in large quantities within the mononuclear cells of the blood during acute infection.

Virology

Influenza virus is part of the genus Orthomyxovirus in the family Orthomyxoviridae. Virus particles are 80–120 nm in diameter. The RNA genome is segmented, with four fragments. The RNA is closely associated with nucleoprotein (NP) in a helical structure. The NP is specific to the three types of influenza virus: A, B and C. The matrix

protein or membrane protein, with a mass of 2 kDa, surrounds the nucleocapsid and is the major protein of the virus particle. This is enclosed by the envelope, which contains two virus-encoded glycoproteins: the haemagglutinin, responsible for attachment of the virus to host cell receptors, and the neuraminidase, of molecular weight 200–250 kDa (Fig. 7.2). Both the haemagglutinin and the neuraminidase are antigenically variable, and this is useful in the classification of the viruses.

Epidemiology

Epidemics of influenza occur in most years during the winter months. These are usually due to type A viruses, although type B epidemics and mixed type A and type B epidemics also occur. Type C is occasionally recognized as causing local outbreaks. Attack rates during epidemics seldom exceed 10% in the general community, but may be much higher — up to 50% — in closed institutions such as boarding schools and nursing homes for the elderly. Extensive pandemics are much less common. This century, pandemics have been recorded in 1918, 1957 and 1968.

These epidemiological findings are mirrored by the changes in the antigenic structure of the virus.

Antigenic drift is responsible for the yearly epidemics as new subtypes of haemagglutinin slowly evolve. Infection with an epidemic strain provides antibody which will cross-react with closely related haemagglutinin types, and confers partial immunity to infection by slowly evolving types from year to year. Antigenic drift arises in the virus because of selection pressure imposed by the partial immunity of the population. Periodically a major change (shift) occurs in the haemagglutinin or neuraminidase antigen. The population has little or no cross-reacting antibody to the 'new' virus, and a pandemic results.

Age-specific attack rates during an epidemic reflect existing immunity from exposure to previously prevalent strains. Attack rates are often highest among school-age children. In contrast, complication rates and mortality are greatest in the elderly and those with underlying chronic conditions. The most severe forms of infection occur during pandemics.

Excess mortality during influenza epidemics
1 During an influenza epidemic, deaths due to respiratory disease may increase by as much as 50%.
2 Deaths due to cerebrovascular and cardiovascular disease also increase.
3 Excess mortality is not usually followed by a deficit during the following year.

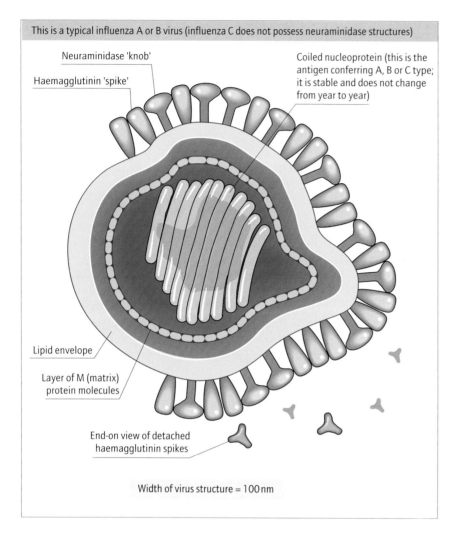

This is a typical influenza A or B virus (influenza C does not possess neuraminidase structures)

Neuraminidase 'knob'

Haemagglutinin 'spike'

Coiled nucleoprotein (this is the antigen conferring A, B or C type; it is stable and does not change from year to year)

Lipid envelope

Layer of M (matrix) protein molecules

End-on view of detached haemagglutinin spikes

Width of virus structure = 100 nm

Fig. 7.2 Structure of influenza viruses.

4 There were an estimated 26 080 excess deaths attributable to influenza in England and Wales during the 1989/90 epidemic.
5 Between 80% and 90% of excess deaths are in people aged 65 years or over.

Clinical features

After an incubation period of 3 or 4 days there is a sudden onset of severe malaise and prostration. Fever may be high, sometimes with shivering and sweating. The malaise and loss of appetite can be so severe that the disease begins with an episode of vomiting. There is dull aching in the muscles and constant or stabbing arthralgia. A variable range of associated symptoms includes headache, sore throat, loose stools and shortness of breath. Uncomplicated influenza usually persists

for 5–7 days before the fever decreases and gradual convalescence begins.

The respiratory tract is the most important target of the infection. There is always a viral pneumonitis, which may be widespread and relatively mild, or may take the form of interstitial pneumonia or a segmental infection. Severe pneumonitis can cause considerable morbidity and sometimes death. Other respiratory features include tracheitis, croupy cough, laryngitis and sometimes sinusitis and conjunctivitis. Influenza C infections are uncommon. They are often mild, and conjunctivitis is a prominent feature.

Other body systems can be significantly affected. There is often a subclinical myocarditis with altered electrocardiogram patterns and variable types and numbers of extrasystoles. Postural or exercise-related hypotension can lead to fainting.

There is a low but definite rate of viral encephalitis or meningoencephalitis in influenza epidemics. This co-incides with viral excretion from the respiratory tract. Cases often present with headache, meningism, irritability, altered personality and drowsiness. Examination of cerebrospinal fluid (CSF) shows excess lymphocytes and slightly raised protein levels. Recovery is slow and fluctuating.

Laboratory findings

Laboratory findings reflect the severity of tissue damage and the response to interferon production. The white cell count is low, often 3 or $4 \times 10^9/l$. The transaminase levels are raised, and are of both liver and tissue origin. Oxygen saturation, measured by pulse oximetry, is often reduced, even when there is no clinical evidence of significant pneumonitis. Some patients with severe myalgia and weakness have elevated creatine kinase levels.

Complications

Secondary bacterial infection

Secondary bacterial infection is a common problem. Influenza predisposes not only to *Streptococcus pneumoniae* and *Haemophilus influenzae* secondary infections, but also to severe *Staphylococcus aureus* pneumonia. Staphylococcal pneumonia often develops quickly, causing purulent sputum and deteriorating lung function, but any increase in the white cell count is slow or absent. Nodular or patchy opacities are seen on chest X-ray; small abscess cavities may develop; and staphylococcal bacteraemia may occur. Secondary bacterial infection should be urgently considered in any patient with deteriorating respiratory function. Blood and sputum cultures should be obtained in all such cases, and antibiotic treatment should be commenced, including drugs effective against *S. aureus*.

Bacterial sinusitis or otitis media can also complicate influenza in both children and adults. The expected pathogens are the same as for pneumonia.

Postviral complications

Postviral complications occur with variable frequency, depending on the characteristics of both the causative virus and the affected population. Prolonged convalescence with fatigue is common, often lasting from 6 to 12 weeks. Neurological effects include Guillain–Barré syndrome, mononeuropathies and occasionally encephalopathy. Persisting encephalopathy is rare, but the encephalitis lethargica cases in 1918 may have been related to the influenza pandemic of that year.

Diagnosis

Mild and sporadic cases may be dismissed as colds, croup, bronchitis or viral meningitis, although virus can later be identified after cell culture of nose or throat swab specimens, nasopharyngeal aspirate, bronchial washings or even CSF. Cases may be identified clinically in epidemics, from the sudden, disabling onset and the variety of systems affected (Fig. 7.3).

Laboratory diagnosis

A rapid diagnosis can be made by demonstrating type-specific antigen in nasopharyngeal cells by direct immunofluorescence.

It is important that virus isolation is carried out so that the changes in the antigenic structure of the virus can be detected for future vaccine preparation. The virus may be isolated by inoculating nasopharyngeal secretions

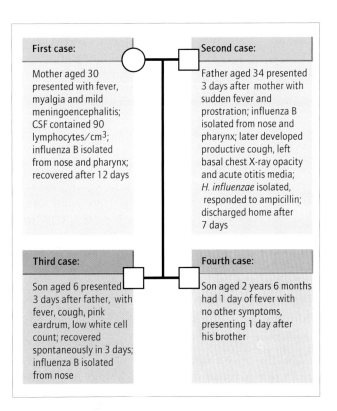

First case:
Mother aged 30 presented with fever, myalgia and mild meningoencephalitis; CSF contained 90 lymphocytes/cm³; influenza B isolated from nose and pharynx; recovered after 12 days

Second case:
Father aged 34 presented 3 days after mother with sudden fever and prostration; influenza B isolated from nose and pharynx; later developed productive cough, left basal chest X-ray opacity and acute otitis media; *H. influenzae* isolated, responded to ampicillin; discharged home after 7 days

Third case:
Son aged 6 presented 3 days after father, with fever, cough, pink eardrum, low white cell count; recovered spontaneously in 3 days; influenza B isolated from nose

Fourth case:
Son aged 2 years 6 months had 1 day of fever with no other symptoms, presenting 1 day after his brother

Fig. 7.3 A family outbreak of influenza B, illustrating the range of presentations and their relationship to the patients' ages.

into primary monkey kidney cells or continuous human diploid fibroblasts. These should be incubated at both 33 and 37°C, as some viruses replicate optimally at a lower temperature. The growth of virus in the cell culture is detected by haemadsorption using guinea-pig and chicken erythrocytes (but guinea-pig erythrocytes do not adhere to cells infected with type C). Virus can also be recovered from nose or throat swabs and occasionally from CSF. After primary isolation, the virus is typed in dedicated reference laboratories.

Alternative techniques include the detection of neutralizing, complement-fixing or haemagglutinin antibodies. Paired sera are required. An alternative is single radial haemolysis which uses a blood agar in which the red cells are coated with influenza antigens. Complement is also included. Serum specimens are placed in wells, and antibody diffuses outwards, forming immune complexes with the antigen on the red cells. The immune complexes activate the complement and there is lysis of the affected red cells. The size of the zone of haemolysis is proportional to the concentration of antibody present. A greater than 50% increase in zone diameter represents a significant increase in antibody and evidence of recent infection.

Laboratory diagnosis of influenza
1 Direct immunofluorescence of respiratory secretions.
2 Cell culture of respiratory secretions or cerebrospinal fluid.
3 Serologically by complement fixing or haemagglutinating antibodies or radial haemolysis.

Management

Non-specific treatment is often helpful. Rest, warmth, adequate hydration and analgesia all give considerable relief. The myocardium is protected from excess work, and oxygen desaturation is limited while the patient rests in bed. Reduction of fever is not usually necessary; indeed virus replication may be reduced at temperatures above 35°C (and aspirin is contraindicated in children because of an association with Reye's syndrome).

Amantadine

Amantadine, given within 48 h of onset, has some effect against clinical influenza A (but not other types), shortening the duration of fever by 24–36 h. It is given in a dose of 100 mg twice daily for 5–7 days. Side-effects include drowsiness, confusion and reticulate rash, and can be difficult for elderly patients to tolerate.

Tribavirin

Tribavirin, given by nebulizer, has been found useful in treating influenza pneumonia, but is not licensed for this indication. The principles of treatment are the same as for infants with RSV infection.

Antibiotics

Antibiotics should be given as soon as culture specimens have been obtained when there is suspicion of secondary bacterial infection. An antistaphylococcal agent should always be included.

Prevention and control

Influenza vaccines are non-replicating virus vaccines with a clinical efficacy of approximately 70%. The vaccine is prepared each year from strains similar to those considered most likely to circulate in the forthcoming season. Some vaccines are composed of purified viral surface antigens; others, called split vaccines, are made by separating viral core material from surface structures, and using the partly purified surface structures as the vaccine antigens. Different strains of antigen are used in different years, to adapt to the changeable antigenic structure of the influenza A virus. Usually there are two type A and one type B virus in the vaccine.

Vaccination is recommended for adults and children with chronic respiratory and cardiac disease, chronic renal failure, diabetes and other endocrine disorders and immunosuppression. It should also be given to residents of nursing homes and other institutions for the elderly. In some countries health care workers are routinely vaccinated. The vaccine is contraindicated in patients with known anaphylactic hypersensitivity to egg products.

Amantadine hydrochloride may be used prophylactically during an outbreak of influenza type A. It is indicated for patients in high-risk groups for whom vaccination is contraindicated, or in the 2 weeks following vaccination, before protective antibodies have developed.

Amantadine for treatment and prophylaxis of influenza A
1 Treatment: 100 mg twice daily orally for 5–7 days (child 10–15 years 100 mg daily).
2 Prophylaxis: 100 mg daily orally for 7–10 days.

Other viral pneumonias

Many viruses are capable of causing localized or generalized pneumonitis. Segmental pneumonia, with a distinct chest X-ray opacity, can be seen in infections with adenovirus, RSV, parainfluenza virus and Epstein–Barr virus. In the south-western USA a severe pneumonitis can be caused by a newly described hantavirus, San Nome virus.

Adenovirus

Adenovirus tends to affect children and young adults. Adenovirus type 5 is often implicated. The chest infection may be accompanied by pharyngitis, conjunctivitis, tender lymphadenopathy or, occasionally, a morbilliform rash. Epidemics of such infections can affect closed communities in barracks or institutions. Vaccines have been used to prevent epidemics in military recruits.

Respiratory syncytial virus

RSV can cause outbreaks of segmental pneumonia, particularly among the elderly. The illness is mild to moderate in severity, with fever, cough and shortness of breath. The mortality is low.

Parainfluenza and Epstein–Barr virus

Parainfluenza and Epstein–Barr virus tend to cause subclinical lung disease, though there may be a cough. The segmental lung disease is often discovered by chance on chest X-ray.

Diffuse pneumonitis can be caused by parainfluenza virus, measles and chickenpox. The lung disease is rarely clinically significant in immunocompetent individuals. Varicella pneumonia is the exception, being potentially severe or life-threatening, but it is accompanied by the characteristic chickenpox rash. Oximetry shows an early decline in capillary oxygen saturation and is a useful early warning of severe lung involvement in chickenpox (see Chapter 13).

> **Viruses causing pneumonitis**
> 1 Adenovirus.
> 2 Respiratory syncytial virus.
> 3 Parainfluenza virus.
> 4 Epstein–Barr virus.
> 5 San Nome virus.

Pyogenic bacterial respiratory infections

ORGANISM LIST

Streptococcus pneumoniae
Haemophilus influenzae
Moraxella catarrhalis
Klebsiella pneumoniae
Staphylococcus aureus
Escherichia coli and other Gram-negative rods
Fusobacterium necrophorum.

Rare bacterial lung infections: *Streptococcus pyogenes*, enteric fevers, anthrax, plague, leptospirosis (see relevant chapters).

Acute-on-chronic bronchitis

Introduction

This is a secondary bacterial infection which arises following bacterial colonization of an abnormal bronchial tree. The commonest abnormality is excessive mucus production and poor clearance of the bronchi. While the underlying disorder is not an infection, the repeated attacks of acute infection cause great morbidity, economic loss and progressive damage to the bronchi, leading to further infectious episodes, often complicated by developing bronchospasm.

Epidemiology

Acute and chronic bronchitis are common. The incidence is greatest in adults, although children are also affected. Patients who smoke and those with dust diseases are particularly prone to infection, probably because ciliary clearance of secretions is impaired. Patients with cardiac disease have poor alveolar clearance due to oedema. Most infective episodes occur during the winter. There is evidence that the incidence is related to levels of atmospheric pollution, particularly sulphur dioxide levels.

Pathology

The infection is superficial, affecting the lining mucosa of the bronchi and the mucus-producing goblet cells. There is oedema and acute inflammatory exudate, both of which exacerbate already-existing chronic obstruction.

Clinical features

The illness develops with gradually increasing cough, respiratory rate, expectoration and sputum purulence. The tendency to bronchospasm increases. Systemic effects are few. There may be a mild or moderate fever and the white cell count may be slightly raised. The chest X-ray rarely shows any definite change unless bronchial obstruction has precipitated a complicating segmental infection.

Diagnosis

This is clinical. The sputum is always colonized with upper respiratory tract flora, and may contain neutrophils. This does not change, except in degree, during acute exacerbations.

Management

General measures are very important. Adjustment of bronchodilator treatment, including temporary increases in topical or systemic corticosteroid dosage, will aid ventilation, coughing and drainage of the bronchi. Physiotherapy may be a valuable adjunct. A modest increase in inspired oxygen concentration may be indicated if hypoxia is severe (high oxygen concentrations should be avoided, as they may reduce respiratory drive in habitually hypercapnic patients).

Oral antibiotic treatment is often adequate for the superficial mucosal infection. Agents suitable for *Streptococcus pneumoniae* and *H. influenzae* include tetracyclines, ampicillin, amoxycillin or clarithromycin. Co-amoxyclav additionally covers for *Moraxella catarrhalis*. Courses of antibiotic should be just long enough to terminate infection, but insufficient to encourage the emergence of new colonizing flora; 5 days is ideal. Patients who have received repeated courses of antibiotics may become colonized with Gram-negative rods such as *E. coli* or *K. pneumoniae*. These may need treatment with antibiotics such as co-amoxiclav, co-trimoxazole or cefuroxime.

In severe episodes, parenteral antibiotics may be indicated. Ampicillin or cefuroxime is often effective.

Cystic fibrosis and bronchiectasis

In cystic fibrosis, abnormal and tenacious mucus accumulates in the bronchial tree. The ciliary clearance process is ineffective, leading to colonization of the bronchi with a resident flora which causes repeated infections.

In bronchiectasis the structure of bronchi is abnormal, either because of congenital conditions (e.g. Kartagener's syndrome) or because of damage from repeated infections. Areas of lung contain saccular or fusiform spaces from dilated bronchi. Cilary clearance is ineffective in these wide spaces. Indeed, the respiratory epithelium may become squamous after many infectious insults.

In both disorders, the affected bronchial tree is chronically obstructed and inflamed, producing large volumes of mucus and mucopus. The effect of chronic infection is debility and, in children, failure to thrive. Progressive respiratory insufficiency adds further debility. The infecting organisms include *S. pneumoniae*

and *H. influenzae*, but others are common, including *Staphylococcus aureus, E. coli* and other Gram-negative rods.

The most-feared organism is *Pseudomonas aeruginosa*, which is not only resistant to many antibiotics, but also produces large quantities of alginate capsule-like material, enabling the organism to form microcolonies within which it is protected from the host's immune defence. Furthermore, it produces a variety of enzymes and toxins, including elastase, proteases, DNAse, lecithinase and exotoxin A. These are extremely damaging to both bronchial structures and defence systems, and contribute to deteriorating lung function. Interestingly, it has recently been shown that azithromycin can completely switch off production of these substances, even though it does not kill the organism (which has high minimum inhibitory concentrations for macrolide drugs). This finding has not so far been put to clinical use.

The lesion in cystic fibrosis affects the whole lung (as well as other organs), so that progression is rapid — patients usually die in early adulthood. In bronchiectasis, long-term complications include amyloidosis, hypertrophic pulmonary osteoarthropathy (HPOA) and late malignant change.

Treatment of both conditions depends on vigorous physiotherapy and postural drainage, usually a lifelong twice-daily burden. This is combined with frequent antibiotic treatment of infections. Cystic fibrosis patients may require almost constant antibiotic therapy, and it is now common to treat exacerbations with intravenous drugs which have an antipseudomonal action, e.g. ceftazidime. Many young patients have indwelling Hickman lines with subcutaneous access so that they can commence their own treatment without delay, avoiding repeated hospital admissions, and limiting the damage which infecting organisms can produce.

Surgical treatment of localized bronchiectasis consists of removing an affected and devitalized segment or lobe. This often permits a marked improvement in general health. Heart–lung transplant may be offered to cystic fibrosis patients. This cures respiratory failure and normalizes lung mucus, but the denervated lungs lack a cough reflex, so the exacting physiotherapy must be continued to avoid aspiration (which carries a risk of chronic infection and even bronchiectasis).

Pneumococcal (lobar) pneumonia

Introduction

Streptococcus pneumoniae, also called the pneumococcus, attacks previously healthy individuals as well as those with predisposing conditions, and causes severe morbidity. It is important because of this, but also because the antibiotic-resistant forms, which have become common in other parts of the world, may soon be common in the UK.

Epidemiology

S. pneumoniae is the commonest bacterial cause of community-acquired pneumonia. One community-based study estimated that 4% of adults aged 60–79 years developed pneumococcal pneumonia each year. Particularly high attack rates have been observed in certain occupational groups and geographical areas, for example South African gold miners and in the highlands of Papua New Guinea. Conditions that predispose to infection include sickle-cell disease, anatomical or functional asplenia, chronic cardiac, respiratory, liver and renal disease, diabetes mellitus, alcohol abuse and immunosuppression. The case fatality rate is 10–20%, and is highest in elderly or compromised patients.

Pathogenesis of *S. pneumoniae* infections

S. pneumoniae is a Gram-positive coccus forming part of the *S. oralis* group together with *S. oralis* and *S. mitis*. There are 83 different serotypes based on polysaccharide capsular antigens.

The capsule is a major pathogenicity determinant, the virulence of the organism is related to the capsular polysaccharide type, and less to the quantity of capsular material produced. The lethal infective dose for a mouse is reduced from 10^5 to 10 cfu for organisms with a capsule. Infection with type 3, which produces copious amounts of a linear polysaccharide, is associated with high mortality, but type 30, which produces a similar amount of capsule, is rarely associated with clinical infection.

Cell wall polysaccharides are increasingly recognized as a source of inflammatory antigens. C polysaccharide activates the alternative complement pathway giving rise to C3a and C5a which are vasoactive and recruit polymorphs to the infected site.

Several toxins have been found in *S. pneumoniae*. Pneumolysin is a cytotoxin analogous to streptolysin O (in *S. pyogenes*), and listeriolysin (in *Listeria monocytogenes*). It acts by forming a ring of toxin molecules which dissolve in plasma membranes leaving a hole. Neuraminidase is an enzyme which removes sialic acid from host glycoproteins. Two forms of this enzyme are present in *S. pneumoniae*. Immunization against these toxins partially protects mice from lethal pneumococcal

infection. Pneumococcal surface protein A is a surface-exposed protein with several serological variants. It too is a partially protective antigen but its biological role is yet to be established.

Like other mucosal pathogens, *S. pneumoniae* possesses an IgA protease. This enzyme assists the organism in achieving colonization in the nasopharynx.

Pathogenicity factors for *Streptococcus pneumoniae*
1 Capsular polysaccharide.
2 Cell wall (C) polysaccharide.
3 Toxins: pneumolysin, neuraminidase.
4 Surface protein A.
5 Immunoglobulin A protease.

Pathology

Pneumococcal pneumonia is an infection of the alveoli. The affected part of the lung is solidified and red, due to the blood-stained acute inflammatory exudate which fills the alveolar air spaces. This is called red hepatization because the solid lung resembles liver. As the action of phagocytic enzymes liquefies the exudate, some of it is expectorated. This produces blood-stained, 'rusty' sputum, full of neutrophils and Gram-positive diplococci. In patients who recover, the exudate resolves completely, and the intact alveolar epithelium resumes its normal appearance.

Clinical features

The onset of illness is sudden, with high fever and a range of non-specific symptoms including vomiting, loose stools, headache or pleuritic chest pain. Sweating is not usually prominent. Respiratory symptoms are usually absent at this stage and physical examination is normal, as is the chest X-ray. The main clue suggesting bacterial illness is neutrophilia, often $15–25 \times 10^9/l$.

After an interval of a few hours to several days, a dry cough suddenly develops. An area of end-inspiratory crepitations is now detectable on chest examination, and here the classical signs of consolidation soon develop. The chest X-ray now shows a typical dense opacity filling all or most of a lobe (Fig. 7.4).

A further interval elapses before sputum is produced, probably reflecting the time during which the solid red hepatization begins to liquefy. If untreated, a proportion of patients would suddenly lose their fever and improve (healing by crisis), this corresponds with the appearance of effective antibodies in the blood. Others would succumb to spreading infection, bacteraemia or respiratory failure, or slowly recover (healing by lysis).

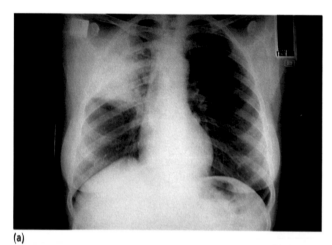

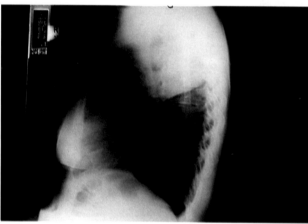

Fig. 7.4 Lobar pneumonia: chest X-ray showing typical consolidation in the right upper lobe; (a) posteroanterior and (b) right lateral views.

Diagnosis

This can be suspected on clinical and X-ray evidence once cough and consolidation develop. Few patients go on untreated to the stage of rusty sputum. In the absence of sputum, bacteriological confirmation may not be possible, but some patients produce sufficient sputum to demonstrate neutrophils and crowds of Gram-positive diplococci. Culture and sensitivity tests are then helpful.

Klebsiella pneumoniae can cause lobar pneumonia in patients with long-standing asthma, debilitating disease or alcoholism. Unlike pneumococcal infection, there is copious sputum containing many neutrophils and large, capsulated Gram-negative rods.

Management

Prompt and vigorous treatment helps to avoid severe complications. Benzylpenicillin is effective, usually highly so, against most pneumococci isolated in the UK. Five to 15% of cases are caused by pneumococci with reduced penicillin sensitivity, but high-dose penicillin may still be effective in these cases (but not in meningitis caused by penicillin-tolerant pneumococci, as it does not reach sufficient concentration in the CSF). Doses of 1.8–2.4 g 6-hourly intravenously are recommended. Erythromycin or cephalosporins such as cefuroxime or cefotaxime are suitable alternatives. Imported pneumococci can be highly resistant to penicillin, erythromycin, cephalosporins and chloramphenicol, requiring treatment with drugs such as vancomycin or teicoplanin.

Treatment for pneumococcal pneumonia
1 Benzylpenicillin i.v. 1.8–2.4 g 6-hourly.
2 Alternatives: cefuroxime 750–1500 mg i.v. 6–8-hourly; cefotaxime i.v. 1–2 g 8-hourly; erythromycin 50 mg/kg i.v. daily in four divided doses.

Treatment should be continued for about 7 days. *K. pneumoniae* is resistant to penicillin and ampicillin. It must be treated with a broad-spectrum cephalosporin such as cefotaxime, or an aminoglycoside.

Complications

Pleural effusion

Pleural effusion on the affected side is the commonest problem. This is often a sterile exudate, containing few white cells. It tends to occur during treatment, and often responds to one or two simple aspirations. In a few cases fluid persistently reaccumulates, and may require operative drainage and pleurodesis.

Extension of infection

Extension of infection to adjacent pleura or pericardium is more likely if the pneumonia is recognized or treated late. It is marked by swinging fever and typical localizing pain, often related to postural changes in endocarditis.

Empyema should be drained as completely as possible, to avoid loculation of pools of fluid. Up to a litre of fluid can be withdrawn each day (withdrawing more may lead to hypotension or reactive pulmonary oedema). An indwelling chest drain can be used if rapid reaccumulation of fluid persists (Fig. 7.5). High-dose intravenous antibiotic treatment should be given. Intrapleural antibiotic offers no advantage, as the antibiotic often becomes trapped at the site of injection, or destroyed by proteases or lysozymes.

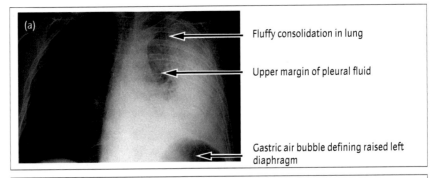

Fluffy consolidation in lung

Upper margin of pleural fluid

Gastric air bubble defining raised left diaphragm

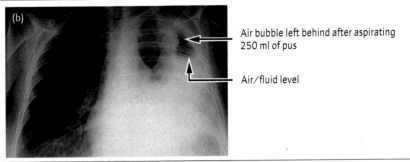

Air bubble left behind after aspirating 250 ml of pus

Air/fluid level

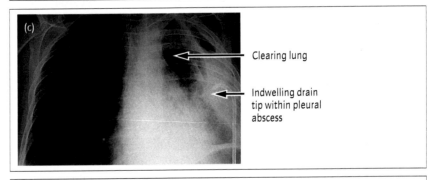

Clearing lung

Indwelling drain tip within pleural abscess

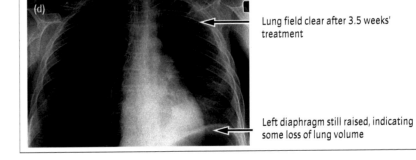

Lung field clear after 3.5 weeks' treatment

Left diaphragm still raised, indicating some loss of lung volume

Fig. 7.5 (a–d) Chest X-ray series showing management of pneumococcal empyema complicating lobar pneumonia: the empyema was first aspirated, but later required drainage with an indwelling catheter before resolution was achieved.

Pericarditis should be treated with maximum anti-biotic dosage. Drainage is hazardous, but must be carried out if there are signs of tamponade (echocardiography is useful in confirming the presence of fluid in the pericardial cavity). The procedure is best performed by an experienced operator.

Bacteraemia

Bacteraemia is a serious complication, which increases mortality to about 20%. It is more likely in infections with type 3,6 or 5 pneumococci. Metastatic infection, such as meningitis, peritonitis or brain abscess, may further complicate bacteraemia.

Prevention and control

Pneumococcal vaccine is a non-replicating vaccine containing purified capsular polysaccharide from each of the 23 types of pneumococcus which together account for over 85% of invasive pneumococcal disease in most western countries. The efficacy is 60–70%, but may be lower in children under 2 years of age and in those with immunosuppression. It is indicated for all those above age 2 with predisposing conditions (see above); in some countries routine vaccination of all elderly people above 60 years of age is recommended. In patients who are undergoing elective splenectomy, the vaccine should be given 2 weeks before the operation.

Revaccination is not normally advised, because of the risk of adverse reactions, except for patients with asplenia or nephrotic syndrome, whose antibody levels are likely to decline more rapidly. Long-term antibiotic prophylaxis with penicillin or amoxycillin is also indicated for patients with sickle-cell disease or other splenic dysfunction, as they can become infected with uncommon types of pneumococci.

Haemophilus influenzae pneumonia

Introduction and epidemiology

H. influenzae rarely causes primary pneumonia in adults, but children are readily colonized by organisms of polysaccharide capsular type b (Hib) which cause serious bacteraemic diseases. Hib disease is common in children below age 4; after age 6 most children have gained antibodies and are immune. Hib diseases are rapidly declining in incidence since imunization became available.

Manifestations of Hib disease include pneumonia, meningitis, epiglottitis, septic arthritis and facial cellulitis. Individual children tend to suffer from one manifestation, but different children in a family or community may develop different manifestations within a few days of each other.

Microbiology

The species *H. influenzae* can be subdivided into two groups depending on the presence or absence of a capsule. Non-capsulate strains are important commensals and secondary pathogens of the upper and lower respiratory tract. There are six different capsular serotypes differing in their polysaccharide composition. Serotype b is the usual cause of invasive infection; other serotypes are rarely implicated.

Clinical features

Illness develops gradually, over a few days. It may appear to follow a simple cold or to complicate croup or bronchiolitis, but is often spontaneous. The child is feverish and listless. Cough may not be prominent, but chest examination usually shows typical features of consolidation. Chest X-ray reveals a segmental, lobar or more widespread opacity, and an air bronchogram is often seen.

There is usually a neutrophilia of $15–20 \times 10^9/l$ in the peripheral blood.

Diagnosis

The diagnosis should be suspected in any small child with a localized pneumonia and neutrophilia. Blood cultures often produce a growth of Hib, which may be identifiable by agglutination test in 18–24 h. Small children do not expectorate their sputum, but samples are often obtainable by pharyngeal aspiration (which stimulates coughing), and are also culture-positive.

The differential diagnoses are pneumococcal and *Mycoplasma pneumoniae* pneumonia, both of which are common in toddlers. Early laboratory diagnosis is difficult in both cases, although an erythrocyte sedimentation rate of 70 mm/h or more, if present, favours a diagnosis of mycoplasmal disease.

Laboratory identification

Haemophilus is a fastidious genus whose growth requires the presence of nicotinamide adenine dinucleotide (NAD) and haematin normally found in blood. This characteristic gave rise to its name — 'blood-loving'. These factors are not available in blood agar, but can be released by adding the blood to the medium at 80°C, which gives the medium a chocolate appearance. If a clear medium is required, as for the study of capsulation, a filtered extract from red cells or a peptic digest of meat may be added. Dependence on NAD and haematin can be tested by inoculating the organism on to nutrient agar and placing paper discs containing the factors; growth will only occur around a disc containing both factors. The presence of a capsule can be demonstrated by slide agglutination with serotype-specific antiserum. This should be performed on all isolates where type b disease is suspected.

Antibiotic resistance is becoming increasingly common, especially to ampicillin and to chloramphenicol. The presence of a beta-lactamase, TEM-1, which had its origin in *E. coli*, is responsible for the majority of cases of ampicillin resistance. This enzyme can be detected by rapid tests using a cephalosporin, nitrocephin, which changes colour when its beta-lactam bond is broken.

Management

It is advisable to treat immediately with an intravenous agent while awaiting more diagnostic data. A broad-spectrum cephalosporin such as cefuroxime or cefotaxime is effective against both Hib and pneumococcal infection. Erythromycin is effective against pneumococci and *M. pneumoniae*, but is not highly active against Hib. Clarithromycin has adequate activity against all three pathogens. Chloramphenicol is an alternative to clarithromycin, but about 13% of Hib are chloramphenicol-resistant.

Hypoxic children easily become restless and distressed. Humidified oxygen should therefore be given at minimum concentrations required to maintain capillary saturations of 90–95%. If resting saturations persistently fall below 85%, ventilation should be considered.

Complications

Provided that there is a response to treatment, complications are unusual. It is rare for a child to have more than one Hib disease simultaneously. However, Hib may persist in the nasopharynx after treatment and can occasionally lead to a second manifestation. Chemoprophylaxis during convalescence should prevent this.

Prevention and control

Polysaccharide conjugate vaccines against Hib have recently been included in the routine infant vaccination programmes in many countries (see also Chapter 25).

They have greatly reduced the incidence of all invasive forms of Hib disease, including pneumonia. Hib vaccines do not protect against pneumonia caused by non-type b strains, or infections due to non-encapsulated strains.

Legionnaire's disease and legionelloses

Introduction

Legionnaire's disease was first recognized and its causative organism identified because of an outbreak of severe pneumonia in 1976. Previous outbreaks of feverish illnesses, with the characteristics of air-borne infections, were then shown to be caused by the same family of bacteria. The disease is important because it is often unrecognized until a late stage, it does not respond well to conventional treatment for community-acquired pneumonia, and it can be life-threatening.

Epidemiology

The infection can be transmitted by inhalation of contaminated aerosols generated from hot-water tap and shower outlets, water-cooling towers of office and industrial sites and domestic or recreational whirlpool spas (Fig. 7.6). Legionellae thrive in water at temperatures between 20 and 50°C, and the organism can often be isolated from water systems in buildings as well as from ponds, streams and soil. Legionellae can exist within and gain protection from the cytoplasm of free-living amoebae.

Person-to-person spread does not occur.

The disease occurs both sporadically and as localized outbreaks. Outbreaks are usually associated with a contaminated water source in a large building. Illness preferentially affects the middle-aged and elderly, particularly males and those who smoke or have underlying chronic respiratory disease. In the UK, there are about 150 cases annually and the case fatality rate is 10%.

The incubation period is 2–10 days for legionnaire's disease and 1–2 days for Pontiac fever, the milder non-pneumonic form of the infection.

Microbiology and pathogenesis

Legionellae are Gram-negative aerobic non-sporing encapsulated bacteria. They are catalase- and oxidase-variable and most species of *Legionella pneumophila* produce beta-lactamase. This organism produces an extracellular acid polysaccharide layer which acts as a capsule.

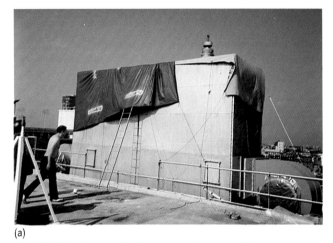

(a)

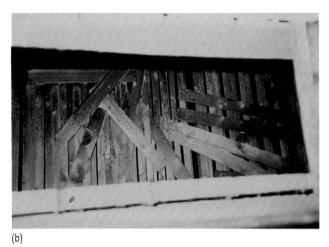

(b)

Fig. 7.6 (a) Poorly maintained rooftop cooling tower which generated a large *Legionella*-containing aerosol: several people contracted legionnaire's disease while passing through nearby streets. (b) Same tower, photographed from above, showing drift eliminator with several damaged slats.

Legionella spp. express a lipopolysaccharide which exhibits some cross-reactions with *Salmonella*. The major surface protein is a protease which is thought to play an important role in the pathogenesis of lung damage associated with legionnaire's disease. Inhalation of organisms within environmental amoebae may enhance invasiveness.

Clinical features

Most of the Legionellaceae are capable of producing a mild or moderate flu-like illness, sometimes with a cough. This condition, when recognized as legionellosis, is often called Pontiac fever, after the first recognized outbreak. A similar illness, accompanied by a rash, was called Fort Bragg fever.

Legionnaire's disease is a severe systemic infection with pneumonia, which is almost always caused by a serotype of *L. pneumophila*. After the incubation period of 2–10 days, there is fever, prostration and cough, often misinterpreted as influenza or bronchitis. In spite of treatment with common antibiotics, fever continues, loose stools are commonly seen, cough and tachypnoea worsen and the patient becomes increasingly confused.

Physical examination shows tachypnoea and purulent sputum in a morose or confused patient. There is usually a distinct area of consolidation or coarse crepitations in the chest, confirmed by demonstrating one or more large opacities on chest X-ray (Fig. 7.7).

Laboratory findings include neutrophilia, an erythrocyte sedimentation rate of 70 mm/h or more, variably elevated urea and creatinine levels and raised transminases. As in many severe chest infections, there may be marked hyponatraemia. A normocytic anaemia may

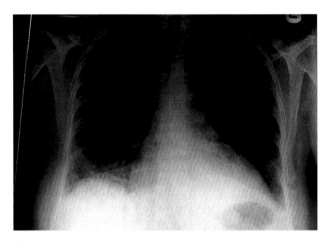

(a)

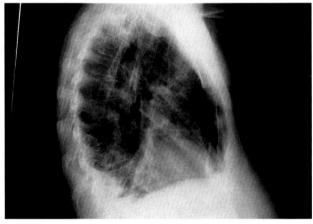

(b)

Fig. 7.7 Legionnaire's disease: extensive lung opacity in a patient with severe symptoms (one of several people infected during a hotel-based group holiday);.(a) posteroanterior and (b) right lateral views.

also develop. Severe respiratory and/or renal failure can develop quickly, especially if treatment is started late.

Diagnosis

This may be suspected on epidemiological grounds. The presence of severe confusion in a previously fit patient is highly suggestive. Few other early pneumonias cause such a wide range of laboratory abnormalities.

Laboratory diagnosis

Direct examination of Gram-stained smears of sputum is not useful as legionellae take up the stain very poorly. A direct fluorescent antibody method is available but in practice is only used for the diagnosis of *L. pneumophila* serotype 1 infection. It has relatively poor sensitivity but a high specificity. *Legionella* spp. are fastidious, growing slowly on a cystine-containing charcoal yeast extract agar. This is made selective by the addition of antibiotics which inhibit other respiratory commensals. Legionellae are identified by their cystine dependence and are serotyped by direct immunofluorescence antibody testing.

Legionnaire's disease can be diagnosed by detecting a fourfold rise in antibody titres or a single high value greater than 1 in 128. Methods such as indirect immunofluorescence and commercial rapid micro-agglutination tests are available. An enzyme-linked immunosorbent assay (ELISA) method for detection of serogroup 1 antigen in urine is also available.

Management

Appropriate treatment should be given on suspicion of the diagnosis, to avoid the danger of respiratory or renal failure. The treatment of choice is intravenous erythromycin in a dose of at least 3 g daily. The addition of ciprofloxacin or rifampicin may speed the response. Chloramphenicol is an alternative additional drug.

Treatment of legionnaire's disease
Erythromycin i.v. 3–4 g daily in four divided doses plus either ciprofloxacin i.v. 200 mg twice daily or rifampicin 600 mg twice daily.

Oxygen is often required, and intensive respiratory support may be needed. Renal failure in late or severe cases demands intensive management.

Complications

Patients who recover usually do so completely, though they may need many weeks' convalescence before their energy returns fully. A few develop lasting, patchy cerebral or bulbar deficit, often attributed to severe hypoxia during the illness. Guillain–Barré syndrome is a rare but recognized complication of acute legionnaire's disease.

Prevention and control

Effective maintenance of building water systems and other potential sources of infection is the key to prevention of legionellosis. This should include adequate chlorination of water supplies and stored cold water, and heating (to above 60°C) of hot water. The design of water systems should avoid stagnation of water in peripheral sections, and permit the achievement of a temperature of 55°C at all hot taps within 15 seconds of turning on. Whirlpool spas should be frequently cleaned and continuously disinfected.

Aspiration pneumonia

This results from failure to cough and protect the airways. It can occur in unconcious or anaesthetized patients, or in those with neuromuscular disease affecting swallowing or breathing. When the chest is erect, the right main bronchus and lower lobe bronchus are nearly vertical, so the right lower lobe tends to be most affected. In a recumbent patient the apical bronchus of the right lower lobe is affected most.

The aspirate contains mixtures of mouth and pharyngeal organisms, mainly penicillin-sensitive streptococci and spirochaetes mixed with anaerobes. These produce a patchy pneumonia, most dense in the vulnerable segment, sometimes leading to abscess formation.

The diagnosis must be suspected in vulnerable patients, and treated with physiotherapy, a penicillin or cephalosporin plus metronidazole. If gastric contents have been aspirated, the inflammatory effect of gastric acid can be inhibited by giving a corticosteroid such as methylprednisolone or prednisolone for the first 24–36 h.

Lung abscess

The commonest cause of a lung abscess is aspiration. Systemic conditions or primary lung infections are rarer causes. Most lung abscesses are polymicrobial, with facultative and anaerobic organisms occurring equally commonly in most series of cases. Staphylococcal bacteraemia is often accompanied by a nodular pneumonitis which can progress to abscesses. Rare infections such as nocardiosis and aspergillosis can cause small abscesses in the lungs.

Hospital-acquired lung abscesses may behave in the same way as community-acquired ones, but in the former, *Klebsiella pneumoniae*, *Pseudomonas aeruginosa* and *Candida* spp. are additional causes, which carry a particularly poor prognosis.

If the abscess can be aspirated, culture and sensitivity testing of the pus are helpful, and healing is promoted. Blood cultures should be obtained before treatment is commenced. Most abscesses can be treated as for aspiration pneumonia, with percutaneous drainage when possible. A minority require surgical drainage.

Anaerobic pneumonia (necrobacillosis)

Introduction and epidemiology

This is a rare condition which tends to affect adolescents and young adults, particularly men. It is a bacteraemic disease, probably arising from infection with *Fusobacterium necrophorum*, which is a colonist of the pharynx and mouth.

Clinical features and diagnosis

Illness begins abruptly with a high fever and very severe sore throat. After 2 or 3 days there is cough and often chest pain. One or more areas of consolidation are detectable on examination and chest X-ray. Standard antibiotic treatment is unsuccessful, the pneumonia extends, renal function deteriorates, hypoxia and hypotension develop. Most cases are fatal unless suspected and treated early.

Blood cultures are often positive, and must always be obtained. Sputum culture may also be positive, but the bacteria are strictly anaerobic, and survive poorly unless maintained in an anaerobic environment. The diagnosis must be considered if the patient is to have a good chance of recovery; the sore throat is a helpful pointer.

Management

Although the pathogen is penicillin-sensitive in laboratory conditions, penicillin has only a slow effect. Metronidazole is more successful, and can be given together with penicillin or broader-spectrum drugs while the diagnosis is confirmed.

Atypical pneumonias

Introduction

The atypical pneumonias are so called because they are so unlike typical lobar pneumonia.

They have a gradual onset, cause prolonged fever and profuse sweating and improve slowly with no point of crisis. There is usually little sputum, and pathogens are not demonstrable by Gram-staining. They are important because they cause morbidity in adults of working age; untreated infections can be prolonged, and epidemics or outbreaks are not uncommon.

ORGANISM LIST

Mycoplasma pneumoniae
Chlamydia pneumoniae
C. psittaci
Coxiella burnetii.

Epidemiology

M. pneumoniae and *C. pneumoniae* are human pathogens whose reservoir of infection is the organism circulating among affected people.

Mycoplasma pneumonia affects all ages but is commonest in school-age children and young adults. Outbreaks occasionally occur, especially in closed institutions. In the UK, epidemics occur at 3- or 4-year intervals. During epidemic years, *M. pneumoniae* competes with *Streptococcus pneumoniae* as the commonest cause of community-acquired pneumonia.

C. pneumoniae has only been distinguished from *C. psittaci* in recent years. The prevalence of seropositivity rises steadily with age until about 60% of individuals have evidence of past infection by the fifth decade of age. Large-scale epidemics have been recognized in Denmark and Canada, and it appears that both primary infection and reinfection can be symptomatic.

C. psittaci is widespread among birds. Infected birds excrete many organisms in their faeces. Infection in humans is acquired by inhaling the organism from desiccated droppings and secretions of infected birds in an enclosed space, or directly from infected birds. Sporadic cases and limited outbreaks have been associated with keepers and fanciers of parrots and parakeets. Larger-scale outbreaks have been associated with duck or poultry farming, and with poultry packing plants, especially with mechanized defeathering processes, which produce heavy aerosols containing faecal organisms. Person-to-person spread is rare. The incubation period is 4–15 days.

Coxiella burnetii is a pathogen of sheep. Transmission to humans occurs by air-borne spread of organisms in dust contaminated from infected placental tissues and faeces. Rarer sources of infection include parturient cats and unpasteurized milk. The infection mainly affects meat workers, farmers and veterinarians. Infection is severe in pregnant women, and often precipitates abortion. No case of infection from a parturient woman has been described.

Microbiology of *Chlamydia* infections

The family Chlamydiaceae consists of one genus including three species. *Chlamydia trachomatis* affects the eye and genital tract and is responsible for trachoma, non-specific urethritis and lymphogranuloma venereum. *C. psittaci* is a causative agent of a zoonotic pneumonia. *C. pneumoniae* causes upper and lower respiratory tract infection, sore throat, laryngitis and pneumonia.

The *Chlamydiae* are obligate intracellular bacteria which exist in two forms: the reticulate body, which is the intracellular vegetative form found inside cells of the hosts, and the infective elementary body which is adapted for extracellular survival and is responsible for transmission (Fig. 7.8). The reticulate body divides by a series of fissions to give intermediate forms and finally elementary bodies. The cycle takes place within a cytoplasmic inclusion body, and ends with the release of infective elementary bodies from the host cell.

Lipopolysaccharide is a genus-specific antigen common to all three species. There are also species-specific polypeptide antigens and in addition *C. trachomatis* exhibits serotype-specific antigens (see p. 221).

The virulence of *Chlamydia* spp. can be correlated with the *in vitro* growth characteristics; more virulent strains tend to grow more slowly. The mechanism whereby this occurs is not fully understood. Cysteine-rich proteins are found in elementary body outer membrane proteins. One of these, a 60 D protein, is thought to be associated with enhanced invasiveness and virulence. Adhesion molecules have also been recognized in *C. trachomatis* and *C. psittaci*.

Clinical features

The acute feverish part of the illness is similar in all types of atypical pneumonia. After an incubation period of 4 days to 2 weeks, there is an insidious onset of irregular, swinging fever, sweating, especially at night, malaise and fatigue. There is often a dry cough. Physical examination is rarely remarkable, except for a patch of crepitations or dullness in the lung fields. The chest X-ray may show anything from a faint, ill-defined segmental opacity to a large and fairly dense consolidation, often much greater than the physical signs suggest. Some patients have a small or moderate pleural effusion, often accompanied by a dull ache or even frankly pleuritic pain on the affected side.

Laboratory findings are variable. There is often a modest, sometimes marked, neutrophilia. Mild elevation of liver transaminases is common. In *Mycoplasma* pneumonia the erythrocyte sedimentation rate is often raised to 70 mm/h or more, but this may not be apparent at the onset of illness. Most patients with *Mycoplasma* pneumonia develop cold agglutinins, but these are usually detectable late, or in convalescence — too late for diagnostic use (but the slight haemolysis which results may be detectable early as a macrocytosis, caused by the presence of excess reticulocytes). A few patients develop severe haemolysis in convalescence. Associated clinical features differ in the different infections.

Chlamydia pneumoniae

C. pneumoniae usually causes acute self-limiting respiratory infections, often mild, rarely presenting to hospital. Other syndromes include moderately severe atypical pneumonia, otitis media, acute-on-chronic bronchitis, persistent or relapsing pharyngitis and the less common myocarditis.

Mycoplasma pneumoniae

M. pneumoniae usually causes pneumonia, but this may be accompanied by tracheitis, bullous myringitis, mild hepatitis or sometimes by a lymphocytic meningitis. Probably at least 25% of infections are feverish illnesses without pneumonia, and it is not uncommon for the illness to present with an associated feature.

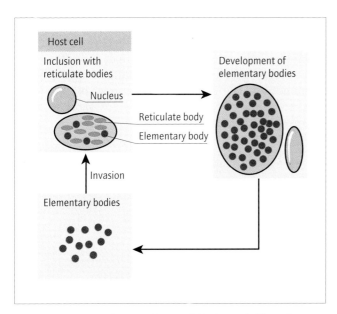

Fig. 7.8 Appearance of intra- and extracellular forms of *Chlamydia* spp.

Pericarditis and myocarditis are rare but recognized features.

Chlamydia psittaci

C. psittaci causes pneumonia in about 60% of infected individuals. The remainder have fever alone. It is debilitating and can be severe and accompanied by respiratory failure. It is a rare cause of culture-negative endocarditis. Occasional cases of myelopathy have been reported, with or without associated pneumonia.

Coxiella burnetii

C. burnetii causes Q-fever. This may be an atypical pneumonia, but just over half of cases are feverish illnesses with hepatocellular disorder. A small proportion of cases, probably less than 1%, become chronic with swinging fever, often clinical jaundice and, in half of cases, endocarditis. In endemic areas this is an important cause of morbidity. Mild to moderate myocarditis may occur in acute or chronic disease.

Diagnosis

The differential diagnosis of many atypical pneumonias can often be inferred from epidemiological circumstances and clinical presentation. RSV and influenza can cause similar illnesses, often in outbreaks.

Patients with *Mycoplasma* infections do not commonly produce sputum. Although *M. pneumoniae* can be cultivated on serum-based artificial media the organism is slow-growing and the diagnostic yield is low. Serology is the mainstay of diagnosis. In many laboratories particle-agglutination tests are used, and a positive result is taken to indicate the presence of immunoglobulin M (IgM) antibodies, and therefore recent infection. IgM-detecting ELISA tests are commercially available. Complement fixation tests are also still used and a positive diagnosis can be made if there is a fourfold rise or fall in antibody titre in two specimens taken 10 days apart. This test has excellent specificity but only provides a retrospective diagnosis. New antigen-detection ELISAs are also available, as is a probe which detects *Mycoplasma* ribosomal RNA.

Chlamydiae

Chlamydiae are often still detected by finding rising titres of complement-fixing antibodies to whole-cell antigen preparations. There is much cross-reaction between antibodies to different species. Species-specific antibodies are detected by microimmunofluorescence techniques, which detect reactions against elementary body antigens. Culture of chlamydiae is not useful in the diagnosis of pneumonias, although it is useful when a diagnosis of *Chlamydia trachomatis* infection is required in cases of sexual abuse or rape. Where a culture diagnosis is required, *C. trachomatis* is readily grown in tissue culture with cyclohexamide-treated McCoy cells.

Q-fever

Q-fever is diagnosed by finding rising titres of complement-fixing antibodies to phase 2 and (in chronic Q-fever) phase 1 antigens. Coxiellae isolated from infected animals express phase 1 antigens, but after passage through embryonated eggs, these are replaced by phase 2 antigens.

In cases of hepatitis, there is a characteristic histological change, with many small granulomata, often with clear centres and always with a halo of eosinophils in their periphery (see p. 198). *Coxiella burnetii* can be demonstrated in silver- or Giemsa-stained smears, or by direct immunofluorescent staining.

Management

The antibiotics of choice are tetracycline or chloramphenicol. Erythromycin is a useful alternative, but may be less effective in Q-fever and some cases of psittacosis. Treatment may be given orally in mild and moderate cases, but should be given parenterally in severe or complicated cases (this is easier with erythromycin and chloramphenicol). Chloramphenicol is considered to be the treatment of choice when Q-fever occurs in pregnancy. Ciprofloxacin is highly active in laboratory testing and may be a valuable alternative but treatment failures have been reported. Ciprofloxacin is not reliably effective in chlamydial and mycoplasmal pneumonias. The response to treatment is not always fast, so courses of 10–14 days are advisable to avoid relapse or recrudescence.

Treatment of *Mycoplasma pneumoniae* and *Chlamydia pneumoniae*
1 Erythromycin orally or i.v. 500 mg 6-hourly.
2 Alternative: oxytetracycline orally 250–500 mg 6-hourly.
   All above regimens for 10–14 days.

Treatment of Q-fever
1 First choice: tetracycline orally — same dose as in previous text note.

2 Alternatives and in pregnancy: chloramphenicol orally or i.v. 500 mg 6-hourly or ciprofloxacin orally 500 mg twice daily (i.v. 200 twice daily).

All above regimens for 14 days.

Treatment of psittacosis
1 First choice: tetracycline orally — same dose as for *Mycoplasma pneumoniae* and *Chlamydia pneumoniae*.
2 Alternative: erythromycin orally or i.v. — same dose as for *M. pneumoniae* and *C. pneumoniae*.

Both above regimens for 10–14 days.

Care must be taken not to miss endocarditis in Q-fever. The presence of phase I antibodies is a warning. Echocardiography, physical examination, repeated C-reactive protein estimations and follow-up assessments for 2 or 3 months are advisable in cases of doubt.

Pertussis

Introduction

Pertussis, or whooping cough, is an epidemic disease caused by *Bordetella pertussis*. Although it is now rare, as immunizaton is widespread, it can rapidly become prevalent if immunization rates drop. Large epidemics occurred in the 1980s after concerns about vaccine safety resulted in low rates of acceptance (Fig. 7.9). The clinical disease is prolonged, severe and distressing. Morbidity is high in infants, and there is a significant mortality in infants and in older children with respiratory or cardiac disease.

Epidemiology and pathology

B. pertussis causes widespread infection of the airways, and is readily transmitted by the air-borne route. It is a small, Gram-negative rod which is typed by its cell-wall proteins, or agglutinogens, designated. 1, 2 and 3. Most clinical isolates are of type 1,3 or 2,3. Antibodies to these are protective. In the absence of immunization, large epidemics occur every 3–4 years.

Clinical features

After an incubation of 14–20 days, illness begins with a simple cough and slight fever. Over 4 or 5 days coughs begin to be grouped into paroxysms, which lengthen until up to 20 or 30 coughs occur with no inspirations between them. During coughing large volumes of thick mucus accumulate in the upper airways and are expectorated in ropy strands. Finally the paroxysm ends with a stridulous inspiratory cry, and often with a vomit. Some patients have little cough, but whoop and vomit; some cough and vomit, but rarely whoop. Adults and a few children may suffer sneezing paroxysms. The paroxysms last for 2 or 3 weeks before gradually improving over 10–14 days.

The effect of the paroxysmal cough may produce cyanosis and, in infants, apnoeic attacks. The venous pressure is raised, there is facial lividity and sometimes conjunctival haemorrhage or facial petechiae (Fig. 7.10). In infants there may be intracranial haemorrhage. A combination of hypoxia and small haemorrhages can cause cerebral impairment or even large focal brain

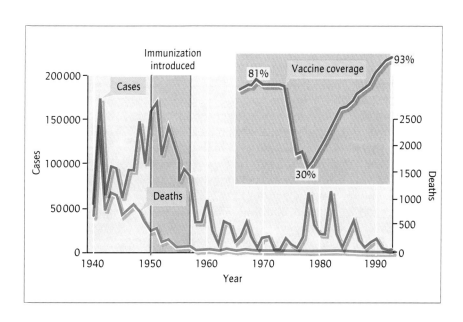

Fig. 7.9 Decline and resurgence of pertussis in England and Wales with changing vaccine coverage.

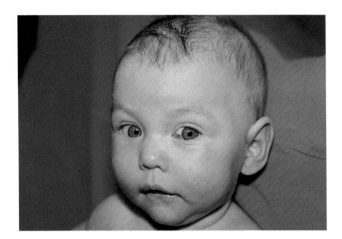

Fig. 7.10 Pertussis in a 6-month-old: subconjunctival haemorrhage produced by severe cough.

lesions. Although secondary or aspiration pneumonia occurs, the rare fatalities are usually caused by cerebral damage.

Diagnosis

This is usually clinically obvious, but mild cases may be similar to croup, bronchiolitis or persisting asthma. A lymphocytosis of $15–25 \times 10^9/l$ is strongly suggestive of pertussis.

Microbiology

B. pertussis is a small Gram-negative coccobacillus. There are three species in the genus Bordetella: B. pertussis, the causative agent of whooping cough; B. parapertussis, which is rarely associated with the whooping cough syndrome; and B. bronchoseptica, which is primarily a pathogen of animals responsible for a destructive nasal infection in pigs.

The pathogenicity of the organism is related to its toxins. A number of antigens are recognized, including fimbrial haemagglutinin, pertussis toxin and a 67 kDa protein. Pertussis toxin mediates the paroxysmal cough and a unique lymphocytosis, affecting all lymphocyte subtypes. Much research has focused on which of these antigens are immunologically protective.

The bacterial agglutinins and fimbrial haemagglutin are the main adhesion antigens.

Other toxins include tracheal cytotoxin, which causes ciliostasis and destruction of ciliated epithelium, and adenyl cyclase which destroys polymorphs and stimulates the cough reflex.

Laboratory diagnosis

A pernasal swab is the optimal method for obtaining a specimen for culture. The cultivation of the organism is difficult because B. pertussis is fastidious and relatively slow-growing, which means that its growth is often inhibited by faster-growing commensal organisms which contaminate clinical specimens.

The organism may be detected by culture of nasopharyngeal swab specimens on Bordet–Gengou or charcoal yeast extract agar with antibiotic supplements. Antigen detection methods have been described. IgM-based ELISAs have also been described but have not yet found a place in routine use.

Management

Although erythromycin is active against B. pertussis in cultures, it has not produced definite improvement in controlled trials. Treatment is therefore largely symptomatic, and directed at limiting the effects of lasting toxin-mediated cough. Antitussives have a limited effect, and care must be taken not to cause sedation. The airway should be protected by postural drainage in infants by holding them face- and head-downwards during paroxysms. Cyanotic or apnoeic attacks can often be helped by gently suctioning the airways to remove tenacious mucus. A humidified atmosphere may help. Severely affected infants may be nursed in a cot oxygen tent. Assisted ventilation is rarely needed.

Paroxysms are easily precipitated by feeding or by breathing cold air. Most children lose weight. Small, frequent feeds are important, and food should be offered after coughing or vomiting. Small children may be fearful of paroxysms, and need sympathetic reassurance.

Prevention and control

Erythromycin treatment does not reliably reduce the infectiousness of the disease, nor afford good post-exposure prophylaxis, though it is often given for its slight beneficial effect. Sufferers expel diminishing numbers of organisms for up to 3 weeks after paroxysms begin. An effective vaccine is whole-cell killed vaccine which forms part of the universally available triple vaccine. Subunit vaccines containing combinations of fimbrial haemagglutinin, pertussis toxin, 67 kDa antigen and agglutinogens have been manufactured and are used in some countries. Fears of severe encephalopathy associated with whole-cell pertussis vaccine have not been supported by extensive studies. The only contraindication to the vaccine is a severe reaction to a previous dose.

Fungal infections of the lower respiratory tract

Introduction

Fungal respiratory infections are rare in immunocompetent patients in the UK, mainly because exposure to highly pathogenic fungi is rare. There is a limited list of pathogens, mostly from endemic areas overseas, which cause diseases requiring differentiation from unusual, nodular or cavitating chest infections.

Aspergillosis

Aspergillus spp. have a worldwide distribution. They inhibit dark areas, such as ventilation ducts, cavities in buildings and spaces behind wall panels. They produce millions of spores which are inhaled and primarily infect the lungs.

Indolent colonization of stagnant bronchioles or old cavities can produce a hypersensitivity reaction with bronchoconstriction. This can precipitate deterioration in patients with pre-existing asthma or chronic bronchitis. Affected patients have precipitin antibodies in their serum, and may respond well to treatment of the *Aspergillus*, although recurrence can be a problem.

In pre-existing cavities fungal hyphae may produce a ball-shaped growth which irritates the cavity wall, causing cough and often haemoptysis (a severe problem in up to 25% of sufferers). A single lesion like this may not produce hypersensitivity, and precipitins may not be present. The X-ray or imaging appearance of this aspergilloma is typically of a round, space-occupying lesion surrounded by a narrow, clear air space. Such lesions are treated surgically by segmental or lobar resection when circumstances permit, but half or more may improve with chemotherapy.

Itraconazole has good activity against the fungus, and is the treatment of choice for disease of moderate severity. Inoperable aspergilloma may respond to this or to intravenous amphotericin.

Histoplasmosis

Histoplasma capsulatum is yeast, widely distributed in dry, hot areas, and is said often to be associated with dried bird droppings. Although it can produce systemic disease, with granulomata in the liver, or granulomatous disease of the skin, it often affects the apex of the lung. The appearance of the lung disease is very like tuberculosis, with nodular apical lesions and often one or more cavities.

The pathogen can be demonstrated in the sputum as typical yeast-like organisms with a very distinct thick capsule. A complement fixation test also provides a means of serodiagnosis.

Treatment is with parenteral amphotericin. Other antiyeast agents such as itraconazole or fluconazole may be useful additional treatment. Mild disease may be treatable with oral agents alone. Surgical resection may be indicated for advanced disease.

Blastomycosis

This is caused by the yeast *Blastomyces*, whose endemic area is confined to the USA. It causes a disease similar to histoplasmosis, but may affect any lung area, not only the apex. Diagnosis and treatment are as for histoplasmosis.

Coccidioidomycosis

The cause of this disease, *Coccidiodes immitis*, is virtually confined to the San Joachim valley of the western USA. It tends to cause a rapidly progressive bronchopneumonia or pneumonia unresponsive to antibiotics but mild cases also occur. The fungal hyphae grow rapidly in standard cultures, and produce segmented chains containing millions of spores. The spores are highly infectious, and patients with suspected coccidioidomycosis should always be isolated.

Treatment is with amphotericin (see Chapter 4).

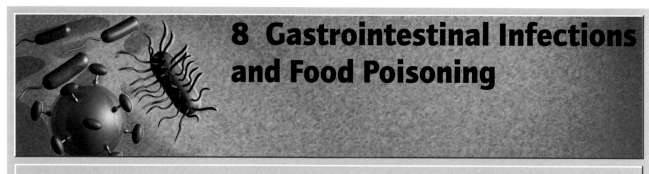

8 Gastrointestinal Infections and Food Poisoning

Introduction

Infections of the gastrointestinal tract are among the commonest infections in all communities of the world. There is little doubt that they cause the greatest morbidity and mortality. Even in the UK, where water supplies, sanitation and education reach high standards, surveys suggest that intestinal infections are causing increasing illness and loss of working days.

Structure and environment of the gastrointestinal tract

The gastrointestinal tract is a tube, open to the environment at both ends, into which a great deal of foreign material is introduced each day. Microorganisms, which may be pathogens, enter every time food, drink or utensils are put into the mouth. The local environments vary widely in different parts of the gastrointestinal tract, and this influences the nature of the local flora and of pathogens which may invade.

The stomach is highly acidic and contains variable amounts of air. Few bacteria survive this environment

for long but many pass quickly through. Boluses of food, especially fats, can protect bacteria during this passage. Chocolate and cheese are thought to enhance survival of salmonellae in this way.

The upper small intestine is alkaline. It has a highly vascular mucosa which is attractive to adherent parasites. It also contains bile, which strongly influences the local flora; almost all flora of the small bowel grow well on bile-containing media, e.g. MacConkey's agar. The highly absorptive mucosa of the jejunum and ileum offers a means of entry for toxins, not only those adapted to adhere to mucosal cells but also systemic toxins which may cause non-intestinal diseases such as botulism. Toxins may be elaborated by bacteria in food or be components of the food itself.

The terminal ileum and colon are the most anaerobic parts of the bowel. They are inhabited by very large numbers of anaerobic bacteria, both Gram-positive and -negative, cocci and rods, including sporing organisms. Facultative organisms such as *Escherichia coli* can also occupy this environment. Faecal streptococci are plentiful.

150

Some organisms, such as the yeast *Candida*, are able to reside throughout the bowel. Others may pass through, being excreted in the faeces for a while, but not causing long-term colonization.

Natural defences of the gastrointestinal tract

Gastric acid

Gastric acid is one of the major first defences of the gastrointestinal tract. While it may not sterilize the stomach contents completely and it has no effect on acid-fast organisms, it greatly reduces the numbers of bacteria which go on to enter the intestines. This is practically demonstrated in patients with achlorhydria, who are easily infected by very small numbers of salmonellae or vibrios, and suffer severe illness as a result.

Bile salts

The bile salts of the duodenum inhibit many organisms, killing some by disrupting their cell surfaces. The exceptions are the family of Enterobacteriacae, for example *E. coli*, which live well in a medium of bile salts. Lower in the bowel, bile salts are reabsorbed and their effect is diminished.

Normal bowel flora

The normal bowel flora confers colonization resistance which is a complicated phenomenon depending on competition between microorganisms. It is more than simply priority of place for the local flora. Bacteria modify their environment by the production of metabolic products which may alter the local pH or redox potential. Some produce poisonous chemicals such as hydrogen sulphide or volatile fatty acids which can inhibit other organisms. Many of the Enterobacteriacae produce natural antibiotics, called enterocines, which are harmful to other species, but not to their own. It has also been shown that faecal streptococci inhibit other organisms, such as *Clostridium difficile*, the cause of pseudomembranous (antibiotic-associated) colitis. All of these factors combine to favour particular types of organisms in the environments of the bowel.

Invading organisms must overcome colonization resistance if they are to invade the bowel mucosa. The protective effect can be reduced by antibiotic modification of normal flora, predisposing a patient to infection by pathogens to which he or she may be exposed. Thus, salmonella infection in exposed people is more likely if they are pretreated with streptomycin or tetracycline.

Immune responses

Immune responses in the bowel are also important protective mechanisms. The bowel mucosa is rich in lymphocytes and contains much lymphoid tissue. Cell-mediated immunity can be demonstrated by finding lymphocytes sensitized to the antigens of recently active pathogens. Humoral immunity is provided by secreted immunoglobulin A (IgA). Plasma cells are often plentiful in established mucosal inflammation. The immune responses of the gut are exploited when oral polio vaccine is given; after immunization the mucosa resists invasion by these enteroviruses which are then deprived of their usual means of entry into the body.

Motility

The motility of the gastrointestinal tract assists greatly in clearing pathogens. This is amply demonstrated when obstruction or stasis alters the local environment. The stagnant stomach becomes colonized by organisms which ferment the contents, quickly losing its acidity. Blind loops or diverticula in the bowel can easily become the foci of abscesses containing bowel flora. Approximately 50% of the weight of faeces is composed of bacteria. The diarrhoea of bowel infections is probably a major mechanism by which the causative pathogens are cleared from the gut.

Protection against toxins

Protection against absorbed toxins is afforded by the portal circulation and the liver. The microsomal enzymes of the hepatocytes detoxify many drugs and other substances. Toxins absorbed from the gut enter the portal circulation and are intercepted by the liver before they can reach the general circulation. The gut flora naturally generate endotoxin, and the portal venous blood contains significant endotoxin concentrations. However, after passage through the liver, hepatic venous blood contains only negligible amounts. It is possible that the hepatocytes are not the only destroyers of endotoxin, for isolated Kupffer cells can also inactivate it *in vitro*.

Normal defences of the bowel
1 Gastric acid.
2 Bile salts.
3 Lymphoid tissue.
4 Enterocines.
5 Normal bowel flora.
6 Secretory immunoglobulin A.
7 Motility.

General principles of managing gastrointestinal infections

Diagnostic tests

The most obvious effects of bowel infections are diarrhoea and vomiting.

Stool specimens

Stool specimens are relatively easy to collect but it is important to include the most liquid part of the stool, which is the most likely location of excreted pathogens. If there is much mucus, some of this should also be obtained (a syringe is a convenient means of collecting liquid or viscous material).

Mucosal specimens

Some parasites and ova are only sparsely excreted and more direct specimens increase the likelihood of positive diagnostic results. Examples include trophozoites of *Entamoeba histolytica* or schistosome ova which may both be more readily detected in scrapings or small biopsies taken from the rectal mucosa at proctoscopy (a small spatula or gloved finger may be used to obtain scrapings). Specimens should be taken from the edge of any ulcer or area of inflammation.

Intestinal fluids

In giardiasis or strongyloidiasis the parasites may not be detectable in stool samples, but are readily demonstrated in duodenal aspirate, biopsy or material obtained by the string test. In the string test the patient is asked to swallow a gelatin capsule into which is coiled a weighted length of soft, absorbent string. The free end of the string is fixed at the mouth: the weighted end unwinds from the capsule as it passes through the stomach and into the duodenum. After allowing 30–60 min resting time, the string is withdrawn and the adherent material is examined for parasites.

Vomitus

Vomitus is rarely obtained but it may contain viruses in acute viral gastroenteritis or bacteria in some types of toxic food poisoning. It is worth attempting to collect specimens, especially in patients who do not have coexisting diarrhoea.

Other specimens

Other specimens which may be useful include blood cultures, which are mandatory in patients with fever. Positive blood cultures are seen in a minority of patients with salmonellosis and on occasions in other gastrointestinal infections. Serum may contain antibodies to toxins or to *Salmonella* O, H and Vi antigens.

Management of gastrointestinal diseases

Principles of oral rehydration

Few gastrointestinal infections disable all of the mucosal absorption function of the bowel. In toxin-mediated diarrhoeas there is no damage to absorption; hypersecretion is the problem. In other diarrhoeas mucosal cells may be damaged, but some survive intact and can function sufficiently to absorb fluid and electrolytes. Absorption of sodium and water can be maximized by giving sufficient of each with the optimum amount of glucose to 'drive' the active transport systems as rapidly as possible. A steady input of this mixture can allow absorption to overtake diarrhoeal fluid loss, even in severely dehydrated patients. At the same time, potassium will flow passively along concentration gradients. This solution can be given until normal hydration is restored, as determined by clinical condition or body weight. Thereafter the sodium intake may be reduced. This is important in small children who excrete sodium loads inefficiently; sodium overload easily causes oedema which may be slow to resolve. The easiest adjustment of sodium intake is achieved by diluting the solution to approximately half-strength or by alternating it with drinks of water, dilute juice or squash.

Recommended composition of oral rehydration fluid	
Sodium:	150–155 mmol/l
Glucose:	200–220 mmol/l
Potassium:	4–5 mmol/l

This solution can be given until normal hydration is restored, as determined by clinical condition or body weight.

Intravenous rehydration

This is indicated for shock, exhaustion precluding oral feeding and for progressive dehydration in spite of oral hydration therapy. The electrolyte solution of choice is half-normal sodium chloride solution (0.45%). This provides adequate sodium, but with less risk of sodium overload than normal saline. Potassium may be added to the solution if required. It is seldom necessary to add any other electrolyte even in children with considerable acidosis; rehydration alone will allow normal homeostasis to restore the acid–base balance. Once hydration is restored to normal, dextrose saline may be included in maintenance treatment, as long as the plasma electrolyte balance remains satisfactory. A guide to children's fluid and electrolyte requirements is given in Table 8.1.

Infant feeding in diarrhoeal illnesses

It is not nowadays the practice to withhold feeding from infants or small children with diarrhoea. Infants who are fed early lose less weight than those who are offered only fluids. Some work in Third World countries suggests that rice-water feeds are associated with earlier improvement of diarrhoea than feeds made with plain water.

Secondary acquired lactose intolerance

This is a particular problem in infants and young children. It is commonest after rotavirus infection and enteropathogenic *Escherichia coli* infections, which can cause severe mucosal damage. Lactose absorption depends on lactase enzyme systems in the mucosal brush border. It takes time for the enzymes to become functional after mucosal healing. Until this happens, the lactose in milk and other dairy foods cannot be absorbed, so it ferments in the bowel lumen, causing abdominal discomfort, flatulence and acid diarrhoea soon after feeding.

Infants with lactose intolerance can be maintained on lactose-free or low-lactose formulae such as soya-based milks, Pregestimil and some of the low-lactose Galactomin preparations. The problem is temporary; once the infant is gaining weight satisfactorily, normal feeding can soon be resumed. Older children, including weaning infants, can be given non-dairy solids to replace milk feeds.

Secondary acquired lactose intolerance must be distinguished from the primary loss of the lactase system, which occurs particularly in adult oriental and Caribbean people. The final loss of the system can be precipitated by a diarrhoeal episode, and lactose absorption will not return in these cases. Fortunately, the lactose absorption system is the only fragile mucosal function; other sugar absorption systems are rarely affected by intestinal infection.

Drug treatment of vomiting and diarrhoea

Antiemetic drugs

Antiemetic drugs are often helpful in the management of severe vomiting, reducing fluid loss to a level at which oral rehydration can be effective. There are three main types of antiemetic drugs — phenothiazines (of which prochlorperazine is popularly used in hospitals), metoclopramide and domperidone. Phenothiazines and metoclopramide are slightly sedative at antiemetic doses, and both occasionally cause dopamine-induced dystonic reactions, especially in children and teenagers. Domperidone has dopaminergic actions, but does not cross the blood–brain barrier, and does not cause such noticeable central effects.

Antidiarrhoeal drugs

Antidiarrhoeal drugs are rarely successful in clinical practice. All of those currently available simply reduce gut motility. This allows fluid faeces to accumulate, but the symptoms resume as soon as the expanded bowel volume is filled. The likelihood of atropine-like side-effects such as dry mouth and a tendency to urinary retention is a further disadvantage. Antidiarrhoeals tend

Age	Daily baseline fluid requirement (ml/kg)	Daily sodium (mmol/kg)	Daily potassium (mmol/kg)	Total daily calcium (mmol)
1–2 days	75–100	2.5	2.5	12.5–17.5
Up to 1 year	150	2.5	2.5	12.5–17.5
1–3 years	100	2.5	2.5	20–25
4–6 years	90	2.0	2.0	20–25
7–10 years	70	2.0	2.0	20–25
10–14 years	60	1.5	1.5	30–38

Table 8.1 A guide to children's fluid and electrolyte requirements

to produce toxic effects similar to those of atropine in small children, and are not therefore recommended for this age group. In general it is better to deal with abnormalities of hydration, using oral or intravenous fluids, than to resort to antidiarrhoeal drugs.

Laboratory diagnosis of diarrhoea

The diagnosis of infective diarrhoea depends on the identification of the pathogen from faeces by electron microscopy, by culture or by demonstration of antigens. In the case of viruses, electron microscopy and culture are most often used. As all bacterial bowel pathogens are closely related, the only reliable diagnosis is made by culture and formal identification of individual pathogens.

At least three specimens should be examined. A faecal suspension is inoculated onto a combination of media. All of the media employed for this purpose are selective. The more selective the medium is, the easier it is to detect the presence of the pathogen sought, but the disadvantage is that highly selective media are also inhibitory to the salmonellae to some extent, which may mean that specimens containing low numbers of pathogens will not be detected. A relatively non-selective medium such as MacConkey agar is usually inoculated in combination with a more selective medium which is designed to facilitate the isolation of particular pathogens (Fig. 8.1).

Managing food-borne disease in the community

In developing countries without safe water supplies, the majority of gastrointestinal infections are water-borne. In developed countries, where water is less likely to be contaminated, food-borne disease is a much more important cause of morbidity. It has been estimated, for example, that more than 50% of all cases of infectious gastrointestinal disease in the UK are food-related. The incidence of several food-borne pathogens has increased considerably in recent years (Fig. 8.2).

Ideally, all food produced for human consumption would be free from pathogenic bacteria. In practice, food is frequently contaminated and measures are required to ensure that it is safe at the point of consumption.

A number of measures are aimed at reducing the level of bacterial contamination at source. These include good animal husbandry and slaughtering of infected livestock. Such measures are normally the responsibility of central government. Further down the chain of supply, a complex legislative framework exists which controls the processing, storage and preparation of food by retailers. The enforcement of these regulations is the responsibility of local government.

At consumer level, prevention of food poisoning depends on good practices for cooking and storing food and on personal hygiene. Food should be cooked thoroughly and eaten immediately. Cooked and raw food should be stored separately. Perishable items should be kept in properly maintained refrigerators. Food not in a refrigerator should be covered to protect it from flies, rodents and other animals. Food-handlers should wash hands before and after food preparation. Any cuts, abrasions or other skin lesions should be covered before preparing food. A food-handler who is ill (particularly with diarrhoea or vomiting) should not prepare food until fully recovered.

> **Prevention of food poisoning**
> 1 Safe food production: healthy flocks and herds, avoiding use of sewage to fertilize food crops.
> 2 Food-manufacturing processes: hygienic slaughtering and meat packing, rodent-free storage of crops, storage at chill or refrigeration temperatures, hygienic packaging, cold chain during distribution.
> 3 Domestic and commercial food hygiene: adequate refrigeration, avoidance of cross-contamination, use within spoilage dates, adequate decontamination of food by washing and/or cooking, personal and kitchen hygiene.

Food poisoning is a notifiable disease in the UK. Outbreaks should be promptly investigated to determine the source and implement any necessary control measures. The principles of outbreak investigation are described in Chapter 25.

Viral infections of the intestinal tract

ORGANISM LIST

Rotavirus
Adenoviruses (high serotype numbers)
Caliciviruses
Small round structured viruses
Small round viruses
Astroviruses
Coronaviruses
(Hepatitis A and E viruses; see Chapter 9).

Rotavirus gastroenteritis

Epidemiology

Rotaviruses are the most common viral cause of acute gastroenteritis in young children. It has been estimated

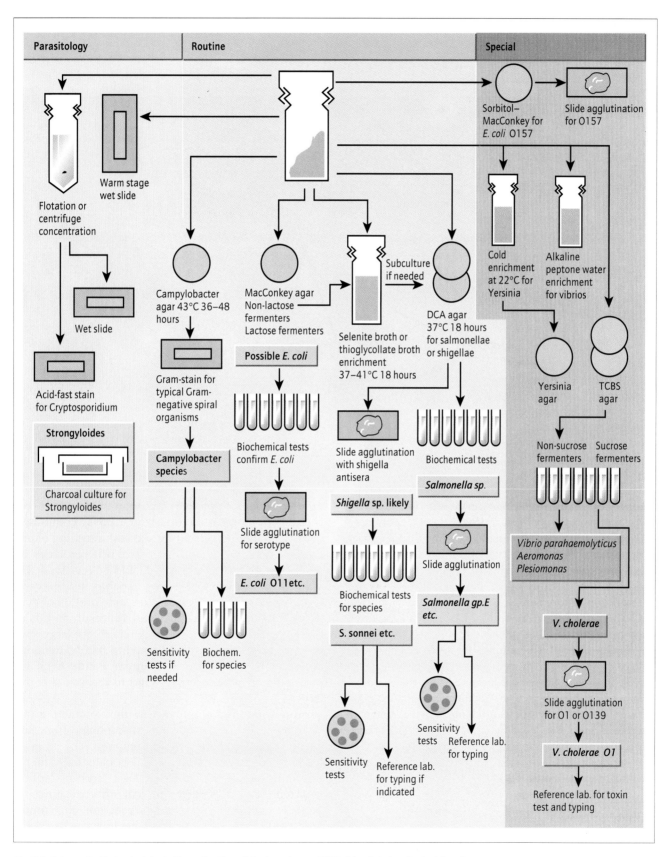

Fig. 8.1 Scheme for the bacteriological investigation of stool specimens. TCBS, thiosulphate–citrate–bilesalt–sucrose.

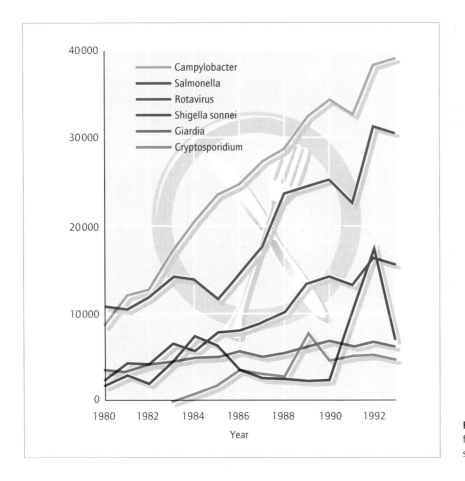

Fig. 8.2 Trends in the incidence of common food-borne infections in England and Wales since 1980.

that up to a million children worldwide die each year from rotavirus diarrhoea. Most deaths occur in developing countries with inadequate medical facilities; however the disease is also an important cause of morbidity in developed countries. It has been estimated in the USA that a third of all hospital admissions for diarrhoea in children are due to rotavirus infection.

Over 10 000 laboratory-confirmed cases are reported each year in the UK; this probably represents only a small fraction of the total. The number of reports has increased in recent years. Some of this increase may be an artefact due to improved virological techniques for the examination of faecal specimens. The peak incidence of infection is between 6 and 24 months. Clinical infection is rare in children over 5 years of age, although subclinical infection is probably common. The sexes are equally affected. The disease has a highly seasonal pattern — most infections occur during the winter months.

Clinical features

The incubation period is about 24 h and is followed by a rather abrupt onset of both diarrhoea and vomiting. A mild to moderate fever is common at the onset, but rarely persists for more than 1 or 2 days. Vomiting is usually moderate, permitting successful feeding of oral fluids. Prolonged vomiting is rare; if it continues for more than 48 h the diagnosis should be reviewed. The severity of the diarrhoea is very variable. In a few cases it is profuse enough to cause gross dehydration or even shock. Blood is occasionally seen, especially in infants under the age of 1. This probably reflects the large-scale destruction of mucosal cells, leaving friable, denuded areas in the duodenum and upper ileum. Even the most severely affected cases tend to recover after 2–4 days.

Adults are often immune to the common group A rotaviruses, but a few are susceptible, often suffering vomiting as their major symptom. The illness is usually transient, but the patient is potentially highly infectious while the vomiting lasts, and susceptible children may be infected by an affected nurse or mother. Group B and C rotaviruses are uncommon, and adults are less likely to be immune to them. They have caused large outbreaks of adult gastroenteritis.

Diagnosis

Electron microscopy of diarrhoea stools will often demonstrate typical rotavirus particles (Fig. 8.3). Human rotaviruses do not grow in cell culture.

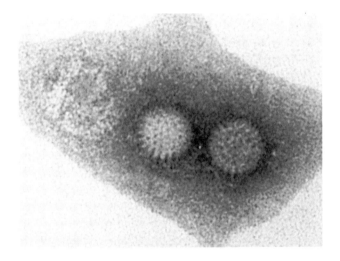

Fig. 8.3 Rotavirus particles demonstrated by negative-stained electron microscopy preparation of a diarrhoea stool. Courtesy of Professor P.D. Griffiths and Ms G. Clewley, Department of Virology, Royal Free Hospital School of Medicine.

Management

Most cases are readily managed with oral rehydration treatment. A minority of cases, however, have persistent diarrhoea, exacerbated by attempts to give milk feeds. This is caused by postgastroenteritis lactose intolerance, and is managed by avoiding milk and yoghurt in the diet, and/or by substituting a low-lactose milk for the child's usual formula.

A few infants have exacerbations of diarrhoea after each feed of oral rehydration fluid, suggesting that there are too few functioning mucosal cells to absorb the glucose in the fluid. This is a transient problem but while it lasts hydration can be maintained with sugar-free electrolyte solution, such as half-normal saline.

Intravenous rehydration is rarely indicated, and can usually be discontinued after 24 h.

Rare effects of rotavirus infection

Some 1–2% of children admitted with rotavirus infection present with collapse, hypotension and peripheral cyanosis. It is impossible to determine the aetiology of the condition until persisting diarrhoea and resolution

of fever point to an intestinal infection. A handful of reports exist of cases whose cerebrospinal fluid contained rotavirus particles during this acute illness.

Rotavirus can cause persisting diarrhoea in immuno-suppressed patients, including those with human immunodeficiency virus infection.

Rotavirus vaccines

Orally administered live rotavirus vaccines are currently being developed, using both animal and human virus strains. The protection afforded by these vaccines is variable.

Other viral infections of the gastrointestinal tract

Epidemiology

Small round structured viruses (SRSVs, including Norwalk virus), adenoviruses, astroviruses, caliciviruses and coronaviruses have all been associated with outbreaks of gastroenteritis. Transmission is usually from person to person by the faecal–oral route; however, several food-borne incidents have been reported recently. Many of these are due to shellfish harvested from sewage-polluted estuaries and eaten raw or without sufficient cooking. Aerosol spread probably also plays an important role in many of these infections, particularly in winter vomiting disease (see below). All age groups are affected.

Clinical features

These viral infections are all marked by short incubation periods, varying from a few hours to 1 day. There is more variation of incubation between individuals with the same infection than between infections. In most cases the illness lasts for 1 or 2 days.

Adenoviruses and caliciviruses tend to affect children, adenoviruses causing mainly diarrhoea and caliciviruses mainly vomiting. Adenoviruses have often been identified during surveys in the stools of asymptomatic children, but this is not the case with calicivirus which usually causes symptomatic infection.

Winter vomiting disease

Calicivirus is thought to be a common cause of this disease. The illness has an incubation period of about 1 day followed by several hours of profuse vomiting. After the vomiting gradually ceases there is a period of 24–36 h of fatigue before recovery is complete. This is an intensely infectious disease which often causes school and family outbreaks, affecting both adults and children.

SRSVs and unstructured viruses are common causes of food-poisoning outbreaks. Their association with particular foods is helpful in leading to the suspected diagnosis, as they cause no distinctive clinical features. They are much more often described as causes of adult disease than of childhood infections.

Diagnosis of viral gastroenteritis

An aetiological diagnosis in viral gastroenteritis is most important in the investigation of outbreaks in closed communities such as nursing homes or hospitals. Diagnosis of individual cases requires a considerable

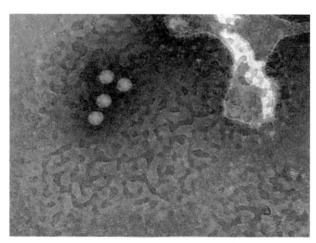

(a)

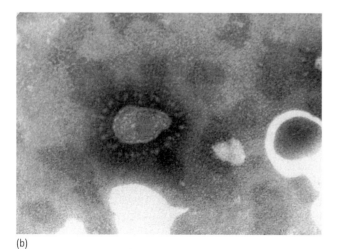

(b)

Fig. 8.4 (a) Small round viruses and (b) a coronavirus in electron microscopic preparation of a diarrhoea stool. Courtesy of Professor P.D. Griffiths and Ms G. Clewley, Department of Virology, Royal Free Hospital School of Medicine.

investment of time and resources, and is of questionable clinical relevance. The principal method of diagnosis is electron microscopy, which enables visualization of the viruses, most of which have characteristic morphology (Fig. 8.4). Enzyme-linked immunosorbent assay tests for the diagnosis of rotavirus are also available.

Bacterial diseases of the gastrointestinal tract

ORGANISM LIST

Common infections
  Campylobacter sp.
  Salmonella sp.
  Shigella sp.
  Escherichia coli
  Clostridium perfringens
  Helicobacter pylori.

Uncommon or rare infections
  Aeromonas sp.
  Vibrio parahaemolyticus
  Plesiomonas sp.
  Yersinia sp.
  Clostridium difficile
  Vibrio cholerae.

Bacteria which elaborate preformed toxins
  Staphylococcus aureus
  Bacillus cereus
  Clostridium botulinum.

Escherichia coli gastroenteritis

Introduction

E. coli are inhabitants of human gut, forming the major part of the facultative anaerobic flora. Their role in human disease has only recently been appreciated due to the difficulties of distinguishing commensal types from those which are behaving as pathogens.

In the 1960s certain serotypes of *E. coli* caused large epidemics of gastroenteritis in infants. Important *E. coli* diseases now include toxin-mediated traveller's diarrhoea (see Chapter 19) and haemorrhagic colitis associated with certain serotypes of verocytotoxin-producing organisms.

Microbiology

E. coli are facultative anaerobes which ferment a wide range of sugars, including lactose, producing acid and gas. They are oxidase-, Voges–Proskauer and citrate-negative, but produce indole and are methyl red-positive. They are actively motile due to the possession of flagella.

Pathogenesis

The capsular K antigens of *E. coli* have been shown to be pathogenicity factors which facilitate adherence. Strains possessing a K1 capsule are the most frequent *E. coli* isolated from cases of neonatal meningitis. The mechanism for this is not understood, although it is known that colonization of neonatal rat gut by K1 strains, which adhere to intestinal epithelium, often leads to bacteraemia and meningitis. The best characterized example of the pathogenicity of capsular adherence is the K88 antigen-bearing strains causing scour in piglets.

Fimbriae also mediate attachment to mucosal surfaces (first recognized in the contribution of P fimbriae to the pathogenesis of urinary tract infection). Fimbriae also play a role in the pathogenesis of enterotoxigenic *E. coli* (ETEC) infections, as no disease is produced by toxigenic *E. coli* which cannot adhere to gut mucosa. Some fimbrial colonizing factor antigens (CFAs) have been identified, and these include CFA/I, 6–7 nm rigid fimbriae, and the CFA/II family of antigens, 2–3 nm fibrillar fimbria which are analogous to the K88 antigens of porcine strains. Other similar CFA families have been described in other strains.

Like other Gram-negative bacteria, *E. coli* has a lipopolysaccharide (LPS) antigen in the outer membrane. This is similar in structure to other LPSs among the Enterobacteraciae with a central lipid A core, an oligosaccharide moiety and polysaccharide chain. The lipid A portion is an endotoxin (see Chapter 1). The polysaccharide chain protects the organism from serum lysis and is the main (O) antigen of the organism. More than 150 O serotypes have been described, many of which are related to other *E. coli* pathogenicity factors. For example, the most common enteropathogenic *E. coli* (EPEC) are serotypes O26, O55, O111, O114, O119, O125-9 and O142. Strains responsible for the haemolytic–uraemic syndrome are usually serotype O157.

Toxins elaborated by *E. coli* are important in the pathogenesis of diarrhoeal and systemic disease. Two main enterotoxins are produced by enterotoxigenic *E. coli* (ETEC), the heat-labile (LT) and the heat-stable (ST) toxins.

The LT toxin consists of two polypeptide subunits, A and B. In the native toxin there are five B subunits which mediate attachment to cells via the Gm1 ganglioside, and one A subunit which enters the cell and activates adenylate cyclase. This toxin is biologically and immunologically closely related to cholera toxin (Fig. 8.5).

The ST toxin exists in several forms. ST mediates its toxic activity by stimulating guanylate cyclase.

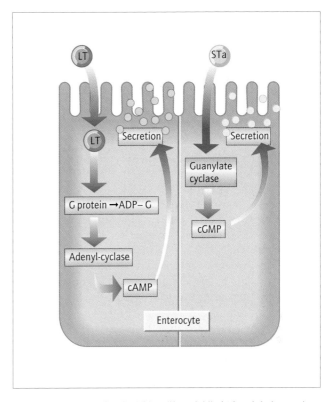

Fig. 8.5 The action of *Escherichia coli* heat-labile (LT) and cholera toxin and of *E. coli* heat-stable toxin (STa).

Some *E. coli* strains, called verocytotoxin-producing *E. coli* (VTEC), make a toxin which kills the cells in vero-cell monolayers. Elaboration of this toxin by O157 and O129 *E. coli* has been implicated in the pathogenesis of haemolytic–uraemic syndrome. This is analogous to the enterotoxin produced by *Shigella dysenteriae* type 1 (the Shiga toxin). Some strains also produce a second cytotoxin, verotoxin 2, which is not neutralized by antibodies to the Shiga toxin.

EPEC have been associated with outbreaks of diarrhoea in institutional settings and in infant diarrhoea in developing countries. These strains lack ST and LT, and have no enteroinvasive properties. Despite this, volunteer studies indicate that these organisms are true pathogens. Electron microscopic studies show that EPEC cause destruction of microvilli without evidence of invasion. It has also been shown that these strains adhere to Hep-2 cells, which is an unusual property for *E. coli*. EPEC adherence factor (EAF) is a 94 kDa protein which is encoded on a plasmid. Infection with EAF-positive strains stimulates production of EAF antibody, which may protect against future infection. Using a DNA probe to detect the EAF gene, studies have indicated that EPEC serotypes must possess the gene to initiate diarrhoeal disease. Another and distinct mechanism whereby EPEC may cause disease is by the elaboration of a Shiga-like toxin.

Another group of *E. coli* responsible for diarrhoea are the enteroadherent *E. coli* (EAEC). These are not classic EPEC serotypes and do not possess the EAF plasmid, or elaborate any of the recognized toxins. It is not yet clear whether the pathogenicity of this organism depends on its enteroadherence property.

Pathogenicity factors for *Escherichia coli*
1 Capsular K antigens (K1).
2 Fimbriae (colonizing factor antigens — CFA/I, CFA/II and others).
3 Lipopolysaccharide O antigens (endotoxin).
4 Enterotoxins (heat-labile and heat-stable).
5 Verocytotoxin (Shiga-like toxin).
6 Enteropathogenic *Escherichia coli* adherence factor (EAF).
7 Enteroadherence (mechanism unknown).

Epidemiology

The routes of transmission and epidemiological features of *E. coli* vary considerably between different pathogenic types and in different geographical locations. In tropical countries where standards of hygiene are poor, ETEC are the commonest bacterial cause of diarrhoea in children. Humans are the main source of infection which is transmitted by contaminated food and water. The disease is uncommon in western Europe and the USA, although ETEC are an important cause of traveller's diarrhoea.

EPEC are usually spread from person to person by the faecal–oral route, although transmission via contaminated baby food also occurs. Most infections occur as outbreaks of infantile enteritis. The incidence of EPEC infections is decreasing in many countries.

Enteroinvasive *E. coli* (EIEC) infections are also rare in developed countries. Infection is usually food-borne but direct person-to-person spread may also occur. All age groups are affected.

VTEC were first described in Canada in the late 1970s. They are associated with several serogroups of *E. coli*, although by far the commonest is serogroup O157. During the 1980s the incidence of VTEC infection and its clinical sequelae (haemorrhagic colitis and haemolytic–uraemic syndrome) increased rapidly in the USA and Canada. VTEC is now the commonest cause of acute renal failure in children in North America. In the UK, VTEC infections are uncommon, but of increasing importance (Fig. 8.6). The infection is spread by contaminated food (notably hamburger meat) and unpasteurized milk. In the USA and many European

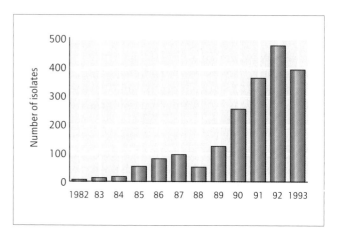

Fig. 8.6 Increasing reports of verocytotoxin-producing *Escherichia coli* infection in England and Wales.

countries, outbreaks have occurred in the community, in nursing homes for the elderly and in children's day-care centres.

Clinical features

The incubation period is usually 1 or 2 days, but may be up to 5 days. The onset is abrupt, with both vomiting and diarrhoea for the first 6–24 h, followed by watery diarrhoea alone. There is often a moderate fever at the onset. There is little abdominal pain in uncomplicated gastroenteritis, and the illness is clinically similar to viral gastroenteritis or salmonellosis. A minority of cases exhibit severe disease with rapid dehydration and collapse, or prolonged illness with persisting diarrhoea and sometimes lactose intolerance.

Haemorrhagic colitis

Haemorrhagic colitis affects both children and adults. It begins as an unremarkable diarrhoeal illness, but quickly progresses to a syndrome of bloody diarrhoea and abdominal pain. In spite of the intense illness, fever is not an important feature. Sigmoidoscopy reveals an acutely inflamed colonic mucosa and the condition can be mistaken for acute inflammatory bowel disease. The majority of cases are self-limiting, with spontaneous recovery within 7–10 days. A handful of cases have proved persistent, requiring prolonged symptomatic support and attempts at specific chemotherapy.

Haemolytic–uraemic syndrome

Haemolytic–uraemic syndrome is mainly a disease of children, but can also affect adults. The adult form in particular is said to overlap with the syndrome of thrombotic thrombocytopenic purpura (TTP). The important features are a rising blood urea and creatinine, microangiopathic haemolytic anaemia and thrombocytopenia (Fig. 8.7). Clinical suspicion can be alerted by a raised blood pressure, persistent vomiting or fits. Although most cases of haemolytic–uraemic syndrome seem to follow a gastrointestinal illness, this may be extremely mild and need not include bloody diarrhoea or abdominal pain.

More than half of clinically apparent haemolytic–uraemic syndrome cases require haemodialysis, but the outlook is good and almost all VTEC-associated cases recover fully in time.

Diagnosis

Apart from haemorrhagic colitis, the gastrointestinal illnesses produced by *E. coli* are non-specific, and must be suspected on epidemiological evidence alone. Outbreaks of disease in travellers or haemolytic–uraemic syndrome outbreaks will alert the clinician to seek appropriate diagnoses, and the public health specialist to seek associated cases.

In haemolytic–uraemic syndrome the diarrhoea is often transient and may be over by the time systemic illness is apparent. VTEC becomes undetectable at an early stage and many specialists find that a search for the pathogen is fruitless after the fifth or sixth day of illness.

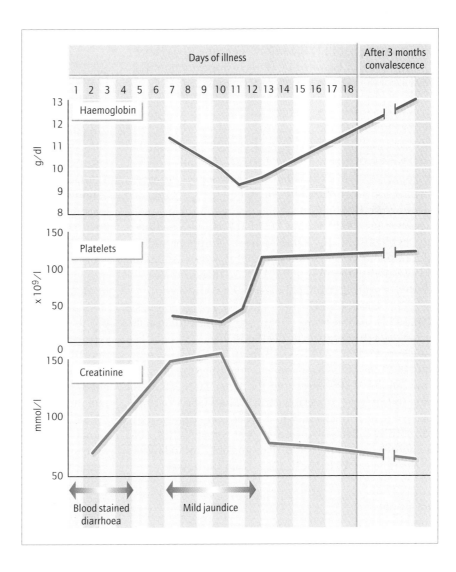

Fig. 8.7 The evolution of haemolytic–uraemic syndrome after an attack of diarrhoea.

Laboratory diagnosis

E. coli pose significant problems for diagnosis in the microbiological laboratory. In most situations in enteric bacteriology, inhibition of a range of species will enable the pathogen sought to be selected. In this instance the pathogen and the normal flora are the same species and the conventional methods of selection cannot be employed.

EPEC are limited to a relatively small number of serotypes. In children under the age of 3 years in whom the diagnosis is suspected, an additional blood or nutrient agar plate is inoculated and several colonies of *E. coli* are 'screened' with polyvalent antisera to the EPEC strains.

VTEC strains are found in several O serotypes, among which O157 predominates. This strain is unusual among other *E. coli* in not fermenting sorbitol. A modified form of MacConkey's agar, incorporating sorbitol in place of lactose, can be used to identify the majority of these strains. In addition to this, toxigenicity must be tested by applying culture supernatant to vero-cell monolayers. Unselected stool cultures can be tested by DNA hybridization for the presence of the verocytotoxin-producing gene.

Management

In most cases symptomatic treatment with adequate hydration is all that is needed. Specific chemotherapy is indicated in cases of severe or prolonged disease, collapse or disease in elderly and debilitated patients.

Pathogenic *E. coli* have become resistant to many antimicrobial agents, including broad-spectrum penicillins and cephalosporins, trimethoprim, sulphonamides, chloramphenicol and even aminoglycosides. Isolation and sensitivity testing of the *E. coli* are therefore recommended if specific treatment must be contemplated.

The agents most likely to be effective are quinolones, as in *Salmonella* infections. Treatment with ciprofloxacin for 3–5 days can be given orally if possible.

It is not clear whether antibiotic treatment will influence the development of haemolytic–uraemic syndrome in VTEC infection. Evidence suggests that some antibiotics stimulate verocytotoxin production, but that quinolones inhibit it. It is very likely that antimotility drugs increase the probability of haemolytic– uraemic syndrome, possibly by delaying the clearance of VTEC or its toxin from the bowel.

Prevention

Prevention of *E. coli* gastroenteritis is by the provision of adequate facilities for disposal of faeces and hand-washing facilities. Scrupulous attention to hygiene is important, particularly in nurseries, where infection is common. Hamburger meat should be cooked thoroughly before eating. Travellers to tropical countries should avoid drinking untreated water and eating high-risk foods such as raw vegetables, salad, unpeeled fruit and undercooked meat (see Chapter 19).

Salmonella infections

Introduction

It is important to appreciate the difference between salmonella food poisoning and typhoid and paratyphoid fevers caused by specific enteric fever salmonellae. The food-poisoning organisms infect both humans and animals, and are both biochemically and clinically different from the enteric salmonellae which are exclusively human pathogens. Enteric fevers are mainly associated with travel, and will be discussed in Chapter 19.

Epidemiology

There are approximately 2200 different serotypes of *Salmonella* which infect animals. Most of these are capable of causing salmonellosis in humans, although only about 200 are reported in any one year in the UK. Currently the most common are *S. enteritidis*, *S. typhimurium* and *S. virchow*.

Poultry is the commonest source of human salmonellosis. Up to 60% of poultry meat may be contaminated with salmonella. Both the shell and occasionally the white of eggs can be contaminated. Other meats such as beef and pork are also well-recognized sources. Transmission is usually by ingestion of inadequately cooked food, or food which has been contaminated during storage or preparation and eaten without further cooking. If contaminated food is stored without adequate refrigeration, the organisms multiply and achieve an infective dose.

Other routes of transmission are less common. Food-handlers are not usually a source of infection unless they remain at work with diarrhoea.

Person-to-person spread by the faecal–oral route sometimes occurs, usually in institutions such as psychogeriatric hospitals and old people's homes.

Many countries experienced an unprecedented rise in salmonellosis during the late 1980s. The commonest epidemic serotype varies between countries, and over a period of years within the same country. In the UK, beef-associated *S. typhimurium* was replaced by poultry- and egg-associated *S. enteritidis* phage type 4 in the 1980s. In mainland Europe the predominant type in the 1990s is *S. enteritidis* phage type 8.

Salmonellosis typically occurs either sporadically or in small outbreaks, often within households. Large outbreaks, although more readily detected, are less common. They usually occur in association with large functions such as weddings or in institutions.

All age groups are affected; however the incidence is greatest in children and in the elderly. Transmission occurs most frequently during late summer and early autumn, especially in hot weather.

Microbiology

Like *E. coli*, this genus is part of the Enterobacteraciae and has the characteristics of this family of organisms. It is a non-lactose fermenter, produces acid and gas from glucose, metabolizes citrate, and produces hydrogen sulphide. These and other biochemical characteristics are used in the identification of salmonella growth in selective media, such as triple sugar-iron medium. In this medium, gas production from glucose causes fractures in the agar column, and hydrogen sulphide production blackens the iron-containing agar layer (Fig. 8.8). *S. typhi*, *S. cholerae-suis*, *S. paratyphi* and *S. arizona* can also be differentiated from other salmonellae on the basis of their biochemical reactions.

Salmonellae possess lipopolysaccharide (LPS), which is their somatic O antigen, and exists in 60 types. These, together with the flagellar H antigens, define the serotype which in this genus is identified by a species name, e.g. *S. enteritidis*, *S. typhimurium*, *S. virchow*, etc. The LPS protects the bacterial cell from the bactericidal activity of serum, influences macrophage interactions, decreases susceptibility to host cationic proteins and functions as endotoxin.

The ten commonest *Salmonella* spp. in the UK
1 *S. enteritidis*.
2 *S. typhimurium*.
3 *S. virchow*.
4 *S. dublin*.
5 *S. bovis-morbificans*.
6 *S. hadar*.
7 *S. newport*.
8 *S. braenderup*.
9 *S. heidelberg*.
10 *S. montevideo*.

Injection of small amounts of *S. typhi* LPS in human volunteers can reproduce typhoid-like symptoms. *S. typhi* (and also *S. paratyphi* C and some *Citrobacter* spp.) possess the Vi antigen, a polysaccharide capsule consisting of alpha-1,4,2-deoxy-*N*-acetylgalacturonic acid. Its effect is to prevent phagocytosis and to mask the O antigen, reducing the minimum infective dose for organisms possessing this antigen.

Pathogenesis

Salmonella food poisoning is an infection of gut epithelium, which does not extend beyond the basement membrane. The salmonellae first digest the mucosal glycocalyx, and then invade the mucosa. This is followed by phagocytosis of the organism by the epithelial cells. Salmonellae which cause invasive disease are thought to be transported through the cells by this route, whereas those strains which cause enteritis remain localized.

In salmonellosis there is excessive fluid secretion from the ileum and jejunum. For invasive salmonellae, survival within macrophages is the main pathogenic attribute. This is probably genetically controlled, depending on the expression of factors which protect the organisms from the effects of neutrophil and macrophage cationic proteins. Intramacrophage survival can be abolished by mutations which make salmonellae more susceptible to oxidative stress.

Clinical features

After an incubation period of 18–36 h, there is an illness of variable severity. The first symptoms are malaise, nausea, vomiting and often fever. Diarrhoea soon follows and becomes the main feature within 24 h. The diarrhoea is watery and brown, often becoming greenish if it persists. In most cases the fever resolves by the first

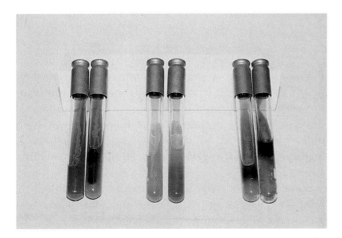

Fig. 8.8 Effect of *Salmonella* growth in triple sugar-iron medium.

or second day and the intestinal symptoms improve soon afterwards. In more severe cases illness may persist for many weeks with low-grade fever, continuing diarrhoea and progressive debility. Abdominal pain is not an important feature of the illness, although discomfort accompanies the call to stool.

Elderly patients often are fare badly. They have insufficient cardiovascular reserve to withstand sudden fluid loss, and may suffer low-output cardiac failure, myocardial infarction or stroke during acute diarrhoea. They tolerate the necessary rehydration poorly and easily develop pulmonary oedema. Confusion, hypostatic chest infections and the risk of deep-vein thrombosis during immobility are longer-term hazards.

Patients with achlorhydria are especially susceptible to salmonellosis. They are infected by small doses of organisms, and are often severely ill with high fever, intense watery diarrhoea and a surprisingly high blood urea — out of proportion with the apparent degree of dehydration. They are more likely than other patients to have salmonella bacteraemia.

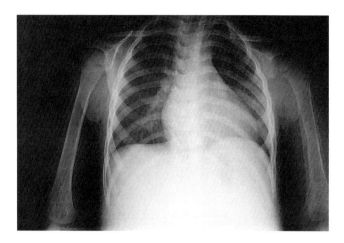

Fig. 8.9 *Salmonella* osteomyelitis in the humerus of a child with sickle-cell disease.

Salmonella colitis

Salmonella colitis occurs in up to 10% of patients, who then complain of colic and bloody stools. Sigmoidoscopy often confirms the presence of colonic inflammation.

Salmonella bacteraemia

Salmonella bacteraemia and metastatic infections are uncommon. They can occur in association with obvious bowel infection, but are almost equally common in patients without preceding bowel symptoms. Some salmonellae are more likely than others to produce bacteraemia; *S. dublin* and *S. cholerae-suis* commonly spread to the blood stream, but fortunately they are rare in the UK.

Sites of tissue damage may become infected by salmonellae, even when bacteraemia has not been apparent. Commonly affected sites are bones and joints, including those of sickle-cell sufferers (Fig. 8.9), and arterial aneurysms. Occasionally a patient presents with a soft-tissue abscess affecting, for example, the skin (Fig. 8.10), the kidney or the ischiorectal fossa, and laboratory investigation reveals salmonellae in the pus. These infections are presumably blood-borne, and there is rarely a convincing explanation for their occurrence.

Diagnosis of salmonellosis

There are few specific features of salmonellosis, especially in the mild presentations which commonly

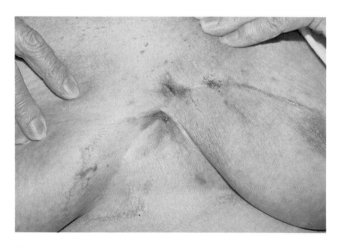

Fig. 8.10 *Salmonella typhimurium* breast abscess: this abscess was unresponsive to treatment with antistaphylococcal agents, but resolved after prolonged co-trimoxazole therapy (there had been no preceding diarrhoeal illness).

occur. It is, however, the commonest cause of persisting diarrhoea without abdominal pain. Recovery of a *Salmonella* sp. from the diarrhoea stool confirms the specific diagnosis. Blood cultures are indicated if fever is high or persists for more than 48 h. A high blood urea, voluminous watery stools or a history of achlorhydria makes blood cultures mandatory.

Stool cultures should always be carried out in patients presenting with extraintestinal salmonella infections, as asymptomatic excretion may be discovered. The bowel is a reservoir of infection in such cases.

Isolation and identification of salmonellae and shigellae

Since the selective procedures to identify salmonellae and shigellae are largely the same, the diagnostic laboratory methods for the two organisms will be described together.

A wide range of media have been described for the isolation of *Salmonellae* and *Shigellae*. All contain selective agents to inhibit the different components of the gastrointestinal flora. These compounds are intended to inhibit the normal faecal flora, but may also inhibit the pathogens to some extent. Thus there is a balance between selection and diagnostic yield. Bile salts will select for organisms which inhabit the bowel. More selective still is sodium desoxycholate, found in xylose lysine desoxycholate (XLD) agar, or desoxycholate citrate agar (DCA). Even more inhibitory are media containing bismuth sulphate, such as Wilson and Blair's medium.

For the best chance of recovering salmonellae (or shigellae) from stool cultures, most microbiological laboratories would use a combination of media — one less selective medium (MacConkey or XLD) for the diagnosis of the more fastidious shigellae, and a more inhibitory medium (DCA or Wilson and Blair) to select for salmonellae.

These media contain indicator systems to aid the selection of colony types for further study. The simplest of these is lactose and neutral red. Organisms which ferment lactose will alter the pH of the medium, changing the colour of the indicator and producing pink/red colonies (Fig. 8.11). As neither salmonellae nor shigellae ferment lactose, these organisms form clear colonies (easily distinguished from the pink colonies of *E. coli* and klebsiellae). In XLD agar more complex changes take place: organisms which ferment xylose include coliforms and salmonellae. This causes a fall in pH, but salmonellae also decarboxylate lysine, causing a counter-balancing rise in pH. Shigellae neither ferment xylose nor decarboxylate lysine. Thus salmonellae and shigellae both appear red in this medium, in contrast to other neutral coliform organisms which only produce acid, and have yellow opaque colonies. Ferric ammonium citrate in this medium and DCA will indicate colonies of hydrogen sulphide producers (salmonellae) which will have a black centre.

The next stage in the diagnostic process is the use of biochemical screening tests to distinguish them from *Proteus* colonies, which have similar appearances. These fermentation reactions utilize combination media such as Kligler iron agar, triple sugar agar or Kohn's tubes. Commercially produced kits also detect the characteristic activity of preformed enzymes (API ZYM). Organisms giving characteristic reactions are then subjected to full biochemical and serological identification. The biochemical tests include sugar fermentation tests, decarboxylation and dehydrogenation reactions and hydrogen sulphide production.

Serological identification of salmonellae and shigellae is unreliable without biochemical confirmation, because of the many cross-reactions with commensal gut flora.

Full typing of *Salmonella* spp. is only indicated for the identification and investigation of outbreaks. Typing methods available include sensitivity testing for agents such as trimethoprim, ciprofloxacin, chloramphenicol and sulphamethoxazole. Phage typing is available for some *Salmonella* spp.

Salmonella spp. which can be phage-typed

1 *S. enteritidis.*
2 *S. typhimurium.*
3 *S. virchow.*
4 *S. typhi.*
5 *S. paratyphi.*

Management of salmonellosis

Most mild cases require only oral rehydration while awaiting spontaneous recovery. Intravenous fluids may be needed for 12–24 h if dehydration or exhaustion dictates. Even bacteraemic patients will often make a rapid recovery with non-specific treatment.

Specific antimicrobial chemotherapy is indicated if no spontaneous improvement is evident after 36–48 h

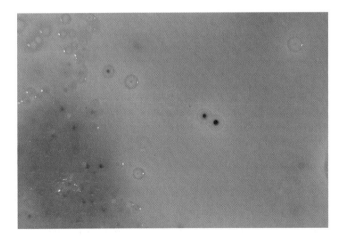

Fig. 8.11 Pink colonies of lactose-fermenting Enterobacteriacae growing on MacConkey agar.

rehydration therapy, or if shock is present. It is also indicated in those at special risk. This includes sickle-cell patients, immunosuppressed patients and the elderly, because of the severe complications of salmonellosis that all of these groups may suffer.

The antimicrobial treatment of choice is limited by the broad spectrum of antibiotic resistance that salmonellae have evolved in recent years. Since food-poisoning salmonellae are natural colonizers and pathogens of animals as well as humans, they have been widely exposed to the antibiotics used in both veterinary and medical practice. They are usually resistant to a wide range of agents, including tetracyclines, sulphonamides, aminoglycosides and broad-spectrum penicillins and cephalosporins. A substantial proportion are resistant to trimethoprim and chloramphenicol. The recently introduced quinolone agents, however, are very active against Enterobacteriaceae and most salmonellae are sensitive to treatment with them.

Recommended regimens include oral ciprofloxacin or norfloxacin. In rare cases of quinolone resistance, trimethoprim, co-trimoxazole or chloramphenicol may be effective, but these agents should not be used before the sensitivity of the organisms has been confirmed. Long courses of treatment are not usually necessary; 4 or 5 days' treatment is usually sufficient.

Patients with shock or bacteraemia should be treated with intravenous antibiotics. Ciprofloxacin or another quinolone remain the treatment of choice. In case of resistance to quinolones, chloramphenicol may be given, pending sensitivity testing to trimethoprim, trimethoprim–sulphonamide mixtures and extended-spectrum cephalosporins.

Treatment of salmonellosis
1 First choice: ciprofloxacin orally 500 mg twice daily for 3–5 days, or norfloxacin or ofloxacin orally 400 mg in the same regimen.
2 Alternatives: trimethoprim orally 200 mg twice daily for 5–7 days, or co-trimoxazole orally 960 mg in the same regimen, or chloramphenicol orally 500 mg 6-hourly for 5–7 days.
3 Invasive salmonellosis: ciprofloxacin or ofloxacin i.v. 200 mg twice daily. Alternative: chloramphenicol i.v. 500 mg 6-hourly.

Sequelae of salmonellae infections

Continuing excretion of the salmonellae

This is demonstrable for a variable time after a salmonella bowel infection, but usually stops within 1–4 weeks. Prolonged or permanent excretion is rare.

Predisposing factors include gut disorders such as diverticulosis, inflammatory bowel disease or ischaemia, and immunological disorders, including acquired immunodeficiency syndrome (AIDS). Treatment with inappropriate antibiotics, particularly aminoglycosides or ampicillin, may also prolong excretion. Excretion probably occurs less often after treatment with ciprofloxacin (but not after norfloxacin).

Salmonella excretion does not compromise the health of an otherwise fit patient, and is only a minimal cross-infection hazard once the diarrhoea has ceased and personal hygiene is easy to maintain. Excretors who are food, water or dairy workers can, however, initiate food-poisoning outbreaks, and are therefore subject to public health legislation.

The progress of excretion may be followed by weekly or twice-weekly stool examinations. Most specialists would declare a patient clear after three consecutive negative tests. This does not necessarily mean that salmonellae are no longer excreted; it simply indicates that the numbers are small. Testing should stop therefore when the required negative specimens have been obtained, to avoid the complication of a further positive test.

Metastatic salmonellae infections

These should be treated with an antibiotic to which the salmonella is sensitive. Long courses of treatment are often needed to clear the salmonellae from the infected site. Abscesses may need 3 or more weeks' treatment; bone and joint infections may require 6 weeks or longer. Clinical progress and the results of follow-up imaging, erythrocyte sedimentation rate or C-reactive protein measurements may be used to decide when treatment can be stopped.

Postinfectious disorders

Salmonella bowel infections are occasionally followed by reactive arthritis (see Chapter 24). This is usually monoarticular, affecting a large joint such as the knee. Gradual resolution should be expected, and symptomatic treatment with non-steroidal anti-inflammatory drugs is helpful.

Prevention and control

General principles for the prevention and control of bacterial food poisoning apply to salmonellosis. In the UK salmonella infections in farm animals are notifiable under the Zoonoses Order, and are investigated by the State Veterinary Service.

Shigellosis (bacillary dysentery)

Introduction

Bacillary dysentery is an important worldwide disease. In western countries the endemic *Shigella* spp. cause self-limiting illnesses which are generally mild. Tropical shigelloses tend to be both more severe and more persistent, causing serious morbidity, especially in children. Malnutrition is gravely exacerbated by the prolonged diarrhoea and fever of shigellosis.

Epidemiology

Shigellosis is spread from person to person by the faecal–oral route. This occurs either by direct contact with faecally contaminated hands, or indirectly from contaminated food, milk or water. Water-borne shigellosis is important in rural tropical areas. Secondary spread within households is common. Outbreaks occur under conditions of crowding and poor sanitation or personal hygiene, for example in prisons, psychiatric institutions and nursery schools. Food-borne outbreaks are less common, but do occur. An incident due to contaminated iceberg lettuce affected several European countries during 1994.

About 3000 cases are reported annually in the UK, of which two-thirds are due to *S. sonnei*. The peak incidence is in children under 5 years of age.

Microbiology

There are four species of *Shigella*: *S. sonnei*, *S. flexneri*, *S. boydii* and *S. dysenteriae*. They share the characteristics of the Enterobacteraceae and are closely related to *E. coli*. They are relatively inert biochemically and are, for example, non-lactose fermenters, and non-motile. *S. sonnei* and *S. dysenteriae* are biochemically distinct but *S. boydii* and *S. flexneri* are very similar. Serological characterization is therefore important for identification and typing. *S. dysenteriae* is divided into 10 serotypes on the basis of O antigens, *S. flexneri* into six types and *S. boydii* into 15. *S. sonnei* is serologically homogeneous, and if typing is required, colicine typing must be performed. For the other species serotyping is sufficient for epidemiological purposes, but phage typing can be performed if necessary. A phage-typing system for *S. sonnei* has recently been developed.

Pathogenesis

Shigellae are enteroinvasive, penetrating the intestinal wall in a similar manner to salmonellae. However, in this instance the burden of disease falls on the large bowel where there is a significant defect in water absorption. Ulceration is a feature of intestinal invasion by shigellae in comparison to salmonellae and this is due to the elaboration of exotoxins.

There is active fluid secretion from the small intestine but this is very much less than occurs in ETEC disease. Thus the clinical features of dysentry are caused by excess fluid loss from the small bowel, together with a major defect in large-bowel water reabsorption. The ulceration and inflammatory process bring about the bloody diarrhoea characteristic of this infection.

Clinical features

After an incubation period of 3 or 4 days there is a prodromal illness of high fever lasting 12–24 h. Non-specific features of this prodrome often occur in children and include meningism, convulsions and confusion. The white-cell count is usually high ($12–16 \times 10^9$/l). However in most cases the fever resolves suddenly, and diarrhoea with colic occurs soon enough to avoid the need for such investigations as lumbar puncture.

S. sonnei and *S. boydii* tend to cause brown watery diarrhoea in which various amounts of mucus are mixed. Blood may be seen in the stool, but the amount is rarely large. The diarrhoea usually subsides spontaneously after 3–5 days.

S. flexneri and *S. dysenteriae* often cause more severe and prolonged disease in which irregular fever continues and increasing amounts of mucus and blood appear in successive stools. Distressing colic accompanies the call to stool and is exacerbated by attempts to eat or drink. Untreated disease of this kind can lead to dehydration and progressive malnutrition.

Both types of illness can be followed by asymptomatic excretion of the pathogen lasting from a few days to several weeks and occasionally longer. Because of the low infective dose of shigellae such excretors can be hazardous, especially in nurseries and children's institutions.

Diagnosis

The clinical syndrome of bloody diarrhoea with colic usually indicates a diagnosis of dysentery. Bacillary dysentery must be distinguished from amoebic dysentery and inflammatory bowel disease. The mainstay of differential diagnosis is laboratory identification of the pathogen (see p. 165).

Management

Mild shigellosis requires only symptomatic treatment. Antispasmodic agents are helpful in relieving colic. In more severe cases antibiotic treatment can terminate the illness, though it often takes 2 or 3 days for diarrhoea to cease completely. Ciprofloxacin is often successful, and tends to eliminate excretion as well as curing disease.

Prevention and control

The infection can be prevented by providing facilities for safe disposal of faeces and clean water for hand-washing, together with education on good hygiene. *Shigella* dysentery is notifiable. Cases should be excluded from handling food until their stools are clear of organisms.

Campylobacter infections

Introduction

Campylobacter infections occur as commonly as salmonella infections in most parts of the world, and add significantly to the burden of childhood gastroenteritis in at-risk communities. In developed communities they do not cause as much morbidity as salmonella infections because they rarely produce metastatic or bacteraemic disease. Asymptomatic excretion is uncommon and campylobacters are not transmitted from person to person, so they cause fewer public health hazards than many other organisms — though large food- and water-borne outbreaks have been documented.

Epidemiology

Campylobacter enteritis is the commonest cause of bacterial food poisoning in the UK. About 40 000 cases are reported each year, and the incidence is increasing. Some of the increase is due to the more widespread availability of sensitive laboratory techniques.

Most cases are sporadic and associated with the consumption of contaminated poultry. Sporadic infection has also been attributed to the contamination of milk by birds that peck through the tops of doorstep milk bottles. Outbreaks are usually due to consumption of unpasteurized milk or untreated water.

The peak incidence of *Campylobacter* enteritis is during the summer months, about 8 weeks earlier than the seasonal increase in salmonellosis (Fig. 8.12). There is a bimodal age distribution with the greatest incidence in infants and young adults. Infection occurs more frequently in rural areas than in cities.

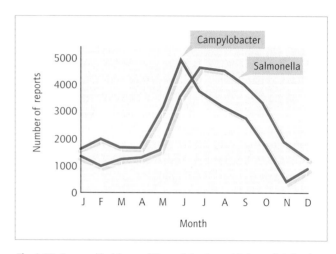

Fig. 8.12 Seasonal incidence of *Campylobacter* and *Salmonella* infections.

Pathogenesis

Campylobacter spp. were recognized as animal pathogens long before their role in human disease was appreciated. This was in part because of difficulties in isolating these organisms from human faeces. They are members of the family Spirillaceae on the basis of the DNA composition. There are four species associated with human enteritis: *C. jejuni*, *C. coli*, *C. fetus* and *C. lari*.

C. jejuni is rapidly killed in the pH found in the stomach, and the chance of infection is increased if the organism is consumed in milk, which may protect it from gastric acid. The infective dose may be as low as 500 organisms.

Campylobacters possess a cell-wall LPS of low molecular weight similar to that found in *Haemophilus* or *Neisseria* sp. This molecule, like other LPSs, contains a lipid A moiety. It is also antigenically diverse with many serotypes being described.

Campylobacters are motile on the basis of possession of flagella. These are thought to play an important role in establishing infection, and convalescent serum contains antibody to flagellin. The surface-exposed flagellar antigens are predominantly strain-specific but species-specific antigens are present.

C. jejuni produces an enterotoxin which causes fluid accumulation in ileal loops, and a cytopathic effect in Chinese hamster ovary cells and Y-1 mouse adrenal cells. Its mode of action is similar to that of cholera toxin and the LT toxin of *E. coli*. Other toxins, including a cytotoxin, may also be implicated in the pathogenesis of *Campylobacter* enteritis.

Adherence of *C. jejuni* to the intestine is thought to be mediated through L-fucose receptors.

Pathogenicity factors for *Campylobacter jejuni*
1 Lipid A — containing lipopolysaccharide.
2 Flagellar antigens.
3 Toxins: enterotoxin and cytotoxin.
4 Enterocyte adherence mediated through L-fucose receptors.

Clinical features

The incubation period is usually 3 or 4 days, but can be up to 8 or 9 days. This is followed by approximately 24 h prodromal illness with fever, headache and prostration. The main illness consists of diarrhoea, which is watery and may be bloody. Vomiting may occur at the onset. Abdominal pain is common, and is constant rather than colicky. Abdominal examination often reveals rebound tenderness which may be severe.

Campylobacter infection occasionally causes very severe abdominal pain with little diarrhoea, or only tiny stools containing mostly mucus and blood. Distinction from acute surgical conditions such as acute appendicitis, salpingitis and ectopic pregnancy may therefore be difficult. The abdominal X-ray shows multiple fluid levels in acute bowel infections, and is often unhelpful. X-ray examination should not be omitted, however, as it may show other diagnostic features such as free gas in the peritoneum or, in children the C-sign of intussusception. Early ultrasound examination may assist diagnosis.

Rare cases of systemic *Campylobacter* infection occur, often affecting children with diseases causing iron overload. The patient is feverish and blood cultures are positive.

Prolonged infection can mimic inflammatory bowel disease, with persistent bloody diarrhoea, abdominal pain and low-grade fever but stool cultures will indicate the infectious aetiology.

Diagnosis

The diagnosis can be suspected clinically if typical abdominal pain and peritonism accompany acute diarrhoea.

Laboratory diagnosis

Special laboratory techniques are required to identify campylobacters from heavily contaminated specimens such as faeces. The first successful method utilized the ability of campylobacters to pass through micropore filters while other enteric organisms were retained. There are now selective media which permit routine isolation of campylobacters from faeces. The selective agents employed are a mixture of antibiotics including vancomycin, polymyxin B, trimethoprim, amphotericin B and cephalothin. Selection is improved if the cultures are incubated at 43°C.

Campylobacters are microaerophilic organisms which grow better at reduced oxygen tension and with an increased concentration of carbon dioxide. Commercially available gas-generating systems make this an easy procedure to carry out.

In most laboratories identification can be confirmed by Gram-staining to demonstrate the characteristic 'gull wing' morphology, and by obtaining a positive oxidase reaction. Biochemical testing can be used to differentiate the species, and disc testing of antimicrobial sensitivities can be performed.

Microbiological characteristics of campylobacters
1 Filterable through micropore filters.
2 Optimum growth at 43°C.
3 Characteristic spiral morphology.
4 Microaerophilic.
5 Oxidase-positive.
6 Resistant to vancomycin, polymyxin B, cephalothin, trimethoprim.
7 Sensitive to erythromycin and ciprofloxacin.

Clinical management

Many mild cases respond readily to symptomatic treatment before the diagnosis is confirmed. Specific treatment is indicated in severe or prolonged illness (and a good response will obviate concerns about surgical or inflammatory conditions). The treatment of choice is a short course of oral erythromycin. Three or 4 days' treatment is usually enough. Ciprofloxacin is often effective, but resistance readily develops with prolonged or repeated use. These drugs can be used parenterally in severe or systemic infections.

Treatment of *Campylobacter* infection
1 First choice: erythromycin orally 250 mg 6-hourly for 3 or 4 days.
2 Alternative: ciprofloxacin orally 500 mg twice daily for 3 days (resistance easily develops).

Prevention and control

Campylobacter enteritis, like salmonellosis, may be prevented by good hygienic practice. Milk-borne spread can be avoided by pasteurization. The most effective long-term measure would be to control infection in poultry, but the existence of many environmental sources of infection makes this difficult.

Infection with 'food-poisoning' vibrios

These members of the family Vibrionaceae, like *V. cholerae*, are all natural residents of water. The range of Vibrionaceae is wide, some living in salt water, some in brackish or fresh estuaries and ponds. None of them produce cholera toxin, but in *V. parahaemolyticus* at least, pathogenicity is probably related to the production of a haemolysin.

Vibrio parahaemolyticus is a natural resident of brackish water, which may be concentrated in the gut of filter-feeding and scavenger shellfish. The most common vehicle of infection is a meal of shrimps or prawns. Most cases occur sporadically, although outbreaks have been reported. The disease is rare in the UK but common in South-east Asia and the USA. Other non-cholera vibrios including non-toxigenic and non-O1 *V. cholerae*, *V. alginolyticus*, *V. fluvialis* and *V. mimicus* are occasionally reported. The main symptoms are watery diarrhoea and colicky abdominal pain.

Aeromonas spp. are also members of the Vibrionaceae family and are natural inhabitants of water. They can be isolated from diarrhoea stools of some cases of 'food poisoning', and may also be contracted directly from water by fishermen or boatmen. *Aeromonas* infection is relatively common in Japan where fresh-water fish is often eaten raw. The number of infections reported in the UK is small (less than 50 per annum), but increasing. Half of all reported infections are in young adults.

Plesiomonas shigelloides is related to *Aeromonas* and is less certainly associated with food poisoning. Between 30 and 60 laboratory reports are received each year in England and Wales.

Diagnosis

If the clinician suspects *Vibrio* infection on epidemiological or other grounds, he or she should make a specific request for the organisms to be sought (see below). Diagnosis is usually of epidemiological rather than therapeutic value, as the associated illnesses are rarely more than moderately severe and a few days' symptomatic treatment is all that is needed.

Laboratory diagnosis

Vibrionaceae cannot be identified in routine stool cultures intended to detect Enterobacteriaceae. They are usually sought by inoculating stool on to a high-pH selection/indicator medium containing bile salts, which inhibit many other bowel flora. The most used medium is thiosulphate–citrate–bile salt–sucrose (TCBS) medium

containing a bromothymol blue indicator. Food-poisoning vibrios grow well on this medium. Most are non-sucrose-fermenters, producing blue-green colonies, which distinguish them from *V. cholerae*, a sucrose-fermenter which produces yellow colonies.

A suitable enrichment medium for vibrios is alkaline peptone water.

Yersinia infections

Yersinia enterocolitica and *Y. pseudotuberculosis* are capable of causing bowel disease. *Y. enterocolitica* is rapidly emerging as an important cause of diarrhoea. In some countries, for example Belgium, the infection is as common as salmonellosis and *Campylobacter* infections. It is still relatively rare in the UK, although the number of reported cases increased more than 10-fold during the 1980s to 580 in 1989.

Transmission occurs from contaminated food, milk and water. Most infections are sporadic. It is thought that many infections are due to consumption of raw or undercooked pork, although raw vegetables have also been implicated. A few milk-borne outbreaks have been reported in the USA.

Most infections occur in children under 5 years of age. There is a seasonal pattern, with more infections during autumn and winter.

The associated illness is a mild-to-moderate gastroenteritis, often with aching abdominal pain. Post-infectious problems, particularly arthritis and erythema nodosum, can be as troublesome as the bowel illness itself, and persist for some weeks (Fig. 8.13).

Diagnosis requires special investigations. Culture of *Yersinia* sp. from stool is possible (see below), but diag-

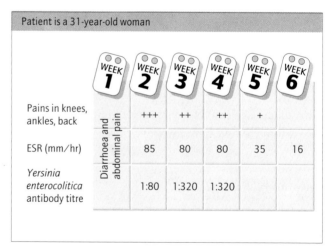

Fig. 8.13 Progress of *Yersinia* food poisoning associated with arthritis. ESR, erythrocyte sedimentation rate.

nosis is often considered late and rising titres of antibodies must then be sought in paired serum samples.

Y. enterocolitica will grow slowly on MacConkey's agar showing pinpoint colonies after 48 h incubation. Specialized *Yersinia* media simplify the isolation of these organisms. Selection is obtained due to the presence of sodium desoxycholate, crystal violet and an antibiotic combination (Irgasan, novobiocin and cefsulodin). *Y. enterocolitica* has translucent colonies with a dark pink centre which may be surrounded by a pale opalescent zone of precipitated bile salts.

Treatment of yersiniosis is possible; tetracyclines may be given orally, e.g. oxytetracycline 250–500 mg three or four times daily or doxycycline 100 mg daily, both for 7–10 days.

Y. pseudotuberculosis also causes human disease, but this is more often mesenteric adenitis than diarrhoea. Fever and right lower quadrant abdominal pain must be differentiated from appendicitis, salpingitis or the onset of Crohn's disease. Ultrasound examination will often reveal oedematous terminal ileitis and groups of enlarged mesenteric lymph nodes. Similar findings, even in the absence of diarrhoea, can occur in *Salmonella* and *Campylobacter* infections, demonstrating the overlapping nature of symptom complexes in intestinal infections. It is therefore worthwhile requesting stool cultures in patients with terminal ileitis and mesenteric adenitis, in case specific treatment can be offered for the distressing symptoms.

Helicobacter pylori and acute gastritis

Helicobacter pylori, like the campylobacters, is a member of the family Spirillaceae. It is found in the gastric mucus and surrounding the apices of gastric parietal cells in patients suffering from acute hypochlorhydric gastritis and chronic gastritis. It is also prevalent in the stomachs of patients with duodenal ulcers.

Diseases associated with *Helicobacter pylori*
1 Acute hypochlorhydric gastritis.
2 Chronic gastritis.
3 Gastric ulcer disease.
4 Duodenal ulcer disease.

H. pylori leads to acute and chronic inflammation in the gastric antrum. The organism elaborates a potent urease, which produces a local alkaline environment. This is thought to upset the natural feedback mechanism for gastric acid, resulting in a high gastrin level and consequent hyperacidity. Humans are the only known reservoir of infection. While its exact role in gastritis and ulcer disease is uncertain, self-inoculation has resulted in symptomatic gastritis. This suggests that it may be a pathogen or at least an important factor in pathogenesis. The origin of the organisms colonizing the stomach is uncertain but possibilities include infected or colonized humans, or perhaps food. In developed countries the prevalence of *H. pylori* infection is between 20 and 40%; however, up to 95% of duodenal ulcer patients may be colonized.

Similar bacteria are known to be commensals of the stomachs of many mammals. A related organism, *Gastrospirillum hominis*, has recently been identified in the human stomach, and may be another cause of peptic ulcer disease.

Treatment with agents such as bismuth salts or ampicillin and metronidazole, which inhibit *Helicobacter*, can relieve symptoms. However, resistance to single-drug treatment develops quickly, making effective cure difficult. The most successful regimen is amoxycillin plus metronidazole plus a bismuth preparation, continued for 1 month. Acid-reducing drugs greatly enhance the effect of antibiotic treatment.

Diseases caused by bacterial toxins

ORGANISM LIST

Staphylococcus aureus
Bacillus cereus and other *Bacillus* spp.
Clostridium perfringens, C. difficile, C. botulinum.

Staphylococcal food poisoning

Introduction

Staphylococcus aureus is able to produce a variety of toxins, among which are enterotoxins (A–E). They are preformed toxins produced during replication of the staphylococci in prepared food. Food poisoning occurs when food becomes contaminated by an infected individual, usually from a skin lesion or nasopharyngeal secretions. The organism subsequently multiplies and produces toxin which is absorbed and travels in the circulation to the vomiting centre, causing vomiting by a central effect. It may also cause bowel irritation, leading to mild, transient diarrhoea.

In some countries, including the USA, *S. aureus* is a leading cause of food poisoning. In the UK it is comparatively rare; approximately 100 cases are reported annually.

Clinical features

The incubation period varies from 30 min to 6 h. Malaise and nausea are quickly followed by vomiting, which may be severe and repeated, causing dehydration or even shock. Occasional deaths are reported. The vomiting lasts from 2 to 6 h and is followed by several hours' exhaustion before recovery is complete.

Diagnosis

The illness is similar to winter vomiting disease and other viral infections. Single cases are rarely extensively investigated. The absence of diarrhoea also limits the availability of specimens, though staphylococci may be recovered from vomitus if this is available, and can then be shown to produce enterotoxin.

Family- and catering-associated outbreaks are relatively common and may indicate a food source. Remaining food can then be examined for the presence of enterotoxin and/or enterotoxin-producing staphylococci.

Diagnosis of staphylococcal food poisoning
1 Demonstration of toxin-producing *Staphylococcus aureus* in suspected food.
2 Demonstration of toxin-producing *S. aureus* in vomitus.
3 Demonstration of an enterotoxin in suspected food.

Management

Management is symptomatic, and may include the necessity for emergency intravenous rehydration.

Prevention

Prevention is by hygienic food preparation, particularly covering skin lesions with a waterproof dressing. Food-handlers with extensive staphylococcal skin infection should be excluded from work.

Bacillus cereus food poisoning

Bacillus cereus is an aerobic Gram-positive rod, which forms spores. It is found in soil and dust, and easily contaminates cereals and some beans. It may also occur in animal faeces and occasionally contaminates meat.

Illness occurs following ingestion of contaminated food that has been kept at ambient temperatures after cooking. The disease is relatively uncommon in the UK; fewer than 500 cases are reported annually.

Food-poisoning serotypes produce spores which resist boiling. Boiled foods, particularly rice, may be stored at ambient temperatures for later rewarming (or frying). The spores germinate during storage and highly heat-resistant preformed toxins accumulate in the food. Occasional outbreaks have also been associated with meat and vegetable dishes. The toxins cause severe vomiting by a central effect, producing an illness just like staphylococcal food poisoning.

B. cereus of the types found in meat more often produce diarrhoea, mediated by locally acting preformed toxins. Some other *Bacillus* spp., e.g. *B. subtilis*, may also occasionally cause food poisoning.

Botulism

Introduction

Botulism is caused by preformed toxins of *Clostridium botulinum*, elaborated during the germination of spores in anaerobic conditions. Different strains of *C. botulinum* produce one of six toxins (A–F). Human disease is usually caused by A or B, derived from soil; occasional cases are caused by type E, derived from estuarine or marine mud.

Home-canned or home-bottled vegetables and salads are the commonest sources of illness, usually causing family outbreaks. In Europe, infection is usually due to smoked or preserved meats. It is a rare disease in the UK because commercial canning is highly controlled, but rare community outbreaks have been caused by commercial products. An outbreak of 27 cases occurred in the north-west of England in 1989, caused by canned hazelnut purée contained in yoghurt (Fig. 8.14).

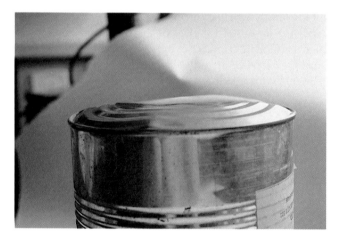

Fig. 8.14 A 'blown' tin of hazelnut purée which had not been properly heat-treated, resulting in the formation of botulinum toxin type b; 27 people developed botulism after eating hazelnut yoghurt prepared from the contents of such a tin. Courtesy of Dr Richard Gilbert, Central Public Health Laboratory.

Clinical features

The toxin causes paralysis by blocking neuromuscular junctions. The incubation period varies from 24 to 48 h or more, depending on the dose of toxin consumed. Malaise and mild gastrointestinal symptoms may precede neurological features. The onset of neurological disturbance is insidious and subtle, often initially dismissed as 'hysteria'. Paralysis develops from the head downwards, aiding differentiation from the opposite process in Guillain–Barré syndrome. Dry mouth and blurred vision are followed by difficulty with swallowing and speech. Respiratory paralysis and generalized weakness soon follow. Once paralysis is established it can last for several weeks, though eventual recovery is usual, if the patient is supported by ventilation in the meantime. Autonomic dysfunction and smooth-muscle paralysis mean that the blood pressure may be unstable and bowel function will be disturbed.

Diagnosis

Initial diagnosis must depend on clinical findings. A history of recent consumption of suspect food may be helpful. The cerebrospinal fluid is usually normal. Electromyography shows features of developing denervation (but in the earliest stages may suggest an axonal lesion). *C. botulinum* is not found in the stool, and toxin is rarely demonstrable in serum. Both the organism and its toxin are demonstrable in left-over food, and sometimes in containers and on utensils. The toxins are destroyed by heating.

Laboratory diagnosis of botulism
1 Demonstration of *Clostridium botulinum* in suspected food.
2 Recovery of *C. botulinum* from unwashed food containers or utensils.
3 Demonstration of *C. botulinum* toxin in food, food containers or patient's serum.

Management

This is supportive, and consists mainly of appropriate intensive care. Polyvalent antiserum is available from regional public health laboratories, and can be given to prevent further fixation of toxin in the nervous system. Antitoxin can also be given prophylactically to others who ate the suspect food.

A minority of cases are mild and can even be self-limiting, but respiratory function should be closely monitored, and measures taken to protect the airway, in case muscular weakness predisposes to aspiration of saliva or stomach contents.

Infant botulism

This is a rare condition with worldwide occurrence. It is cased by rapid replication of *C. botulinum* in the infant bowel. Both the bacteria and high concentrations of the toxin are found in the stool of affected infants. The source of the *C. botulinum* is unknown, but may be direct from soil or derived from food. Some affected infants have consumed honey before their illness.

Affected infants are aged between 6 weeks and 3 months (suggesting that infant botulism and cot death are related, at least). The onset is insidious, with weak suckling, constipation and shallow respirations. Many infants recover with supportive measures only, including postural drainage, careful feeding or tube feeding and careful observation of respiratory function. Less than half require ventilation. No secondary case has been reported following exposure to the stool of an affected infant.

Clostridium perfringens food poisoning

Clostridium perfringens is an anaerobic Gram-positive rod which inhabits the bowel of many animals, and may contaminate meat during butchery and storage. Its spores survive boiling and will germinate in the anaerobic conditions in stored stews, soups, gravies and large joints of meat. The infection is usually food-borne and occurs when contaminated food such as meat is allowed to stand at room temperature for long periods.

Replicating bacteria are then eaten with the food. They multiply in the large bowel, elaborating toxin locally. After 18–36 h incubation the toxin causes watery diarrhoea with colicky abdominal pain which may last for 3–5 days. Outbreaks typically occur in association with large-scale catering with inadequate facilities for cooling and storing food.

C. perfringens can be recovered from the diarrhoea stool and identified as a 'food-poisoning' serotype. It is also possible to demonstrate toxin in the stool.

Clostridium difficile and pseudomembranous colitis

Pseudomembranous colitis is almost always antibiotic-associated, though rare cases occur apparently spontaneously. A milder version of the disease, without severe colitis, is recognized as antibiotic-associated diarrhoea. Antibiotics which most commonly precipitate the condition are those which strongly inhibit normal gut flora, especially faecal streptococci. These include clindamycin, ureidopenicillins and very broad-spectrum cephalosporins. However ampicillin, rifampicin and ciprofloxacin have also been associated with a few cases.

Watery diarrhoea occurs abruptly, usually 3 or 4 days after antibiotic treatment commenced. Abdominal pain and soreness accompany the diarrhoea, and low-grade fever is common. *C. difficile* and its toxin can both be demonstrated in stool specimens. Colonic biopsies show typical changes, with focal inflammation in lymphoid tissue expanding and erupting through the muscularis mucosae to emerge in the mucosa. Mucosal destruction and inflammatory exudate produce a thick pseudomembrane. Slow improvement may follow discontinuation of antibiotics, but progressive inflammation and perforation can occur in some untreated cases.

The isolation of *C. difficile* from stools does not make the diagnosis of pseudomembranous colitis as this organism is carried by up to 30% of hospital patients. The diagnosis is supported by the demonstration of toxin in patients' stools and confirmation of the toxic effect on cells in tissue culture. A positive result is reported if the effect is inhibited by *C. difficile* antitoxins. An enzyme-linked immunosorbent assay method for the detection of toxins has been developed. A pathological diagnosis can be made by showing typical histological

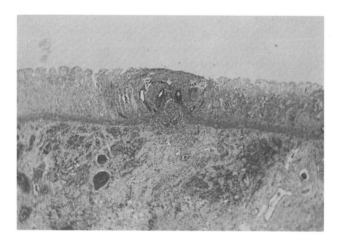

Fig. 8.15 Pseudomembranous colitis: intense inflammation erupts from beneath the muscularis mucosae, producing an accumulation of necrotic debris in place of the damaged mucosa.

changes on biopsies of affected colonic mucosa (Fig. 8.15).

The treatment of choice is oral vancomycin 250 mg three times daily for a week. Relapse sometimes occurs and can be treated by repeating this course. Metronidazole is often, but not always, effective. Parenteral treatment may be given, with good effect, if oral treatment is impossible.

Non-bacterial toxins and food poisoning

TOXIN LIST

Bean haemagglutinins
Scombrotoxin
Shellfish toxins (diarrhoetic and paralytic)
Ciguatera toxin
Cyanobacterial toxins (blue-green algae).

Bean haemagglutinins

These haemagglutinins are found in varying amounts in many species of beans. Red kidney beans contain large amounts and are the commonest cause of clinical problems. The toxin is destroyed by vigorous boiling; when the beans are soft they are also safe to eat. Incomplete cooking is particularly likely if beans are insufficiently soaked, or if they are cooked as a casserole ingredient. Illness, consisting of severe vomiting followed by profuse diarrhoea, develops very quickly after consumption of as few as five or six beans. In severe cases the patient has been ill before finishing the meal. Haemagglutinin intoxication is uncommon. Most incidents in the UK are caused by red kidney beans, although one outbreak was attributed to a haricot bean product.

Scombrotoxin

Scombrotoxin is a substance which develops during spoilage of scombroid fish, such as mackerel, tuna and bonito. Sardines have also been implicated in cases of food poisoning. It is thought that the toxin is either histamine or a closely related substance. Even mildly spoiled fish can be toxic and, since the toxin is highly heat-resistant, neither cooking nor canning can make the affected fish safe to eat.

Symptoms of intoxication follow 1–4 h after eating fish. They are identical to the symptoms of histamine toxicity, with headache, flushing, urticarial rash and swelling or tingling of the lips and mouth. Spontaneous recovery takes 4–6 h.

Diarrhoetic shellfish poisoning

Diarrhoetic shellfish poisoning is caused by a toxin produced by the shellfish themselves. Some shellfish are well-known to be toxic (for instance, the red whelk) but are occasionally mistaken for edible species. The resulting illness is a short-incubation acute diarrhoea whose severity is proportional to the dose of toxin.

Paralytic shellfish poisoning

Neurotoxins are elaborated by dinoflagellates which are low in the food chain of many sea creatures. The dinoflagellates multiply rapidly when the sea is warm and nutrients are plentiful. They sometimes form a visible 'bloom', often red or brown in colour (the so-called red tide). Shellfish and other filter feeders consume large quantities of this and the toxin accumulates in their bodies. Humans become poisoned by eating affected clams or crustacea. In tropical waters fish such as groupers can accumulate very large amounts of ciguatera toxin, becoming more poisonous with increasing age and size.

Symptoms of poisoning are caused by interference with neuromuscular junctions. Bradycardia, tingling of the lips and fingers and muscle weakness are common, and can continue for many hours in severe cases. Rare cases of death have been reported in patients who consumed large quantities of shellfish.

Ciguatera poisoning can be life-threatening. It is mainly seen in the Caribbean, where it is well-recognized. Local people do not eat large fish (and they often test prospective meals on family pets). Bradycardia and hypotension can be severe; profound muscle weakness also occurs and can affect respiratory muscles. It may take days or weeks for the symptoms to abate, and persistent compromise of neuromuscular transmission may mean that for many weeks afterwards even a meal of 'safe' fish can precipitate weakness. Intensive support may be required for such severely affected patients. Many less severe cases also occur, with gradual recovery from mild weakness and bradycardia.

Cyanobacterial toxins

These are produced by the blue-green algae which thrive in fresh water when the weather is warm and nitrates or other nutrients are plentiful. An algal 'bloom' is visible in the water. The toxins are extremely irritant, and cause erythema, burning and even blistering of exposed skin and mucosae. Ingestion affects mainly animals, but occasional human cases of diarrhoea, vomiting and abdominal pain are reported. Abnormal liver function tests and sometimes jaundice also occur. Species of cyanobacteria can readily be identified by direct microscopy of affected water.

Poisoning incidents have been reported from many countries, but only rarely in the UK. In 1989 10 young army recruits were affected following canoeing and swimming exercises through a scum of algal bloom in Staffordshire.

Parasitic infections of the gastrointestinal tract

ORGANISM LIST

Protozoa
Giardia intestinalis
Cryptosporidium parvum
Entamoeba histolytica.

Helminths
Enterobius vermicularis
Trichuris trichiura
Ascaris lumbricoides
Hookworms
Strongyloides stercoralis
Tapeworms.

Laboratory diagnosis

The simplest means of diagnosing parasitic infections of the gastrointestinal tract is to examine a saline-wet preparation of stool microscopically under the × 10 and × 40 objective. To improve the diagnostic yield, concentration techniques are employed. These include flotation methods such as the zinc sulphate, magnesium sulphate and sucrose flotation techniques or the formol ether centrifugation technique. Flotation methods vary in their ability to concentrate different species whereas the formol ether technique effectively concentrates helminth ova and protozoal cysts. Individual parasites are identified on the basis of their size as measured by an eyepiece graticule calibrated against a stage micrometer, and their characteristic morphology. Some examples of protozoan and helminthic parasites are demonstrated in Fig. 8.16.

In patients with acute amoebic dysentery the transit time in the large bowel may be increased to such an extent that motile amoebae may be identified in the stool by microscopy. These organisms are very susceptible to cooling and desiccation, and therefore should be processed as soon as possible. Microscopic examination should be performed on a heated stage so that trophozoite motility may be preserved as long as possible. Scrapes from the base of ulcerative lesions demonstrated on proctosigmoidoscopy may show motile trophozoites.

The larvae of *Strongyloides stercoralis* are infrequently seen in the stools. The diagnostic yield is increased if the stool is placed in a Petri dish, mixed with activated char-

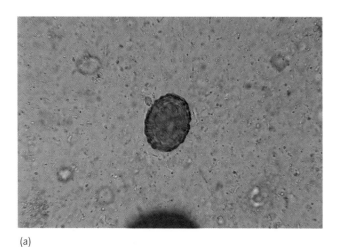

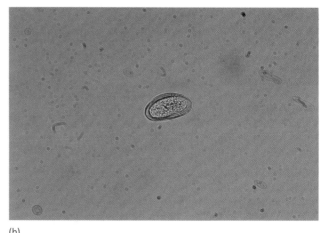

(a)   (b)

Fig. 8.16 Examples of parasitic infections demonstrated by microscopy of unstained faeces: (a) ovum of *Ascaris lumbricoides*; (b) ovum of *Enterobius vermicularis*. (See also Fig. 3.1.)

coal and incubated at room temperature for 5 days inside another dish. Larvae differentiate and migrate into the second dish and can be detected using a plate microscope. The diagnosis may be aided by performing a string test, although there are differing reports of its efficiency. The patient swallows a weighted string which passes into the upper small intestine where it remains for approximately 2 h. It is then retrieved and the juice and attached material are concentrated by washing and centrifugation before examination using the × 10 and × 40 objectives. This technique does have the advantage that *Giardia intestinalis* can also be diagnosed by this means.

Giardiasis

This diarrhoeal disease is caused by *G. intestinalis*, a flagellate protozoan. Infectious cysts are passed in the faeces of both sick patients and asymptomatic carriers. Cysts survive for many days in sewage-contaminated water, and infect a new host when the water is consumed. Direct faecal–oral spread is possible but less common. Large outbreaks can occur when water treatment procedures are defective or when breakage of water pipes allows contamination after treatment. Dogs may carry the organism and also excrete infectious cysts.

The disease is common in areas of poor sanitation and in institutions such as nurseries. Children, especially under 5 years, are affected more frequently than adults. The infection also occurs in travellers to countries with inadequately treated water supplies. The number of reports is increasing in the UK, probably due to more widespread examination of faecal samples for cysts, leading to better diagnosis.

The effects of infection vary from asymptomatic cyst passage to severe acute diarrhoea. *Giardia* adheres to the mucosa of the jejunum and upper ileum, using a ventral 'sucker'. In heavy infections the whole mucosa may be occluded, leading to malabsorption and steatorrhoea with rapid weight loss. Chronic cases are common; flatulence and passage of greasy, loose stools are particularly noticeable in the mornings and may persist for weeks or months.

Diagnosis is made by demonstrating cysts in the faeces, or by finding trophozoites in string test specimens, duodenal aspirate or biopsy specimens. Treatment is with metronidazole 400 mg three times daily for 1 week or a single dose of tinidazole. Either treatment may be repeated in the occasional event of relapse.

Cryptosporidiosis

Cryptosporidium parvum is a member of the family Sporozoa. Infectious oocysts are excreted by cattle, contaminating pasture and surface waters. Surface water can contaminate broken water mains, causing large outbreaks. Human cases are also infectious, and family outbreaks are quite common.

The disease may be spread in a number of ways. Several outbreaks have been reported in children's nurseries, probably spread by the faecal–oral route. Waterborne transmission is increasingly being recognized as an important cause of both community outbreaks (Fig. 8.17) and sporadic infection. Transmission also occurs between animals and humans by the faecal–oral route. Agricultural and veterinary workers are infected by this route. Children who come into close contact with animals during farm visits are also at risk.

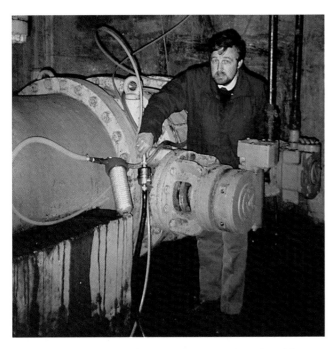

Fig. 8.17 Leakage from this drainage system contaminated a public swimming pool, causing a large outbreak of cryptosporidiosis. Courtesy of Dr David Casemore, Rhyl Public Health Laboratory.

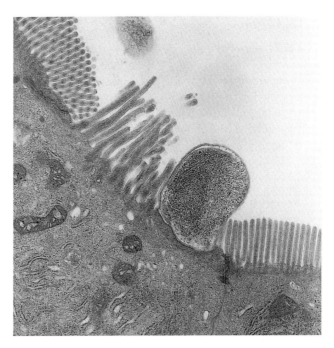

Fig. 8.18 Electron micrograph of a developing trophozoite of *Cryptosporidium parvum*, attached to mucosal cells in the small bowel. The parasite is within a vacuole formed from the host-cell brush border membrane. Courtesy of Dr David Casemore, Rhyl Public Health Laboratory.

The organism was first identified in the UK in 1983. Since then, the number of laboratory reports has risen steadily as the number of laboratories testing for the organism has increased. *Cryptosporidium* is now the fourth most commonly identified cause of gastro-intestinal infection in the UK. Seasonal peaks occur in spring and late autumn.

The parasite attaches to the small-bowel mucosa, damaging the brush border of the enterocytes (Fig. 8.18). After an incubation period of 3–6 days there is an acute onset of diarrhoea, often with abdominal pain and colic. The average duration of illness is about 3 weeks.

Diagnosis depends on demonstrating oocysts in the faeces, by acid-fast stains such as modified Ziehl–Nielsen or auramine techniques. No effective specific treatment exists but azithromycin treatment has been reported to ameliorate the symptoms. Most patients can benefit from a light diet while awaiting recovery.

Amoebiasis

Introduction

Entamoeba histolytica causes infection and disease in many parts of the world where sanitation is poor. The effects of infection range through asymptomatic ex-cretion of cysts to chronic intestinal infection, sometimes with granuloma formation, to acute amoebic dysentery. Extraintestinal abscesses may also occur, and can threaten life if untreated.

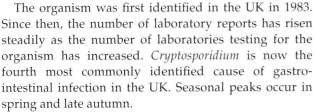

Manifestations of amoebiasis
1 Asymptomatic cyst passage.
2 Chronic intestinal symptoms.
3 Caecal granuloma (amoeboma).
4 Amoebic dysentery.
5 Amoebic liver abscess.
6 Rare other extra-intestinal disease.

Epidemiology

Amoebiasis is mainly spread via contaminated food, especially raw vegetables, and water. Infection is common in areas of poor sanitation and personal hygiene, for instance tropical countries, children's homes and psychiatric hospitals. The disease occurs principally in adults and is rare in children below 5 years of age.

Up to 1000 cases are reported annually in the UK. Half of these are known to be acquired overseas, principally in the Indian subcontinent.

Pathogenesis

Cysts of *E. histolytica* are passed in the stools of affected individuals. After ingestion the trophozoites excyst and attach to the mucosa of the large bowel. The amoebic surface membrane carries the glycoprotein galactose *N*-acetyl-D-galactosamine which acts as a lectin and mediates binding to the mucosal cells. Amoebae secrete a pore-forming enzyme, amoebapore, of which there are three closely related types, a, b and c. These all contain six cystine residues in a similar structure to that found in saponins and pulmonary surfactant.

Clinical features

Amoebic dysentery has a variable incubation period, from a few days to 4–6 weeks. Watery diarrhoea then presents and rapidly becomes bloody. A swinging fever develops. Colicky abdominal pain increases and may be replaced by constant pain as disease progresses. The stool is replaced by mucus in which are mixed large quantities of blood. Severe, untreated cases can progress to acute colonic dilatation, with risk of perforation.

Diagnosis

Acute amoebiasis is always a differential diagnosis of dysentery. Other causes of bloody diarrhoea include VTEC infection, pseudomembranous colitis, ulcerative colitis and Crohn's colitis. Inflammatory bowel disease should be suspected if repeated stool examinations reveal no pathogens. Sigmoidoscopic biopsy is helpful if typical changes of inflammatory bowel disease or pseudomembranous colitis are present. Even in acute amoebiasis it may be difficult to demonstrate amoebae or cysts in the stool; biopsies from ulcer edges will usually show undermined (flask-shaped) ulcers with amoebae packed in their eroded borders.

Laboratory diagnosis

Intestinal amoebiasis is diagnosed by detection of amoebic trophozoites containing red cells. This form is only present in fluid diarrhoea where the specimen must be examined with minimum delay so that motile amoebic trophozoites can be visualized. In specimens which are examined after a delay or in semiformed or formed stools, amoebic cysts should be sought by the formal ether technique. Less than half of patients with amoebic dysentery produce antibodies to *E. histolytica* but these antibodies are almost invariably present in patients with invasive amoebiasis. Immunofluorescence antibody and enzyme-linked immunoabsorbent assays have been described. These tend to remain positive after an attack of systemic amoebiasis. A rapid technique using cellulose acetate precipitation is the first to become positive in amoebic liver abscesses and should be used for urgent diagnosis. This positivity is rapidly lost after successful treatment. Species-specific diagnosis has been described detecting antibody to the surface-binding lectin.

Management

This consists of specific treatment, pain relief and the maintenance of hydration, which usually requires intravenous fluid therapy. The treatment of choice is metronidazole 800 mg three times daily, initially given intravenously, then by mouth when the patient can tolerate oral intake. Treatment should be continued for 7–10 days, depending on the speed of response.

Once cured of the acute disease, many patients continue to excrete infectious cysts. This can be terminated by treatment with an intestinal amoebicide. Diloxanide furoate is the best available choice; the dose is 500 mg every 8 h for 1 week (this may be omitted if the patient is soon to return to an endemic area, as reinfection and resumption of excretion are then inevitable).

Prevention

The disease can be prevented by providing water that has been treated by filtration, and adequate disposal of human faeces. Travellers to tropical countries should avoid drinking water that is not known to have been properly treated and unpeeled fruit and raw vegetables. Known carriers should be given instruction in thorough hand-washing after defecation.

Chronic intestinal amoebiasis

This is extremely common in endemic areas. Chronic infection causes fluctuating symptoms of abdominal pain and mild diarrhoea. *E. histolytica* preferentially affects the caecum, so right iliac fossa pain and tenderness occur, and must be differentiated from appendicitis. Persisting mucosal inflammation stimulates granuloma (amoeboma) formation. Large amoebomas may produce the same problems of bowel obstruction as caecal carcinomata, and appear the same on barium studies. Stool examination will reveal the amoebic cysts in such cases. The condition responds to treatment with intestinal amoebicides, but surgery may still be needed for obstructing amoeboma.

Amoebic abscess

This is a complication of intestinal amoebiasis, which may follow apparent or subclinical bowel infection. The liver is by far the commonest site affected; others include pleura, pericardium and occasionally excoriated perineal or abdominal skin. The localized infection causes intense inflammation and tissue damage which is visible as dark necrosis in advancing skin lesions.

Clinical features

The patient usually presents with high fever, leukocytosis and a raised erythrocyte sedimentation rate. Many patients have palpable enlargement and tenderness of the liver, but some have a paucity of physical signs. An elevated right diaphragm, small right-sided pleural effusion or slight collapse of the lower lung segment should direct attention to the liver in a case of pyrexia of unknown origin.

Diagnosis

Useful investigations include ultrasound examination and computed tomographic (CT) scanning, which will demonstrate the space-occupying lesion in the liver. The abscess is usually a single lesion in the right lobe, accessible to diagnostic aspiration and drainage. Left-sided abscesses are rare and difficult to localize on physical examination or ultrasound scan. CT scanning is the investigation of choice for this and other unusual sites.

Amoebae are rarely demonstrable in aspirate, as they are closely adherent to the abscess wall. However, the pus has a typical pinkish (anchovy-sauce) appearance which is diagnostically helpful.

Serological tests are usually positive and permit rapid diagnosis.

Management

Metronidazole is the treatment of choice. It readily penetrates the abscess wall and can allow such rapid healing that aspiration is unnecessary. The dose is 800 mg three times daily for 10–14 days (see Chapter 9).

Helminth infections of the bowel

Introduction

These infections are among the commonest chronic conditions found in humans. They are endemic wherever there is environmental contamination with human or animal faeces, and some are directly transmitted by the faecal–oral route.

Helminths with direct person-to-person transmission

Some species, *Enterobius vermicularis* (threadworms) and *Trichuris trichiura* (whipworms), inhabit the large bowel and rectum, deriving nutrients from the faeces. They release ova which are detectable by microscopic examination of unstained faeces. Whipworms fix themselves to the bowel wall by their narrow head end; their wider body may be seen on proctoscopy, dangling from the mucosa.

Threadworms are freely motile and may even be seen lying in the appendix on histology of surgical specimens. They emerge from the anus, particularly at night, to deposit ova on the perineal skin. This causes irritation which may spread into the vagina, especially in children. Worms can be seen macroscopically as tiny moving threads in the faeces or on the skin. Adults or their ova can be trapped by pressing the sticky side of transparent adhesive tape on to the anal margin at night or just after waking. Microscopy of the tape, stuck to a glass slide, can then be performed to make the diagnosis.

These worms are readily treated with mebendazole, which is given as a single oral dose of 100 mg. This kills the worms and terminates the infection. Threadworms can be paralysed by treatment with piperazine. This is usually given as a mixture of piperazine phosphate and senna in powder form. The senna ensures that worms are passed in the faeces before regaining motility.

> **Treatment of threadworm infection**
> 1 First choice: mebendazole single oral 100 mg dose (not recommended in pregnancy or for children under 2).
> 2 Second choice: Pripsen (piperazine 4 mg and sennoside 15.3 mg per sachet). Adult and child over 6 years: one sachet stirred into milk or water and repeated after 14 days (age 3 months to 1 year, one-third of a sachet; 1–6 years, two-thirds of a sachet); each sachet contains 7.5 ml of powder.

Ascaris lumbricoides

Epidemiology

Ascariasis is transmitted by ingestion of soil that contains infective eggs, or vegetables that have been contaminated by soil or sewage. In tropical countries, up to 50% of children may be infected. Children who eat soil are most at risk. The peak incidence of infection is between 3 and 8 years of age. Between 500 and 1000 cases are reported each year in the UK, although the incidence is declining.

Clinical features

At the onset of infection ova germinate in the upper gastrointestinal tract and the larvae migrate through the tissues to the lungs. A sufficiently large number of larvae can cause clinically evident lung irritation. Cough, wheezing and mild fever are associated with an eosinophilia; the whole syndrome is called pulmonary eosinophilia.

Uncomplicated infection causes no systemic features, though the occasional passage of a worm *per rectum* can be unpleasant and distressing. Worms may also be expelled orally if vomiting occurs. They are incidental findings in contrast studies of the gastrointestinal tract, when they are outlined and their gut is filled by radiopaque medium.

Very heavy worm loads can cause complications, as small ducts, such as the bile and pancreatic ducts, can be entered and obstructed by worms. Closely entwined masses of worms can even obstruct the small bowel (especially when the worms are irritated in the early stages of piperazine intoxication). These conditions may resolve spontaneously, but without treatment there is a risk of recurrence.

Diagnosis

Clinical diagnosis is based on seeing worms in stools, vomitus or contrast X-rays. Eosinophilia without other cause may raise suspicion, especially in the presence of respiratory symptoms.

A laboratory diagnosis is made by demonstrating ova in wet preparations or concentrates of faeces.

Management

The treatment of choice is single-dose mebendazole, which kills the worms without making them hyperactive first. Combinations of piperazine and purgatives are also effective (see text note p. 177), but are less pleasant to take, as piperazine causes significant nausea at effective doses, and may also provoke hyperactivity of the worms. In endemic situations it may still be worthwhile offering treatment as this will reduce the worm load, lessening the likelihood of complications and reducing the 'stealing' of nutrients from the bowel (which may be important in an undernourished child).

Prevention

The infection can be prevented by education of children in hand-washing after defecation and safe disposal of human faeces.

Hookworms

Introduction

Hookworm infection is not endemic in westernized countries, but is often present in recently immigrated individuals. Hookworms feed on blood, and heavy worm loads can cause significant anaemia, especially in children and others whose diet is low in iron.

Epidemiology

The infection is transmitted via faecally contaminated soil. In this infection, eggs hatch into larvae which become infective and penetrate the skin, especially of the feet. All ages are affected, although infection is commonest in children.

The disease is common in the tropics, and rare in temperate climates. About 500 imported cases are reported annually in the UK.

Pathogenesis

Hookworm ova are passed in faeces and infective larvae develop in an extracorporeal soil life cycle. The larvae can attach to and penetrate human skin, from where they migrate through the tissues to the lungs. They then pass to the pharynx and are swallowed, producing intestinal infection. In the intestine they attach to the bowel wall by their grinding mouth parts, damaging mucosa and releasing blood, which is their source of nutrition.

Clinical features

Larval migration in the early stages of infection causes both local skin irritation (ground itch) and pulmonary eosinophilia. Once the intestinal infection is established there are no specific features other than those of iron-deficiency anaemia.

Larva migrans

Larva migrans is a condition of abortive human infection by animal hookworms, usually those of dogs. The larvae penetrate human skin, but continue to migrate aimlessly through the tissues until they die. Eosinophilia and persisting skin irritation result, often with transient urticarial rashes and sometimes with respiratory symptoms.

Management

The treatment of choice is mebendazole. Dietary iron supplements may be needed in anaemic children. In rare cases of severe anaemia, transfusion may be given.

Prevention

Prevention is by wearing shoes and safe disposal of human faeces.

Strongyloidiasis

Strongyloides stercoralis has a life cycle similar to that of hookworms, except that rhabditiform larvae rather than ova are excreted in the faeces. While many such larvae will undergo a developmental stage in soil before penetrating the skin of a subsequent host, some of them become infectious before being excreted. These may reinvade the original host by penetrating the bowel wall or perianal skin. Strongyloidiasis is therefore a persistent infection, even after the host has left the endemic area.

The infection is transmitted when infective larvae penetrate the skin. The disease is common throughout tropical countries, but also occurs in temperate zones. Fewer than 100 cases are reported annually in the UK.

Intermittent migration of larvae causes the syndrome of larva currens. A local urticarial rash (Fig. 8.19) appears several times a week in various sites, usually on the trunk or thighs. Eosinophilia is usually present, and larvae may be demonstrated in faeces, duodenal aspirate or string-test material.

Immunosuppressed patients may suffer massive tissue invasion by larvae, without the tell-tale eosinophilia. Sometimes immunosuppression has been caused by in-

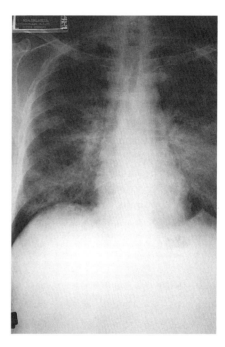

Fig. 8.20 Chest X-ray of an Asian patient who had received increasing doses of prednisolone for 'asthma'; he had *Escherichia coli* bronchopneumonia secondary to massive migration of *Strongyloides stercoralis* larvae.

creasing doses of prednisolone given to control 'asthma', which may have been missed pulmonary eosinophilia. The migrating larvae often carry bowel bacteria with them, and may enter the lungs (Fig. 8.20) or the meninges, causing secondary coliform infections.

The diagnosis must be considered in immunosuppressed patients who originate from the Far East, Africa, Asia or other endemic areas (transplanted organs may also contain larvae and cause infection if the donor had strongyloidiasis).

Treatment consists of albendazole 400 mg daily for 3 days, with a second course after 3 weeks if indicated. Thiabendazole daily for 3 days is an alternative, but has a significant incidence of gastrointestinal side-effects. Immunosuppressed patients may need both larger doses and longer treatment, depending on their response. Nausea, diarrhoea and sometimes fever limit the dose of thiabendazole.

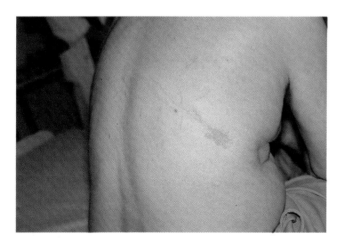

Fig. 8.19 Strongyloidiasis: recurrent urticarial rash of larva currens in a man infected as a prisoner of war in Burma in the 1940s.

Treatment of strongyloidiasis
1 First choice: albendazole orally 400 mg daily for 3 days. (May be repeated after 3 weeks.)
2 Second choice: thiabendazole orally 25 mg/kg (maximum 1.5 g) 12-hourly for 3 days.
In immunosuppressed patients, albendazole may be given in doses of 400 mg twice daily for up to 4 weeks. These courses may be repeated up to three times with intervals of 14 days.

Toxocariasis

Introduction

This is usually a mild disease, predominantly of children, caused by *Toxocara canis* and *T. cati*. The natural hosts for these two organisms are dogs and cats respectively, who excrete eggs in faeces. After 1–3 weeks' incubation, the eggs are infectious. Children become infected directly by eating contaminated soil, or indirectly by eating contaminated raw unwashed vegetables. After ingestion, embryonated eggs hatch in the intestine, larvae penetrate the wall and migrate to the liver and lungs. From the lungs, organisms spread to the abdominal organs (visceral larva migrans) or the eyes (ocular larva migrans).

Clinical features

Clinical features are variable and may include fever, chronic abdominal pain, a generalized rash, pneumonitis, hepatomegaly and focal neurological lesions. Ocular larva migrans may cause endophthalmitis with loss of vision in the affected eye.

Diagnostic tests

Diagnostic tests include an enzyme-linked immunosorbent assay and demonstration of *Toxocara* larvae by liver biopsy, although this is seldom justified. Anthelminthic therapy is of doubtful value.

Trichinellosis

This is a disease caused by a systemically invading roundworm, *Trichinella spiralis*. Infection occurs from eating raw or undercooked pork or bear containing larval cysts. It is rare in the UK.

Symptoms are variable, although conjunctivitis, oedema of the eyelids and retinal haemorrhages are characteristic early features. This may be followed by thirst, sweating, chills and remitting fever. Cardiac and neurological complications may occur after 3–6 weeks. There is a marked eosinophilia, which may assist in the diagnosis. Serological tests are available. Thiabendazole and mebendazole are both used in treatment.

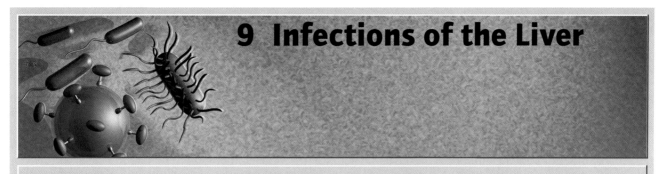

9 Infections of the Liver

Introduction

The liver is a complex organ. It receives blood from the intestinal tract via the hepatic portal system, and is sustained by 'systemic' blood via the hepatic artery. The liver cells perform many functions. They are the site of detoxification and metabolism of many intrinsic and extrinsic substances, including ammonia, complex amines, endotoxin and many drugs. They are the main site where glycogen is manufactured, stored and eventually reconverted to glucose, and they are the only important source of blood glucose. They are the only site of synthesis of urea, and of several proteins, including albumin and the clotting factors III, VII, IX and X.

The biliary system is the route of excretion of bilirubin, derived from the metabolism of haem substances. It is also important in the enterohepatic circulation of bile salts. Several drugs are excreted to a greater or lesser extent, and therefore concentrated, in the bile; these include penicillins, cephalosporins and rifampicin. Bile also contains cholesterol, which easily crystallizes, and may form gallstones. Patients with a high turnover of haem excrete high bilirubin loads, and are at risk of pigment stones.

Infections of the liver tend to affect either the cells, producing typical hepatocellular disorder, or the biliary tract, producing cholestasis together with the features of infection in a hollow organ. Space-occupying lesions in the liver (e.g. abscesses or granulomata) tend to produce the biochemical changes of cholestasis, but rarely cause clinically important jaundice.

Viral infections of the liver

ORGANISM LIST

Hepatitis A virus
Hepatitis B virus
Delta virus (Hepatitis D)
Hepatitis C virus
Hepatitis E virus
Other hepatitis viruses including GB types A, B and C
Epstein–Barr virus
Cytomegalovirus
Yellow fever (and other arboviruses).

Hepatitis A

Introduction

This a common disease worldwide. It is highly infectious to close contacts and therefore spreads easily among children. Many cases are subclinical; others cause moderate morbidity. Mortality is very low — less than 0.1% — but this means that about 1% of hospital admissions with hepatitis A suffer severe or life-threatening disease.

Epidemiology

In the developing world where sanitation is poor, hepatitis A is endemic. Most individuals become infected in childhood when the disease is mild or asymptomatic. Immunity is lifelong and outbreaks in adults are uncommon.

In more developed countries, infection in children is less common and many older children and young adults are susceptible. Three distinct patterns of disease occur: (i) sporadic infections among adult travellers to endemic countries; (ii) epidemics affecting mainly school-age children; and (iii) explosive common source outbreaks (Fig. 9.1)

Epidemics of hepatitis A in developed countries tend to evolve slowly, last for several months and affect large geographical areas. The infection is spread from person to person, mainly by the faecal–oral route. Transmission occurs within households, nurseries, schools and other institutions.

Common-source outbreaks are usually associated with food contaminated by an infected handler or undercooked molluscan shellfish harvested from contaminated waters. Water-borne outbreaks occur occasionally.

In the UK over 7000 laboratory-confirmed cases of hepatitis A are reported each year. The highest incidence

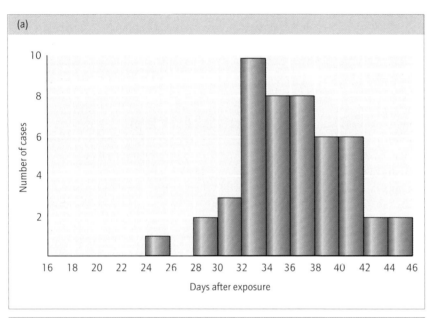

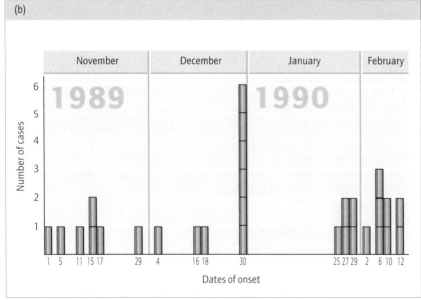

Fig. 9.1 (a) Rapidly evolving or explosive epidemic of hepatitis A, originating from a common source — in this case raspberries which were contaminated with human excreta before packaging. (b) Slowly evolving community outbreak of hepatitis A, spreading by the person-to-person route.

is in children aged 5–9 years of age. The proportion of cases acquired abroad varies from year to year, but may be as high as 20%. The overall incidence is declining, although large epidemics occurred in 1982 and 1990.

Virology

Hepatitis A virus (HAV) was previously classified as an enterovirus. It has now been reclassified as a hepatovirus in the family Picornaviridae. It is a small RNA virus with a single-stranded genome of positive-sense RNA, approximately 7.5 kb in length. A single polypeptide is synthesized and cleaved by viral proteases. The virion is 27 nm in diameter. The capsid consists of three major polypeptides, VP1, VP2 and VP3 ranging in size from 220 to 330 amino acids. The virus particle is more stable to heat, detergents and proteases than the other picornaviruses and this may explain the ease with which it is transmitted. Neutralizing antibodies are directed against groups of closely clustered epitopes on the virus surface.

The virus does not grow readily in tissue culture but has been adapted to growth in a wide range of primate cells. Adaptation to growth in cell culture occurs after serial passage.

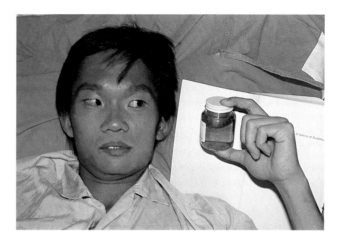

Fig. 9.2 Hepatitis A: typical appearance of jaundice and dark urine in viral hepatitis; the patient is no longer suffering from fever or malaise

Clinical features

The incubation period is 15–45 days. This is followed by a typical viral-type illness with malaise, lassitude, myalgia, arthralgia and variable fever. Features of hepatitis gradually replace the prodromal illness after 2–7 days. Many patients complain of nausea or vomiting and a few, especially children, may have loose stools. The urine darkens as bilirubinuria increases, and the stools may be noticeably pale. Jaundice then develops, first seen in the sclerae and later in the skin (Fig. 9.2).

The fever resolves as jaundice becomes established. At this stage virus excretion ceases and the patient is no longer infectious. Most patients feel better once the jaundice appears. After a few days the appetite returns and the jaundice begins to resolve.

Only non-specific changes of viral infection are observed during the prodrome; the white-cell count is normal, with a few atypical mononuclear cells. As the prodrome ends, rising plasma transaminases indicate hepatocellular damage, and conjugated bilirubin appears in blood and urine. The early transaminase levels are often 2000–3000 IU but these fall rapidly in most cases, and are often below 100 IU after 7–10 days.

Unlike the other viral hepatitides, hepatitis A commonly causes cholestasis, with a rise in alkaline phosphatase to 250–400 IU during convalescence. Abnormality of bile salt excretion may then cause itching. Occasionally cholestasis is prolonged, with deepening jaundice and severe pruritis, persisting for months if untreated. This does not indicate prolonged infection — it is a postinfectious event.

Diagnosis

Clinical suspicion depends on a typical history of malaise followed by jaundice and accompanied by bilirubinuria, and the absence of risk factors for other types of viral hepatitis. Prolonged vomiting in an otherwise well child might be due to anicteric hepatitis and should prompt a test for bilirubinuria or estimation of transaminases, particularly if the epidemiological history is compatible with hepatitis A. Risk factors for other types of viral hepatitis are not always present, however, and it is important that laboratory investigations include a search for evidence of hepatitis B and C (see pp. 190 and 192).

Glucose-6-phosphate dehydrogenase deficiency can cause sufficient haemolysis to produce clinical jaundice, often following an acute infection, ingestion of proprietary antipyretic drugs or eating beans (favism). In travellers, malaria is a common cause of haemolysis, usually accompanied by fever. Haemolytic (acholuric) jaundice is not accompanied by bilirubinuria; urinalysis will therefore suggest this alternative diagnosis.

Persistence of fever in viral hepatitis is unusual once jaundice has developed. In febrile hepatitis a diagnosis of Epstein–Barr virus (EBV) infection, or even of leptospirosis, may need to be excluded.

Acute cholecystitis can cause jaundice with fever. Pain in the right hypochondrium is a common accompaniment. Gallstones may cause pain and obstructive jaundice. Painless cholestatic jaundice is often a feature of biliary or pancreatic carcinoma. It should be considered in all middle-aged or elderly patients with jaundice. An elevated alkaline phosphatase is a useful warning sign of obstructive pathology.

Some drugs cause hepatocellular damage. Alcohol is the most common, but paracetamol toxicity must not be forgotten. A history of drug treatment or overdose must be sought in jaundiced patients.

Differential diagnosis of viral hepatitis
1 Other infections: Epstein–Barr virus infections, cytomegalovirus, leptospirosis.
2 Infections of the biliary system: acute cholecystitis, acute cholangitis, acute pancreatitis.
3 Obstructive jaundice: gallstones, tumours of the pancreaticobiliary system.
4 Haemolysis, e.g. glucose-6-phosphate dehydrogenase deficiency, malaria.
5 Drug jaundice, e.g. alcohol and paracetamol (hepatocellular), phenothiazines (cholestatic).

Laboratory diagnosis

Immunoglobulin M (IgM) antibodies become detectable when jaundice develops and persist for approximately 3 months, and occasionally for up to 2 years. IgG antibodies increase steadily after the onset of symptoms, and confer lifelong immunity. The basis of diagnosis is the demonstration of specific IgM by antibody-capture enzyme immunoassay (EIA). An EIA to detect specific IgG may be employed to determine immune status before or after vaccination.

Treatment

Specific treatment is rarely required. Bed rest and simple analgesics ameliorate severe prodromal symptoms. Antiemetic drugs can safely be given. Antipruritic drugs may be helpful in convalescence, but cholestyramine is more effective for severe pruritus. There is little evidence that bed rest is necessary once the transaminases have shown a significant fall.

Prolonged severe cholestasis responds to treatment with corticosteroids. Initial dosage with prednisolone 30–40 mg/day can be reduced over 2–4 weeks depending on the rate of fall of the alkaline phosphatase.

Complications

Liver failure

Liver failure is the most common complication. In some cases it is fulminant and early, presenting with altered consciousness before jaundice develops; in others it is subacute and progressive, appearing as an inexorable deterioration in liver function and deepening of jaundice.

Clinical indicators of liver failure are persistent vomiting, disturbed behaviour, flapping tremor of the outstretched hands and increasing drowsiness. Poor cerebral function is classically demonstrated by showing the patient's inability to copy a drawing of a five-pointed star, although he or she may be able to copy a square (constructional apraxia).

The earliest biochemical changes are the disappearance of blood constituents whose levels are maintained by the liver. These are glucose, clotting factors and urea (albumin has a longer half-life of 14 days and falls late in liver failure). The transaminase levels may not accurately reflect hepatocellular damage as they inevitably fall when few liver cells remain; however initial levels above about 7000 IU may alert the clinician to the possibility of failure developing (Fig. 9.3). In established hepatic coma the electroencephalogram shows characteristic 3/s slow-wave patterns.

Treatment. Treatment is initially supportive, and is based on four main objectives:
1 Maintaining the blood glucose to avoid hypoglycaemic convulsions or cerebral damage. This often requires constant infusion of 10% dextrose solution, and occasionally further glucose supplementation.
2 Minimizing amine production by avoiding protein loading and by emptying the bowel of replicating bacteria. Oral magnesium sulphate is commonly given to empty the bowel. It is no longer considered necessary to add non-absorbable antibiotics to this regimen.
3 Minimizing the likelihood of bleeding while clotting factors are deficient. This is achieved by nursing the patient quietly with minimum movement, avoiding vigorous or traumatic procedures. The risk of bleeding from gastric erosions is reduced by giving H_2-receptor blockers (cimetidine or ranitidine), or hydrogen–potassium pump blockade (omeprazole).
4 Avoiding exacerbation of the condition by drugs or protein loads. Some drugs cause marked deterioration in liver function. These particularly include diuretics, opiates, major tranquillizers and drugs whose side-effects include hepatotoxicity.

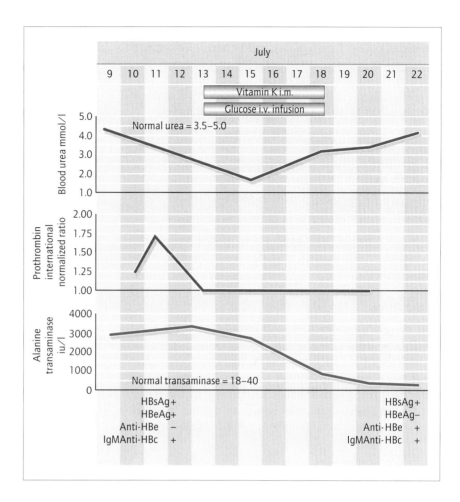

Fig. 9.3 Development of liver failure in a patient with a severe attack of hepatitis B; the patient made a spontaneous recovery with supportive treatment.

Short-acting benzodiazepines may be given for sedation. Paracetamol is a useful analgesic, as its toxic metabolite is not produced during liver failure. Transfusions of fresh plasma constitute a protein load, and should be reserved for treating haemorrhagic events (in any case, the clotting factors are quickly consumed and do little to prevent longer-term widespread oozing). Small doses of vitamin K may be given to avoid deficiency during a catabolic state, but large or frequent dosage should be avoided.

Specialist liver units

Specialist liver units not only offer experienced management, but may also be able to arrange a life-saving liver transplant. In hepatitis A, infection is often over by the time liver failure is established, so the outlook for a successful transplant is good. Early referral to an appropriate unit gives the best chance of arranging such treatment.

Prevention and control

The most effective prevention for hepatitis A is good sanitation and personal hygiene. Adequate facilities for hand-washing and sanitary disposal of faeces are very important, particularly in nurseries and schools were spread is likely to occur. The risk of common-source outbreaks can be minimized by proper education of food-handlers and adequate cooking of shellfish.

Human normal immunoglobulin (HNIG) is available for pre- and postexposure prophylaxis. An intramuscular injection provides passive protection which lasts for 6–8 weeks. It should be given to travellers to endemic areas, particularly younger adults and those travelling rough. Individuals who travel frequently should be tested for hepatitis A antibody as they may have naturally acquired immunity. HNIG can also be used to prevent or attenuate infection after exposure to a case. To be effective it must be given within 1 week of exposure.

A killed vaccine against hepatitis A has recently become available. It is most likely to be useful for regular travellers to endemic areas. Its role in the control of outbreaks is not yet certain.

Cases of hepatitis should be isolated until 1–2 days after the onset of jaundice. The disease is notifiable.

Prevention of hepatitis A
1 Safe water supplies.
2 Effective sanitation.
3 Personal hygiene.
4 Safe food-handling.
5 Pre-exposure prophylaxis: human immunoglobulin and inactivated vaccine.

Hepatitis B

Introduction

This disease causes much morbidity and mortality in some parts of the world where it is highly endemic. The importance of hepatitis B lies in its ability to cause prolonged or permanent infectious carriage, leading eventually to cirrhosis and malignant change in the liver. Vertical and horizontal infection from mother to child can produce successive generations of infectious carriers.

Virology and pathogenesis

Hepatitis B is a small enveloped virus containing partially double-stranded DNA (Fig. 9.4). The DNA contains four major genes which each code for more than one protein. The surface protein gene codes for three polypeptides (including hepatitis B surface antigen; HBsAg) which make up the viral envelope. The C gene codes for the core or capsid protein (hepatitis B core antigen; HBcAg) and the precore protein. The P gene codes for the reverse transcriptase and RNAase, and the X gene for transactivator proteins. HBsAg is the major protein of hepatitis B virus. The major antigenic determinant of HBsAg is the a antigen; antibodies to this antigen confer protection after infection or vaccination. In addition there are a pair of mutually exclusive subdeterminants d or y and w or r, giving four phenotypes, adw, adr, ayw and ayr. The frequency of these phenotypes varies in different parts of the world.

HBcAg is the major component of the nucleocapsid. Hepatitis B e antigen (HBeAg) may be generated from this antigen by proteolytic cleavage.

Hepatitis B virus typically causes an acute hepatitis which is characterized by liver cell necrosis and periportal histiocytic infiltration. The necrosis is centri-

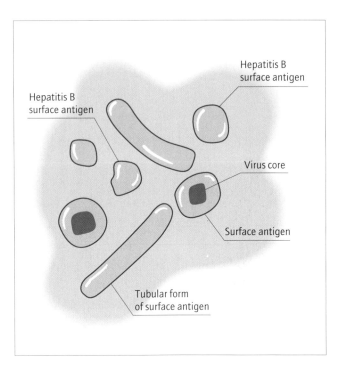

Fig. 9.4 The structure of hepatitis B virus showing excess surface antigen.

lobular and multifocal. Rarely, massive necrosis occurs associated with considerable disruption of the reticulin framework of the liver. In a proportion — estimated at approximately 10% — of patients, chronic hepatitis occurs, associated with chronic persistent infection. Liver carcinoma is an important complication of chronic hepatitis with an excess risk of 100-fold.

Hepatitis B virus DNA is integrated into host cell DNA. This insertion is random and may affect important genes near to the site of integration.

Epidemiology

It is estimated that there are 300 million chronic carriers of the hepatitis B virus worldwide. The incidence of acute disease and prevalence of carriage varies considerably from country to country (Fig. 9.5). In some parts of South-east Asia, 10–20% of the population may be carriers, whereas most countries in Europe and North America have carriage rates below 2%.

Where carriage rates are high, acute infection occurs mainly in infants and young children. The most important routes of spread are intrapartum and horizontally within households. Skin disease and arthropods may be important factors in horizontal disease transmission

Global distribution of HBsAg

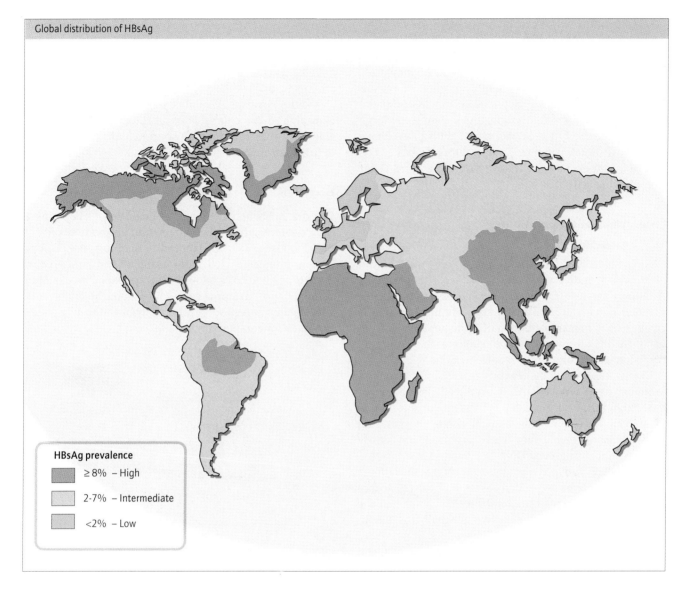

HBsAg prevalence

- ≥ 8% – High
- 2-7% – Intermediate
- <2% – Low

Fig. 9.5 The varying prevalence of hepatitis B surface antigenaemia in different regions of the world. Courtesy of Dr Julia Heptonstall, Communicable Disease Surveillance Centre.

between children in developing countries, because they allow the transfer of body fluids from person to person.

In low-prevalence countries most infections are sporadic and arise in adults. Transmission occurs by inoculation through needlestick injuries, shared syringes, bites and scratches or by sexual contact. Those most at risk of infection include intravenous drug abusers, homosexual men, residents and staff of institutions for the mentally handicapped, surgeons and dentists, laboratory workers and morticians, renal dialysis patients and recipients of unscreened blood and blood products.

Risk groups for hepatitis B in developed countries
1 Intravenous drug abusers.
2 Homosexual men.
3 Sexual contacts of antigen-positive persons.
4 Residents in long-stay homes for mentally handicapped people.
5 Renal dialysis patients.
6 Recipients of multiple blood products.
7 Surgeons, dentists and morticians.
8 Infants of e antigen-positive mothers.

The infection is relatively uncommon in the UK. Approximately 500 confirmed cases are identified each year, mostly in adults belonging to high-risk groups. The prevalence of HBsAg carriage is less than 0.5% overall, although this may be considerably higher in certain ethnic subgroups of the population and in long-stay institutions for mentally handicapped people. A large outbreak occurred in 1984, associated with intravenous drug abuse. Small common-source outbreaks have been reported in association with tattoo parlours and other skin-piercing activities.

Clinical and laboratory features

The incubation period is long — from 3 to 6 months. It is followed by a prodromal viral illness and then a period of afebrile jaundice very similar to that of hepatitis A. Although it is said that a serum sickness-like prodrome can occur, with mild arthritis and a faint rash, this is rarely seen. Clinical distinction of acute hepatitis A from hepatitis B is rarely possible but cholestasis, common in convalescent hepatitis A, is rare in hepatitis B.

During replication of hepatitis B virus in the liver, a large excess of viral HBsAg is produced. This becomes detectable in the serum 2–8 weeks before any elevation of transaminases. As the clinical illness begins and transaminases rise, other viral products are easily detected, including viral DNA polymerase and HBeAg, a blood-borne derivative of core or c antigen; the latter is found only in liver cells. As recovery and convalescence progress, antibodies to the viral proteins appear in the blood, and the proteins themselves gradually disappear. IgM anti-HBc is detectable at the onset of clinical disease. Anti-HBe usually appears in the first 1–3 weeks and HBeAg then becomes undetectable. Anti-HBs appears late in convalescence, after 6 weeks to 6 months, and HBsAg then disappears.

The process of antibody development and antigen clearance can cease at any stage, leaving the patient with persisting antigenaemia. During the state of HBeAg carriage, patients' blood and body fluids contain potentially replicating virus components and are highly infectious. If anti-HBe antibodies fail to develop, the patient's blood remains significantly infectious, even if HBeAg disappears. Patients whose blood is only HBsAg-positive are much less infectious.

If antigens remain detectable after 6 months the patient is considered to be a carrier of hepatitis B antigen. The incidence of carriage is probably in the range of 5–10% of cases. Carriage is more likely in infants and in patients with defective immunity. Many carriers have normal liver function and are well, but those with persisting e antigenaemia, or lack of e antibody, are at risk of chronic persistent hepatitis, chronic active hepatitis, cirrhosis and eventual hepatocellular carcinoma. They are also at risk of infecting their infant during or soon after its birth.

As with hepatitis A, many cases of hepatitis B are subclinical, and the course of clinical disease is very variable. However, this does not seem to affect the likelihood of future carriage or clearance of virus.

Diagnosis

The diagnosis and the stage of evolution of hepatitis B can be inferred from the antigen and antibody profile of the blood (Fig. 9.6). The laboratory diagnosis uses EIA or radioimmunoassay (RIA) for antigens and antihepatitis B virus antibodies. IgM anti-HBc appears 2 weeks after HBsAg and disappears a few months after uncomplicated infection. Anti-core IgG antibody persists for much longer, perhaps for life.

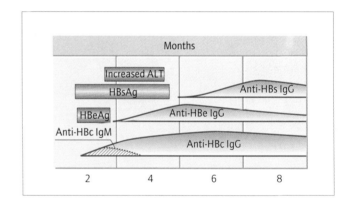

Fig. 9.6 The evolution of hepatitis B: occurrence of hepatitis B virus markers and antibodies in the blood of infected patients. Courtesy of the Communicable Disease Surveillance Centre.

Treatment

There is no specific treatment of acute hepatitis B. Cases are therefore managed symptomatically, as for hepatitis A.

Treatment of e antigenaemia

Treatment of e antigenaemia is helpful, both in reducing the infectiousness of the patient's blood and body fluids, and in reducing the future likelihood of liver disease. The only effective treatment is with parenteral interferon-alpha, which is given in a dose of 10 MU three times weekly for about 3 months. If treatment is effective there is often a short illness with abnormal transaminases followed by e antigen clearance. In different series 15–40% of patients have become HBeAg-negative, but few also clear HBsAg. Higher doses of interferon are probably more effective, but dosage is limited by influenza-like side-effects. Interferon treatment is not effective in patients who were infected perinatally. The new antiviral drug lamivudine may be useful in reducing antigenaemia.

Complications

Liver failure

Liver failure is the most important early complication. Its presentation and management are the same as for hepatitis A. However, liver transplantation is a less attractive treatment because replicating virus may persist in pancreas and other tissue, and can infect the new liver.

Rare complications

Rare complications include rash (more common in children, affecting the peripheries early in the illness), renal failure and, exceptionally, rare aplastic anaemia.

Prevention and control

Immunization

Both active and passive immunization against hepatitis B is possible. Hepatitis B vaccines contain HBsAg either derived from human plasma, or produced from yeast cells using recombinant DNA technology. A course of three injections provides active protection which lasts for 3–5 years. As approximately 10% of recipients do not produce an antibody response, postvaccination screening should be done and a booster dose given if necessary. The proportion of non-responders increases with age. The response may also be reduced if the vaccine is given intradermally or in the buttock.

In low-incidence countries such as the UK, vaccination is indicated for pre-exposure prophylaxis of high-risk groups (see above). In higher-incidence countries mass immunization in infancy is justified.

A specific immunoglobulin (HBIG) prepared from the plasma of selected donors provides passive protection against hepatitis B. It is normally used in combination with vaccine to provide passive/active immunity: (i) for infants born to mothers who are HBsAg-positive

(particularly those who are also HBeAg-positive and/or anti-HBeAg-negative); (ii) following percutaneous or mucosal exposure to infected body fluids; and (iii) for sexual contacts of acute cases.

Immunoglobulin must be given within 1 week of exposure, and preferably within 48 h. A course of vaccine should be started at the same time.

Other measures

Hepatitis B can also be prevented by ensuring that all blood and blood products are screened and that blood is not collected from donors at risk of infection. All syringes, needles and skin-piercing equipment should be thoroughly sterilized after each use; wherever possible disposable equipment should be used. Carriers of HBsAg may be restricted from certain occupations. The disease is notifiable.

Prevention of hepatitis B
1 Pre-exposure prophylaxis with non-replicating vaccine.
2 Postexposure prophylaxis with specific immunoglobulin and vaccine.
3 Universal testing of donated blood products.
4 Use of condoms.
5 Use of clean needles and other skin-piercing equipment.
6 Safe disposal of hospital sharps.
7 Use of disposable haemodialysis equipment.

Delta hepatitis

Introduction

Delta hepatitis, or hepatitis D, is caused by a satellite virus which cannot invade cells in the absence of HBsAg. It therefore only affects patients during the antigen-positive stages of acute hepatitis B, or long-term HBsAg carriers. Simultaneous infection with hepatitis B and D is thought to cause more severe disease than hepatitis B alone.

Virology and pathogenesis

Hepatitis D virus, the delta agent, is an enveloped RNA virus of similar size to hepatitis B virus (38–41 nm compared to 42 nm for hepatitis B). The envelope consists of the same three surface proteins as hepatitis B virus, although the relative amounts are different. The virus core contains only one known protein, the delta antigen. Replication occurs in the nucleus of the cell via a host RNA polymerase. Two complementary strands of RNA are synthesized from the circular genome. One, the antigenome, is an exact complement of the genome. The second, a smaller fragment, is polyadenylated and acts as the messenger RNA for the delta antigen. Infected liver cells become packed with several hundred thousand copies of hepatitis D virus genome.

The delta agent is thought to be directly cytotoxic. Although *in vitro* studies are not conclusive, there is evidence that asymptomatic infection is common. The presence of hepatitis B virus is required to provide the envelope proteins, enabling hepatitis D virus to spread from cell to cell, and to express its pathogenic potential. The coexistence of hepatitis D and hepatitis B virus is associated with an accelerated progression to carcinoma. Delta antigen and IgM antibody are detectable in the blood during infection.

Epidemiology

Infection due to hepatitis D is always associated with a coexistent hepatitis B infection, sharing its routes of transmission. The distributions of the two diseases are therefore similar. Infection occurs endemically among infants and children in areas of high HBsAg prevalence and sporadically among adults exposed to blood and body fluids in low HBsAg prevalence areas.

Prevention and control

Control measures are the same as for hepatitis B, although no specific immunoglobulin or vaccine exists. Controlling the spread of hepatitis B prevents the occurrence of hepatitis D.

Hepatitis C

Introduction

Hepatitis C virus has not yet been isolated, but is an RNA virus similar to some togaviruses. Its genome has been fully characterized. It is a common cause of blood-borne non-A non-B hepatitis. Following the acute infection the liver function tests may fluctuate for many weeks, and, while the majority of cases eventually recover, 20–40% may have persisting hepatitis with the risk of late cirrhosis or hepatocellular carcinoma. HCV exists in a number of serotypes, which have different potential for causing persisting viraemia.

Virology

The story of hepatitis C is intriguing: its existence was long predicted on epidemiological grounds, as a cause of short-incubation posttransfusion hepatitis. Its existence was proven, and antigens for immunoassay were developed, when viral messenger RNA was purified from the serum of infected patients. Complementary DNA was prepared by reverse transcriptase and the phage, lambda gt11, was used to produce proteins for screening against sera from cases of non-A non B hepatitis.

The virus possesses a single, positive RNA strand. Its genome is similar to that of flaviviruses and animal pestiviruses.

Epidemiology

Hepatitis C has been found in every country where it has been sought. The disease is transmitted by exposure to blood and blood fluids, probably contaminated blood transfusions. However, spread through contaminated needles and syringes is also important. Sexual transmission probably occurs, but much less readily than with hepatitis B. Vertical transmission from an infected mother is uncommon. The incidence in the UK is not known at present, but 1 in 1400–2000 blood donors possesses antibodies, and most of these have hepatitis C RNA, demonstrable by polymerase chain reaction (PCR) in their blood.

Clinical features

The incubation period of blood-borne hepatitis C is usually 3 or 4 weeks. A typical illness with malaise followed by jaundice is usual. Many cases are subclinical; the likelihood of early liver failure is not yet quantified.

Diagnosis

The diagnosis of hepatitis C depends on the detection of antibodies to recombinant antigens. The different assays used include antibody capture and antibody competition EIA. Reactivity in these may not indicate infection as cross-reactions readily occur, for instance during EBV infection. This is particularly important when large populations such as blood donors are screened. A positive test must be confirmed by an alternative method, for instance an antibody-capture-positive could be confirmed by recombinant immunoblot assay, or antibody competition EIA. Patients in the acute phase of infection may be seronegative or give weak responses, as seroconversion is usually delayed for up to 12 weeks. Similarly, false-positive results may be obtained in patients who have recently received blood products containing antihepatitis C virus antibodies.

In chronic hepatitis C virus infection, detection of antibodies is not sufficient to make a diagnosis. As the virus cannot yet be cultured, the only methods to detect persisting virus are detection of hepatitis C virus RNA by dot-blot hybridization or by PCR.

Treatment

There is no specific treatment. Tribavirin therapy can cause a temporary reduction in transaminases, but this is not maintained when the drug is discontinued.

Interferon treatment reduces elevated transaminase levels in up to 80% of patients with chronic hepatitis C. This effect is gradual, unlike the effect in hepatitis B when an exacerbation of hepatitis may herald rapid improvement. It is thought that interferon has an antiviral action in hepatitis C, while its effect is mainly immunological in hepatitis B. Half of patients who respond to interferon treatment will relapse when therapy is stopped. Different HCV serotypes have differing responses to interferon.

Complications

A rare, severe type of aplastic anaemia occasionally follows hepatitis C. Most affected patients are in the convalescent stage, and have had a non-A non-B infection. The aplasia is profound and permanent. As bone marrow transplant offers the best hope of cure, blood and platelet transfusions should be avoided as far as possible, so that antihaemocyte antibodies are not induced. Expert haematological advice should be sought. Cryoglobulinaemia, with acrocyanosis and renal failure, is a rare complication of hepatitis C.

Prevention and control

General measures for the prevention of hepatitis B (see above) apply also to hepatitis C. There is no vaccine or specific immunoglobulin available. Screening of donated blood has been carried out since 1991. The role of HIG in postexposure prophylaxis has not been assessed.

Hepatitis E

Introduction

At least one more type of hepatitis virus causes disease in humans. In parts of the Middle East, and limited areas of the Far East and Africa, cases of non-A non-B non-C hepatitis occur. The disease behaves rather like hepatitis A, but is unaccountably severe in pregnancy, causing a

mortality of 10–20%. Jaundice is often prolonged, lasting 4 or 5 weeks. The possible existence of other hepatitis viruses has not been discounted.

Virology

Hepatitis E is a small (32–24 nm) non-enveloped RNA virus, of uncertain classification. It possesses a single-stranded, polyadenylated RNA of approximately 7.5 kb with three open reading frames. Two putative proteins are predicted, one of which is an RNA polymerase. Structural proteins are coded on the second of the three open reading frames. The virus is unstable in storage and has not yet been cultivated artificially.

Epidemiology

The epidemiology of this disease is not well-described. Epidemics have been identified in several countries, particularly in South-east Asia. In these outbreaks, young adults, especially males, are predominantly affected. The source of infection is usually contaminated water; person-to-person spread by the faecal–oral route also occurs.

Diagnosis

Tests for the diagnosis of hepatitis E are in development. Examination of stool by immuno-electron microscopy may reveal the presence of virus-like particles. An antibody-capture EIA has been developed using recombinant proteins. Methods to detect hepatitis E virus in stools by PCR have been reported.

Prevention and control

General sanitary measures and personal hygiene are effective in limiting spread. No vaccine or immunoglobulin is available.

Epstein–Barr virus

The virus is transmitted in saliva by person-to-person contact. Under conditions of crowding and poor hygiene, most children are infected early in life when the disease is usually mild or asymptomatic. In less disadvantaged populations, infection occurs principally among adolescents and young adults, giving rise to a more debilitating illness. Approximately 15% of clinically recognized cases of EBV infection have clinical hepatitis. This is usually accompanied by fever, atypical lymphocytosis and positive heterophile antibody tests (see Chapter 6).

Cytomegalovirus

Cytomegalovirus infection is very common. In developed countries 40% of adults have evidence of immunity; this figure rises to 100% in some developing countries. About 1800 (3%) of the 600 000 children born each year in England and Wales are congenitally infected with cytomegalovirus and 10% of these are likely to develop severe permanent handicap as a result of the infection. Infection is almost always asymptomatic in the immunocompetent. On rare occasions fever, mild jaundice, low-grade atypical lymphocytosis and a negative heterophile antibody test are accompanied by sero-conversion to cytomegalovirus (see Chapters 12 & 21).

Yellow fever

Introduction

Yellow fever is endemic in parts of the tropics, including Africa, and tropical South America (Fig. 9.7). It is hardly ever imported into European countries because of the International Health Regulations' requirements for immunization of travellers.

The cause is a flavivirus which is transmitted by mosquitoes of the *Aedes* sp.

Epidemiology

Two epidemiologically distinct patterns of disease transmission occur. In Africa, the disease is transmitted from monkeys, the main host, to humans (and from human to human) by the bite of the *Aedes* sp. of mosquito (principally *A. aegypti*). These mosquitoes breed mainly in small water containers such as discarded coconut shells, and inhabit villages and towns. Periodic explosive outbreaks of urban yellow fever occur, often in association with a breakdown in mosquito control measures. Countries between 15°N and 10°S are affected.

In South America, the vector is a forest-dwelling mosquito of the genus *Haemagogus*. The disease occurs endemically among young adult male forest workers. This pattern of transmission is known as sylvan yellow fever. Almost every country in South America has been affected at some time.

The disease has never been reported outside Africa or mainland South America, with the exception of Trinidad.

(a) Yellow fever in Africa	(b) Yellow fever in South America
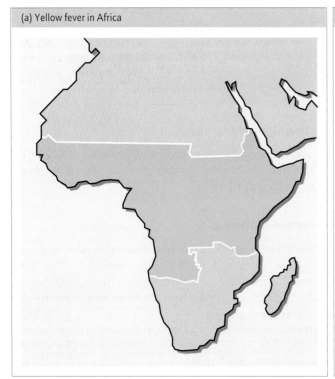	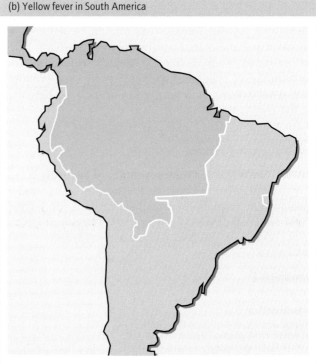

Fig. 9.7 Yellow fever: world map showing affected countries. (a) In Africa; (b) in South America. Courtesy of the World Health Organization.

The incidence of yellow fever has risen sharply in recent years. Between 1986 and 1988, 5395 cases and 3172 deaths were reported to the World Health Organization — the highest in any 3-year period since 1948. Large outbreaks occurred in Peru and Nigeria. Official figures represent only a small fraction of the total cases.

Clinical features

After an incubation period of 6 or 7 days, symptoms appear abruptly, with fever, myalgia and prostration. As with many arboviral infections, a remission of fever and symptoms often occurs after 4 or 5 days. Sometimes the illness ends here, but severe cases progress, with further fever, clinical jaundice, bleeding characterized by haematemesis and progressive collapse.

Diagnosis

The diagnosis can be suspected in unvaccinated patients who have recently visited endemic areas. Virus can be demonstrated in the blood in the first few days of illness. Serology is the main means of diagnosis, and is carried out by arbovirus reference laboratories.

Prevention and control

Yellow fever vaccine is prepared from the attenuated 17 D strain of yellow fever virus. One dose protects for at least 10 years. As with other live vaccines, it may not be given to pregnant women or the immunocompromised. Human immunoglobulin contains no significant yellow fever antibodies and can be given at any time in relation to the vaccine. Several countries in endemic zones of Africa and South America require certification of vaccination before entry.

In endemic areas, the disease is preventable by mass immunization and vector control programmes.

Bacterial infections of the liver parenchyma

ORGANISM LIST

Leptospira spp.
Coxiella burnetii
Brucella spp.
Mycobacteria.

It can be seen from this list that bacterial hepatitis is rare. These bacterial infections are really multisystem diseases in which liver disorder or jaundice is an important or predominant part of the clinical picture. They are important in the differential diagnosis of infectious liver disorders.

Leptospirosis

Introduction

Leptospirosis is a zoonotic disease produced by infection with a variety of *Leptospira* spp. Infections in humans are often due to *Leptospira* of small rodents, cattle, pigs or occasionally dogs. The organisms survive in water, and inoculation of contaminated water infects humans. The disease is important economically among farming communities.

Epidemiology

Transmission occurs when skin or mucosa is exposed to fresh water contaminated by the urine of infected animals or by direct contact with animals. In the UK, the principal animal reservoirs are rats (*L. interrogans* var. *icterohaemorrhagiae*) and cattle (*L. hebdomadis* var. *hardjo*). Approximately 50 cases are reported each year, the majority of which are due to these two serotypes. Two groups are affected: those exposed occupationally, and those infected during recreational exposure. In both groups the disease occurs mostly in men. Farmers, vets and sewer workers are the main occupational risk groups. Recreations associated with infection are swimming, canoeing, windsurfing and fishing.

People at risk of leptospirosis
1 Farmers.
2 Sewage workers.
3 Vets.
4 Water sport enthusiasts.
5 River fishermen.

Microbiology

The genus *Leptospira* is divided into two morphologically identical species: *L. interrogans*, which contains all mammalian pathogens, and *L. biflexa*, containing environmental organisms which are not human pathogens. *L. interrogans* is divided into more than 200 serovars on the basis of agglutination reactions. For simplicity, the names of these serovars are shortened, giving the apparent status of a species, so that *L. interrogans* var. *icterohaemorrhagiae* is more commonly known as *L. icterohaemorrhagiae*.

The organisms usually have a preferred mammalian host but can infect a wide range of species, including humans. Thus, *L. icterohaemorrhagiae*, the causative agent of Weil's disease, has its reservoir in the rat, and *L. hebdomadis*, another common human pathogen, occurs in cattle. *L. canicola*'s preferred host is the dog, while in humans it causes canicola fever.

Clinical features

The clinical picture is quite variable, comprising a combination of fever, hepatitis, meningitis, nephritis and rash. In severe cases there may be a marked bleeding tendency. Mild and subclinical infection is common with all types of leptospirosis. While the full severe picture of Weil's disease is commonly seen in *L. icterohaemorrhagiae* infections, it can also occur with other types.

The incubation period is from 1 to 3 weeks, occasionally shorter or longer, and is followed by an illness which may evolve through two or three phases:
1 First, a phase of acute infection lasting up to a week with fever, malaise and (unusually in a bacterial infection) widespread myalgia; at this stage there is bacteraemia and bacteriuria, and a polymorph leukocytosis gradually develops.
2 Second, the appearance of conjunctival suffusion. This may overlap both the preceding and subsequent phase.
3 Finally, the phase of immunopathology with liver, central nervous system and kidney involvement, and the appearance of antibodies in the blood; fever persists throughout the illness (Fig. 9.8).

The meningitis is associated with moderate elevation in the cerebrospinal fluid protein level and lymphocyte count; the glucose level is not altered. Meningitis is more associated with canicola fever, while hepatorenal disturbance is marked in *L. icterohaemorrhagiae* infection.

Bleeding is due mainly to widespread vasculitis, which is the most damaging feature of the disease. While thrombocytopenia is quite common, other features of disseminated intravascular coagulation are rare. A rare but well-recognized feature of severe disease is a widespread nodular pneumonitis which may even be life-threatening.

In practice the evolution of the disease is rarely as distinct as this and patients may be thought to have viral hepatitis or meningitis at presentation. Warning signs are the association of red eyes and fever with hepatocellular liver disturbance, or of hepatocellular disorder with meningitis. Most cases have significant proteinuria and many have microscopic or macroscopic haematuria with or without casts.

The rash is often maculopapular in the early stages, and its presence, particularly if petechiae or bruising develops, is a helpful sign. A few severely ill patients present with pyrexia of unknown origin with liver disorder; many of these have thrombocytopenia.

Important clinical features of leptospirosis
1 Early myalgia.
2 Hepatitis with fever.
3 Renal impairment.
4 Lymphocytic meningitis.
5 Conjunctivitis.
6 Rash, sometimes haemorrhagic.
7 Thrombocytopenia.
8 Blood, protein and/or bilirubin in the urine.
9 Rare, nodular pneumonitis.

There is a 5–10% mortality in severe cases. Fatalities are due to cardiovascular collapse, often with haemorrhagic myocarditis, and usually associated with renal failure and haemorrhage.

Diagnosis

Clinical diagnosis can be strongly suspected on the basis of epidemiological and clinical features. A useful pointer in flu-like presentations with only fever and myalgia is the finding of protein, blood and/or bilirubin on stick-testing the urine.

Laboratory diagnosis

Leptospira can be visualized in the blood of patients on the occasions when they present during the primary

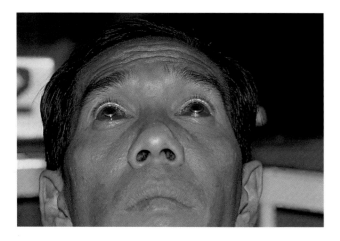

Fig. 9.8 Leptospirosis: jaundice and haemorrhagic conjunctivitis in a feverish farmer. Courtesy of Dr D. Lewis.

phase of the illness, but false-positive results are common. Freshly voided urine can be examined by dark-ground microscopy but this must be done quickly before the organisms die in the acidic environment.

Leptospira can be cultivated from the blood during the first week of illness and from the urine later in the course. The diagnostic yield is often low, as shedding may be intermittent. A specialized medium such as the semisolid agar of Ellinghausen and McCulloch is required for successful culture. *Leptospira* are micro-aerophilic and grow beneath the surface of the medium. Suspensions of cultures can be examined by dark-ground microscopy to confirm the presence of the organisms, which can be identified by slide agglutination, using panels of antisera.

Diagnosis is usually made by serology. Two alternative techniques are used: the first is the *Leptospira* agglutination technique, in which *Leptospira* of various serogroups (groups of closely related serovars) are agglutinated by patient's serum. More recently, an enzyme-linked immunosorbent assay (ELISA) technique which detects specific IgG and IgM has been described. This makes it possible to confirm the diagnosis on a single serum specimen.

Diagnostic methods for leptospirosis
1 Dark-ground microscopy of blood or urine.
2 Cultures of blood or urine.
3 Serum *Leptospira* agglutination tests.
4 Serum immunoglobulin M enzyme-linked immunosorbent assay.

Treatment

Many cases make a spontaneous recovery in 10–14 days. Even after the bacteraemic phase, antibiotic treatment can modify the course of severe leptospirosis. The organisms are sensitive to many antibiotics, and the usual treatment of choice is benzylpenicillin. A course of 7–10 days is usually sufficient. Tetracycline, sulphonamides and erythromycin are all likely to be effective, but the effectiveness of cephalosporins is unpredictable and chloramphenicol is useless.

Treatment of leptospirosis
Benzylpenicillin i.v., 1.2–2.4 g, 6-hourly *or* oxytetracycline orally, 500 mg 6-hourly, both for 10 days.

Complications

Recovery from leptospirosis is usually complete. Some 1–2% of cases develop late uveitis some weeks after recovery. This can be treated with standard ophthalmological anti-inflammatory preparations.

Prevention and control

The most important preventive measure is to ensure that proper protective clothing is worn during occupational and recreational exposure. Cuts and abrasions should be covered with a waterproof dressing before exposure to river water. Rodent control measures may further reduce the risk of infection on farms. Vaccines which provide some protection against the most common serotypes are available for use in animals. Human vaccines have also been developed, but are associated with a high incidence of adverse reactions and give only limited protection.

Causes of granulomatous hepatitis

Granulomatous hepatitis may be caused by a number of infections, most of which are chronic or subacute. They have to be distinguished from non-infectious causes of parenchymal granuloma, including sarcoidosis, vasculitides, and occasionally drugs such as quinine.

ORGANISM LIST

Coxiella burnetii
Brucella spp.
Mycobacterium spp.
Histoplasma capsulatum.

Chronic Q-fever (*Coxiella burnetii*)

This can follow acute Q-fever, or can commence without previous illness. It usually presents with swinging fever, abnormal liver function tests with a cholestatic picture, and often clinical jaundice. Half of patients with chronic Q-fever also have *Coxiella burnetii* endocarditis (see Chapter 14).

Acute Q-fever is a zoonosis which occurs in those exposed to sheep and sheep products at work. It often presents as atypical pneumonia (see Chapter 7).

Chronic Q-fever can be confirmed by demonstrating phase I antibodies to *C. burnetii*. Liver biopsy shows a characteristic histological picture, with many small, non-caseating granulomata which have a peripheral zone of eosinophils (Fig. 9.9).

Tetracycline or chloramphenicol is the treatment of choice. Two or 3 weeks' dosage is sufficient in uncomplicated cases. If endocarditis is present, a course of 6 weeks must be given, and chloramphenicol is then inadvisable.

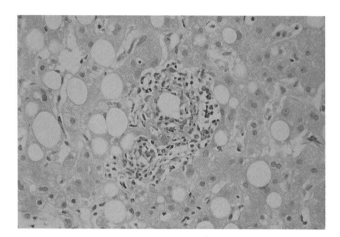

Fig. 9.9 Q-fever: liver biopsy showing small granulomata with a peripheral zone of scattered eosinophils.

Brucellosis

Brucellosis is a zoonosis (see Chapter 20). There is probably some granulomatous change in the liver of most patients with clinically evident brucellosis, which is a multisystem disease often with low-grade bacteraemia. It is rare for liver disorder to be the main feature of brucellosis, but liver granulomata may be discovered during the investigation of pyrexia of unknown origin and should prompt consideration of the diagnosis.

In acute brucellosis blood cultures are often positive, though prolonged culture may be required. Serodiagnostic tests can demonstrate IgG or IgM antibodies to *Brucella* spp.

The treatment of choice is 6 weeks' treatment with tetracycline (doxycycline is useful in a once-daily dose, but some experts favour twice-daily demeclocycline). Streptomycin or rifampicin is recommended during the middle or last 2 weeks to ensure a bactericidal effect. Streptomycin is probably the better choice (see Chapter 20).

Tuberculous granulomata of the liver

Granulomata are always present in miliary tuberculosis. They are often small and non-caseating, and must be distinguished from the identical granulomata of brucellosis, sarcoidosis, autoimmune diseases and rare fungal infections. Much confusion can be spared by ensuring that biopsy material is cultured for mycobacteria, fungi and pyogenic organisms.

Serum should also be obtained to permit diagnosis of brucellosis, yersiniosis or autoantibody-positive conditions. The serum angiotensin-converting enzyme level will be elevated if pulmonary sarcoidosis coexists with liver disease, as is often the case.

Abscesses of the liver

Introduction

Liver abscesses are a relatively common cause of pyrexia of unknown origin, and sometimes present with a complete lack of localizing physical signs. Before the advent of accurate imaging techniques, half of all abscesses were diagnosed at postmortem examination. Nowadays they can be readily demonstrated, and modern antibiotics permit effective treatment.

Pyogenic liver abscess

ORGANISM LIST

Escherichia coli
Klebsiella spp.
Serratia spp
Other Enterobacteriaceae

Faecal streptococci
Streptococcus milleri
Staphylococcus aureus

Bacteroides spp.
Other bowel anaerobes.

Many abscesses, especially those related to abdominal or biliary sepsis, contain a mixture of two or more organisms.

Pyogenic abscesses may be a result of bacteraemia (when other abscesses may also exist, for example, in the brain). They may complicate or follow abdominal sepsis, or they may be apparently spontaneous. They vary from single large lesions to multiple moderate or small ones, and may even be widespread and microscopic.

Clinical features

Patients usually present with high, swinging fever, marked neutrophilia and a high erythrocyte sedimentation rate. Large abscesses may produce tender enlargement of the liver, even progressing to fluctuant lesions pointing between the ribs. Even without abdominal signs, inflammation below the diaphragm will often produce a small right-sided pleural effusion, visible on chest X-ray (Fig 9.10).

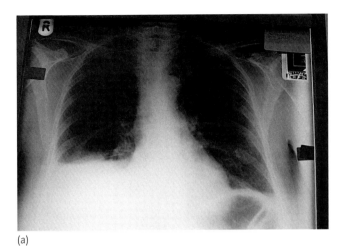

(a)

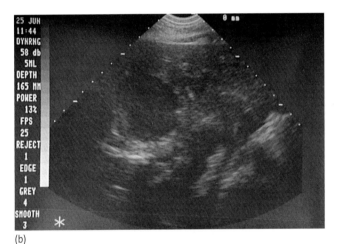

(b)

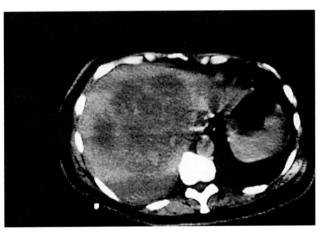

(c)

Fig 9.10 Liver abscess: (a) pleural reaction at the right lung base; in the absence of significant liver tenderness, the combination of this opacity with neutrophilia and a raised erythrocyte sedimentation rate can lead to the erroneous diagnosis of atypical pneumonia; the huge multilocular abscess is demonstrated by (b) ultrasound and (c) computed tomographic scan.

The liver function tests are usually abnormal, showing a moderate elevation of alkaline phosphatase. Clinical jaundice is rare.

Diagnosis

The investigation of choice is imaging. Ultrasound examination will demonstrate most large or moderate-sized lesions. Small lesions, or those whose sonic density is near to that of liver, are best demonstrated by computed tomographic scan. Gallium scan or magnetic resonance scan are excellent for demonstrating inflammation, and will show moderate to small lesions. Liver biopsy may be necessary to demonstrate multiple small or microscopic lesions.

The most accurate microbiological information is obtained from aspiration of the abscess and culture of pus. When the liver lesions complicate bacteraemia, a microbiological diagnosis can often be made from blood cultures. In bacteraemic cases caused by *Streptococcus* 'milleri', the likelihood of abscess formation in the brain must be remembered.

Patients who have visited endemic tropical areas may have amoebic liver abscesses (see below). Immuno-compromised patients may have abscesses caused by unusual organisms, e.g. *Nocardia* spp. (see Chapter 21).

Management

A liver abscess is a serious problem. Treatment should be commenced as soon as blood cultures and pus have been obtained, and should be designed to cover the likely range of causative organisms. The choice of anti-microbials can be adjusted later in the light of cultural evidence.

A third-generation cephalosporin or a broad-spectrum penicillin will be effective against Enterobacteriaceae. Faecal streptococci are also common, however, and the addition of an aminoglycoside will enhance the effectiveness of beta-lactams in this case. Metronidazole may be added to account for anaerobic organisms. If blood-borne infection is suspected, it may be worth including an antistaphylococcal drug in the initial treatment regimen.

Basic treatment for pyogenic liver abscess
Ampicillin i.v., 1 g 6-hourly *or* cefotaxime i.v., 2–3 g 8-hourly; *plus* gentamicin i.v. or i.m., 2–5 mg/kg daily in three divided doses (providing peak blood levels up to 10 mg/l, trough levels less than 2 mg/l); *plus* metronidazole i.v. or rectally, 500 mg 8-hourly.

An adequate response to treatment is indicated by reduction in size of the lesion or lesions, reduction in fever and a falling erythrocyte sedimentation rate.

Drainage of pyogenic abscesses

Drainage of pyogenic abscesses is advisable for moderate or large lesions. Diagnostic aspiration may be sufficient drainage if it is followed by a good response to antimicrobial therapy. Repeated image-guided needle aspiration may speed the healing of large lesions or improve a slow response to treatment.

Failure to respond to adequate chemotherapy or repeated reaccumulation of pus requires the insertion of an indwelling drainage catheter and prolongation of chemotherapy, until satisfactory resolution is demonstrated by temperature response and imaging. Some large or persistent abscesses are inaccessible to needle aspiration or drainage, and there is then no alternative to formal surgical evacuation.

Complications

Rupture of a liver abscess into the peritoneal or pleural cavity causes a sudden deterioration in the patient's condition, and may lead to endotoxaemia and collapse. The aim of treatment is to prevent this by controlling the infection and draining abscesses at risk. In western countries patients almost always seek medical help before rupture is imminent.

Amoebic liver abscess

Introduction

Exposure in endemic areas may lead to amoebic abscess, the commonest complication of *Entamoeba histolytica* infection of the bowel (see Chapter 8). Amoebic abscesses tend to be large and single, usually in the right lobe of the liver (Fig. 9.11).

Diagnosis

The presentation is identical to that of pyogenic liver abscess, except that the patient may have preceding or coexisting features of dysentery. However, over half of patients have no bowel symptoms at any time. Diagnostic aspiration is useful, as amoebic abscesses contain brownish-pink, thick (anchovy-sauce) pus which is quite different from greenish or yellow-grey pyogenic pus. Amoebae are rarely seen in the pus, as they are firmly fixed deep in the wall of the abscess. Bacterial culture of the pus should also be carried out, as pyogenic and amoebic infections occasionally coexist.

The mainstay of diagnosis is serology. Patients with current or recent systemic amoebiasis have positive fluorescent antibody tests (FAT). Residents of western countries are unlikely to have positive FATs from previous amoebiasis. Residents of endemic areas may have pre-existing FAT responses, but a gel precipitin test is also positive in acute systemic amoebiasis, and quickly

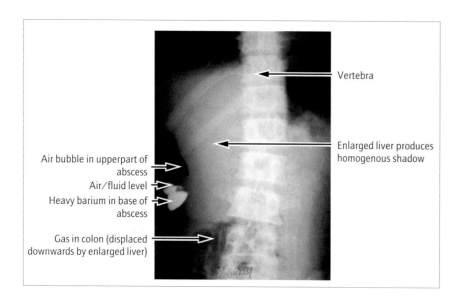

Air bubble in upperpart of abscess

Air/fluid level

Heavy barium in base of abscess

Gas in colon (displaced downwards by enlarged liver)

Vertebra

Enlarged liver produces homogenous shadow

Fig. 9.11 Amoebic liver abscess: needle aspiration has been followed by injection of contrast dye, outlining the large abscess in the right lobe of the liver. Courtesy of Dr D. Lewis.

becomes negative when the condition is cured. A positive gel precipitin test is strongly suggestive of amoebic abscess.

Treatment

The treatment of choice is metronidazole 800 mg three times daily until satisfactory healing has been demonstrated — usually at least 2 weeks. Many small and moderate-sized abscesses will heal without requiring drainage once metronidazole has been commenced. A few very large lesions, or ones which continue to enlarge after treatment is established, may require further episodes of drainage.

It is very unusual for metronidazole to fail, but occasionally an amoebic abscess appears to resist treatment. In such cases the addition of chloroquine 600 mg daily may induce a response. Chloroquine readily penetrates the abscess wall and has an additive effect to that of metronidazole. If the abscess still fails to resolve, the possibility of coexisting or complicating bacterial infection must be considered, and broad-spectrum antibiotic treatment may be indicated.

Complications

Rupture of an amoebic abscess

Rupture of an amoebic abscess may release pus into the peritoneum, the pleura or even the pericardium. The resulting widespread infection causes severe inflammation and may result in shock and collapse, or in secondary abscesses which themselves require drainage. Rupture is unusual if the abscess is easily accessible to percutaneous drainage, as single right-lobe abscesses usually are. Abscesses in the left lobe of the liver are more difficult to approach. Failure to respond promptly to treatment is indicated by persisting fever and unchanging or increasing size on imaging. Surgical drainage should be considered in such cases.

Secondary pyogenic infection

Secondary pyogenic infection is uncommon, but well-recognized. It should be considered in all cases of poor response to metronidazole treatment. Serology usually suggests acute amoebic infection, but the pus may not have the typical appearance. Gram-negative rods, faecal streptococci and/or anaerobes may be recovered on culture. Presumptive treatment should be commenced with broad-spectrum antimicrobial chemotherapy pend-

ing culture results. Metronidazole must be given to cover both amoebae and anaerobes.

Prevention and control

See Chapter 8.

Cholangitis

Introduction and epidemiology

Cholangitis is infection of the biliary tree. It is often associated with surgical disorders of the gallbladder or bile ducts. Typical examples include gallstones, chronic cholecystitis, benign and malignant strictures of the bile duct or of larger hepatic ducts and, occasionally, pancreatitis. It can complicate instrumentation of the common bile duct, for instance endoscopic retrograde cholangiopancreatography, for which antibiotic prophylaxis should always be given.

Pathology

The causative organisms almost always colonize the biliary tree by ascending from the duodenum. Coliforms such as *Escherichia coli*, *Klebsiella pneumoniae* and *Serratia* spp. are common pathogens. Enterococci and anaerobes, particularly *Bacteroides fragilis*, are also often found. Debilitated patients and those who have received broad-spectrum antibiotics can occasionally develop candidal cholangitis.

Clinical features

The common presentation is with right hypochondrial pain, fever, often rigors, and a variable degree of jaundice, which is not always clinically apparent. Laboratory tests show a neutrophil leukocytosis, a raised alkaline phosphatase level and a raised bilirubin.

Many patients have a past history suggestive of biliary or pancreatic disease.

Diagnosis

This is often made on clinical and laboratory information. Contrast and isotope imaging of the biliary tree is difficult when the biliary pressure is raised by infection. Ultrasound or computed tomographic scanning may show gallstones and/or a dilated duct system.

Blood cultures should be obtained, but are not always positive. Bile may be obtained for culture, either by cannulation of the bile duct or by image-directed percutaneous aspiration from dilated intrahepatic ducts. Bile duct cannulation may carry a risk of introducing further organisms, but this should be weighed against the therapeutic advantage of draining the infected bile.

Management

This is usually commenced 'blind', with an appropriate range of antibiotics. Gentamicin or other aminoglycoside, or a broad-spectrum cephalosporin, is appropriate for coliform infections. Ampicillin or amoxycillin, plus an aminoglycoside, will provide effective treatment for enterococcal infection. Metronidazole is the treatment of choice for anaerobes. The antibiotic regimen can be modified if the response is unsatisfactory or the bacteriological results suggest a need for change.

Surgery or drainage may be an important part of treatment if purulent bile is trapped or loculated. An early surgical opinion is therefore of value.

Complications

The most important of these are Gram-negative bacteraemia and shock, abscess formation and erosion of the gallbladder. Clinical vigilance must be maintained to ensure that treatment reduces pain and fever, that the blood pressure is maintained, and that the abdominal pain does not become generalized or peritonitic.

Colonization of the biliary tree

Colonization of the biliary tree with intermittent bacteraemias can be a difficult situation to manage. A patient with one or more strictures in the biliary tree can acquire colonization of the bile without symptoms of infection. At varying intervals there are transient bacteraemias. The patient describes sudden fever, severe rigors and then sweating and defervescence. The episodes may last anything from 15 min to several hours.

It is often difficult to obtain blood cultures at the correct time for a positive result. Some patients become debilitated and lose weight because of frequent fevers, some have laboratory signs of cholestasis. The diagnosis depends on suspicion, and imaging should be performed to identify the cause of the condition. Sometimes this is a single stricture, and is amenable to correction; at others a condition such as sclerosing cholangitis is responsible. There is then a choice of treating bacteraemias as they arise, or of attempting chemoprophylaxis. Culture of the colonized bile will identify the organism and its sensitivities.

Parasites of the liver

ORGANISM LIST

Schistosome species (*Schistosoma mansoni* most important)
Hydatids, especially *Echinococcus granulosus*
Fasciola hepatica and other flukes.

Schistosomiasis

Introduction

Schistosomes are trematodes which derive their name from the large genital cleft in the body of the male, in which the longer, slimmer female lies throughout its adult life. The adult forms live in the visceral veins of humans; *Schistosoma mansoni* mainly lives in the veins of the small bowel but also in the portal veins of the liver, *S. japonicum* in the veins of the small bowel and *S. haematobium* in the vesical plexus. The paired schistosomes produce many fertile ova, some of which lodge in the tissues, causing an intense inflammatory response, and some of which penetrate the mucosae and are released into the environment in faeces or urine. They 'hatch' on contact with fresh water.

Free ova release motile parasitic stages which invade fresh-water snails. They are eventually released from the snails as cercariae, which use their motile tails to swim in the water. The cercariae die in a few hours if they are unable to attach to a host's skin and penetrate it. They shed their tails on entering the skin, and become invasive schistosomules. These migrate through the tissues causing an inflammatory reaction and eosinophilia, until they mature and settle as mating pairs in their favoured venous site, where they live in pairs, producing up to 2000 eggs per day (Fig. 9.12).

The pathology of schistosomiasis is directly related to the worm burden. Eggs are normally passed outwards into the lumen of the gut or bladder to complete the life cycle. Some ova pass through the portal veins to reach the liver, where they cause inflammation leading to fibrosis and portal hypertension. Egg deposition in the lungs (usually in *S. japonicum* infections) can cause lung fibrosis and cor pulmonale. Ectopic eggs in the spinal cord or central nervous system can result in transverse myelitis or epilepsy. Eggs in the bladder wall can result in fibrosis, and chronic heavy infection is associated with bladder malignancy.

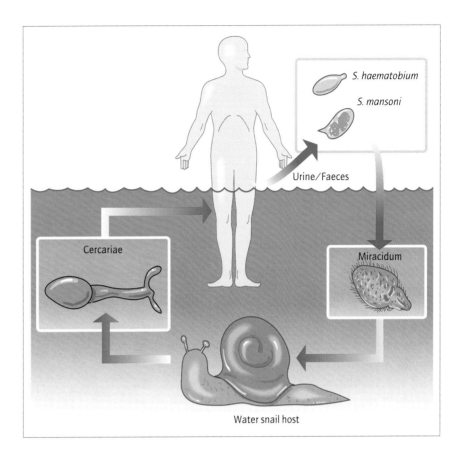

Fig. 9.12 Schistosomiasis: the life cycle of the parasite.

Epidemiology

It is estimated that 200 million people are infected worldwide. Transmission occurs wherever there is exposure to water inhabited by infected snails. This occurs when fresh-water rivers are used for washing, or in rice-growing areas. The peak prevalence of infection is in children aged 5–15 years.

The reservoir of infection for *S. haematobium* and *S. mansoni* is humans, although domestic animals are also a reservoir for *S. japonicum*. The geographical distribution of disease follows that of the infected snails, which are species-specific. The vector snail for *S. haematobium* occurs throughout the Middle East and Africa, particularly along the Nile valley. *S. mansoni* has a wider distribution in Africa, the Middle East, Brazil, Surinam and the West Indies. *S. japonicum* occurs in the Far East and South-east Asia.

Two patterns of disease are seen: focal (associated with small water sources) and non-focal (associated with large marshy areas, mainly in South-east Asia). In some areas, the disease incidence has increased in recent years due to the construction of reservoirs. Transmission is greatest during the rainy season.

Clinical features and diagnosis

The severity of clinical disease depends on the numbers of invading parasites. Slight infections are rarely symptomatic. More intense invasion may cause a sequence of symptoms and signs, while massive parasite loads can cause severe or even fatal disease. Heavy or repeated infections can lead to chronic and progressive ill health.

There are several stages of schistosomal infection, as detailed below.

Swimmer's itch

Swimmer's itch results directly from cercarial invasion of the skin. It happens within a few hours of exposure and clears up in 24–48 h. A rash may affect the exposed skin.

Invasive stage

The invasive stage begins after about 24 h as schistosomules migrate through veins and lymphatics to the lungs and viscera. The patient may complain of dry cough and abdominal discomfort. The spleen may be palpable and there is eosinophilia in the blood.

Toxaemic phase

A toxaemic phase, often called Katayama fever, follows significant infection after about 15–20 days. A prostrating illness includes fever, lymphadenopathy, splenomegaly, diarrhoea and eosinophilia. Severe cases can be life-threatening, especially in completely non-immune travellers.

Acute disease

Acute bowel disease begins after 6–8 weeks as ova are deposited in the bowel wall. The main effects are dysentery-like diarrhoea and weight loss, which may persist for as long as 6–12 months.

Chronic disease

Chronic disease may take several forms. The bowel may show fibrotic, polypoid or granulomatous lesions. The liver may become firm and large. Severe cases develop severe portal fibrosis and hypertension, with splenomegaly, hypersplenism and risk of variceal bleeding (hepatocellular function is usually well-preserved).

S. mansoni can cause rarer effects, of which two are important: one is nephrosis, and the other is a type of granulomatous transverse myelitis following ovum deposition in the spinal cord.

S. japonicum tends to cause more intense invasion and more severe or widespread disease. Chronic features include cardiac involvement with cor pulmonale and alterations in the electrocardiogram.

In all types of schistosomiasis, adventitious ova may be deposited in many tissues, including the brain, but overt tissue damage is rare.

Diagnosis

Clinical diagnosis is important up to, and sometimes for 2 or 3 weeks after, the stage of Katayama fever. From then on, antibodies begin to appear and serodiagnosis is possible. Ova appear in the stool from 6 to 8 weeks after infection.

If ova are scanty, rectal snips (fragments of mucosa teased off the rectal wall with a needle or biopsy forceps) may be squashed on a microscope slide and examined. These often prove positive.

Management

Praziquantel is the treatment of choice. It is given as a single dose of 40 mg/kg, preferably after an evening meal as this minimizes the side-effects of abdominal discomfort or vomiting. Treatment must be given without delay in suspected neurological cases.

For *S. japonicum* 60 mg/kg is given in two divided doses on the same day.

Treatment is not fully effective unless given *after* the deposition of ova has begun. This is important, as Katayama fever responds poorly. In severe Katayama fever prednisolone is helpful in limiting inflammation and controlling tissue damage. An initial dosage of 40–60 mg/day should be reduced as rapidly as the patient's condition allows.

The faeces can be examined 1 month after treatment, when ova will still be seen, but they should now all be dead. Death is demonstrated by diluting the stool with distilled water. This stimulates any live ova to hatch rapidly, releasing active miracidia.

Prevention and control

The most effective method is to provide safe water and sanitation for communities in infected areas, together with education on avoiding contact with potentially infected water. Snail control is expensive and only likely to suceed in small focal areas of infection. An alternative approach is to reduce egg excretion of the human reservoir by chemotherapy. In high-prevalence areas, it may be necessary to treat the whole population, whereas in low-prevalence areas it is more cost-effective to treat children (who are high egg excreters) and clinically affected adults. Tourists to infected areas should be advised of the risks of swimming in fresh water.

Hydatid disease

Introduction and epidemiology

Hydatid disease is the illness caused by the cystic phase of the small tapeworms *Echinococcus granulosus*, whose host is the dog, and the rarer *E. multilocularis*, whose host is usually the fox.

E. granulosus is the commonest cause of human disease. Tapeworm eggs passed by infected dogs are often deposited in fields, where they are consumed by their natural secondary host, the sheep. The eggs migrate from the gut to parenchymal organs, usually the liver and occasionally the lung, where they develop into cysts containing several tapeworm scolices (heads, capable of attachment to the gut wall when they are released from the cysts). The usual life cycle is completed when a dog eats cyst-infected sheep tissue, allowing the establishment and maturation of a tapeworm in the dog's gut. This cycle is common where dogs and sheep exist together; sheepdogs are particularly at risk.

Human disease occurs when tapeworm ova are ingested by humans, often as a result of close contact with a working or pet dog. Tapeworm cysts then develop, and may enlarge for many years before they become clinically apparent.

Clinical features

E. granulosus infection usually causes a solitary cyst in the liver, or occasionally the lung. The enlarging cyst may produce abdominal pain or swelling, or may obstruct the biliary system, leading to jaundice. Lung cysts can cause partial bronchial obstruction, with repeated chest infections. Rupture of cysts is rare, and are more often related to attempted surgery than spontaneous. Eosinophilia is not seen, unless leakage of cyst contents causes an allergic reaction.

E. multilocularis is more invasive then *E. granulosus*. It tends to produce multiple and complex cysts, and also to invade a variety of organs, including the brain.

Diagnosis

Cysts may be visible as thin-walled, fluid-filled structures in plain radiographs, especially of the lungs, and in liver ultrasound scans. Computed tomographic scans may reveal that they contain smaller, daughter cysts, and on magnetic resonance scans magnified images may demonstrate scolices within them.

A number of reliable serological methods are available, which will confirm infection on examination of a single serum. Complement fixation and ELISA are the commonest.

Management

Albendazole is effective in hydatid disease. It is given in a dose of 400 mg twice daily for 4 weeks, and this may be repeated up to four times, with intervals of 1 or 2 weeks between courses. Liver and renal function should be checked during treatment.

As the cysts die, they may become painful and inflamed for a time. Anti-inflammatory analgesics are then helpful. Corticosteroids are not usually required.

Surgery without prior chemotherapy is undesirable, as rupture of the cyst may cause an anaphylactic reaction, and can also seed the peritoneum and other tissues with many living daughter cysts (Fig. 9.13). Cystectomy may be performed after treatment; it is usual to inject formaldehyde into the cyst before manipulating it, to ensure that the scolices within are dead.

It is impractical to excise multiple cysts, or some of those in the brain. Albendazole offers a good chance of disease regression in such cases.

Liver flukes

Introduction

Liver flukes are trematodes which live in the intra-hepatic bile ducts. Like other trematode parasites, they have a life cycle which includes multiple hosts. *Fasciola hepatica* is the only liver fluke endemic in the UK. It has fresh-water snails as its second host. Cercariae migrate on leaving the snail's body, and become attached to vegetation, existing as non-motile metacercariae until eaten by humans or sheep. Wild watercress is the commonest source of human infection. In oriental countries

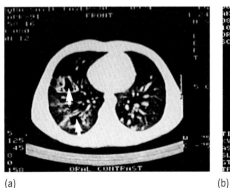
(a)

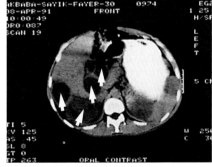
(b)

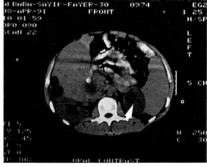
(c)

Fig. 9.13 Hydatid disease: computed tomographic body scan showing: (a) two thin-walled cysts in the right lung (arrows); (b) several cysts in the liver (arrows); and (c) a large cyst in the spleen (arrow). The patient's abdominal pain and the size of the cysts improved dramatically with albendazole therapy.

Clonorchis (opisthorchis) sinensis is common. This fluke affects humans, dogs, pigs, cats and even rodents. Its next host is the snail; cercariae then invade fish (especially fresh-water carp) or shrimps which are again eaten by humans and other animals.

Ingested metacercariae excyst in the duodenum, penetrate the bowel wall, cross the peritoneum and eventually migrate through the capsule and parenchyma of the liver to reach the bile ducts.

Clinical features

These can be divided into two phases.

Acute

The acute presentation is with fever, abdominal pain and liver tenderness and eosinophilia. These features occur as the parasites migrate and invade the liver. They vary from mild to severe, depending on the parasite load, and may last for 3 or 4 months. Episodes of obstructive jaundice may occur as flukes settle in the biliary tree.

Chronic

Chronic fascioliasis reflects persisting irritation of bile ducts. Upper quadrant pains, fevers, cholangitis and persisting eosinophilia may occur. Localized stasis and infection can produce liver abscesses. Over a period of years the flukes may die, being passed in the faeces or becoming calcified in the liver.

Diagnosis

Eggs are passed in the faeces once adult flukes are established in the liver. They are often scanty and are best demonstrated by concentration techniques. Serological tests are positive early in *Fasciola* infections, but are not helpful in early *Clonorchis* cases.

Management

The treatment of choice is praziquantel 20 mg/kg daily for 3 days. The drug is best taken at night to avoid abdominal discomfort and nausea in waking hours. Treatment is not always completely effective and may need repeating after an interval, if egg excretion continues.

Prevention and control

Fascioliasis can be prevented by avoiding consumption of wild watercress, especially if grown on land grazed by sheep. The use of sheep faeces for fertilization of water plants should be avoided. Snail control is technically feasible, but not economically justified.

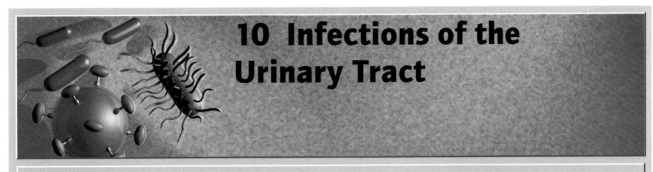

10 Infections of the Urinary Tract

Introduction

Urinary tract infections are common in most communities. Both the collecting system of the urinary tract and the kidneys themselves may become infected.

The collecting system is usually bacteriologically sterile, but the urethra opens to the exterior at the perineum, a site rich in potentially pathogenic flora. Protection from ascending infection is derived from the regular flow of urine, diluting and expelling pathogens; from the mucosal defence mechanisms of the urinary tract; from the antibacterial properties of the urine itself and from the integrity of the sphincters separating the urethra from the bladder and upper tract. Disturbance of any of these mechanisms predisposes to ascending infection. Examples of such predispositions include the following:

1 Mechanical abnormalities of the urinary tract, which may cause stagnation of urine, and bacterial replication behind strictures or in residual pools of urine.

2 Disruption of the urothelium, spoiling its mucosal defence mechanisms and allowing the establishment of epithelial infection.

3 Abnormal chemical constituents in urine, e.g. glucose, which may encourage the survival and replication of organisms.

4 Foreign bodies, such as stones, tumours or, rarely, schistosome eggs and associated granulomata, which may become colonized with pathogens and act as a reservoir of infection.

5 Loss of sphincter function (including that due to indwelling catheters), which destroys an important barrier to ascending colonization of the bladder.

Pregnancy causes dilatation of the collecting system with reduced motility and a greater than usual volume of stagnant urine, predisposing to colonization and ascending infection.

The kidneys have a complex glandular structure of tubules and blood vessels. They receive about one-third of the cardiac output and are therefore susceptible to infection by blood-borne pathogens, as well as to damage from severe ascending infections. Previously healthy kidneys may show only a temporary decline in excretory function during bacteraemic disease, but localized infection in the form of renal abscesses can also occur. This is more likely if the kidney has a pre-existing abnormality such as one or more cysts, areas of scarring or infarcts.

Pathogenesis

Uropathic strains of *Escherichia coli* possess fimbriae. This subject is discussed in more detail in Chapter 1. Type I mannose-sensitive fimbriae appear to be important in strains colonizing the bladder. Type P fimbriae favour colonization of the kidney. Also, organisms may undergo phase variation after attachment to the host's epithelium, changing their expressed antigens to those less readily recognized by phagocytes.

Symptoms

These are classically divided into symptoms of urethral irritation, bladder irritation or upper tract symptoms originating in the pelvicaliceal system and/or the kidney. Obstruction or severe inflammation of a ureter may also produce typical ureteric pain, felt in the flank and radiating to the lower abdomen and perineum (or the testicle in men).

Urethral symptoms

Urethral symptoms are burning or stinging at the meatus and in the perineum, with a continuous desire to micturate, causing marked frequency. There is often severe dysuria.

Bladder symptoms

Bladder symptoms include an unpleasant, heavy feeling in the suprapubic area, which may be relieved somewhat by micturition. Suprapubic tenderness is common. Urethral symptoms often coexist.

Pyelonephritis

Pyelonephritis is represented by loin pain, which can be confirmed by demonstrating tenderness in the renal angle on the affected side. Rigors are a common accompaniment to renal symptoms. An obstructed or hydronephrotic kidney may produce a tender palpable or ballottable mass in the upper abdomen.

In clinical practice, symptomatic localization of disease correlates poorly with the true site and extent of infection. Any or all of the classical symptoms may be present in infections of various parts of the urinary tract, and many urinary infections occur without specific symptoms. Spurious symptoms are common, particularly in children but also in young adults. These include failure to thrive, episodic nausea and vomiting, and symptomless fever. Without a high index of suspicion, persisting infection can cause impaired health or, in infants, long-term renal damage. Acute or severe urinary infections may present with watery diarrhoea, spurious meningism or febrile convulsions. Unlike many infections, urinary infection can exist in the absence of fever or significant neutrophilia.

Non-specific symptoms of urinary tract infections
1 Failure to thrive.
2 Episodic nausea.
3 Diarrhoea.
4 Meningism.
5 Pyrexia of unknown origin.
6 Febrile convulsions.

Diagnosis

The urinary tract above the urethra is normally bacteriologically sterile, but the urethral meatus and surrounding perineum are colonized with a mixture of skin and bowel flora. In women vaginal flora or pathogens may contaminate the urethra.

Three-glass test

The three-glass test is a classic way of using urine to demonstrate the presence of inflammation in the urinary tract. Urination is commenced into the first container; when the flow is established, the midstream urine (MSU) is directed into the second container; the last few millilitres are passed into the third container, making an effort to expel all urine from the bladder and urethra.

The first urine passed contains debris, cells and organisms from the urethra. Visual inspection often reveals strands of mucus if urethritis is present. The MSU contains bladder urine. A normal specimen appears clear and transparent, while cloudiness indicates the presence of cells, bacteria or crystals. The final (terminal) sample contains matter from the clefts of the trigone or from glands adjacent to the pelvic urethra. Mucus strands are often seen in cases with prostatitis. Schistosome ova from the bladder wall are best recovered from terminal urine (Fig. 10.1).

Other useful investigations

A number of screening techniques have been developed for the rapid detection of urinary tract infection. These techniques usually use dipsticks. Glucose can usually be detected in overnight fasting urine in normal subjects. In patients with urinary tract infection, the glucose is typically metabolized by the organism and is undetectable. Absent glucose may indicate active urinary infection. A proteinaceous exudate from the urinary epithelial surface arising as the result of an inflammatory process may give a positive reading on a protein strip. Many urinary

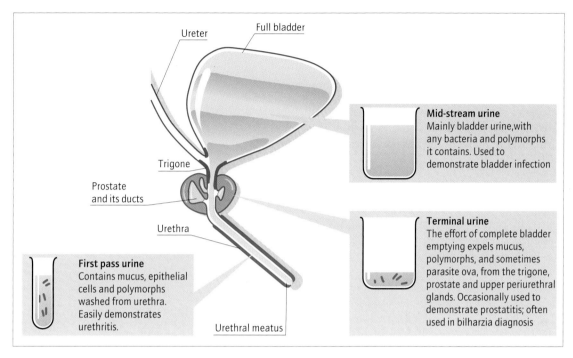

Fig. 10.1   The three-glass procedure for examining urine.

pathogens catalyse the reduction of nitrate to nitrite and this may be detected, indicating urinary infection.

The presence of a large number of white cells provides indirect evidence of urinary tract infection: however, it must be remembered that white cells are a normal part of the urine. It is only when they are present in an excess ($>10/\text{mm}^3$) that disease is indicated. Raised concentrations of white cells in the urine may arise as a result of fever, exercise or contamination from a vaginal discharge. The absence of white cells does not exclude infection as they may rapidly lyse in acid urine.

Bacteriuria and its relationship to infection

Although bladder urine is usually sterile, it has been repeatedly shown that bacterial colonization of the bladder is common in girls and women, and that it also occurs in boys and men. Because both colonization and asymptomatic infection are frequently encountered, criteria are required to decide whether infection is truly present.

The most helpful test is semiquantitative bacterial culture. Epidemiological studies show that infection is likely to be present if colony counts suggest a bacterial concentration of more than $10^8/l$ in women. A concentration of less than $10^7/l$ suggests that infection is unlikely, while intermediate concentrations require fur-

ther investigation. It is widely accepted that the different anatomy of the lower urinary tract in men affects this principle. Infection is considered likely in men and boys when the bacterial count in the MSU is $10^6/l$ or greater.

When the significance of bacteriuria is in doubt, urine can be obtained from the bladder by catheterization using an aseptic technique. Suprapubic aspiration of urine is possible in infants, in whom the full bladder is an abdominal organ. Numerical criteria are not applied to these specimens in which any bacteria are taken to indicate infection.

Microbiological diagnosis of urinary tract infection

Handling the specimen

If a specimen is contaminated at the time of collection, the number of organisms is likely to be small, assuming, of course, it has been kept at a temperature at which bacteria do not multiply and the specimen has been processed quickly. A rigid view of results must not be taken when interpreting the results of semiquantitative culture; the specimen may have been taken later in the day, so that organisms have not had the opportunity to multiply in the bladder. The urine may be more dilute than that found in an early-morning specimen. In addition, if the specimen is delayed in transit, organisms which were present in non-significant numbers may have multiplied sufficiently to give a positive result. Despite the potential pitfalls, examination of MSU is the most useful method for investigating urinary tract infection.

The laboratory diagnosis of urinary tract infection is divided into three stages: (i) microscopy; (ii) semiquantitative culture; and (iii) sensitivity testing. Each of these has a contribution to make to the interpretation of clinical diagnosis.

Microscopy

The presence of pyuria (neutrophils in the urine) is useful evidence of infection when accompanied by bacteriuria. White cells are normally found in the urine, but numbers above 10 cells/mm^3 are considered abnormal. In most laboratories, an unspun specimen of urine is examined either in a counting chamber (disposable chambers are commercially available) or by using a microtitration tray and an inverted microscope.

A number of non-infectious conditions also cause pyuria; these include urinary stones, tumours of the urinary tract and reactions to drugs and chemicals such as cyclophosphamide. Pyuria in apparently sterile urine can also be caused by tuberculosis, rarer conditions such as brucellosis, chlamydial infections, and when bacterial growth has been suppressed by antibiotic therapy.

Causes of sterile pyuria
1 Urinary stones.
2 Urinary tract tumours.
3 Drug reactions.
4 Tuberculosis.
5 Brucellosis.
6 Chlamydial infections.
7 True urinary tract infection partly suppressed by antibiotics.

Bacteria may be seen readily in unstained uncentrifuged preparations of urine. This is often associated with significant bacteriuria and some laboratories will inoculate a primary sensitivity plate (see below). This approach is justified on the basis that the smallest number of bacteria which can be seen is 10^4 cfu/ml, which is similar to the significance level.

Microscopy also enables the quality of the specimen to be evaluated. The presence of epithelial cells indicates skin contamination, indicating that the specimen should be repeated, or the results interpreted with caution.

In addition, white cell casts may indicate renal infection and red cells or red cell casts may be seen in glomerulonephritis or endocarditis.

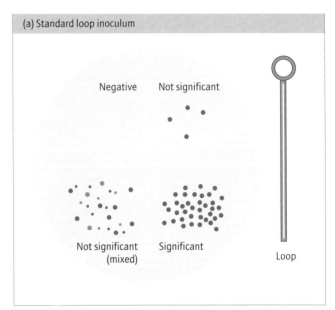

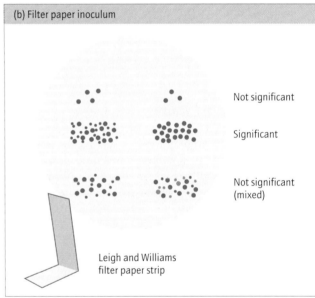

Fig. 10.2 Methods of semiquantitative urine culture. (a) Standard loop inoculum; (b) filter paper inoculum: the filter paper is dipped into the urine and then pressed onto the agar plate.

Culture

Many methods have been developed for semiquantitative culture of urine. The simplest of these is to inoculate a standard loop of 1 µl. The presence of more than 100 cfu will be the equivalent of >10^5 cfu/ml. It is usual to report cultures with 10^4 cfu/ml as indicating significant infection (see above). A method using filter paper strips to deliver a standard inoculum has been described (Fig 10.2).

In all culture systems it is important to inhibit the motility of *Proteus* spp. Itself a common pathogen of urine, its swarming growth may obscure other organisms (Fig. 10.3). Bile salts effectively inhibit swarming, and these are incorporated into MacConkey agar. Most urinary pathogens will grow in the presence of bile salts, but some fastidious organisms (see p. 40) are inhibited. Electrolyte-deficient media such as cysteine lactose electrolyte-deficient (CLED) medium prevent swarming and support the growth of more fastidious organisms.

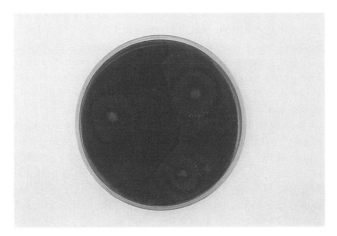

Fig. 10.3 *Proteus* sp. swarming on a blood agar plate after overnight incubation; the same inoculum on a MacConkey's agar plate forms discrete colonies.

Ascribing significance to a culture is the most important problem. Most laboratories use a protocol method to do this.

The adequacy of the specimen is indicated by the absence of epithelial cells on microscopy. Excess neutrophils support a diagnosis of infection.

Most important is the number of organisms (see above) and the purity of culture: organisms present in lower numbers may be significant if present in pure culture, whereas larger numbers of enterococci and coliforms present together probably indicate a contaminated specimen and the need for a repeat specimen.

The identity of the organism is also important. Isolation of an organism usually present on the skin but recognized as a common urinary pathogen may indicate the need for a repeat specimen.

Indicators that bacteriuria is significant
1 Adequate specimen (no epithelial cells).
2 Excess neutrophils.
3 Purity of culture.
4 Number of organisms (appropriate for type of urine specimen).
5 Identity of the organism.

Automated methods

Several automated methods have been described which rapidly identify specimens containing a significant number of organisms for subculture. Growth detection methods are based on changes in optical density, or electrical impedance. Subculture is then performed by conventional techniques.

A semiautomated system uses a series of microtitration trays containing different identification and sensitivity test media. Specimens are inoculated by multipoint inoculator and the plates incubated at 37°C for 18 h. The changes in the media are read by a computer-driven image analyser. Contaminated cultures are detected by visual inspection of the reactions of test media included in the trays. As isolation, identification and sensitivity testing occur in parallel rather than sequentially, a final result is usually available within 24 h.

Identification and sensitivity

For most clinical situations, simple or presumptive identification is all that is necessary. The laboratory methods utilized usually reflect this. Thus, a lactose-fermenting organism capable of indole production will be labelled a coliform. Urease-positive organisms will be reported as *Proteus* sp., and enterococci diagnosed on the basis of their characteristic colonial morphology and hydrolysis of aesculin. Automated and semiautomated methods produce a species or genus diagnosis by use of a computer database.

Sensitivity tests should be performed on all potentially significant isolates. Antibiotics used in the treatment of urinary tract infection include ampicillin and co-amoxiclav, co-trimoxazole, nalidixic acid, nitrofurantoin, and 4-fluoroquinolones such as ciprofloxacin. In addition, inpatient specimens should be tested against the injectable penicillins, e.g. azlocillin, cephalosporins, e.g. cefotaxime, and the aminoglycosides.

Urethritis and the urethral syndrome

Introduction

Infection of the urethra often occurs as part of a more extensive urinary tract infection. However, the urethra is also intimately concerned with the genital tract, and is often involved in sexually transmitted diseases. In women, it is also often affected by genital infections such as candidiasis and non-specific vaginitis.

Herpes simplex
Escherichia coli
Coagulase-negative staphylococci
Other Enterobacteriaceae
Neisseria gonorrhoeae
Chlamydia trachomatis
Gardnerella vaginale
(Lactobacilli)
(Diphtheroids)
Candida albicans.

Epidemiology

This varies according to the infecting organism. Urethritis occurring as part of a general urinary tract infection is commoner in females than males and increases with age. More than two-thirds of urinary tract infections are due to *E. coli*.

Urethritis associated with sexually transmitted disease is usually due to *Chlamydia trachomatis* or *N. gonorrhoeae*, less commonly herpes simplex or *Trichomonas vaginalis* (see also Chapter 11). Males are affected more commonly than females because of the higher preponderance of asymptomatic infections among females and the higher incidence of infection in male homosexuals. The incidence of gonorrhoea and trichomoniasis declined throughout the 1980s, especially among older patients who modified their sexual behaviour in response to the acquired immunodeficiency syndrome (AIDS) epidemic. Since 1989 there has been a slight increase in reported levels of gonorrhoea. In contrast, the incidence of both genital herpes and *Chlamydia* infection has been increasing since the early 1980s in both sexes but especially among females for genital herpes.

Clinical features

The main features are frequency and urgency of micturition, with burning dysuria. In men, particularly those with sexually transmitted diseases, there may be a urethral discharge. This is mucoid, mucopurulent or occasionally frankly purulent. Mild urethral discharge is most noticeable first thing in the morning.

Slightly more than half of all cases are associated with bacterial cystitis, with pyuria and a diagnostic growth of bacteria from the urine. In most cases the pathogen will be a coliform, but in women it may be a coagulase-negative staphylococcus.

Both chlamydial infection and gonorrhoea affect the urethra, and on occasions both conditions coexist. In women with sexually transmitted urethritis there is often an associated vaginal infection and there may be a discharge. The meatus of both the male and female urethra may be affected by genital herpes simplex, in which case the typical vesicular lesions are usually evident and painful inguinal lymphadenopathy may occur.

Urethral syndrome

The urethral syndrome in women is the presence of symptoms without significant bacterial growth or demonstrable vulvovaginal infection. About half of sufferers have midstream bacteriuria of less than $10^7/l$. Surveys show that these women have positive growth in catheter specimens of bladder urine, and probably have low-grade urinary infection which can be treated conventionally. About half of the remainder will have positive investigations for *Chlamydia*.

Among the rest it is sometimes possible to demonstrate fastidious organisms such as lactobacilli or *Gardnerella*. The clinical significance of these findings is uncertain, but appropriate treatment is sometimes helpful. Finally, *Candida albicans* can affect the vulva, especially in pregnancy or after antibiotic treatment. It should be treated if swabs are positive.

There are some non-infectious causes of severe urethral irritation. In middle-aged women urethral caruncle produces a small, red swelling at the meatus. This responds to surgical treatment. Irritants in the urine may include drugs such as rifampicin, warfarin and cyclophosphamide. Dietary irritants such as cayenne or chilli may also cause urinary symptoms when excreted.

Diagnosis

This depends on a combination of adequate history, appropriate urinary specimens and including swab tests for viral, bacterial and chlamydial cultures when indicated.

Management

Many patients can be managed with simple antimicrobial chemotherapy, as for urinary tract infection. Coagulase-negative staphylococci are usually sensitive to flucloxacillin. A 5–7-day course is usually sufficient. Chlamydial infection responds to tetracycline or erythromycin given in conventional doses for 2 weeks. Other organisms may be treated according to laboratory sensitivity tests.

Relapse or failure to respond should prompt a careful search for predisposing factors such as prolapse or atrophic vaginitis, surgical conditions such as caruncle, or carriage of an organism by a sexual partner (even *Candida* infections can recur for this reason).

> **Reasons that urethral symptoms may fail to respond to antimicrobial therapy**
> 1 There is a predisposing factor (atrophic vaginitis, urethral caruncle, small anterior prolapse).
> 2 There is chemical irritation from drugs or strong spices excreted in the urine.
> 3 There is herpes simplex infection.

Cystitis and ascending urinary infections

ORGANISM LIST

Adenoviruses
Escherichia coli
Coagulase-negative staphylococci
Klebsiella pneumoniae
Other coliforms
Proteus mirabilis
Other Proteaceae
Candida albicans.

Introduction

Cystitis is infection of the bladder and often of the upper urinary tract. It is extremely common, but affects the sexes and age groups differently, depending on the prevalence of bacteriuria in each group. Thus, among infants, boys are more commonly affected, particularly those who are uncircumcised. Among children and young adults, females outnumber males by as much as 10 to 1. In the older age groups the occurrence of infection is favoured by prostatism in men, and by incontinence in the frail or disabled of both sexes.

Clinical features

It is impossible to distinguish clinically between infection confined to the bladder and that which has ascended to involve the ureters and renal calyces. Symptoms of frequency, urgency, dysuria and suprapubic discomfort are common. The urine is often cloudy or even pale pink or frankly blood-stained. Proteinuria and microscopic haematuria are the rule. Spurious or non-specific symptoms are also common, especially in young patients.

Symptoms tend to resolve spontaneously in many cases, but this is misleading, concealing the presence of continuing low-grade infection. Fever may be slight or absent; neutrophilia is not the rule in simple urinary infections. Continuing infection may be harmful in patients at risk of renal damage or of severe exacerbations of infection (see below).

When infection affects the renal parenchyma there is often pain and tenderness in the renal angle, upper abdomen or loin. Nausea is common; vomiting or loose stools may occur. Abscesses, either renal or perinephric, may form; warning signs are increasing pain, fever and neutrophilia.

Some urinary tract infections are associated with intermittent or continuous bacteraemia. High fever and rigors are signs of this, and endotoxaemic shock may follow. Bacteraemia is made more likely by foreign bodies in the urinary tract, and is very likely to occur if instrumentation or catheterization is performed while untreated infection exists.

Diagnosis

A high index of suspicion is needed to detect less obvious cases. Laboratory examination of the urine should be requested whenever the diagnosis is a possibility and the blood urea or serum creatinine should be checked. Feverish patients in hospital should always have two blood cultures before chemotherapy is commenced.

Urine examination is sometimes unexpectedly negative, either when a patient has strongly suggestive signs of urinary infection, or when severe infection has failed to respond to initial appropriate therapy. Microbiological reasons for this have already been discussed. However, pus and organisms from an infected kidney may be trapped behind an obstruction at the pelviureteric junction or in the ureter. This prevents microbiological diagnosis, and prevents drainage and healing of the loculated infection. A renal excretion scan or intravenous urogram will show reduced excretion from the affected kidney, which may also be swollen or frankly hydronephrotic.

Management

The immediate requirement is the abolition of the acute infection. Mild or uncomplicated infections are usually caused by Gram-negative rods. A suitable choice of antibiotic for initial treatment would be nitrofurantoin, trimethoprim, cephalexin or co-trimoxazole. All of these agents are concentrated in the urine, and reach adequate therapeutic levels when given orally. Cloxacillin and flucloxacillin are usually effective against coagulase-negative staphylococci. *Klebsiella* and some other unusual urinary pathogens are uniformly resistant to ampicillin. Very broad-spectrum agents are rarely required, and should only be given when indicated by laboratory test results.

Oral treatment of urinary tract infection
1 First choices: cephalexin 250–500 mg 6-hourly (child 25–50 mg/kg daily in three divided doses); trimethoprim 200 mg 12-hourly (child 2–5 months, 25 mg; 6 months to 5 years, 50 mg; 6–12 years, 100 mg, all twice daily; contraindicated in pregnancy and in neonates).
2 Second choices: co-trimoxazole 960 mg 12-hourly (child 6 weeks to 5 months, 120 mg; 6 months to 5 years, 240 mg; 6–12 years, 480 mg; contraindicated in pregnancy and under 6 weeks of age); nitrofurantoin 50 mg 6-hourly with food (child over 3 months, 3 mg/kg daily in four divided doses). Nitrofurantoin has many side-effects, including occasional severe nausea. Co-trimoxazole carries a risk of severe skin reaction or neutropenia, especially in the elderly. It should only be used if there is no satisfactory alternative.
  All of the above regimens for 7 days.

Severe infections with high fever, neutrophilia or shock should be treated initially with parenteral antibiotics. Broad-spectrum cephalosporins such as cefotaxime are useful and have low toxicity. When fever is controlled, treatment may be continued orally, with any effective antibiotic.

The duration of treatment is controversial. Although treatment with single large doses of amoxycillin is possible, a substantial proportion of infecting organisms are now resistant to this drug. Most specialists recommend 5–7 days' treatment for uncomplicated infections, but some feel that longer courses are needed to eradicate bacteriuria. It seems reasonable to treat severe infections for a total of 10–14 days.

Infection behind an obstruction usually demands surgical treatment. Debris or a ureteric stone can often be removed via a ureteric catheter, but if the obstruction is impassable the kidney must be drained by nephrostomy and formal surgery carried out when the infection is controlled.

Prophylaxis of urinary tract infection

Some individuals suffer repeated attacks of urinary infection and often have continuing bacteriuria between attacks. Low-dose antimicrobial chemoprophylaxis will often suppress bacteriuria, improving both the patient's health and quality of life. Temporary prophylaxis may also be indicated, for instance while awaiting treatment of a predisposing condition.

Prophylaxis of urinary tract infection
1 First choice: trimethoprim 100 mg at night (child 1–2 mg/kg) or nitrofurantoin 50–100 mg at night (child over 3 months, 1 mg/kg).
2 Alternatives: cephalexin 250 mg at night (child 125 mg at night) or co-trimoxazole 480 mg at night (child 6–12 mg/kg).

Urinary tract infections in children

Urinary infections in children are often associated with abnormalities of the renal tract. These may predispose to further infections. Examples include urethral valves in boys, bladder outflow obstruction, duplex drainage systems and stones (which may themselves be associated with metabolic disorders such as renal tubular acidosis). Many children have ureteric reflux, which allows infection to ascend to the kidneys. This is thought to cause renal scarring. As 20% of all cases of chronic renal failure have evidence of scarring, it is important to detect childhood infections and to manage them vigorously. A consensus view of experts in childhood infections may be summarized as follows.

1 Detect the infection. Urine should be collected and cultured from all feverish children, unless there is an obvious alternative cause.
2 Treat promptly. Antibiotic treatment should be commenced as soon as specimens have been obtained (it can be modified later, if necessary). At this stage all children should have at least a good-quality renal ultrasound examination to outline the kidneys, and a plain abdominal radiograph to detect stones.
3 Maintain prophylactic chemotherapy and investigate further. Suitable prophylaxis includes trimethoprim 1–2 mg/kg daily or nitrofurantoin 1 mg/kg daily. Co-trimoxazole may also be used as a single daily dose. Once the infection is controlled an excretion scan should be performed to demonstrate excretory function and to outline the collecting system (children over 1 year old may have an intravenous urogram instead).

All infants, and older children with abnormalities of the other tests, should have a cystourethrogram to search for ureteric reflux. Cystourethrograms may be direct (contrast or isotope is introduced into the bladder) or indirect (the bladder and urethra are imaged using contrast or isotope which has been excreted via the kidneys). Direct studies are necessary to demonstrate small degrees of reflux confined to the lower urethra. Indirect studies are useful for follow-up of major reflux, and avoid the need for repeated catheterization.

Prophylactic antibiotics may be discontinued if bacteriuria has ceased and all investigations are normal.

Repeat urine cultures should be performed every 3 or 4 months until the age of 2, following which culture need only be performed if infection is suspected.

Urinary tract infections in men

Urinary infections are relatively common in infant boys, who are four times more likely than girls to have bacteriuria, and in elderly men, when prostatism predisposes to stagnation of residual urine in the bladder. In later childhood and adult life, males are only one-tenth as likely to have bacteriuria as are women.

Men with classic Gram-negative urinary infections should therefore be investigated, as the likelihood of urinary tract abnormality is high. Imaging studies which outline the renal pelvis, calyces and ureters should be performed, to demonstrate deformities or reduplications of the collecting system. If there is evidence of back-pressure the possibility of partial urethral obstruction should be considered. This may be due to bladder exit obstruction or to urethral valves persisting into adulthood.

If no pyogenic organisms are found on urine culture, the patient should be investigated for sexually transmitted or other genitourinary infection, even if urethral discharge is not evident.

Urinary tract infections in pregnancy

This is one of the commonest complications of pregnancy. Nearly half of all women who have bacteriuria detected at the first antenatal assessment will develop overt infection. Even asymptomatic bacteriuria should therefore be treated. A further discussion of infections in pregnancy is found in Chapter 12.

Chronic pyelonephritis

This is thought to be the result of damage to the growing kidney from ascending urinary tract infections in childhood. It is often nowadays called reflux nephropathy. It finds a parallel with chronic bronchitis in that a mechanical or anatomical abnormality predisposes the normally sterile organ to bacterial colonization. Recurrent infections then cause further damage and impair function.

Reflux nephropathy, with scarring of the kidney, is associated with a 10% risk of renal failure in later adult life and with a 20% risk of hypertension. Each successive urinary infection causes a dip in renal function which never quite returns to its previous level. About half of all renal scars are present when the first urinary tract infection is diagnosed.

Treatment is directed at controlling infections and preventing recurrences. Prophylactic antimicrobial chemotherapy may have a place in the prevention of further episodes. Recurrent infections are often with the same organism, having the same antimicrobial sensitivities. Nitrofurantoin is a useful prophylactic drug, as it is concentrated in the urine while attaining only very low levels in the blood and other systems. Its general side-effects are therefore few (confined to nausea or mild gastrointestinal symptoms). Trimethoprim also produces few side-effects, and its spectrum is such that it causes little significant disturbance of the bowel flora.

Surgery is important in relieving obstruction and removing stones. Its place in correcting ureteric reflux is more controversial, but many would advocate surgery for gross reflux through a patulous ureteric orifice.

In established reflux nephropathy the treatment of hypertension is important, as raised blood pressure can damage the kidneys further, as well as causing hypertensive atheroma and heart disease.

Bilharzia

In endemic areas, bilharzia is a common cause of chronic urinary tract disease. The disease occurs throughout Africa and the Middle East, but especially along the Nile valley (see Chapter 9). The adult *Schistosoma haematobium* resides in the venous plexus of the bladder wall. The spiked ova penetrate the mucosa to be excreted in the urine. Haematuria is common in heavy infections which cause severe inflammation. Inflammatory granulomata, fibrosis and calcification distort the bladder and lower ureters, causing repeated infections and progressive reflux nephropathy.

Early invasive schistosomiasis can present with Katayama fever (see Chapter 9). Serological tests become positive 2–4 weeks after the original fever and eosinophilia.

Haematuria and acute urinary symptoms follow invasion of bladder wall venules by schistosomes. Following this, typical ova are excreted. These are best demonstrated in the pellets from centrifuged early-morning or terminal urine specimens. Serology is usually positive by this stage.

The treatment of choice for bilharzia is praziquantel. For prevention and control, see Chapter 9.

Acute epididymo-orchitis

ORGANISM LIST

Mumpsvirus
Coxsackievirus
Escherichia coli

Other coliforms
Neisseria gonorrhoeae (rare)
Chlamydia trachomatis (rare).

Acute epididymo-orchitis usually has a sudden onset. There is pain, swelling and redness of one or both testicles, with or without symptoms of cystourethritis. Fever and other systemic symptoms are common. It must be distinguished from acute torsion of the testis, which requires urgent surgical correction.

There may be obvious features of the underlying systemic disease, e.g. parotitis in mumps or severe muscle pain in coxsackie B infections.

The first step in diagnosis is to exclude torsion of the testis, which is common in fit young men. Testes which undergo torsion often have abnormal anatomy, with the testis hanging horizontally, below the epididymis instead of lying anterior to it. This may be demonstrable by clinical or ultrasound examination. In cases of doubt a surgical opinion must be sought.

Bacterial pathogens may be demonstrable on MSU examination or by urethral swab. Viral infections are diagnosed initially on clinical grounds and ultimately by the cultural and serological methods applicable to the individual viruses.

Treatment is that of the underlying condition. Antimicrobial chemotherapy, as for urinary infections, is appropriate for bacterial infections, and should also be attempted if the aetiology is not obvious. A short course of prednisolone treatment will alleviate oedema and inflammation in viral infections, and will not prolong the natural course of the disease. A well-fitting scrotal support or underpants will reduce discomfort. Anti-inflammatory analgesics, such as soluble aspirin, diclofenac or ibuprofen, are helpful. Stronger analgesics may be required early in the disease.

Chronic or persisting epididymo-orchitis is a rare feature of tuberculosis (particularly of the renal tract), and of brucellosis.

Bartholin's abscess

Bartholin's glands open into the posterior part of the vulval vestibule via a duct on each side. Infection is usually unilateral, causing intense pain, swelling and tenderness deep to the labia on the affected side. Common causative organisms include *Staphylococcus aureus* and *E. coli*, which probably ascend from the perineal skin and then become trapped as oedema obstructs the duct. Broad-spectrum antibiotics may be effective, but surgical drainage is often required.

On rare occasions the abscess contains chlamydiae or mycobacteria. Culture of the pus obtained at surgery is therefore advisable, to confirm the aetiology.

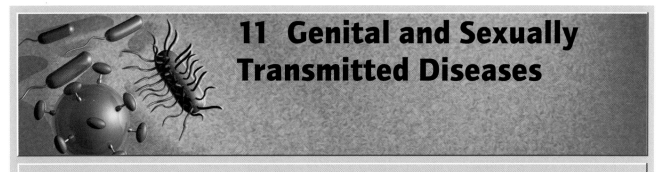

11 Genital and Sexually Transmitted Diseases

Introduction

The structures of the male and female genital tract differ greatly, but they have their pelvic position and perineal connections in common. Both the vagina and the urethra are lined with squamous epithelium and, in both sexes, the upper genital tract has unique structures which are both germinal and secretory.

In men the genital tract flora tend to reside on the glans of the penis and the urethral meatus. Chronic colonizing and infecting organisms may exist in the normally sterile upper urethra, prostate and epidydimis.

In women the vulva and vagina have a complex flora partly derived from the perineal skin, and partly dictated by the acidic environment of the adult vagina, which is maintained by a large population of lactobacilli. The normal vaginal flora help to maintain the health of the mucosa and to inhibit the establishment of *Candida* infections, to which this site is especially vulnerable.

The female urethra and cervix are vulnerable to acute and chronic invasion by pathogens. Infection may ascend the female genital tract to cause endometrial and tubal infections, and even to affect intra-abdominal organs.

In both sexes the genital tract can act as the portal of entry for systemic or bacteraemic disease. Disease at distant body sites may originate from the genital tract. Fastidious organisms are carried and protected in genital secretions, and may be deposited in the mouth, the eye or the rectum, depending on the type of sexual activity, and the use or availability of protective or hygienic measures. It is important to remember these associations when investigating possible sexually transmitted infections.

Trends in incidence of the commonest sexually transmitted diseases are shown in Fig. 11.1. There is a difference in incidence between different ages and sexes. This is because women become sexually active at an earlier age than heterosexual men, and homosexual men at a later age (Fig. 11.2). The incidence of gonorrhoea and trichomoniasis declined throughout the 1980s, especially among older patients who modified their sexual behaviour in response to the acquired immunodeficiency syndrome (AIDS) epidemic. Since 1989 there has been a slight increase in reported levels of gonorrhoea. In contrast, the incidence of both genital herpes and *Chlamydia* infection has been increasing since the early 1980s in both sexes but especially among females for genital herpes.

Viral infections of the genital tract

ORGANISM LIST

Papillomaviruses
Herpes simplex viruses.

Human papillomaviruses, warts and intraepithelial neoplasia

Introduction

Human papillomaviruses (HPVs) are small DNA viruses, with a circular genome of double-stranded

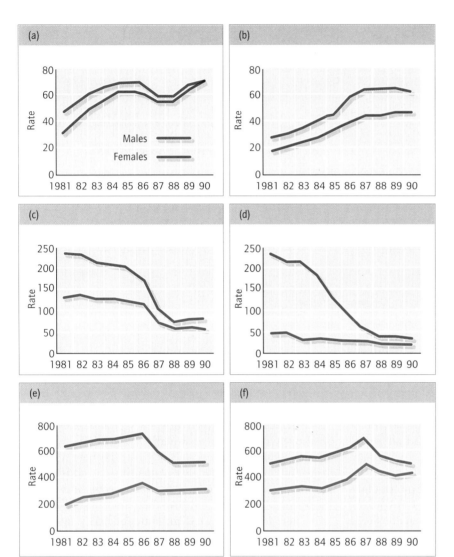

Fig. 11.1 Diagram showing trends in the incidence of common sexually transmitted diseases in the UK. (a) Genital herpes; (b) genital warts; (c) gonorrhoea; (d) infectious syphilis; (e) non-specific genital infection; (f) other conditions not requiring treatment. Courtesy of the Communicable Disease Surveillance Centre.

DNA, which cause warts. There are at least 60 types of papillomavirus, loosely associated with types of cutaneous, genital and laryngeal warts. Approximately half of papillomavirus types have only been identified in lesions affecting the skin in epidermodysplasia verruciformis.

Genital warts, like all warts, are spread by contact. The clinical result can be anything from one or two lesions on the shaft of the penis, the glans, vulva, perineum or anal margin, to large areas of moist, shaggy lesions. Genital warts are a major problem in pregnancy, when they become very extensive and hypertrophic, even sufficient to interfere with vaginal delivery.

The diagnosis is clinically obvious, and rarely needs other confirmation. The best treatment is daily topical podophyllin resin, in the form of a paint. The surrounding skin should be protected with soft paraffin ointment and the paint should be washed off after 6 h, as podophyllin is irritant, and toxic if absorbed. Extensive warts should be treated in successive small areas. Podophyllin is contraindicated in pregnancy but after delivery the warts shrink somewhat, and can be treated conventionally.

Cervical intraepithelial neoplasia and papillomavirus types 16 and 18

Recent investigation by hybridization studies and polymerase chain amplification has shown the presence of papillomavirus genome in neoplastic cells of the cervix significantly more often than in normal epithelium.

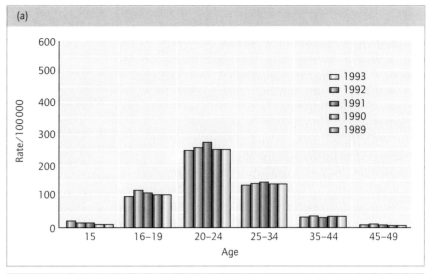

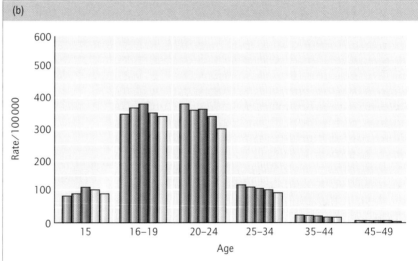

Fig. 11.2 (a) Male and (b) female age- and sex-related incidence of chlamydial genital infection in the UK.

Typing studies show that type 16, and to a lesser extent type 18, predominate in neoplastic cells; other papillomavirus types do not show such markedly different distributions in malignant and non-malignant cells. This suggests association of a sexually transmitted viral infection with a disease known to be associated with sexual activity at a young age, and with multiple sexual partners.

Vaginal intraepithelial neoplasia

Vaginal intraepithelial neoplasia has been extensively studied recently, and it has been possible by hybridization to demonstrate papillomavirus DNA in the lesions. HPV type 6 has been most commonly found. HPV types 6 and 11, and sometimes 18, 16 and other types, have been found in vulval and penile intra-

epithelial neoplasias. Whether the virus is a cause or effect of the mucosal change is not clear. Nor is it known whether the mild intraepithelial lesions progress to frankly neoplastic disease or whether they resolve spontaneously. Nevertheless, HPV is under investigation as a possible initiator of genital malignancy.

Genital herpes simplex infections

Pathology and epidemiology

Genital herpes simplex is a common infection which spreads by direct contact, usually but not always sexual. It used to be caused mainly by herpes simplex virus type 2 (HSV 2), but in the last two decades type 1 has become more common in genital infections. Both types of infection can be associated with HSV infection in other sites, particularly cold sores and other cutaneous infections. The incidence of both genital herpes and genital warts has increased in recent years, particularly among females. Some of this increase is due to the recurrence of both diseases among patients with human immuno-deficiency virus (HIV) infection; it is also likely that ascertainment has improved considerably.

As with other herpesvirus infections, there is a primary and postprimary type of disease, and periods of asymptomatic excretion of virus from the previously affected genital tract. Virus has been demonstrated in the urethra and the vas deferens of asymptomatic men. Antiviral treatment of acute disease prevents neither relapses nor asymptomatic excretion, so that contact-tracing is an ineffective means of controlling genital herpesvirus infections.

Clinical features

Primary infection

Primary infection is often clinically obvious, painful and distressing. The incubation period averages 4 or 5 days, but varies very widely. Illness begins with mild fever and malaise, and tender inguinal lymphadenopathy, which is usually unilateral and rarely severe. After a day or two, tense superficial vesicles appear and quickly break to become painful ulcers. The commonest site for the vesicles is the coronal sulcus or glans of the penis, the vulva or the anal margin. On occasions the soreness is so severe that it inhibits micturition and causes acute urinary retention. Rare cases of faecal impaction are seen when the perianal area is involved.

Associated neurological problems

Associated neurological problems can occur in primary HSV 2 infections.

Viral meningitis is not uncommon, and may be missed if mild. Lumbar puncture reveals typical cerebrospinal fluid (CSF) changes with lymphocytosis, and HSV 2 can be isolated from the CSF. The meningitis is benign, and resolves in a few days.

Radiculitis of the pelvic nerve roots can also occur. There is pain and stiffness of the lower back, sometimes with associated meningism. The neurological lesion is asymmetrical, and may produce paraesthesia or anaesthesia of the buttock, thigh or perineum. This interferes with the initiation of urination and defecation. Weakness of the sphincters of both bladder and rectum and reduced detrusor function can also occur. Occasionally,

other muscles of the perineum or thigh are affected. The course of the disorder is variable, but is often 5–10 days or more. Recovery is gradual, but almost always complete.

> **Clinical presentations of primary genital herpes**
> 1 Painful inguinal lymphadenopathy.
> 2 Painful genital ulcers.
> 3 Lymphocytic meningitis (herpes simplex virus type 2 only).
> 4 Pelvic radiculitis (herpes simplex virus type 2 only).

Postprimary genital herpes

Postprimary genital herpes is like a cold sore. It may affect the buttock, thigh, perineum or the genitalia. The appearance of a group of vesicles is heralded by mild malaise, with local pain or burning. The vesicles last for 2 or 3 days before healing by drying and epithelialization. Abortive attacks, with transient appearance of a few papules, also occur. These recurrences can be very frequent, and in women may occur premenstrually for month after month. Although there is little fever or systemic change, women particularly may feel fatigued and suffer radiation of pain to the thighs and back.

Recurrences are unlikely to decline in frequency if they persist for more than a year after the first attack.

Diagnosis

This is often clinically obvious. Herpesvirus particles can be demonstrated by electron microscopy of vesicle fluid or scrapings. Both HSV 1 and HSV 2 grow rapidly in routinely used cell cultures, producing typical cytopathic effects in 48–72 h. Seroconversion is demonstrable in primary attacks.

Management

Aciclovir is effective against HSV. Oral medication is sufficient in many cases. The recommended dosage for primary and postprimary attacks is 200 mg five times daily for 1 week. Topical treatment may have a weak local effect, but is ineffective against virus in the lymph nodes and nervous system.

Severe primary infections are best treated with intravenous aciclovir 5 mg/kg 8-hourly, and usually require courses of 5 days, occasionally longer. Meningo-radiculitis may respond better to 10 mg/kg doses.

Frequent recurrences can be prevented by suppressive therapy with oral aciclovir 400 mg twice daily. When recurrences are confined to the premenstrual days, treatment need only be taken at this time. Unpredictable or more frequent attacks require continuous suppression.

> **Treatment of genital herpes**
> **1** Acute attacks: aciclovir orally, 200 mg five times daily for 7 days; or valaciclovir 1 g twice daily; or famciclovir 250 mg twice daily.
> **2** Meningoradiculitis: aciclovir i.v., 10 mg/kg 8-hourly for 5–10 days.
> **3** Suppression of recurrences: aciclovir orally, 400 mg twice daily continously, or in the week before menstruation every month.

Famciclovir has recently been licensed for treating herpes genital. Valaciclovir is effective against HSV 1 and HSV 2.

Complications and cautions

True complications are rare; staphylococcal secondary infection of the lesions is the most likely. This is marked by increasing inflammation and exudation, often of yellowish pus. It responds to treatment with an antistaphylococcal antibiotic such as cloxacillin or flucloxacillin. Oral medication for 5 or 6 days is often sufficient.

Herpes simplex infection is severe in the neonate and in immunosuppressed patients. In pregnancy it can be transmitted during delivery and (rarely) transplacentally, causing extensive, life-threatening disease in the neonate (see Chapter 12).

HSV infection is a trying and damaging infection in AIDS when it is often persistent, extensive and rather invasive. It is justifiable to offer prolonged aciclovir prophylaxis in such cases. However, aciclovir-resistant organisms sometimes emerge and cause continuing lesions in highly immune-deficient patients.

Erythema multiforme accompanies herpes simplex attacks and recurrences in a small group of people, among whom particular tissue types (DQW3 and/or DRW53) predominate. HSV DNA can be demonstrated in erythematous skin but not in normal skin. The severity of attacks diminishes over a period of 24–36 months, and eventually the erythema does not occur. Suppression of the herpes simplex recurrences prevents the erythema multiforme attacks.

Bacterial infections of the genital tract

ORGANISM LIST

Chlamydia trachomatis (serogroups D–K)
Neisseria gonorrhoeae
Treponema pallidum
Gardnerella vaginale
Actinomyces spp.
Haemophilus ducreyi
Lymphogranuloma venereum (*Chlamydia trachomatis* serogroups L1, L2, L3)
Mycoplasma hominis
Ureaplasma urealyticum.

Chlamydial genital infections

Introduction

These infections form a large group of the non-specific or non-gonococcal genital infections, which are now the commonest genital infections throughout the world. Diagnosis of chlamydial infections has increased steadily over the past 20 years. It has been estimated that up to 50% of cases of non-gonococcal urethritis in the USA are caused by *Chlamydia trachomatis*. Chlamydial genital infections are important not only because of the high transmission rates and high morbidity that they cause, but because of their contribution to infertility due to chronic pelvic infection and their ability to cause significant intrapartum infection of neonates.

Pathology

C. trachomatis is an obligately intracellular bacterium which lacks a cell wall. It is a member of the genus *Chlamydia* which contains two other species, *C. psittaci*, a zoonotic pathogen, and *C. pneumoniae*, a respiratory pathogen of humans (see Chapter 7).

C. trachomatis exists in several serotypes: A, B, Ba and C, which are associated with ocular trachoma (see Chapter 5); D–K, associated with oculogenital infections and neonatal infections (see Chapter 12); and L1, L2 and L3, the causes of lymphogranuloma venereum.

Chlamydia are discussed in more detail in Chapter 7.

Clinical features

In men the commonest manifestation of infection is urethritis, causing dysuria, urethral and meatal soreness and urethral discharge, which is most noticeable in the morning, before micturition. This may occur alone, or cause persisting symptoms after treatment of gonorrhoea. Ascending infection can cause epididymitis, acute prostatitis and chronic prostatitis. Chlamydial infection can also cause non-specific proctitis, possibly after anal intercourse.

In women urethritis and cervicitis are common, with symptoms of soreness, dysuria and mucoid discharge, though without significant systemic features. Ascending infection typically causes acute salpingitis. This presents as fever, neutrophilia and lower abdominal pain. It must be distinguished from appendicitis. Wider invasion can occur, producing a picture of perihepatitis (Curtis–Fitz-Hugh syndrome), with high fever, upper abdominal pain and guarding, and abnormal liver function tests. Rare cases of perihepatitis are seen in men, though the route of infection is uncertain.

Many lower genital tract infections are asymptomatic, particularly in women. Pelvic or abdominal disease can therefore occur without preceding genital symptoms. Occasionally, the occurrence of chlamydial infection in a neonate reveals the presence of asymptomatic infection of the parents.

Ocular infection can coexist with genital symptoms in both sexes, usually as a persisting conjunctivitis.

Clinical presentations of chlamydial infections
1 Urethritis.
2 Cervicitis.
3 Proctitis.
4 Conjunctivitis.
5 Salpingitis.
6 Prostatitis.
7 Perihepatitis.
8 Infected neonate.

Diagnosis

Urethritis and cervicitis are often clinically apparent. Diagnostic tests must be performed (see also Chapter 7), as gonorrhoea is the differential diagnosis and may also coexist with chlamydial disease.

Salpingitis does not have the distinctive evolution of appendicitis, and may be accompanied by vaginal discharge, which can be examined microbiologically. Pain and guarding are suprapubic. Swelling, induration and tenderness in one or both fornices are often found on vaginal examination.

Perihepatitis must be differentiated from gallbladder disease and liver abscess. Ultrasound or computed tomographic imaging may help by showing a healthy gallbladder and/or oedema and brightness of the liver capsule.

Laboratory diagnosis of chlamydial genital infections is usually made by antigen detection. Swabs are taken from the urethra, cervix or rectal mucosa. Direct immunofluorescent (IF) or enzyme-linked immunosorbent assay (ELISA) methods are used to detect chlamydial group antigen in the cellular material obtained. The results of IF tests are highly process- and observer-dependent, and are slightly less reliable than ELISA or cultural methods.

C. trachomatis can be cultured from swab specimens in cultures of cycloheximide- or idoxuridine-pretreated McCoy cells. HELA cells are also suitable for *Chlamydia* cultures. Positive results are demonstrated by the presence of chlamydial inclusion bodies on Giemsa- or iodine-stained cells, or by antigen demonstration using direct IF or ELISA techniques.

Serology is not helpful in the diagnosis of chlamydial genital infections.

Management

The usual treatment is a 2-week course of a tetracycline such as daily doxycycline or twice-daily Deteclo. The simplest regimen possible is chosen to encourage compliance. Erythromycin 2 g daily in divided doses is an alternative. Azithromycin in a single dose of 1 g is at least as effective as tetracycline, but expense prohibits its widespread use.

Systemic infections require parenteral treatment. Erythromycin is then the treatment of choice.

Treatment of chlamydial infections
1 First choice: doxycycline orally 200 mg on day 1, then 100 mg daily for 2 weeks; or Deteclo one tablet 12-hourly for 2 weeks.
2 Alternatives: erythromycin orally 2 g daily in two to four divided doses for 2 weeks; or azithromycin orally 1 g single dose.
3 Systemic infections: erythromycin i.v. 500 mg to 1 g 6-hourly for 5–7 days.

Surgery for acute salpingitis is avoided if possible, as salpingectomy reduces fertility. Fibrosis of the lumen can still affect tubal function if healing is slow or incomplete.

Role of Ureaplasma urealyticum in non-specific genital infection

Some non-specific genital infections are not associated with *C. trachomatis*. *U. urealyticum* can be detected by cultural techniques (using media suitable for mycoplasmata; see Chapter 7) in a substantial proportion of these. The importance of this is that *U. urealyticum* is often resistant to tetracycline. It is usually sensitive to erythromycin.

Complications

The most important complication of non-specific genital infection is Reiter's syndrome. This is a postinfectious condition affecting mainly men, and associated with the human leukocyte antigen (HLA) B27 tissue-type. It causes prolonged synovitis and connective tissue inflammation (see Chapter 24).

Lymphogranuloma venereum

This is a tropical sexually transmitted disease caused by the serotypes L1, L2 and L3 of *C. trachomatis*. It has an incubation period of 2–30 days. A small, shallow ulcer or ulcers may appear at the site of inoculation on the genitalia, but most patients present with a slowly enlarging, usually bilateral lymphadenopathy in the inguinal or femoral region. Suppuration is common, with one or more draining sinuses and slow healing. There are many systemic features, such as fever, meningism, pericarditis, keratitis and skin rashes, all of which slowly resolve. Years later, perineal and inguinal fibrosis may occur, causing rectal strictures in women and genital lymphoedema in men.

Diagnosis can be made by serological testing, or by demonstrating the typical histology of the primary lesion or lymph nodes.

The treatment of choice is tetracycline, which must be given for at least 3 weeks. Treatment of early disease prevents late fibrosis, which is not amenable to antibiotic therapy.

Gonorrhoea

Introduction and epidemiology

Although less common than non-specific genital infection, gonorrhoea still causes millions of infections worldwide. As well as local infection, it can also cause bacteraemic disease which is easily mistaken for other conditions, often being recognized and treated late.

In contrast to viral infections of the genital tract, the incidence of gonorrhoea has fallen in many developed countries in recent years. The decline has been mainly among patients over 25 years of age. In younger age groups, particularly young homosexual males, the incidence has started to increase again after a period of decline during the late 1980s. This trend suggests poor response to prevention initiatives among adolescents.

Clinical features

Gonorrhoea most often causes local genital infection, with urethritis and/or cervicitis, and relatively few systemic effects. Subclinical infection has always been recognized in women, but is increasingly described in men also. The most common clinical presentations are urethritis in men and cervicitis in women. The throat or the rectum can be affected, often asymptomatically.

Ascending infection occurs in a minority of cases, causing prostatitis, epidydimitis, salpingitis and occasionally perihepatitis.

Gonococcal bacteraemia

Gonococcal bacteraemia tends to present with local inflammatory lesions, rather than a simple fever. The accompanying genital infection may be mild or subclinical.

Arthritis is common, frequently affecting both knees, but the ankle or the wrist are also vulnerable (Fig. 11.3). The patient is feverish; the joint or joints are painful and swollen, and may be surrounded by considerable erythema. There is usually an effusion, which can be large in the knees.

Many patients have a rash, which is often very sparse. It is vasculitic, with individual, painful lesions, often vesicles with an intensely inflamed halo (Fig. 11.4). These lesions look very like herpes simplex vesicles but are found on extensor surfaces, particularly of the fingers, the elbow or the foot. A few patients have a bruising or haemorrhagic component to the rash, making it similar to a meningococcal rash.

Clinical presentations of gonorrhoea
1 Urethritis.
2 Cervicitis.
3 Proctitis.
4 Pharyngitis.
5 Salpingitis.
6 Prostatitis.
7 Perihepatitis.
8 Septic arthritis.
9 Bacteraemia (often with rash).

Diagnosis

Urethritis and cervicitis are clinically apparent. Gram stain of the pus, of urethral and/or cervical swabs shows many neutrophils and both intracellular and extracellular Gram-negative diplococci. This test is more sensitive in men than in women.

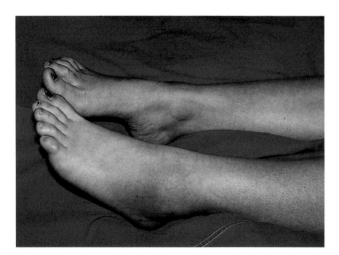

Fig. 11.3 Gonococcal arthritis affecting the ankle 1 week after contact with a new sexual partner.

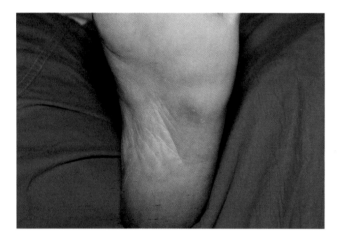

Fig. 11.4 Gonococcal skin lesion: an intensely inflamed, rather vasculitic lesion; the same patient as in Fig. 11.3.

Salpingitis usually presents surgically, as a differential diagnosis of appendicitis or acute abdomen. Suprapubic tenderness and guarding, the absence of the usual evolution of appendicitis, adnexal swelling and tenderness and vaginal discharge point to the diagnosis.

Gonococcal bacteraemia should be suspected in any young patient with a fever and arthritis. Aspiration of the affected joint shows many neutrophils, but demonstration of gonococci is difficult until late in the illness. Blood cultures are the main diagnostic test. Gonococci are present in the skin lesions, and can be recovered from vesicle fluid.

When genital swabs are taken, it is important to take rectal and throat swabs also, as one of these may be the only site yielding positive cultures. Specimens obtained by prostatic massage may also be positive.

Neisseria gonorrhoeae is a delicate organism and does not survive for long outside the body. Specimens from the male urethra may be obtained using a platinum loop as many swab materials are inimical to the survival of this organism. Ideally specimens should be examined in a side room by microscopy and inoculated on to culture medium and incubated locally, or transported with the minimum delay to the microbiology laboratory.

Specimens in which *N. gonorrhoeae* is sought are usually heavily contaminated with other bacteria. Antibiotics must therefore be added to the medium to aid selection. The organism is also delicate and fastidious, so the medium must be very nutritious, containing lysed blood and additional growth factors such as yeast extract. The usual medium inoculated is a modified New York City medium or Thayer–Martin medium in parallel with a non-selective medium such as chocolate agar. The plates should be incubated in 5–10% carbon dioxide and increased humidity, and inspected after 24 and 48 h. Suspect colonies are identified by the oxidase test and sugar oxidation tests. Confirmation of identification can be made by serological agglutination tests. The presence of a beta-lactamase enzyme can be detected rapidly using the commercial kits based on a cephalosporin which changes colour when the beta-lactam bond is broken. Susceptibility to penicillin, tetracycline, spectinomycin, ciprofloxacin and a third-generation cephalosporin should be tested.

Several systems of typing have been developed based on monoclonal antibodies or auxanograms. They are not in routine clinical use.

Management

To ensure compliance, on-the-spot treatment is offered, as far as possible, for simple genital infections. For penicillin-sensitive organisms this consists of amoxycillin orally 3 g as a single dose, or ampicillin 2 g plus probenecid 1 g (a further dose of the latter treatment is given to women, with an interval of 8–12 h). Penicillin-allergic patients can be given cefuroxime 1.5 g intramuscularly (half the dose in each of two sites) or oral ciprofloxacin 250 mg as a single dose.

Penicillin-resistant gonorrhoea is treated with single-dose ciprofloxacin 250–500 mg orally or with spectinomycin 2 g, given by deep intramuscular injection. A further dose of spectinomycin 1 or 2 g can be given at another site in difficult cases. Cefuroxime is often effective against penicillin-resistant organisms. Ceftriaxone 250 mg intramuscularly is effective but expensive.

Salpingitis, perihepatitis and bacteraemia require admission to hospital and treatment with intravenous penicillin (or a cephalosporin if cultures indicate penicillin-resistance). A week's course is usually sufficient. Care must be taken that complications of bacteraemia, such as endocarditis, are not overlooked; the erythrocyte sedimentation rate and C-reactive protein usually remain raised during convalescence if complications exist.

Treatment of gonorrhoea
1 Penicillin-sensitive organisms: ampicillin orally 3 g single dose, or ampicillin 2 g plus probenecid 1 g orally. Single dose for men, repeated after 12 h for women.
Alternative: cefuroxime i.m. 1.5 g single dose (half the dose in each of two sites).
Systemic disease: benzylpenicillin i.v. 1.2–2.4 g 4–6-hourly for 7 days.
2 Penicillin-resistant organisms: ciprofloxacin orally 250–500 mg single dose, or spectinomycin i.m. 2 g single dose, or azithromycin orally 1 g single dose, or ceftriaxone i.m. 250 mg single dose.
Systemic disease: cefuroxime i.m. or i.v. 750 mg 6–8-hourly for 1 week.

Complications

The commonest complication of gonorrhoea is re-infection. This is important because repeated infections, severe infections, or those in which treatment is delayed or complicated by penicillin resistance can all lead to tissue damage. In men urethral strictures may need repeated dilatation or even operative intervention. Prostatic damage and chronic inflammation may also follow. In women tubal damage and obstruction can cause infertility, and predispose to chronic pelvic inflammation.

Syphilis

Introduction and epidemiology

Syphilis, caused by the spirochaete, *Treponema pallidum*, is now relatively uncommon in British genitourinary clinics. It remains important, however, because it is prevalent in some places overseas and in travellers, and remains more common in homosexual men than in other social groups. Early cases must be detected and treated to avoid the problems of congenital infection and of damaging, late manifestations which cause great morbidity and dependence.

Although now uncommon in most developed countries, the incidence has started to rise again in some countries, notably inner cities in the USA. This increase has occurred mainly among intravenous drug abusers and prostitutes.

Clinical features

Primary syphilis

Primary syphilis is a local infection which involves mucocutaneous sites and their draining lymph nodes. The incubation period can vary from about 10 days to 10 weeks or more. Then the typical primary lesion or chancre develops. This is usually a single, painless ulcer with a border and base of induration. The common sites of the chancre are the foreskin, coronal sulcus, vulva, fourchette, uterine cervix or adjacent structures such as the urethra or penile shaft. There is painless enlargement of local lymph nodes. About 5% of chancres are extragenital, affecting the lips, mouth or nipple.

Atypical chancres are common, often taking the form of multiple or painful lesions. They can be mistaken for herpes simplex, chancroid or small malignant lesions.

Secondary syphilis

Secondary syphilis develops 6–8 weeks after the primary manifestations, though a small proportion of patients have no history of chancre, and present with secondary disease. It is a spirochaetaemic disease with fever, rash and generalized lymphadenopathy.

The rash is usually generalized, maculopapular or papular, extending to the palms and soles. It is notorious for variability, however, and serpiginous or discoid lesions can occur, making differential diagnosis difficult. Other cutaneous and mucous membrane lesions are common. There may be superficial erosions in the mouth: when covered with greyish exudate these are called mucous patches. Serpiginous mouth ulcers are called snail-track ulcers. Flat, moist, warty lesions, condylomata lata, may occur on the perineum, especially around the anus. These must be distinguished from the drier, pedunculated simple warts which are common in these sites.

Other systemic manifestations include meningitis, arthritis, arthralgia, mild nephrotic syndrome, patchy alopecia and, in about 5% of cases, iritis or retinitis.

Latent syphilis

Latent syphilis is an asymptomatic state which may persist for years if the early infection is not cured. Slow tissue damage probably occurs throughout this stage, and a few patients have elevated CSF protein levels or mild pleiocytosis, suggesting central nervous system involvement. An unknown proportion of patients maintain this state without further problems, but many will develop late manifestations of the disease.

Late syphilis

Late (tertiary) manifestations of syphilis can affect many systems of the body. The underlying lesion is the gumma, an indolent, granulomatous lesion which may undergo central mucoid degeneration.

In the nervous system, meningovascular syphilis, tabes or syphilitic paresis (general paralysis of the insane) may occur.

Meningovascular syphilis develops sooner than many late manifestations. It causes vasculitis and lepto-meningitis, particularly at the base of the brain and the upper spinal cord. It can present as a frank meningitis, often with papilloedema, or more often with focal neu-rological disorder, such as cranial nerve palsy, weakness and wasting of the hands, transverse myelitis or ataxia. The vascular disease can produce strokes, which must be differentiated from thrombotic or embolic strokes. Epilepsy can also occur. There is a moderate lympho-cytosis and a raised protein level in the CSF.

Tabes is now exceptionally rare. It is caused by selective degeneration and demyelination in the posterior columns of the spinal cord and the dorsal nerve roots. It presents with a triad of dysaesthesia and anaesthesia, pains and ataxia. The pains are typically shooting girdle or limb pain, sometimes accompanied by abdominal pain and vomiting (gastric crisis), which may be prolonged or repetitive. Ophthalmoplegia is common. The pupils may be small and fail to react to light, while retaining the reaction to accommodation (Argyll Robertson pupil). Hypoaesthesia leads to severe trophic changes in the joints of the legs and feet (Charcot joints).

Syphilitic paresis usually presents as slowly pro-gressive dementia, with or without some tabetic features. Some patients are euphoric and grandiose, but this diminishes as memory and judgement decline. The CSF contains many lymphocytes and the protein content is high, helping to differentiate the condition from Alzheimer's disease or psychosis.

In the cardiovascular system the important lesion is aortitis, occurring 20–30 years after the original infection.

There is intimal thickening and loss of elastic tissue from the root and ascending part of the aorta. The aortic valve ring is dilated, the orifices of coronary arteries may be occluded and an aortic aneurysm commonly develops.

In other systems there may be single gummas or gummatous infiltration, causing chronic osteomyelitis or periostitis, nodular liver enlargement or skin lesions which may ulcerate, producing a sticky discharge.

Laboratory diagnosis

The protean manifestations of syphilis mean that it is part of many differential diagnoses, especially of neurological conditions.

In primary syphilis a rapid diagnosis can be made by dark-ground microscopy of exudate from the chancre or of aspirate from enlarged inguinal lymph nodes. The spirochaetes can be identified by their typical, tightly coiled, 'watch-spring' morphology. They also have typical motility, rotating about their long axis, or bending at an angle.

The organism of syphilis, T. pallidum, has not been cultivated in artificial medium and therefore diagnosis is by serological means. Antibodies may be detected by their interaction with cardiolipin-based reagin antigens, treponemal antigens or T. pallidum itself. The cardiolipin-based assays are derived from the original Wassermann reaction, although modern tests are more specific. The test used in most laboratories is the VDRL (Venereal Disease Research Laboratory) test which uses a stand-ardized antigen to perform an agglutination test. Carbon particles can be incorporated to simplify reading of the test — the rapid plasma reagin (RPR) test. These tests are subject to biological false-positive results due to cross-reacting antibodies in patients with connective tissue disease, or malaria. However, their value is that they become positive early in the course of infection and become negative after treatment. They are useful there-fore for establishing the duration of infection and the treatment status.

Specific treponemal tests use a cultivatable treponeme, the Reiter's treponeme, as the antigen and are therefore less subject to false reactions. Positive results appear later in the course of infection but remain positive for life. The commonest test of this type is the T. pallidum haemagglutination assay (TPHA). This test is technically simple to perform and large numbers of specimens can be handled with ease. Positive results can be titrated and confirmed using a T. pallidum-based test.

The most specific test available for routine laboratories is the fluorescent treponemal antibody absorption (FTAABS) test. T. pallidum is bound to a glass slide and patient serum is first absorbed to remove group-reactive antibody, then placed on the slide and incubated. After washing, the binding of specific anti-*T. pallidum* antibody is detected using a fluorescent antihuman immunoglobulin. By changing the isotype specificity, either immunoglobulin G (IgG) or IgM may be detected. The IgM test is especially useful for detecting acute and congenital infection. The other specific *T. pallidum* test is the *T. pallidum* immobilization (TPI) test which uses live treponemes. The difficulty of providing reagents for this test and for controlling it mean that it is a reference technique (Table 11.1)

More recently enzyme immunoassay (EIA) tests have been described and are now reaching routine use. These are capable of detecting specific IgG or IgM and are suitable for all of the uses for which traditional tests have been employed. In addition, because of their format, they are capable of a degree of automation.

Management

Penicillin is the treatment of choice for all forms of syphilis. Primary syphilis should be completely curable, with eradication of spirochaetes from the body. It can be treated with daily or twice-daily intramuscular procaine penicillin injections for 10–14 days. Long-acting penicillins are no longer routinely available in the UK. A suitable alternative may be to give amoxycillin in standard doses with probenecid 500 mg 6-hourly to maintain tissue levels. For penicillin-allergic patients, a variety of alternatives exist, including cephalosporins and tetracyclines, but these and the variety of new antibiotics on the market are not well-tried in treating syphilis.

Secondary syphilis can be treated in the same way as primary. It remains controversial whether every spirochaete is eradicated after a bacteraemic disease, but adequate treatment seems to abolish almost all risk of late manifestations.

Follow-up

Careful follow-up is essential after treatment is completed. Cure is followed by a gradual decline in the VDRL titre, which should show significant decline after 6 months and become undetectable after 18–24 months. A persisting positive test is an indication for retreatment. More specific tests such as the TPHA remain positive indefinitely. After secondary syphilis or neurological involvement it is advisable to perform a lumbar puncture after 6 months. If the CSF has not returned to normal, retreatment is indicated.

Treatment

Treatment of late syphilis may not always reverse established tissue damage, but it can provide dramatic improvement in meningovascular syphilis. Other late manifestations can be prevented from progressing or at least slowed significantly, and in some cases worthwhile improvement is achieved. Prolonged treatment may be required to obtain the best result.

Jarisch–Herxheimer reaction

The Jarisch–Herxheimer reaction is important in treating late syphilis. Within hours of the first antibiotic dose, there is an exacerbation of swelling and inflammation, with significant fever in most cases. This can be a serious problem if, for instance, a coronary ostium is further occluded, or if epilepsy or stroke is precipitated. The reaction can be minimized by starting with low doses of penicillin and/or by adding corticosteroid such as prednisolone 30–40 mg daily during the first few days of treatment.

	VDRL/RPR	TPHA	FTA-abs	IgM (ELISA or FTA)
Congenital infection	+	+	+	+
Primary infection	+	–/+	–/+	+
Untreated secondary	+	+	+	+
Treated or late disease	–	+	+/–	–

VDRL, Venereal Disease Research Laboratory; RPR, rapid plasma reagin; TPHA, *Treponema pallidum* haemagglutination assay; FTA-abs, fluorescent treponemal antibody absorption; IgM, immunoglobulin M; ELISA, enzyme-linked immunosorbent assay.

Table 11.1 Results of serological tests for syphilis at different disease stages

Complications

The most important complications of syphilis are related to infection in pregnancy. Early untreated syphilis often results in abortion, but succeeding pregnancies are increasingly likely to proceed to term. Transplacental infection of the fetus is likely, causing both early and long-term disease (see Chapter 12).

Chancroid

This is a local genital infection caused by *Haemophilus ducreyi*, a Gram-negative rod. It is uncommon in the UK, but widely prevalent in the West Indies, south-east USA, North Africa, the Middle East, China and parts of the Mediterranean. It is therefore often an imported disease.

Its importance is that it is often mistaken for syphilis, which may coexist. It can be transmitted by asymptomatic carriers of the organism. Small abrasions are especially susceptible to infection with chancroid which, in turn, increases the chance of infection with other sexually transmitted pathogens.

After an incubation period of 2–5 days, the typical, soft sore lesion quickly develops. This is a large, irregular, painful ulcer, almost always on the genitalia. The local lymph nodes become enlarged, inflamed and very painful. A suppurating lymph node may discharge via the skin, leaving a large ulcer crater.

The diagnosis can be made by Gram stain and culture of scrapings from lesions or discharge from lymph nodes. A suitable specimen must be taken from the lesion, which should be thoroughly cleansed. A cotton wool swab should be applied vigorously and the swab plated on to isolation medium with the minimum of delay. Mueller-Hinton and enriched gonococcal medium with the addition of charcoal has recently been shown to improve the isolation rate. There is considerable research interest in the rapid diagnosis of chancroid by EIA and other techniques but no method has yet gained acceptance in routine use. The ulcers have a characteristic histological appearance, so biopsy is useful in cases of doubt. Syphilis should always be excluded by dark-ground microscopy and serological testing.

Chancroid responds readily to treatment with sulphonamides, which are ineffective against syphilis. A convenient treatment is a single 2 g dose of sulfametopyrazine (Kelfizine W), which can be repeated after a week if necessary. Side-effects are fewer with 7–10 days' treatment with co-trimoxazole or a short-acting sulphonamide.

Chancroid is sometimes confused with a condition called granuloma inguinale, an indolent, progressive ulcerating condition confined to the genital skin and subcutaneous tissues. It is a *Calymmatobacterium granulomatis* infection usually seen in tropical climates where poor hygienic conditions prevail. While it may spread by sexual contact, it is only slightly infectious, and is possibly mainly an autoinfection of faecal origin. Tetracycline, erythromycin and co-trimoxazole are all effective treatments.

Bacterial vaginosis and *Gardnerella vaginale*

Bacterial vaginosis is an inflammation of the vagina for which no direct cause is apparent. There is variable irritation, soreness and sometimes a slight discharge. Examination of material obtained by swabbing shows the presence of neutrophils and sometimes of clue cells (squamous epithelial cells covered with adherent bacteria).

Gardnerella vaginale can be recovered in culture from 60–80% of cases. Its presence is often predictable because of the offensive odour produced when the vaginal secretions are alkalinized. This occurs naturally when semen is introduced into the vagina, or when the introitus is washed with soap. Many women present with a main complaint of odour.

Cases from which *Gardnerella* is not recovered may be infected by other bacterial pathogens, such as *Mycoplasma hominis* or *Ureaplasma urealyticum*, but the role of these organisms in pathological conditions is uncertain and they are seldom specifically sought. Viruses may also play a part, but no viral species has been recognized as regularly associated with vaginosis and herpes simplex is rarely isolated from such cases.

Although *G. vaginale* is not an anaerobe, the condition usually responds to a 1-week course of metronidazole. On the occasions that the infection recurs, it is worth taking swabs from the coronal sulcus or urethral meatus of the woman's partner, where the organism is occasionally found.

Pelvic inflammatory disease

Introduction

This is an ill-defined condition of women in which there is chronic gynaecological symptomatology, with evidence of inflammation in intrapelvic organs, and often in vaginal and cervical swab specimens. Occasionally there is extensive oedema, fibrosis or abscess formation, with much distortion of pelvic structures.

Although prolonged or recurrent infection with *Neisseria gonorrhoeae* or *Chlamydia trachomatis* may be responsible, a single causative organism is often not identified. *M. hominis* is an uncommon cause of urinary tract infections, and of bacteraemia or sepsis associated with pelvic surgery or malignancy. It probably contributes to a significant proportion of pelvic infections. The condition causes morbidity and infertility throughout the world.

Clinical features

These are pain, malaise and often slight vaginal discharge. The pain may be suprapubic, radiating to the thighs or referred to the lower back. There is often aching discomfort or tenderness on intercourse. Dysmenorrhoea or excessively heavy menstrual periods are common. In severe cases there is chronic fever and/or weight loss.

Pelvic examination shows tenderness and sometimes swelling or induration in the vaginal fornices. Discharge is variable, but is often seen and may be mucoid or mucopurulent. There may be a coexisting condition which makes infection more likely. These include anatomical distortion due to varying degrees of prolapse or previous disease of the cervix or fallopian tubes. Intrauterine contraceptive devices can also predispose to endocervical and ascending infections.

Diagnosis

Material obtained from vaginal and cervical swabs often contains low or moderate numbers of neutrophils. Specific pathogens are rarely recovered, though *Actinomyces* spp. are commonly found when infection is associated with intrauterine devices. Tuberculosis should be borne in mind as a differential diagnosis, and appropriate samples should be examined for mycobacteria (see Chapter 18). Endometriosis and malignancy should be excluded. Urinary tract infection should also be sought.

Pelvic ultrasound scan may show fluid in the pouch of Douglas, distortion of the fallopian tubes or inflammatory masses in the pelvis. Cervical cytology and uterine curettage are useful tests, with histological examination, and microbiological tests for bacteria, including mycobacteria. Laparoscopy permits direct examination of the pelvic organs, and small biopsies or other sampling may be possible. Actinomycosis can produce granulomatous infiltration of the pelvis, with loss of tissue planes.

Management

This is usually empirical, based on the assumption that this secondary type of infection is likely to be polymicrobial. The organisms involved may be coliforms, anaerobes and/or a variety of flora from the genital tract. The patient is offered a broad-spectrum treatment, often consisting of metronidazole plus ampicillin, erythromycin, azithromycin or tetracycline. Courses as short as 2 weeks may be successful, but more prolonged treatment may be needed if infection is loculated or surrounded by chronic oedema.

Removal of any intrauterine device is essential, at least until the inflammation has recovered. Surgical correction of anatomical problems may help to avoid recurrence. In severe cases, removal of an affected tube or ovary or even hysterectomy may offer the best chance of long-term cure. In severe actinomycosis antimicrobial chemotherapy will often reduce the bulk of the infection and restore tissue planes. Prolonged treatment may be needed before surgery can safely be undertaken.

Candida albicans genital infections

Candida albicans is a resident of moist skin and mucosae in many parts of the body. The squamous epithelium of the vagina and vulva or the glans of the penis are susceptible to candidal infection. Inflammation and maceration of the affected surface are often accompanied by a soft, white exudate which tends to form plaques or spots. Itching and marked oedema are common. Predispositions include diabetes, antibiotic treatment, hypercalcaemia and disorders of cell-medicated immunity.

The genitalia of adult women are protected from candidal infection by lactic acid (and probably by peroxides) produced by most strains of *Lactobacillus acidophilus*, with which the vagina is heavily colonized. This protective colonization is lost in pregnancy and after antimicrobial chemotherapy. The inflammatory symptoms of vulvovaginal candidiasis are often accompanied by a voluminous, cheesy vaginal discharge with little odour. Itching and oedema of the mucosa are common.

The diagnosis is often clinically apparent. Microscopy of the exudate shows many budding yeasts, and extensive formation of pseudohyphae, a mark of aggressive candidal growth. Positive cultures are readily obtained.

Superficial infections respond to topical treatment with nystatin cream or with nitroimidazoles such as clotrimazole or econazole creams. Vaginal candidosis is better treated with pessaries or vaginal cream. Clotrimazole or econazole pessaries are well-tolerated in courses of

1–5 days, depending on the preparation used. Single-dose clotrimazole vaginal cream is also effective. Nystatin pessaries must be given for up to 2 weeks, and tend to soil the underwear more than the other preparations.

Persistent or recurrent infections can be treated with oral triazole drugs. Itraconazole can be given as a 1-day course. Fluconazole is more often used as a 1- or 2-week course in extensive disease or in the immunosuppressed.

Treatment of vaginal candidiasis

1 Clotrimazole vaginal tablets 500 mg one at night as a single dose, or econazole pessaries 150 mg one at night as a single dose, or clotrimazole 10% vaginal cream 5 g at night as a single dose.

2 Alternative: nystatin pessaries one or two at night for 14–28 days.

3 Systemic treatment: itraconazole orally 200 mg twice daily for 1 day.

4 Additional treatment for vulval involvement: clotrimazole 1% cream or econazole 1% cream twice daily, or nystatin cream to anogenital area three or four times daily.

Trichomonas vaginalis

Trichomonas vaginalis is a flagellate protozoan that thrives in the low oxygen tension of the female lower genital tract. It produces symptoms of soreness and irritating serous or mucoid discharge. It can also colonize the male urethra where it may cause mild symptoms, but is rarely clinically evident.

Smears of vaginal discharge will often contain motile or dying protozoa, readily demonstrable by light microscopy of wet preparations. The organisms can also be transported and cultured in *Trichomonas* medium. Smears can be made from the incubated medium to demonstrate the organisms. This is useful in mild infections when examination of direct vaginal smears may be negative.

It is quite common for cytologists to see *Trichomonas* on Papanicolaou-stained cervical smear preparations. This suggests that even in women, infection may be trivial or inapparent.

Treatment with oral metronidazole 400 mg 8-hourly for 1 week is usually successful. Rare cases of metronidazole resistance have been described.

Other infections transmissible during sexual contact

Introduction

Sexual contact usually includes prolonged skin-to-skin contact, as well as significant exchange of body fluids,
particularly saliva and genital secretions. Minor trauma or small skin lesions can permit exchange of blood, or inoculation of blood on to a partner's mucosae. Some less common practices, often among homosexual men, involve anal and rectal contact, or contact with urine droplets. These contacts increase the likelihood of transmission of several infections whose main means of spread are not by sexual contact.

- Infections spread by skin contact:
  Scabies
  Pubic lice
  Impetigo
- Infections spread by body fluids:
  Hepatitis B
  Cytomegalovirus
  Epstein–Barr virus
- Infections spread by blood:
  Hepatitis B
  HIV (see below)
  Human T-lymphotropic virus I (HTLV I, see below)
- Infections spread by faeces:
  Shigellosis
  Giardiasis
  Amoebiasis.

HIV infection and AIDS

Introduction and epidemiology

AIDS was first recognized as a clinical entity in the early 1980s among homosexual men in USA, although the causal agent and routes of transmission were not identified for some years. The number of cases has risen exponentially, and it is now estimated that over 3 million cases have occurred worldwide (although less than a million have been officially reported). Two-thirds of AIDS cases have occurred in Africa. It is also estimated that there are 11–12 million adults infected with HIV. The World Health Organization has projected that there will be 30–40 million cases of HIV infection in the world by the year 2000.

Two major patterns of disease transmission have emerged during the course of the AIDS pandemic. In Africa and some other developing nations, the predominant modes of spread are through heterosexual intercourse and by vertical transmission to infants from infected mothers. In developed countries, the major routes are through sexual intercourse between men and sharing of contaminated drug-injecting equipment. Receipt of contaminated blood and blood products was an important route of spread in the early stages of the epidemic, although this has largely stopped since most countries now screen blood donations.

All countries of the world are affected, although the greatest impact of the disease is in Africa (Fig. 11.5). Only 5% of cases reported have occurred in Europe. In some European countries, for example Switzerland, the incidence of AIDS may have reached a plateau.

Virology

HIV is an enveloped RNA virus belonging to the lentivirus subfamily of Retroviridae. It was originally designated HTLV III as it was thought to be related to the viruses responsible for tropical spastic paraparesis and adult T-cell leukaemia. Alternative early names were LAV (lymphadenopathy-associated virus) or ARV (AIDS-related virus). HIV 2 is a closely related strain which has been identified from patients in West Africa. There is considerable homology between HIV 2 and simian immunodeficiency virus (SIV). Recently HIV 1° has been described. This is a rare variant of HIV 1 which does not exhibit sufficient antigen to produce a positive anti-HIV 1 antibody test in infected individuals.

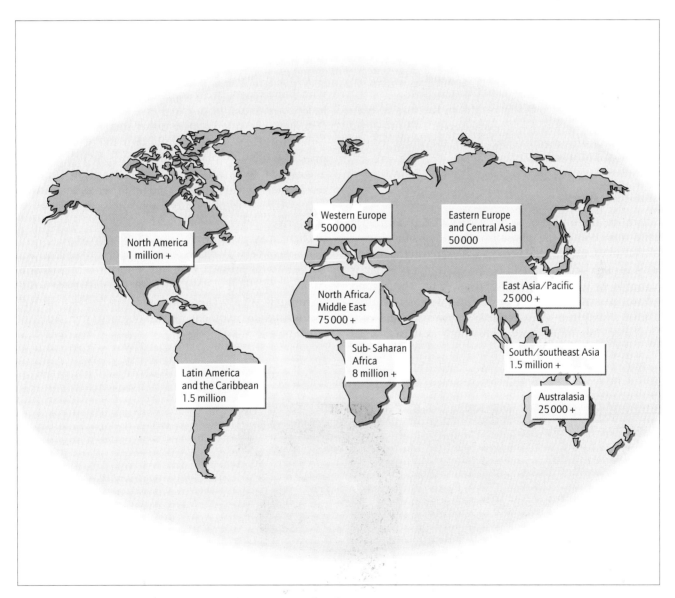

Fig. 11.5 Global distribution of acquired immunodeficiency syndrome (AIDS) cases.

The genetic information of HIV 1 and HIV 2 is found on a single strand of RNA. The genome encodes for a number of proteins essential for viral replication. These include *pol* which encodes reverse transcriptase. This is responsible for generating complementary DNA which is incorporated into the host genome. The *gag* gene encodes a precursor protein which is cleaved to form the core protein p24 which is detectable in early infection. The *env* gene codes for a 160 kDa glycoprotein which is cleaved to form the envelope glycoprotein responsible for the attachment of HIV to the target cells.

Once the virus has entered a target cell its complementary DNA enters the host genome and leads to constant production of viruses. It is thought that the immune system maintains a vigorous antiviral response until it is eventually exhausted and depleted. Coinfection with herpesviruses such as cytomegalovirus or human herpesvirus 6 and 7 may hasten the onset of immunodeficiency. HIV is capable of causing the formation of multinucleate cells.

HIV infection eventually results in the loss of both the total numbers of CD4 lymphocytes and impaired function of those remaining, with inevitable consequences for host immunity.

Clinical features

There are three phases to the course of infection with HIV. The first is the phase of seroconversion during which antibodies to HIV become detectable in the serum. This is often accompanied by a feverish illness which is variable in its presentation and severity. The second phase is a period of asymptomatic, latent infection. During this phase virus replication proceeds and cell-mediated immunity deteriorates until the last, symptomatic phase of the infection is reached. During the symptomatic phase the patient eventually develops serious opportunistic diseases, and is then said to fulfil the definition of AIDS.

Seroconversion illness

Seroconversion usually occurs 6–8 weeks after infection, but incubation can range from 4 to 12 weeks. Individuals exposed to HIV infection may recognize a feverish illness, which can persist for 2–8 weeks. Not all of those affected need to stop working. Those who seek medical advice may have a mild generalized lymphadenopathy and many have a few atypical mononuclear cells in the blood, suggestive of acute viral infection. This is called the glandular fever-like presentation.

A minority of those infected have a more specific seroconversion illness. Some of these have 2–4 weeks' fever with lymphadenopathy and an unusual rash. The skin lesions are ovoid, from 1 to 3 or 4 cm in their long axis (Fig. 11.6) and often appear rather scuffed, a little like a rope burn. They are not painful or itchy. A few patients present with a lymphocytic meningitis, which may last a week or two. All of the seroconversion illnesses resolve without specific treatment. Progression to AIDS occurs sooner in individuals who have illness during seroconversion.

There may be transient immunosuppression during the seroconversion phase. This is apparent in occasional patients who present with an opportunistic infection, such as candidal oesophagitis or *Pneumocystis carinii* pneumonia (PCP). These illnesses usually respond well to appropriate treatment, and do not recur until after the latent phase.

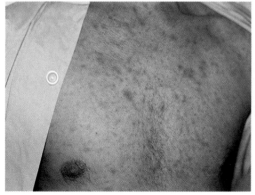
(a)

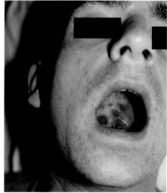
(b)

Fig. 11.6 (a) Rash of large, erythematous lesions and (b) oral lesions in human immunodeficiency virus (HIV) seroconversion illness.

Latent phase

The latent phase of HIV infection may last from 18 months to 15 years or more, with an average of about 8 years. For much of this time the individual is well, not unduly susceptible to infections and recovers apparently normally from common and seasonal infections. The total CD4 (T4) helper-cell population slowly declines, and CD4 helper function is increasingly impaired. This decline is probably exacerbated by each intercurrent infection.

Before they become truly symptomatic many patients develop generalized lymphadenopathy. Rubbery, mobile nodes from 1 cm upwards in diameter are easily palpable. Occasionally these are biopsied, and they have a characteristic histological appearance of reactive histiocytosis. The lymphadenopathy persists through the symptomatic stages.

Symptomatic HIV infection

A sudden increase in the loss of CD4 cells heralds the end of the latent phase. Certain infections may occur at about this time. Herpes zoster is common; it often recovers spontaneously, but can be severe, sometimes even leading to scarring of the skin or eye. It therefore deserves treatment with aciclovir unless it is trivial.

Some bacterial infections are troublesome, most importantly pneumococcal and *Salmonella* infections. Pneumococcal pneumonia is often bacteraemic, but with a misleadingly low white cell count, as neutrophilia is mild or absent. The infection responds to vigorous treatment with penicillin or an appropriate alternative (see Chapter 7). *Salmonella* infections may also be bacteraemic, requiring treatment with ciprofloxacin or a similar drug. In spite of this there may be repeated recurrences of both diarrhoea and of bacteraemia.

Skin and mucosal infections become increasingly common; these include seborrhoeic dermatitis, molluscum contagiosum, relapsing herpes simplex infections, and oral and genital candidiasis. Proliferative disorders, such as oral hairy leukoplakia, also occur. These conditions, which also occur in immunocompetent patients, are not themselves diagnostic of immunodeficiency so they do not fulfil the diagnosis of full-blown AIDS.

Full-blown AIDS

Full-blown AIDS does not coincide exactly with any absolute level of CD4 cell count, but is likely to develop when the count falls to 0.4–$0.2 \times 10^9/l$. Many AIDS patients have counts far below this, and may have undetectable counts for months before their death.

Many cases present with conditions which are so characteristic of cell-mediated immunodeficiency that AIDS can be definitively diagnosed, even without obtaining serological confirmation of HIV infection. Others require the additional confirmation of HIV antibody and/or antigen testing. Clinically evident opportunistic diseases may not require laboratory confirmation; a clinical diagnosis alone fulfils the diagnostic criteria for a presumptive diagnosis of AIDS (Table 11.2).

Some presenting conditions are malignancies, such as Kaposi's sarcoma, lymphomata or invasive carcinoma of the cervix. These may have an infectious aetiology, and represent a defect of immune surveillance of potentially oncogenic infections. A herpesvirus, provisionally called Kaposi's sarcoma herpes virus (KSHV), has been detected in lesions of Kaposi's sarcoma.

Staging of HIV infection

Staging schemes have been described which allow comparison of the severity or progress of the disease in different patients. The most widely used is the Centers for Disease Control (CDC) classification. The main use is to classify patients in research projects. As HIV infection progresses a patient may accumulate many opportunistic conditions of different types, a situation modified by anti-HIV drugs and chemoprophylaxis regimens. Staging is not often used, therefore, in managing individual cases. Research is nowadays more often related to the CD4 count and the presence or occurrence of any HIV-related conditions than to a particular stage.

Centers for Disease Control staging of human immunodeficiency virus (HIV) disease	
Group I	Acute infection, including seroconversion illnesses.
Group II	Asymptomatic infection with or without abnormal laboratory findings.
Group III	Persistent generalized lymphadenopathy.
Group IVA	Constitutional symptoms, including fever or diarrhoea lasting >1 month; weight loss of >10%.
Group IVB	Neurological conditions including encephalopathy, myelopathy or neuropathy.
Group IVC1	Symptomatic infection diagnostic of acquired immunodeficiency syndrome (AIDS).
Group IVC2	Symptomatic infection not diagnostic of AIDS, but related to impaired immunity (e.g. herpes zoster, oral candidiasis).

| Group IVD | HIV-related neoplasia including Kaposi's sarcoma, intracranial primary lymphoma, non-Hodgkin's lymphoma. |
| Group IVE | Other HIV-related disease not classified elsewhere. |

AIDS in infants and children

There are several differences between adults and children in both the presentation of AIDS and the apparent degree of CD4 cell depletion. The CD4 cell count is much higher in infants and young children than in adults.

Disease	Diagnostic criteria
Bacterial infections; multiple or recurrent (child <13 years)	D: culture, antigen detection, CSF microscopy
Candidiasis (trachea bronchi or lungs)	D: endoscopic or post-mortem inspection, cytology, histology
Candidiasis (oesophagus)	D: as above P: oesophageal pain or radiological appearance plus confirmed oral *Candida*
Cervical carcinoma (invasive)	D: histology
Coccidioidomycosis (disseminated or extrapulmonary)	D: microscopy, culture, antigen detection
Cryptococcosis (extrapulmonary)	D: as above
Cytomegalovirus retinitis	P: loss of vision, characteristic ophthalmoscopical appearance
Encephalopathy	D: cognitive and/or motor dysfunction or milestone loss in HIV-infected person (no other identified cause)
Herpes simplex; ulcers for > 1 month, or bronchial lung, oesophageal lesions	D: culture, microscopy, antigen detection
Histoplasmosis (disseminated or extrapulmonary)	D: microscopy, culture, antigen detection
Isosporiasis (diarrhoea > 1 month)	D: cytology, histology
Kaposi's sarcoma	D: cytology, histology P: characteristic skin or mucosal lesions
Lymphoid interstitial pnemonia (child < 13 years)	D: cytology, histology P: typical pulmonary infiltrates for > 2 months (no pathogen found, no antibiotic response)
Lymphoma (Burkitt's, immunoblastic, cerebral)	D: histology, cytology
Mycobacteriosis (disseminated, including extrapulmonary TB)	D: culture P: AFB seen in stool, CSF, urine, blood
Mycobacteriosis: (pulmonary TB)	D: culture or other definitive method P: clinical diagnosis leading to anti-TB treatment
Pneumocystis carinii pneumonia	D: cytology, histology P: hypoxia, symptoms and typical X-ray changes (no other cause)
Pneumonia (recurrent within 1 year)	D: two proven episodes P: two episodes with X-ray or clinical diagnosis
Progressive multifocal encephalopathy	D: EM findings, antigen detection (brain or urine), antibody in CSF or serum
Salmonella (non-typhoid) septicaemia, or recurrent	D: culture
Toxoplasmosis (cerebral: onset > 1 month old)	D: histology, cytology, culture P: neurological abnormality, lesion on scan; serological evidence or treatment response
Wasting syndrome	D: weight loss (> 10% of baseline with > 30 days' fever or diarrhoea; no other cause)

AFB, Acid-fast bacilli; CSF, cerebrospinal fluid; D, definitive diagnosis; EM, electron microscopy; P, presumptive diagnosis; TB, tuberculosis

Table 11.2 Conditions defining a clinical diagnosis of acquired immunodeficiency syndrome (AIDS). In the USA a total CD4 lymphocyte count below 0.2 × 10^9/l is also considered diagnostic

Adult reference values are not reliable indicators, either of CD4 cell loss or of immunosuppression in children.

Adults have usually been exposed to many common infections before acquiring HIV infection, and therefore possess humoral immunity to a wide range of pathogens. Young children do not have this advantage. Furthermore, in those under 2 years old, T-cell-independent antigens are ineffective immunogens. Children are therefore at risk from bacterial infections to which they cannot mount an effective immune response without CD4 helper cells. They are also harmed by viral infections which, instead of being terminated or maintained in a latent state, become persistent, relapsing or progressive.

The occurrence of repeated bacterial infections, including pneumonias, gastroenteritis, skin and upper respiratory infections, is a common presentation of childhood AIDS.

Common viral infections such as measles, chickenpox and especially Epstein–Barr virus infection can cause severe disease and persisting fever. Epstein–Barr virus cannot be terminated and results in lymphocytic infiltrative disease, particularly lymphocytic interstitial pneumonitis (LIP), which is progressive and fatal.

Staging for paediatric human immunodeficiency virus (HIV) infections

P0 Antibody-positive (may be transplacental antibody); unconfirmed infection.
P1 Asymptomatic infection.
   A Normal immune function tests.
   B Abnormal immune function tests.
   C Not tested.
P2 A Constitutional features including delayed growth, delayed milestones, weight loss.
   B Encephalopathy, myelopathy or neuropathy.
   C Lymphoid interstitial pneumonitis.
   D HIV-related infections.
      1 Infections diagnostic of acquired immuno-deficiency syndrome (AIDS).
      2 Recurrent bacterial infections.
      3 Infections suggestive of immunological deficit, including herpes zoster and candidiasis.
   E HIV-related malignancies, including Kaposi's sarcoma, intracranial primary lymphoma and non-Hodgkin's lymphoma.
   F Other diseases not classified elsewhere.

Attempts are made to protect children from these problems by immunization, prophylaxis and early treatment of feverish illnesses. Even measles vaccine should be given to HIV-infected children, whether they have HIV-related symptoms or not, because the risk from measles is much greater than that from the live attenuated vaccine.

Diagnosis

The diagnosis of HIV infection is made by finding HIV antigen or anti-HIV antibody in the blood. The combination of antibody, antigen, clinical condition and serial measurements of the CD4 count can indicate the stage of progression at which the patient has presented (Fig. 11.7).

The diagnosis of HIV infection causes a number of problems for the diagnostic laboratory. There is a need to examine a large number of specimens and the poor prognosis associated with a positive diagnosis means that diagnostic tests must be not only sensitive but also highly specific. All positive results must be subject to strict verification procedures.

The main tests employed in the diagnosis of HIV are antibody tests. A wide range of different formats have been used, including antibody capture EIA, competitive EIA and rapid agglutination tests. These may incorporate HIV 1 and HIV 2 peptides or recombinant antigens. Indeterminate and positive results must be checked by alternative methods, usually by performing two other screening tests which utilize different virus antigens, in parallel with the original test. If all the tests are positive it indicates a positive result which should then be confirmed with a single test taken from a second serum. One positive result associated with two negative results is indicative of a false-positive, and a negative report should usually be issued unless the patient falls into a high-risk group, in which case a second serum should be obtained in 14 days to rule out recent sero-conversion. If one of the three positive results is a weak competitive EIA, HIV 2 infection may be suspected. Discrepant results and suspected HIV 2 infections should be confirmed by a reference laboratory. In the USA, laboratories make more use of a Western blot for confirmation of positive results. HIV antigens are run on a sodium dodecyl sulphate-polyacrylamide gel electrophoresis (SDS-PAGE) and blotted on to nitro-cellulose. The patient's antibody binds to the different antigens, which are clearly separated. A positive result is indicated if two or more of the bands p24, gp41 and gp120/160 are positive.

For a short period immediately after infection, patients may test HIV antibody-negative — the window period. This may prove a problem for patients seeking to check their serological status after an individual exposure. A test may be performed on presentation but a negative result cannot be confirmed until a further negative result

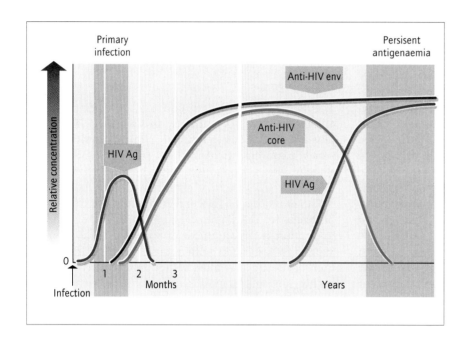

Fig. 11.7 The progression of antigen (Ag) and antibody appearance in the blood of a person infected with human immunodeficiency virus (HIV).

is obtained 3 months after the last exposure to the virus. Other diagnostic tests are available, including HIV culture, polymerase chain reaction (PCR) and p24 antigen testing. Each of these has been in vogue at different times. Some of these tests, notably PCR, p24 antigen EIA and anti-HIV IgA, may be of value in detecting maternofetal transmission, but otherwise have only a limited contribution to routine diagnosis.

Management

Zidovudine and other nucleotide analogues active against HIV can delay the progression of HIV infection, reduce the occurrence of opportunistic infections in AIDS and improve the patient's clinical condition by abolishing malaise and weight loss. They are not sufficiently effective to eradicate HIV infection. With prophylactic therapy against severe opportunistic infections, they have contributed to a prolongation of survival from between 8 and 10 months to 20–30 months from the onset of AIDS-defining conditions. Unfortunately, the effect does not seem to be greatly enhanced by giving antivirals at early stages in HIV disease. This may be partly caused by the gradual emergence of resistance in the patient's HIV virus population during antiviral therapy. The main side-effect of zidovudine is anaemia, and sometimes other cytopenias. These are less likely at dosages of 1.0 g daily or below, and in less severely ill patients.

Zidovudine has recently proved effective in reducing the likelihood of vertical transmission of HIV in pregnancy (see Chapter 12).

Strategies for delaying the development of resistance or increasing the effectiveness of zidovudine with other antiviral drugs are currently under investigation. Newer dideoxynucleotide analogues are now used, either together with zidovudine or after zidovudine has lost its effectiveness in an individual patient. Didanosine (ddI) alone, or combined with zidovudine is as effective, or more so, than zidovudine alone. Zalcitabine (ddC) is a similar drug. ddI can cause peripheral neuropathy, severe pancreatitis, and raised uric acid levels, while ddC causes peripheral neuropathy in over 40% of recipients. As with zidovudine, side-effects are less severe at lower dosage and in less severe ill patients. Lamivudine is a new drug with activity against HIV.

Lymphokines, such as interleukins, have not proved beneficial as additives to antiviral treatment.

A major part of management is prophylaxis and treatment of opportunistic conditions. Prophylaxis is usually given after a first episode of the condition (secondary prophylaxis). Primary prophylaxis is rarely offered as it might encourage infection with resistant organisms, for instance when dealing with mycobacterial infections. However, PCP is so common and serious that patients are offered primary prophylaxis when their CD4 count is consistently below $200 \times 10^9/l$.

Common regimens of prophylaxis include co-trimoxazole or nebulized pentamidine for PCP, aciclovir for herpes simplex, fluconazole for oesophageal candidiasis (which may also prevent cryptococcal meningitis) and ganciclovir to suppress cytomegalovirus retinitis (Table 11.3). Children often receive regular intravenous immunoglobulin to prevent recurrent pyogenic infections. Rare infections have occurred with aciclovir-resistant herpes simplex and fluconazole-resistant fungi.

Prevention and control

The most effective control measure is the use of condoms. Despite extensive health education campaigns, this has failed to control the spread of HIV infection, particularly among heterosexuals who tend not to perceive themselves at risk. Other preventive measures include screening of blood donations, needle exchange schemes for intravenous drug abusers and antenatal screening. Individuals in high-risk categories should be encouraged to be tested for HIV, so that they know their diagnosis,

and can participate in prevention and control measures. No postexposure prophylaxis is effective and even large doses of zidovudine have failed to prevent transmission. No vaccine is currently available.

> **Strategies for the prevention of human immunodeficiency virus (HIV) infection**
> 1 Safe sex: condom use.
> 2 Screening of blood products.
> 3 Needle exchange schemes.
> 4 Antenatal screening.
> 5 Voluntary testing of those in high-risk categories.
> 6 Vigorous control and treatment of genital ulcer diseases.

Human T-lymphotropic virus I

HTLV I is a retrovirus which infects T lymphocytes. Infection spreads by the sexual route, and also vertically

Opportunistic infection	Prophylaxis	Treatment
Pneumocystis carinii pneumonia	Co-trimoxazole orally 960 mg 12-hourly (rash may compel use of alternative) Pentamidine isethionate by nebulizer 150 mg every 2 weeks or 300 mg every 4 weeks	Co-trimoxazole 120 mg/kg daily in divided doses for 14 days (may be given i.v. 1.44 g 12-hourly) Pentamidine isethionate i.v. 4 mg/kg daily for 14 days: by nebulized inhaler 600 mg daily for 21 days
Cytomegalovirus retinitis (suppression)	Ganciclovir by i.v. infusion 5 mg/kg daily or 6 mg/kg on 5 days per week (check blood count frequently) Oral ganciclovir 1 g 8-hourly (2 g 8-hourly after a recrudescence)	Ganciclovir by i.v. infusion (over 1 h) 5 mg/kg 12-hourly for 14–21 days Foscarnet by i.v. infusion 20 mg/kg over 30 min, then 20–200 mg/kg daily (according to renal function) for 14–21 days (check blood count, liver and renal function)
Cryptococcal meningitis	Fluconazole orally 100–200 mg daily	Amphotericin up to 1 mg/kg daily by i.v. infusion (depending on renal function, plasma potassium, blood count, febrile reaction) for 8–12 weeks Liposomal amphotericin up to 6 mg/kg daily if amphotericin fails, or is intolerable Fluconazole i.v. or orally 400 mg, then 200–400 mg daily for 8–12 weeks
Mucocutaneous *Candida*	Fluconazole 50 mg/day orally	Amphotericin orally (suspension) 200 mg 6-hourly Fluconazole 50 mg daily orally for 7–30 days Itraconazole 200 mg daily orally for 15 days
Mycobacterium avium-intracellulare	Rifabutin 300 mg/day orally	See Chapters 18 and 21
Herpes simplex (mucocutaneous)	Aciclovir 200 mg 6-hourly orally	Aciclovir orally 200–400 mg five times daily; i.v. 5 mg/kg 8-hourly (reduced in renal impairment: check blood urea)

Table 11.3 Prophylaxis and treatment of opportunistic conditions in acquired immunodeficiency syndrome

during breast-feeding, and to a lesser extent during parturition.

HTLV I is most common in southern Japan, where the seroprevalence is up to 16%, and in the Caribbean, where it ranges from about 2.5 to 6%. The seroprevalence in native Europeans is probably below 0.5%.

Seroconversion is probably symptomless, but two serious diseases can follow infection: (i) tropical spastic paraparesis, after an average interval of about 4 years (lifetime risk approximately 0.25%); and (ii) acute T-lymphoblastic leukaemia, after an average interval of about 30 years (lifetime risk 2–5%).

Prevention depends on safe sex, and on avoidance of breast-feeding by infected mothers. No satisfactory screening test is yet available for transfused blood, but family screening of affected individuals permits effective identification and counselling of cases.

Other retroviruses

Human T-lymphotropic virus II

This is a retrovirus which has been identified in T lymphocytes less commonly than HTLV I. It has been recovered from the lymphocytes in a case of hairy-cell leukaemia, but an aetiological association has not been established.

Animal retroviruses

A number of retroviruses have been identified in animals. Some, such as SIV and feline immunodeficiency virus, can cause immunological disorders. Others, such as the bovine immunodeficiency virus, have not so far been associated with disease. More distantly related viruses infect other animals. There is no evidence that these viruses infect humans, with the possible exception of rare causes of SIV infection (not shown to be symptomatic) in monkey handlers.

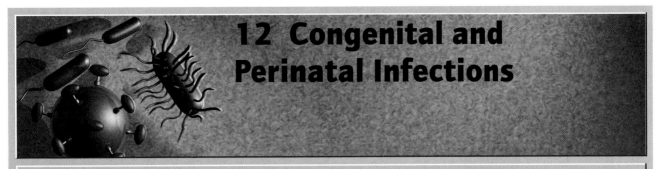

12 Congenital and Perinatal Infections

Introduction

The fetus and neonate can be exposed to infection in a variety of ways (Fig. 12.1). Some maternal infections cause viraemia or bacteraemia during pregnancy; there is then a chance that organisms will cross from the maternal to the fetal circulation, causing transplacental infection. The fetus may die of the infection, may recover *in utero* and be born with or without long-term sequelae, or may be born with continuing infection (so-called congenital infection).

A pregnant woman may be infected with organisms transmissible via blood or body fluids, or her genital tract may be colonized by potential pathogens. In such cases the neonate may be infected during birth, because of contact with infectious maternal blood or genital secretions. The signs of such intrapartum infections usually appear in the first 2–6 weeks of life. If the membranes rupture prematurely, organisms can ascend from the maternal genital tract, colonizing the amniotic sac and sometimes causing amnionitis. The infant is then exposed to a kind of intrapartum infection a few days before delivery.

Once delivered, the neonate enjoys very close contact with its mother, ingesting her breast milk and having intimate face-to-face contact. Older children may eat food from their mother's spoon or have food chewed for them by their mother; the mother may clean a dropped comforter or dummy by licking it. Infants may occasionally ingest maternal blood if breast-feeding from cracked nipples. The duration and extent of such contacts vary in different cultures. Some infections, particularly those spread by saliva, breast milk or other body fluids, can be transmitted from mother to child by these contacts in early infancy. Occasionally infections are transmitted via intimate contact with other family members.

General effects of transplacental and intrapartum infection

These are comparable in most of the infections mentioned.

Transplacental infection

Transplacental infection may put the fetus at risk during the acute stage, but does not necessarily cause any long-term effect. After intrauterine infection with varicella or parvovirus, most fetuses have recovered completely by the time of delivery, and few either die *in utero* or have permanent sequelae.

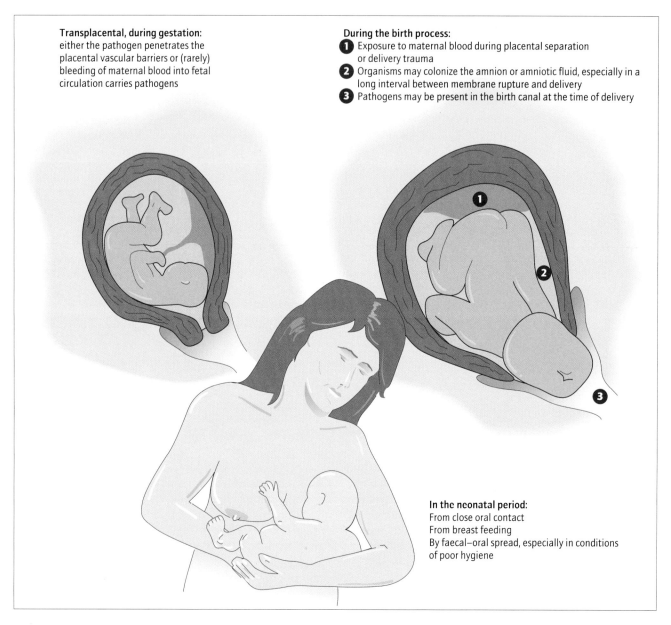

Transplacental, during gestation:
either the pathogen penetrates the
placental vascular barriers or (rarely)
bleeding of maternal blood into fetal
circulation carries pathogens

During the birth process:
1 Exposure to maternal blood during placental separation
  or delivery trauma
2 Organisms may colonize the amnion or amniotic fluid, especially in a
  long interval between membrane rupture and delivery
3 Pathogens may be present in the birth canal at the time of delivery

In the neonatal period:
From close oral contact
From breast feeding
By faecal–oral spread, especially in conditions
of poor hygiene

Fig. 12.1 The three common routes of mother-to-child transmission of infections.

Congenital infections

Children born with congenital infections often have a multisystem disease. Hepatitis, pneumonitis, meningoencephalitis and blood disorders are common, thrombocytopenic purpura is often seen, and the infant often excretes large amounts of the causative pathogen. Many of these acute problems will resolve if the infant survives, but permanent tissue damage may also be present.

The brain, the heart and the inner ear are the tissues most often permanently affected, causing microcephaly, epilepsy, heart murmurs and deafness which can be progressive. Retinopathy is also common, but may not affect sight severely. Isolated nerve deafness is probably the commonest result of intrauterine infection.

Intrapartum and perinatal infections

Intrapartum and perinatal infections rarely cause severe or multisystem disease; indeed with a few exceptions they are often inapparent. Because they take time to develop there is an opportunity for prophylaxis or early treatment, which is particularly important in those few infections which can cause delayed effects or complications.

Outcomes of intrauterine and intrapartum infection
1 Intrauterine infection and recovery.
2 Intrauterine infection and fetal death or stillbirth.
3 Born infected but no disease develops.
4 Born infected, disease develops later.
5 Born infected with active disease.
6 Born with permanent or progressive tissue damage.

Transplacental, intrapartum and postnatal infections

ORGANISM LIST

Transplacental
  Rubella virus
  Cytomegalovirus
  Human parvovirus B19
  Herpes simplex virus
  Human immunodeficiency
    virus
  Varicella-zoster virus
  Vaccinia virus
  Listeria monocytogenes
  Treponema pallidum
  Toxoplasma gondii.

Intrapartum
  Cytomegalovirus
  Herpes simplex virus
  Hepatitis B virus
  Escherichia coli
  Group B *Streptococcus*
  Chlamydia trachomatis
  Neisseria gonorrhoeae
  Listeria monocytogenes.

Postpartum
  Cytomegalovirus
  Hepatitis B virus
  Varicella-zoster virus
  Human T-lymphotropic virus I
  Human immunodeficiency virus
  Herpes simplex virus
  Enteroviruses (e.g. echovirus type 11).

It will be seen that many of these pathogens can infect the fetus and infant by more than one route. The organisms will therefore be discussed, mentioning for each their routes of transmission and the different clinical disorders produced.

Congenital rubella

Introduction and epidemiology

The risk of congenital rubella depends on the stage of pregnancy at which maternal infection occurs. If it occurs during the first trimester, between 80 and 90% of pregnancies carried to term will result in congenital rubella. The risk approaches 100% for infections in the first month. It declines to around 50% during the second trimester and approaches zero after 30 weeks' gestation.

Before the introduction of rubella vaccine, outbreaks of congenital rubella occurred every 5–7 years, following the natural epidemic cycle of rubella (Fig. 12.2; see also Chapter 13). In a typical epidemic year over 1000 infections in pregnant women were reported in the UK. Approximately 90% of these pregnancies were terminated; however, in countries where termination of pregnancy is not readily available, the impact of these epidemics was much greater.

Following the introduction of rubella vaccination, congenital rubella is now rare, and has almost been eliminated in many developed countries, including the UK. There is a residual risk among immigrant women, mainly of Asian origin, who come to the UK from countries that have not yet implemented rubella vaccination programmes.

Clinical features

Rubella in pregnancy approximately doubles the risk of fetal death. Among survivors the effect varies from severe infection and multiple permanent defects to an apparently normal, but infected, neonate. The severity and nature of the clinical problems depend critically on the stage of pregnancy when infection occurred.

Reversible effects

Reversible effects of active infection are often present at birth. These tend to involve several systems, particularly the liver, the blood and the nervous system. The baby often has hepatitis and jaundice. Haemolysis and thrombocytopenic purpura are common, and there is often a low-grade meningoencephalitis. Some have metaphyseal dysplasia with patchy mineralization of the ends of the long bones. Most affected infants are of low birth weight and fail to attain their expected developmental milestones. There is a high mortality in severely affected infants, but these reversible effects resolve in the first 2–6 months of life in those who survive.

Permanent effects

Permanent tissue damage is most severe after infections in the first month of pregnancy, when over half of those born will have multiple defects. Patent ductus arteriosus is the commonest defect, and occurs both with and with-

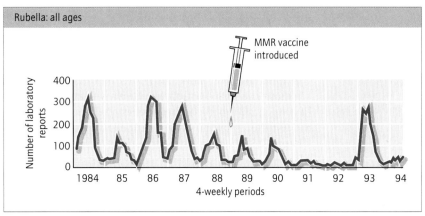

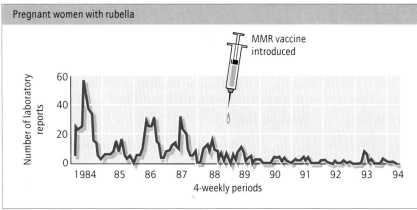

Fig. 12.2 Epidemics of rubella, and their relation to rubella infections in pregnancy; the numbers decline after the introduction of mass immunization.

out pulmonary stenosis. Deafness may be profound, or only detectable by audiometry. Dense cataracts are common after infection in the first month; smaller or faint opacities may occur after second-month infections. Retinal pigment dysplasia is often evident on ophthalmoscopy. The most distressing problem is a severe brain syndrome inhibiting motor, sensory and intellectual development. This can result in a severely disabled child, further impaired by defective vision and hearing.

Hearing defects are probably the commonest effect of infection in the second and third trimesters. Impairment may increase during the early years of life.

Permanent or progressive effects of congenital rubella infection

1 Cardiac: patent ductus arteriosus with or without pulmonary stenosis.
2 Cataracts.
3 Other dysplasias of the retina or uveal tract.
4 Increasingly delayed motor and sensory development.
5 Nerve deafness.

Diagnosis

Exposure during pregnancy should be confirmed, if possible, by serological testing of the suspected case, as the clinical diagnosis of rubella is extremely unreliable (see Chapter 13). A positive immunoglobulin M (IgM) antibody test confirms recent rubella and indicates that the suspect has been infectious. The serological status of the exposed pregnant woman should have been ascertained at her booking appointment. Immunity to rubella does not absolutely protect from reinfection, however, as just under 10% of congenital rubella cases in England are shown to follow maternal reinfection during pregnancy.

The pregnant woman who was seronegative at booking, or whose immune status is unknown, should have an immediate test for IgM rubella antibodies. If negative, the test should be repeated after 2 weeks, or sooner if a feverish illness develops. A final test may be performed after a further week or 10 days. A woman who previously possessed antibodies may not develop an IgM response, but should be followed up to detect a secondary rise in IgG antibody levels. The aim is early detection of rubella infection, so that termination of pregnancy can be offered.

A rubella-infected neonate will have a positive IgM rubella antibody test, which persists until the third month of life. The absence of IgG antibodies excludes the diagnosis of congenital rubella, as neither mother nor child can have been infected.

Laboratory diagnosis of rubella
1 In pregnant woman: serum immunoglobulin G (IgG) at booking; IgM after suspected exposure or illness (repeat after 2 weeks).
2 In fetus: culture of rubella virus from amniotic fluid; fetal blood sampling for serology (only worthwhile after 20 weeks).
3 In neonate: positive IgM (absence of IgG excludes the diagnosis).

Management

Pregnant women with possible rubella infection should be isolated from other antenatal patients.

Most women opt for termination of pregnancy if infected during the first trimester; in later pregnancy there is a balance between the likely fetal damage and the desirability of termination.

Human normal immunoglobulin has been given to exposed women, but rubella infection and fetal damage have occurred even after large doses. Immunoglobulin does not offer reliable postexposure prophylaxis.

The rubella-affected neonate remains highly infectious for several months, and should be isolated from pregnant women. Supportive treatment during the active infectious phase often includes blood or platelet transfusions, sometimes with treatment for immune thrombocytopenia.

The extent of permanent defects should be ascertained by detailed examination. Hearing tests are difficult to perform in infants; observational tests can be complemented with audiometry when the child is old enough. Cataracts can be treated surgically during the first year of life, allowing normal visual development. Cardiac abnormalities often require correction in the early months. Those with severe physical and intellectual disabilities need constant support for both themselves and their families throughout their shortened lives.

Prevention

Rubella vaccine is a live attenuated vaccine produced from the RA 27/3 strain of virus. A single dose elicits protective antibodies in over 95% of recipients. The duration of protection is not yet known, as the vaccine was first produced less than 30 years ago; however, long-term follow-up shows that vaccine-induced antibodies wane at a similar rate as those acquired from natural infection. This suggests that, for most individuals, protection will be lifelong.

Two approaches to the use of rubella vaccine have been adopted. In the UK, selective immunization of susceptible women of child-bearing age was adopted initially. The aim was to provide direct protection to the fetus. This approach was highly successful, reducing susceptibility levels in the antenatal population to between 1 and 2%. Total elimination of congenital rubella is not possible with this strategy as rubella continues to circulate among the non-immunized population. In the USA, and other countries, mass immunization of both sexes early in life (usually as combined measles/mumps/rubella (MMR) vaccine) was adopted from the outset. The aim here is to provide indirect protection, by interruption of rubella transmission among children. Success of this strategy depends upon achieving high coverage (greater than 90%). Since 1988, the UK has adopted this approach.

Prevention of congenital rubella
1 Universal immunization in childhood.
2 Antenatal screening for immunity.
3 Postpartum immunization of susceptibles.
4 Isolation of cases in antenatal units.
5 Active attention to diagnosis in pregnancy.
6 Counselling in pregnancy.

Rubella vaccine is contraindicated in those with immune suppression. It is also contraindicated in early pregnancy because of theoretical damage to the fetus. Follow-up of several hundred babies whose mothers were accidentally vaccinated in early pregnancy has however failed to demonstrate any increased risk of congenital abnormalities. Termination of pregnancy following inadvertent rubella vaccination is no longer indicated.

Congenital and neonatal cytomegalovirus infections

Epidemiology

Cytomegalovirus is the commonest cause of congenital infection in the UK, occurring in 3 per 1000 live births. Although most babies have no symptoms at birth, about 10% of these asymptomatic babies will subsequently develop deafness and neurological impairment. In the

USA, an estimated 2500 infants a year are born with symptoms.

Clinical features

Congenital infection

Congenital infection is apparent at birth in about 10% of cases. It presents with prematurity, low birth weight, hepatomegaly, splenomegaly, thrombocytopenia and prolonged jaundice. About 25% of clinically affected neonates have cerebral irritability, fits or abnormal muscle tone or movement. Pneumonitis is less common, and ventilation is rarely required.

Permanent defects occur in about half of all symptomatically affected infants. Microcephaly and sensorineural deafness are the commonest problems, and often coexist. Microcephaly improves or disappears with growth in a third to a half of those affected. Deafness is a solitary finding in about 10% of cases. Other problems include cerebral calcification, hemiplegia, diplegia or quadriplegia and psychomotor retardation. Choroidoretinitis and myopathy have also been reported.

> **Permanent effects of congenital cytomegalovirus infection**
> 1 Microcephaly.
> 2 Nerve deafness.
> 3 Cerebral calcification.
> 4 Upper motor neurone disorders.
> 5 Psychomotor retardation.
> 6 Choroidoretinitis (rare).
> 7 Myopathy (rare).

The prognosis for later childhood development is poorest in those who have neurological defects at birth. Microcephaly alone does not confer such a poor prognosis as hard neurological signs. Children without neurological defects at birth have a good prognosis, but it is not known whether deafness or other defects may become apparent in late childhood or adulthood.

Intrapartum and perinatally acquired infection

Intrapartum and perinatally acquired infection is often inapparent, although fever, poor growth, pneumonia or late-onset jaundice occasionally occur. It is common for an infant to contract cytomegalovirus infection from its seropositive mother; the majority of all seroconversions occur before school age.

Diagnosis

Infection in pregnancy

Cytomegalovirus infection in pregnancy is rarely apparent, and almost never diagnosed, except by finding congenital infection in the neonate. In the rare situation of a symptomatic primary infection in pregnancy, seroconversion would be demonstrable. Demonstration of IgM antibodies is not completely reliable, as these can appear in postprimary infections, which rarely if ever affect the fetus.

Diagnosis in the neonate

The diagnosis of congenital infection in the neonate depends on demonstrating IgM antibodies or cytomegalovirus excretion during the first 20 days of life. Urine culture and throat swabs are the best sources of virus isolation.

Intrapartum and perinatal infection

Intrapartum and perinatal infection produces positive IgM and cultures after 20 days. Infants who are not tested before 20 days of age cannot have a certain microbiological diagnosis of congenital infection because infection in early infancy is extremely common.

> Immunoglobulin M and cytomegalovirus excretion up to 20 days of age indicates intrauterine infection; after 20 days it indicates intrapartum or perinatal infection.

Management

In pregnancy

If new infection is diagnosed during pregnancy, counselling is based on the knowledge that only 10% of children have any detectable disorder at birth, and that a proportion of these will recover. There is no specific treatment.

Neonatal

The infected neonate needs no active treatment if it appears normal; supportive treatment is needed for temporary acute problems. Future follow-up to detect possible sensorineural deafness is important. Those who present with neurological disorders require more intense follow-up with regular assessments and physiotherapy, rehabilitation and/or educational support as appropriate. It is important not to overlook deafness, which may be difficult to detect in these children.

Prevention

Opportunities for prevention are limited. Blood transfusion and organ donation from cytomegalovirus-seropositive donors to seronegative recipients should be avoided. Since cytomegalovirus in adults is often asymptomatic, screening in pregnancy would require repeated blood sampling. It has been suggested that susceptible pregnant women can reduce their risk by avoiding contact with the urine and saliva of young children, although this is not practical and of unproven benefit. No vaccine is available.

Occupational exposure to young children has not been shown to carry additional risk of cytomegalovirus infection.

Congenital parvovirus infection

This is probably quite common during parvovirus B19 epidemics, when children and adults may develop slapped cheek syndrome or arthralgia and rash (see Chapter 13). It is important to undertake laboratory tests to exclude rubella, which it may closely resemble.

Fetal infection will occur in about half of maternal infections during pregnancy. In almost all cases both mother and fetus recover from the infection and a normal birth follows.

Infection in the second trimester can cause significant damage to the rapidly developing fetal red blood cells. It is estimated that about 9% of all parvovirus-infected pregnancies are at risk of this damage.

Human parvovirus B19 can only infect cells during the S phase of mitosis. Rapid fetal growth in the second trimester must be paralleled by equally rapid production of red blood cells if the fetus is not to become anaemic. Parvovirus infection of the actively dividing red cell precursors causes temporary aplasia, which can be severe enough to produce fetal anaemia and hydrops. In some cases fetal death occurs; in others it seems that the fetus recovers and a normal haemoglobin is restored. Some severely affected cases may be treatable by intrauterine blood transfusion.

Congenital and intrapartum herpes simplex infections

Primary herpes simplex infections may be accompanied by viraemia and, if this occurs in pregnancy, transplacental infection can result.

Congenital infection

Infants born with congenital infection tend to have severe disease with a high mortality. The commonest features are pneumonitis, meningoencephalitis with fits and neurological signs, hepatosplenomegaly and cytopenias. A minority of infants have herpetic lesions of the skin or mucosae.

Diagnosis of congenital infection is important, as treatment of the infant with aciclovir reduces mortality from 80–90% to 10–15%, and can be begun while laboratory results are awaited. An intravenous dose of 10 mg/kg 8-hourly is appropriate. Virus particles can be seen on electron microscopy of throat swabs, bronchial secretions and scrapings from lesions. The virus grows well in cell culture, producing early and diagnostic cytopathic effects.

Intrapartum infection

Intrapartum infection can occur when a mother is excreting herpes simplex virus at the time of the baby's birth. In this case the infant develops skin, conjunctival, oral or genital lesions within a few days of birth. The condition should be treated vigorously, as half of cases will develop disseminated disease. Intravenous aciclovir is the treatment of choice.

Varicella embryopathy and neonatal varicella

Varicella embryopathy

Varicella embryopathy is a rare deformity following varicella infection, usually during the 13th to 20th week of pregnancy. About 12% of adults are susceptible to varicella, so maternal infection during pregnancy is not uncommon during epidemics of chickenpox. Large surveys suggest that varicella embryopathy occurs in about 1 in 200 infected pregnancies.

The usual deformity is cicatricial contracture of a limb, with hypoplasia and reddened scars suggestive of old, zoster-like lesions. If the head is affected, microcephaly and unilateral microphthalmia may occur. There is no evidence that immunoglobulin or aciclovir treatment affects the likelihood of embryopathy after the mother has developed chickenpox.

If a woman with no history of chickenpox is exposed to infection during pregnancy, she should have her anti-varicella antibody titres estimated. If antibodies are present, no further action need be taken. If she is not immune, the woman may be offered postexposure prophylaxis with zoster immune globulin (ZIG). This can prevent or ameliorate infection if given within 10 days of exposure.

Neonatal varicella

Neonatal varicella is a life-threatening, disseminated disease, with a mortality of up to 40%. It occurs in neonates born to women with no immunity to varicella. The neonate has no protective maternal antibodies. It can acquire infection from its mother if she develops chickenpox within 1 week of delivery; if before delivery, she cannot develop antibodies in time to confer transplacental protection, and if after delivery the infant may develop disease in the neonatal period.

The neonate should be offered postexposure prophylaxis with ZIG. If the mother has had chickenpox for less than 8 days, this should be given as soon after birth as possible. If the mother's disease appears within 1 week of birth, ZIG should be given to the infant as soon as possible, preferably within 48 h. Immunoglobulin given to the pregnant mother will not protect the infant.

Maternal varicella

Chickenpox in pregnancy is not necessarily more severe than in the non-pregnant. As in other adults there is a risk of pneumonitis, which is greater in smokers. The severe or highly feverish illness can precipitate early or premature labour.

Aciclovir is not officially recommended in pregnancy, but there is no evidence of adverse effect in those cases where it has been given. It should be used when clinically indicated to treat maternal disease (see Chapter 13). It is not likely to influence the occurrence of embryopathy, though firm evidence for this is lacking.

Congenital HIV infection

Epidemiology

Congenital human immunodeficiency virus (HIV) infection is rare in the UK, where the prevalence of infection in the antenatal population is low (0.4% in London, 0.01% outside London). Between 1982 and 1994 only 127 cases of congenital acquired immunodeficiency syndrome (AIDS) were reported. By contrast, in some parts of Africa the prevalence reaches 25% and HIV 1 is the most important cause of congenital infection. The risk of vertical transmission also varies — from 17% in Europe to almost 30% in Africa. The prevalence of HIV infection in the UK is continuing to rise in the antenatal population, thus congenital infections will become more common in future.

These figures are well-established for HIV 1 infection. It is likely that they differ for the less common HIV 2 infection, which appears to be less easily transmissible. There are insufficient data from which to deduce the probable risk.

Clinical features

A variable percentage of infants born to HIV-positive mothers are premature or of low birth weight. This may be related to the mother's health and does not inevitably mean that the child is infected.

Some infected infants begin to have severe infections and fail to thrive in the first 12–18 months of life, while others have remained persistently antibody-positive for several years without any adverse effect. It is tempting to think that the former have been infected early in gestation and the latter acquired the virus during or shortly before birth, but the true reasons for the different presentations are uncertain.

Diagnosis

All infants of infected mothers will have HIV antibodies in the blood at birth. In the majority these will be passively acquired, transplacental antibodies, and will decline in titre, eventually disappearing between 6 weeks and 6 months of age. HIV antigen, if present, is diagnostic of true HIV infection but may be absent for weeks or years before becoming detectable in the later stages of infection.

The most reliable diagnostic test is the persistence of HIV antibodies, with no decline in concentration by 6 months of age.

Management

Zidovudine has recently been shown to reduce the risk of vertical transmission of HIV 1 by a factor of 60–70%. The optimum regimen is uncertain, but current treatment includes maternal therapy for the last 11–12 weeks of pregnancy and during labour. The infant is treated for 6 weeks after birth. There is no evidence that zidovudine has a teratogenic effect, but information is scanty to date.

Other methods for reducing the risk of mother-to-infant transmission include: the avoidance of breast-feeding; elective Caesarean section; or elective termination of pregnancy after appropriate counselling. The World Health Organization continues to recommend breast-feeding by HIV-positive mothers in developing countries. This is because of the protective effect of breast milk against other opportunistic infections, which outweighs the small additional risk of HIV transmission.

In pregnancy

HIV infection during pregnancy can safely be treated with zidovudine; no teratogenic effect or adverse effect on the fetus has been demonstrated. Some other drugs, including sulphonamides, some antifungal drugs and systemic pentamidine are contraindicated in pregnancy; others, such as rifampicin, are not recommended but are not known to produce adverse effects. Care should therefore be taken with drugs given prophylactically or electively, though life-saving treatment should be given as in the non-pregnant.

The HIV-infected infant

The HIV-infected infant may need no specific treatment for months or years. The normal programme of infant immunization should be followed, including measles vaccine, even in symptomatic children, as the risk from childhood infection is far greater than that from the vaccines.

There is no reason to exclude HIV-positive children from nursery or school; their body secretions do not contain enough virus to pose a danger of infection from casual contact. Cuts and grazes should be cleaned with water, soap or mild disinfectant and covered with a simple dressing. Spillages of blood or body fluids should be absorbed with wadding or absorbent granules, and the area cleaned with soapy solution or a mild household disinfectant/cleanser; the wadding or granules may be placed in a plastic bag for disposal (commercial spillage kits are convenient for this purpose).

Gonococcal ophthalmia neonatorum

Neisseria gonorrhoeae is an uncommon cause of ophthalmia neonatorum. Gram stain of the purulent conjunctival discharge shows many Gram-negative diplococci, confirming the diagnosis. Chloramphenicol eye ointment, applied three times daily for 7 days, is the treatment of choice.

If a mother is known to be infected with *N. gonorrhoeae* at the time of delivery, gonococcal ophthalmia can be prevented by treating the infant with an effective antibiotic. Benzylpenicillin is effective for sensitive gonococci; cefuroxime or cefotaxime is recommended for penicillin-resistant gonococci.

As with chlamydial neonatal infections, both parents should be offered investigation and treatment for gonorrhoea and other sexually transmitted diseases.

Congenital and neonatal listeriosis

Introduction

Both congenital and neonatal *Listeria* are rare in the UK. Fewer than 100 cases a year are reported. Outbreaks occur from time to time, due to consumption of contaminated foods such as soft cheese or pâté (Fig. 12.3).

Clinical features

Congenital listeriosis

Congenital listeriosis is the result of transplacental infection with *Listeria monocytogenes* during maternal bacteraemia. The bacteraemic infection in the mother is usually trivial or inapparent. Features such as transient fever, backache and pruritis are described, but these are common in pregnancy and rarely lead to specific diagnosis. The first sign of a problem is usually recognition of the disease in the offspring.

Listeriosis in early pregnancy often results in fetal death. Other affected infants may be born prematurely, or at term, with severe disease. Characteristically this is a bacteraemic multisystem disease with granulomatous infiltration of parenchymal organs. There is often a purplish, nodular rash on the lower body and legs. Hepatosplenomegaly is common, and the other features of congenital infection are seen, including meningoencephalitis, thrombocytopenia and variable pneumonitis.

Neonatal listeriosis

Neonatal listeriosis follows intrapartum exposure to maternal birth passages colonized by *L. monocytogenes*. The infant becomes ill within the first 2 weeks of life, usually with meningitis and bacteraemia.

Diagnosis

In congenital listeriosis the presence of an unusual rash may suggest the diagnosis. Disease presenting in the neonatal period must be distinguished from the more common *Escherichia coli* or group B streptococcal meningitis and bacteraemia. The recent occurrence of a case or cases in a delivery unit should increase the index of suspicion greatly.

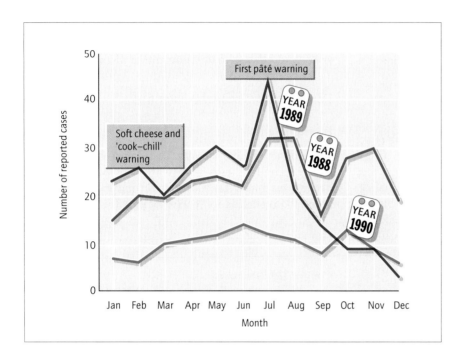

Fig. 12.3 Recent trends in mother/infant listerial infections in the UK; effect of health education and food hygiene measures following epidemics in the 1980s. Courtesy of Dr Jim McLauchlin, Central Public Health Laboratory.

Blood and/or cerebrospinal fluid cultures will provide the definitive diagnosis. In the congenitally infected infants, meconium, urine and gastric aspirate may also be submitted for culture at the time of birth. Products of conception may yield positive culture after abortion.

If the mother is feverish, blood cultures should also be obtained from her. Positive cultures may also be obtained from placental tissue or lochia.

Serological tests may demonstrate listerial antibodies, but these often originate from remote infections or infections by strains of low pathogenicity. Serology is unreliable in making a diagnosis of recent or current listeriosis.

> **Diagnosis of neonatal and congenital listeriosis**
> **1** Culture of meconium, urine and gastric aspirate at birth.
> **2** Culture of blood and cerebrospinal fluid at birth or in neonatal fever or meningitis.
> **3** Culture of products of conception (placental tissue or lochia).

Management

Affected mothers and their infants can be a source of secondary infections, and should be managed in isolation.

L. monocytogenes is sensitive *in vitro* to many antibiotics, including penicillin, ampicillin, tetracyclines, aminoglycosides, imipenem, trimethoprim and co-trimoxazole. It is also sensitive to rifampicin, ciprofloxacin and vancomycin, which are either contra-indicated in pregnancy or the neonate, or penetrate the cerebrospinal fluid poorly. Most cephalosporins are ineffective or only weakly effective.

The response to treatment is not always as satisfactory as expected from laboratory tests. Improvement may be transient, and relapses often occur. This is common with penicillin alone, and can also occur during treatment with other drugs. Some recommend high-dose ampicillin or amoxycillin; others favour the synergistic combination of ampicillin plus gentamicin. The usual penicillin plus gentamicin treatment for neonatal meningitis or septicaemia is also likely to cure, or at least ameliorate, neonatal listeriosis.

When the response to standard treatment is suboptimal, chloramphenicol may produce a good response. It should not be used in combination with other drugs, as there is the possibility of antagonism. If used in the neonate, whose liver detoxifies the drug inefficiently, it must be given initially in a divided dose of 25 mg/kg per day, and plasma concentrations must be monitored. The therapeutic range is 15–25 mg/l; levels above these may cause the grey baby syndrome.

Treatment should not be discontinued too soon because of the risk of relapse. If a good response is obtained, 2–3 weeks' treatment may be sufficient, but extension to 4 or even 6 weeks may be wise after initial slow response.

Prevention and control

Pregnant women should be discouraged from eating foods likely to contain high counts of *L. monocytogenes*. These include soft, ripened cheese such as Brie and Camembert and pâtés. Other food that may contain significant bacterial counts include cook-chilled meals and ready-to-eat poultry: pregnant women should reheat these types of food before consumption. They should also avoid contact with potentially contaminated material such as aborted animal fetuses on farms.

Congenital syphilis

This is now an extremely rare condition. Untreated syphilis in a pregnant woman often causes fetal death and early abortion. However, succeeding pregnancies are more likely to survive to term. The infant may have signs of disease at or soon after birth. If untreated, later manifestations can occur, appearing in childhood, the teens and even in adulthood.

The affected baby is often feverish and has features similar to those of secondary syphilis: rash, condylomata, and mucosal fissures and inflammation. Osteochondritis may cause pain. Persistent rhinitis ('snuffles') is evident, even in mildly affected babies.

Early diagnosis is best made by dark-ground microscopy of material from mucosal or skin lesions. Serology may demonstrate maternal antibodies; only antibodies persisting after 3–6 months of age indicate true infection. The fluorescent treponemal antibody-absorption (FTA-ABS) test is unreliable in the neonate.

Late manifestations tend to appear between the ages of 12 and 20 years. Neurological disorders such as nerve deafness, optic atrophy or pareitic neurosyphilis respond poorly to treatment. Interstitial keratitis often causes damaging corneal opacity, and synovitis of the knees (Clutton's joints) commonly accompanies this protracted

inflammatory condition. Other features include bossing of the frontal bones, chronic periostitis of the tibias (sabre tibia), notching of the incisors (Hutchinson's teeth), 'mulberry' deformity of the first permanent molar and a high arched palate.

The treatment of choice is benzylpenicillin. Neonates can be treated with 300 mg 6-hourly for 10 days, and a good response should be expected. Neurological disease may respond slowly to high-dose treatment, and courses of several weeks may be justified. Interstitial keratitis and Clutton's joints also respond slowly. There seems to be a hypersensitivity component to the keratitis, which can be suppressed by topical corticosteroids; this treatment should be continued until spontaneous remission occurs.

Congenital toxoplasmosis

In the UK toxoplasmosis is a rare infection in pregnancy, affecting between 1 in 1000 and 1 in 2000 pregnancies. It is much more common in France and other continental countries, where attack rates of 2–6% of pregnancies are reported. The great majority of these infections are subclinical.

Transplacental infection occurs in about a third of affected pregnancies, and has only been reported in primary infection. The result of infection depends on the trimester during which infection occurred. Infections in the first and second trimester are more likely to cause significant fetal disease, with the greatest risk between the second and sixth month. Most infections during the third trimester cause only seropositivity in the neonate.

Severely affected neonates may be stillborn or die soon after birth. Others have cerebral calcification, cerebral palsy or epilepsy. Choroidoretinitis is usual, but may not be evident until some months after birth. This may be the only feature in mildly affected infants.

Diagnosis of toxoplasmosis in the pregnant mother is confirmed by the presence of IgM antibodies or by seroconversion. IgM antibodies may also be demonstrated in affected neonates. High titres of antibodies in the infant's cerebrospinal fluid are strongly suggestive of congenital infection. *Toxoplasma gondii* can be recovered from products of conception or from the infant's cerebrospinal fluid by culture in mice or cell cultures.

Intervention is possible if the maternal infection is recognized. Management is expectant in third-trimester infections. Termination may be considered for infections in the second to sixth month of pregnancy. Treatment with spiramycin, a macrolide antibiotic, is thought to reduce the incidence of transplacental infection by reducing maternal parasitaemia. However, fetal infections still occur after spiramycin treatment, and the risk of clinical disease in an infected fetus is unchanged by spiramycin treatment. Spiramycin does not cross the placenta, so cannot cure an already infected fetus. It is not known whether newer macrolides and azolides are more effective.

Diagnosis of *Toxoplasma* infection in mother–infant pairs
1 In the pregnant woman: immunoglobulin M (IgM) antibodies or seroconversion in other antibodies (indication to perform fetal sampling).
2 In the fetus: culture of amniotic fluid; culture of fetal blood samples; serodiagnosis on fetal blood samples (from 20 weeks).
3 In the neonate: IgM antibody in blood; positive culture of blood, cerebrospinal fluid, placenta or products of conception.

Women who have toxoplasmosis are advised to wait until the IgM antibodies have disappeared before attempting to conceive. A small minority have persisting IgM antibodies; after a year it is unlikely that they have persisting parasitaemia, and further delay is not usually recommended.

Treatment of mothers and infants with toxoplasmosis
1 For the infected pregnant woman: spiramycin 3 g/day in divided doses for 3 weeks (perform fetal sampling after).
2 If fetal infection is confirmed in the first 6 months, and termination is not contemplated: sulphadiazine 3 g daily in three or four divided doses *plus* pyrimethamine, single dose, 50 mg daily *plus* yeast tablets eight daily for 3 weeks *alternating with* spiramycin 3 g daily in divided doses for 3 weeks. Continue alternating therapy until delivery.
3 For the infected neonate: suphadiazine 50–100 mg/kg daily in two divided doses *plus* pyrimethamine, single doses 1 mg/kg daily *plus* folinic acid supplement for 3 weeks, *alternating with* spiramycin 100 mg/kg daily in two divided doses for 3 weeks. Continue alternating therapy for 1 year.

Infections which spread only by the intrapartum and perinatal routes

Neonatal and perinatal hepatitis B

Epidemiology

In the UK, the prevalence of hepatitis B surface antigen carriage in the general population is less than 0.5%. Both neonatal and perinatal infection are very uncommon. The risk of infection is between 10 and 25% for infants born to mothers who are e antigen-negative, but rises to 90% for those born to e antigen-positive mothers.

In some parts of the world, notably South-east Asia, the prevalence of infection in the antenatal population exceeds 10%, and neonatal and perinatal infections are very common.

Clinical features

Infants who have been infected by hepatitis B at birth rarely suffer significant illness; they simply develop the antigen and antibody sequence characteristic of acute hepatitis B infection. In the great majority (70–90%) healing is arrested at the stage of e and s antigenaemia, leaving the child at risk in later life of cirrhotic or malignant complications.

Children in whom infection at birth is avoided or prevented may still be exposed during intimate contact with an antigen-positive mother during nursing and early childhood. Other infectious family members can also pose a lesser hazard to the susceptible infant. Hepatitis B infection in early childhood is not often severe, but may be icteric and in exceptional cases can be life-threatening or fatal. The risk of antigen positivity after the acute infection is greatest when seroconversion occurs below 6 months of age; after the age of 9 months the risk is no higher than in older age groups.

Diagnosis

The important aspect of perinatally acquired hepatitis B is the recognition of infectious potential in the pregnant mother. This is done by screening pregnant women from populations with a significant prevalence of e antigenaemia. The main populations concerned are Mediterranean, Far Eastern, Asian and Caribbean people. It is usually unproductive to screen western populations as they have a very low prevalence of antigenaemia, and those who are positive usually carry surface antigen only.

It is pointless to perform any diagnostic tests on the newborn infant of an antigen-positive mother, as the mainstay of management is to provide prophylaxis for hepatitis B infection before antigenaemia can occur, and to ensure protection against future infection in childhood. Effective postexposure prophylaxis is possible because the infant's infection is contracted at the time of birth, and almost never *in utero*.

Management

The labour and delivery should take place in a single-occupancy suite, as the blood and body fluids of the mother present an infection hazard to other mothers and infants.

As soon as possible after birth the neonate should receive hepatitis B immune globulin (HBIG). This prolongs the incubation period of the infection and allows time for active immunization with hepatitis B vaccine. The first dose of vaccine should be given at the same time as HBIG, but in a different intramuscular site. Neonates and infants mount a good immune response to the vaccine. This type of passive–active immunization is now the management of choice, rather than repeated doses of HBIG, which may prevent persisting antigenaemia but do not protect against infection later in childhood. Passive–active immunization reduces the incidence of permanent antigenaemia to about 5% in infants exposed to perinatal infection.

Human T-lymphotropic virus type I infection in infancy

Human T-lymphotropic virus type I (HTLV I) is a retrovirus which infects human T lymphocytes. Seropositivity for this virus is associated with the occurrence of T-cell leukaemia and with a rare acquired neurological disease called tropical spastic paraparesis. The populations in which HTLV I is prevalent include negroes of African and Caribbean origin, and Far Eastern populations, particularly from southern Japan.

The main route of transmission from mother to infant is via breast milk (which contains significant numbers of lymphocytes). Infants of infected mothers are many times more likely to acquire infection if breast-fed than if they are given artificial feeds. Avoidance of breast-feeding, if possible, offers important protection to the child.

Serological tests for HTLV I are currently unreliable, as there are many false-positives for each true positive result. Only Western blotting offers dependable results, and this is unsuitable and far too expensive to use as a screening test. It is hoped that screening for at-risk populations will soon be available.

Neonatal and infant chlamydial infections

Introduction

Chlamydial infections are among the commonest now encountered in both the developed and the developing worlds. They have superseded gonorrhoea and syphilis, which are more readily detected and treated before and during pregnancy. Many pregnant women shed increasing numbers of chlamydiae from the genital mucosa as term approaches, so many neonates are exposed to intrapartum infection.

Clinical features

Chlamydial ophthalmia neonatorum

Chlamydial ophthalmia neonatorum is a severe conjunctivis which appears within 3 or 4 days of birth. It may appear first in one eye, but usually becomes bilateral. There is oedema of the lids, closing of the eye and a purulent exudate which runs from the palpebral fissure. Parting the lids reveals a swollen, bulging conjunctiva.

Neonatal chlamydial pneumonitis

Neonatal chlamydial pneumonitis is a moderately severe, persistent infection which is often, but not always, preceded by ophthalmia. It presents at 3–6 weeks of age with tachypnoea and a repetitive, staccato cough. The chest X-ray is often abnormal, showing streaky or radiating perihilar opacities with or without areas of frank consolidation and air bronchograms. Untreated, it can last for many weeks, producing debility, failure to thrive and significant respiratory impairment.

Diagnosis

Differential diagnosis

Differential diagnosis of ophthalmia neonatorum is important, as both parents may be colonized by the causative organism, and should be offered appropriate examination and treatment. An identical ophthalmia is caused less often by *Neisseria gonorrhoeae*. Staphylococcal or pneumococcal infections are also an occasional cause of purulent neonatal conjunctivitis.

Swabs should be obtained for bacteriological examination, and should include swabs in appropriate transport medium for isolation of gonococci. Scrapings from the inflamed conjunctiva can be examined for typical chlamydial inclusions in the epithelial cells by direct immunofluorescence for elementary bodies, or cultured in McCoy cells for isolation of *Chlamydia trachomatis* or by enzyme-linked immunosorbent assay (ELISA) for the presence of antigen. Serology is unhelpful in the diagnosis of mucosal infections.

Chlamydial pneumonitis

Chlamydial pneumonitis can be confirmed by the diagnostic presence of IgM antibodies to *C. trachomatis* in the infant's blood.

Management

Chlamydial ophthalmia neonatorum

For chlamydial ophthalmia neonatorum the treatment of choice is tetracycline eye ointment applied three times daily for 10–14 days. Chloramphenicol drops or ointment are not recommended as relapse can follow apparently effective treatment. Systemic treatment should also be given with oral erythromycin 125 mg 6-hourly for 10 days, as there is a high probability of coexisting early chlamydial pneumonitis.

Mild 'sticky eye' without conjunctival redness or positive cultures is often non-infectious, caused by sticky secretions from an engorged lacrimal sac, and relieved by twice-daily massage of the sac to empty it.

Chlamydial pneumonitis

For chlamydial pneumonitis the treatment of choice is erythromycin. It may be given orally in a dose of 125 mg 6-hourly for 10–14 days.

Prevention

This depends on detection and treatment of maternal (and paternal) infection before the birth of the infant.

Neonatal bacteraemias

Epidemiology

The epidemiology of neonatal bacteraemia is markedly different from that in other age groups. Approximately 60% of infections are caused by *Escherichia coli* and group B streptococci. The remainder are due to other Gram-negative bacteria, staphylococci, *L. monocytogenes*, *Neisseria meningitidis*, *Haemophilus influenzae* and *Streptococcus pneumoniae* (Fig. 12.4).

Neonatal infection is closely related to colonization of the maternal genital tract. Bacteraemia tends to occur in the first week of life. Meningitis often occurs later, at 2–3 weeks. It is more likely in cases where there is a long interval between rupture of the membranes and delivery, which allows colonization of the amniotic sac with maternal genital flora.

Clinical features

In the first few days of life there are few specific clinical features of bacteraemia. There is often a fever. The infant

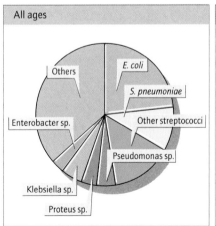
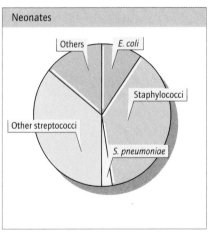

Fig. 12.4 Pie charts comparing the aetiology of neonatal bacteraemia with bacteraemia in other age groups.

is listless, with poor or absent muscle tone (floppy baby) and is uninterested in feeding. The neutrophil count may rise, though in very small babies this is not always a reliable finding.

Meningitis also presents non-specifically, with features of bacteraemia. There may also be vomiting, drowsiness, convulsions or a strange, high-pitched cry.

These presentations should be taken seriously, especially if convulsions occur in the absence of a biochemical cause. All cases of doubt should be investigated. Blood cultures, urine cultures and cerebrospinal fluid examination should all be performed. Gastric aspirate, meconium and urine may also be cultured in the first days of life. Treatment for bacteraemia and meningitis should be commenced while results are awaited.

Management

Intravenous antimicrobial chemotherapy should be given, with a spectrum broad enough to cover both *E. coli* and group B streptococci. Traditionally this has been with a mixture of benzylpenicillin and gentamicin. The use of this mixture for meningitis is not easy, however, as gentamicin penetrates the cerebrospinal fluid poorly, necessitating daily intrathecal injection. Careful monitoring of gentamicin pre- and postdose levels is mandatory in treating both bacteraemia and meningitis.

Broad-spectrum cephalosporins penetrate the cerebrospinal fluid readily, have low toxicity and do not require blood-level monitoring. Drugs such as cefotaxime or ceftazidime are convenient and effective. Treatment should be continued for about a week, with high doses for the first 2–3 days. The choice of antibiotic can be modified if indicated when the results of cultures are available.

Prevention of neonatal sepsis

This depends largely on hygienic and expeditious delivery of an infant. Delayed delivery (longer than 48 h) after rupture of the membranes should be avoided. Attempts to screen mothers for group B streptococcal colonization immediately before delivery have not proved reliable in identifying all cases at risk.

Neonatal staphylococcal infections

The commonest neonatal infection with *Staphylococcus aureus* is umbilical infection. The cut end of the umbilical cord easily accepts colonization and infection, leading to an impetiginous or weeping lesion. Spread to surrounding skin and subcutaneous tissues can occur.

Any area of broken skin may also become infected, as may the conjunctiva.

Bullous impetigo (Lyell's syndrome)

Although *S. aureus* bacteraemia is rare, the effects of staphylococcal toxins are more common. Exfoliative toxins can cause superficial blisters or bullae which quickly break, leaving extensive raw areas. Damage in the layers of the epidermis allows the surface layers to separate and form the blisters. The surface of non-blistered skin can be rubbed off with gentle shearing stress (Nikolsky's sign). The resulting bare patches closely resemble scalds, and the condition is often called the scalded skin syndrome.

The inflamed or weeping lesions are heavily colonized with staphylococci, which can be recovered by culture from swabs. Most cases will recover readily on treatment with oral cloxacillin or flucloxacillin; severe infections need parenteral treatment. Lyell's syndrome can present with very extensive exfoliation. This needs vigorous treatment with antibiotics; the infant requires warmth, humidity, ample fluid replacement, and strict hygiene to avoid superinfection of the bare areas.

Staphylococcal skin lesions are highly infectious. The infant and mother should be separated from others in the neonatal nursery. Control of infection measures should always include hand-washing after each contact with affected individuals. Chlorhexidine is often applied topically to the umbilical stump in the first day or two of life, but this does not preclude the need for strict hygiene generally in the nursery.

Maternal infections related to childbirth

Introduction

Around the time of delivery a woman may have increased susceptibility to conditions such as urinary tract infections because of her changed anatomy and physiology. She may also be more severely affected than others by certain infections such as genital warts, candidiasis or malaria because of altered physiology during pregnancy. Any acute feverish illness can cause premature labour, particularly in the third, and sometimes the first trimester.

There are other susceptibilities in pregnancy and the puerperium because of the presence of tissues or body functions which do not occur at any other time. The placenta is unique to pregnancy; it can be invaded and damaged by some pathogens causing severe maternal morbidity and putting the pregnancy at risk. This is important in some unusual infections including brucellosis, enzootic ovine abortion and, in exposed populations, falciparum malaria. After parturition the placental bed provides a portal of entry for pathogens, which can invade the blood via this route, causing puerperal fever. Finally the breasts become highly vascular and filled with secreted milk. Engorgement and stasis are not uncommon, and occasionally lead to the formation of breast abscesses.

Puerperal fever

ORGANISM LIST

Escherichia coli
Streptococcus pyogenes
S. pneumoniae
Staphylococcus aureus
Other coliforms
Mycoplasma hominis
Clostridium perfringens
Bacteroides fragilis.

Introduction and epidemiology

Any significant feverish illness occurring within 14 days of childbirth, miscarriage or termination of pregnancy may be defined as puerperal fever. It is a severe, usually bacteraemic infection caused by entry of pathogens through either the bare placental bed or through traumatic lesions of the cervix, vagina or perineum.

Clinical features

Most cases begin within 4–7 days of delivery. Fever may be the only sign, but back pain, offensive lochia, faintness or frank shock are sometimes early features. Disseminated intravascular coagulation is a real risk, especially if there are retained products of conception.

There may be clinical features particular to the causative organism. Erysipelas-like lesions on the trunk or arms or a scarlatiniform rash may occur in streptococcal infection. The rash and shock of toxic shock can accompany staphylococcal cases. Intravascular haemolysis, jaundice and even crepitation of vulval tissues may indicate clostridial infection.

Management

Fever in the early puerperium should be taken seriously. If it is not obviously due to a local infection of the skin,

breast or urinary tract, investigations should be carried out and initial treatment begun without delay.

Cultures of blood, urine, lochia and genital swabs should be obtained. The possibility of retained products of conception should be considered; ultrasound examination may help to exclude this. Any retained products should be evacuated (by an experienced operator, as the uterus may be oedematous or friable). Evacuated products should be submitted for microbiological examination.

Initial antibiotic treatment should be active against Gram-negative rods, *Streptococcus pyogenes* and anaerobic organisms. A reasonable regimen would be a mixture of an aminoglycoside, high doses of benzylpenicillin and metronidazole. A broad-spectrum cephalosporin could be substituted for the aminoglycoside and penicillin, but large doses are needed for an adequate antistreptococcal effect. Treatment may be modified when microbiological information becomes available.

Few antibiotics are contraindicated during lactation. Important precautions apply to tetracycline, which is excreted in breast milk and may affect the infant's teeth and bones; sulphonamides, which may exacerbate kernicterus, cause skin rashes or rare haemolysis in glucose-6-phosphate dehydrogenase deficiency; and chloramphenicol, which may cause neutropenia in the infant.

Some patients need intensive support, including treatment for shock, renal failure, adult respiratory distress and disseminated intravascular coagulation (see Chapter 15).

Prevention and control

Delivery should be as hygienic and atraumatic as possible. The placenta should be delivered without undue delay, and retained products should be promptly evacuated. Similar attention should be afforded to premature deliveries, stillbirths and terminations of pregnancy.

When a mother has a severe infection, her infant should be observed closely in the neonatal period as it is at increased risk of bactereamia or meningitis caused by the same organisms.

Breast abscess during lactation

This is a distressing and painful condition, usually caused by a *Staphylococcus aureus* infection. Bacteria probably ascend via the milk ducts, and replicate in an area of stagnation. The abscess often develops soon after breast-feeding commences when the milk flow is relatively intermittent, and difficulties with cracked or infected nipples are commonest. Avoiding breast engorgement and nipple trauma reduces the risk of breast abscess.

A typical hot, tender lesion is palpable in the affected breast, and may point towards the surface as a red fluctuant area. 'Blind' treatment with moderate oral doses of cloxacillin or flucloxacillin is justified in early cases, and may permit early resolution without significant interruption of breast-feeding. The antibiotics are safe for the infant, though rare cases of penicillin rash can occur.

In more severe cases pain may prevent continued feeding; aspiration or drainage of fluctuant lesions may afford relief, and antibiotic treatment will clear residual infection. Lactation can be maintained by gently expressing milk from the affected side and by allowing the infant to feed from the other.

Rare zoonoses in pregnancy

These are brucellosis, Q-fever and enzootic ovine abortion (a chlamydial disease of sheep). All cause abortion in their primary bovine or ovine hosts, and severe infection with placental damage and abortion in pregnant women. However, if both mother and fetus survive, the baby is not permanently harmed.

Farmers, farmers' wives or women working with animals are the population at risk. Q-fever has also spread from cats during the birth of kittens. The diagnosis may be suspected on epidemiological grounds. Urgent serodiagnosis should be sought (see Chapter 7).

Early treatment is essential, and should not harm the fetus. Q-fever and enzootic ovine abortion may be treated with intravenous erythromycin, to which chloramphenicol can be added if a prompt response is not obtained. Q-fever may also respond to treatment with ciprofloxacin, which is highly active against *Coxiella burnetii*. It is not recommended in pregnancy, but its use may be justified in this serious situation.

Brucellosis is difficult to treat, as tetracycline, by far the best choice, may harm the fetus. The risk of co-trimoxazole plus rifampicin is small, and is justified in this situation. Treatment should be continued for at least a month, and retreatment with tetracycline should be given to the mother after delivery to avoid the high risk of relapse after co-trimoxazole treatment (see Chapter 20).

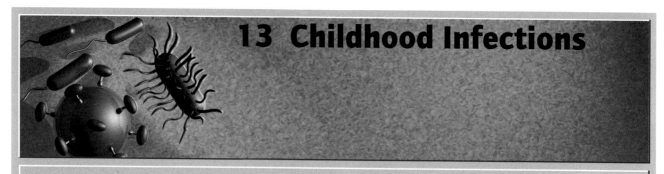

13 Childhood Infections

Introduction

Many infections, both bacterial and viral, are more common in childhood than in adulthood. Examples include primary herpes simplex, hepatitis A and meningococcal disease. Although they can cause considerable morbidity in individuals, these diseases do not cause fast-moving epidemics and they are clinically important in only a small minority of children. In contrast, the epidemic diseases of children discussed in this chapter are almost all highly infectious, have a high rate of significant clinical morbidity, and affect up to 90% of all individuals by the end of childhood.

Nowadays, some have been made uncommon by immunization programmes (Fig. 13.1), but a high rate of immunization must be maintained to prevent their resurgence. Others remain common and are capable of causing large epidemics. In epidemics, the few non-immune adults are at risk of infection, and often suffer more severe disease, with more complications, than those infected in childhood.

A few diseases mentioned here are not highly infectious, but are important differential diagnoses of epidemic diseases with rashes. It is convenient to present them in this context.

Measles

Introduction

Measles is a systemic viral infection whose main features are respiratory disease and rash. It is highly infectious among susceptible individuals and almost always produces clinical disease in those infected. In unprotected populations it tends to occur in large epidemics mainly affecting children, but the recent introduction of effective immunization programmes has made it much less common in many parts of the world.

The important impact of measles is threefold:
1 It can be a severe and debilitating illness.
2 Secondary bacterial respiratory disease is common and may be severe.
3 Post-measles encephalitis is life-threatening and can leave severe sequelae.

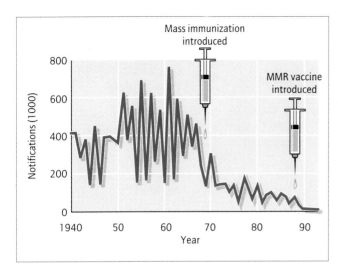

Fig. 13.1 The progress of control of measles after commencement of immunization in the UK.

Epidemiology

The disease is highly infectious with a reproduction rate (see Chapter 1) of 15–17. The attack rate in a susceptible population is usually 95% or greater. Transmission occurs mainly by droplet spread or by direct person-to-person contact, less commonly by air-borne spread or by articles freshly soiled with secretions of the nose and throat. The maximum period of communicability is during the prodromal period and in the first 2 days after the appearance of the rash. The average incubation period is 10 days (range 8–13 days) from exposure to the onset of fever, and 14 days to the onset of rash. Human beings are the only reservoir of infection. Immunity following the disease is usually lifelong.

In the absence of an effective immunization programme, most people are infected in early childhood. The average age at infection is 4 years. Maternal antibody provides protection in young infants; however this is usually lost by about 6 months of age. An unvaccinated person has very little chance of going through life without becoming infected.

In the UK, large epidemics occurred at regular 2-yearly intervals before the introduction in 1968 of a mass vaccination programme (Fig. 13.1). Initially, the coverage of the vaccine was low (about 50%), and epidemics continued to occur every 2–3 years, although the number of cases dropped by 80%. Vaccination coverage has improved to over 90% in recent years and the epidemic cycle has been broken. Many of the cases reported in recent years are in older unvaccinated children. The case fatality ratio has declined from 1 per 100 in 1940 to 0.02 per 100 in 1989. Deaths from measles are now extremely rare. In epidemic years, the disease has a marked seasonal pattern, with a peak incidence in spring and early summer.

Virology

The measles virus is a paramyxovirus of a single serological type related to canine distemper and rinderpest viruses. The measles virus can only infect primates. Its helical nucleocapsid is made up of a single strand of RNA coated with a protein and associated with an RNA-dependent RNA polymerase. The virus is enveloped and varies in diameter from 120 to 200 nm. The envelope contains three major antigens: (i) the matrix or M protein; (ii) H protein, a glycoprotein responsible for haemagglutination and adsorption of the virus to host cell receptors; and (iii) F protein, a glycoprotein which mediates fusion with the host cell membrane and haemolysis. Unlike other paramyxoviruses, the measles virus does not contain neuraminidase.

Like other enveloped viruses, measles is sensitive to ether and is readily inactivated. Despite its high attack rate for the human host it is difficult to culture artificially but it may grow in primary human or simian cells, in which its characteristic cytopathic effect (CPE) is production of multinucleate giant cells. In contrast, vaccine strains produce a spindle-cell CPE.

Clinical features

After 8–13 days' incubation, illness begins with fever and a catarrhal respiratory infection. The high fever is accompanied by extreme irritability, and febrile convulsions are common at this stage. There is conjunctival inflammation, running eyes and nose, persistent croupy cough, mucoid sputum and often coarse crepitations on auscultation of the chest.

The buccal mucosa is also inflamed and Koplik's spots appear. These are raised white lesions which look rather like breadcrumbs or grains of salt on a red, inflamed background (Fig. 13.2). They are reliably present, for a short time during the prodromal period, on the mucosa of the cheek, adjacent to the upper premolars and molars, but can be much more extensive in some cases.

The rash starts in the hairline and behind the ears on the third or fourth day. It reaches the hips on the next day and then the lower legs. On the face it appears as large, swollen blotches (Fig. 13.3) but elsewhere it is maculopapular with largish elements of 1–2 cm in the greatest diameter (Fig. 13.4). It is not pruritic but the skin feels hot and uncomfortable. The Koplik's spots fade as the skin rash evolves.

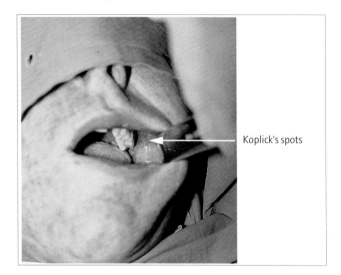

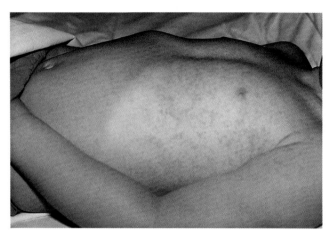

Fig. 13.4 Measles: evolution of the maculopapular rash. By the second day the rash has reached the hips.

Fig. 13.2 Measles: Koplik's spots during the prodrome.

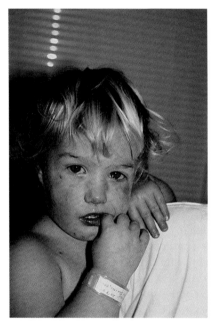

Fig. 13.3 Measles: facies on development of the rash.

Diarrhoea is common at the onset of measles, especially in small children. When the skin rash reaches the lower legs the temperature begins to fall. In the next few days the rash fades to a café-au-lait colour (often called staining); the cough should then subside and the fever resolve. The staining rash fades gradually away within a week or 10 days.

Differential diagnosis

In countries where measles is still common the evolution of the illness is so characteristic that a confident clinical diagnosis is usually possible, even in mild or immunized cases. The absence of respiratory features or Koplik's spots makes the diagnosis unlikely, although Koplik's spots are transient, and their absence may not be significant. The rash of rubella does not spread from the head downwards, and its maculopapular elements are much smaller. Allergic rashes are usually pruritic, unaccompanied by respiratory features and spread in a random way.

Laboratory diagnosis

The laboratory diagnosis of measles is rarely sought, except in countries such as the UK close to eliminating the disease, as the natural history and clinical features are usually so characteristic. Diagnostic difficulty might be encountered in patients with deficient cellular immunity in whom the classic clinical features may be absent.

The white cell count is often normal unless secondary bacterial infection develops, but patients may exhibit a profound leukopenia. Smears may be made of Koplik's spots, and aspirated nasopharyngeal secretions. Demonstration of multinucleate giant cells would support the diagnosis of measles. These preparations may also be examined by an immunofluorescent technique to detect viral antigen. Blood, nasopharyngeal secretions, conjunctival secretions and urine may be taken for culture. Specimens should be transported to the laboratory at 4°C with the minimum of delay due to lability of virus infectivity. Specimens may be inoculated into primary human or simian cells, or continuous-line Vero cells. Isolated virus is identified by the giant-cell CPE, and intranuclear inclusions. Definitive identification can be made by immunofluorescence or virus neutralization.

Complement-fixing, neutralizing and haemolysis-inhibiting antibodies may be sought; they appear with the rash, and reach a peak within 10 days. Thus the first of paired sera should be taken as soon as possible. Immunoglobulin G (IgG) and IgM antibodies may be detected by enzyme-linked immunosorbent assay (ELISA). Antibodies of both classes rise in parallel, but IgM antibodies fall within 3 months, enabling a diagnosis of acute infection to be made. Patients with subacute sclerosing panencephalitis (SSPE) can have persistently elevated IgM concentrations, but this is unlikely to cause diagnostic confusion.

Since the disease has become uncommon, it is usual to confirm the diagnosis by IgM ELISA. Measles IgM can now reliably be detected in a saliva specimen, provided this is collected between 1 to 6 weeks after the onset of symptoms.

Diagnosis of measles
1 Cytology of Koplik's spots or respiratory mucosal cells (shows multinucleate giant cells).
2 Immunofluorescent staining of cells to demonstrate measles antigen (a rapid diagnostic method).
3 Culture if rapidly transported to the laboratory.
4 Demonstration of measles immunoglobulin M by enzyme-linked immunosorbent assay.
5 Rising titres of various antibodies in paired sera.

Treatment

There is no specific treatment for acute measles. In most cases the risk of severe secondary bacterial disease is greater than that from the viral infection itself. Bacterial bronchitis should be easily suspected, sputum culture should be obtained if possible and antimicrobial therapy should include an antistaphylococcal agent.

Problems and complications

Unusually severe measles

Danger signs are the occurrence of severe respiratory disease when the rash is only beginning, or of widespread petechial or haemorrhagic components in the rash. Giant-cell viral pneumonitis, usually trivial in ordinary cases, can cause severe or fatal respiratory failure.

The antiviral drug tribavirin may have some effect in severe measles pneumonitis. A nebulized preparation is obtainable in the UK. Small trials suggest that it may influence the course of myxoviral and paramyxoviral respiratory diseases, though the evidence is not strong enough to make firm recommendations.

A rare effect of the infection is a clinically apparent keratitis, which usually presents as blurred vision in one or both eyes. Cloudy oedema of the cornea is apparent on slit-lamp examination. It is usual to offer antibiotic drops or ointment to protect the inflamed tissue from secondary bacterial infection. The disorder is self-limiting over a period of 3 or 4 weeks.

Measles is a dangerous disease in the immuno-suppressed (see Chapter 21).

Secondary bacterial respiratory infections

Acute otitis media and lower respiratory infection are the commonest complications of measles. Otitis media occurs during the catarrhal phase of the disease, while bronchitis or bronchopneumonia are indicated by persisting cough and fever when the rash is staining (Fig. 13.5). While the usual secondary invaders *Streptococcus pneumoniae* and *Haemophilus influenzae* are common causes of this, *Staphylococcus aureus* is also a real likelihood, as in influenza.

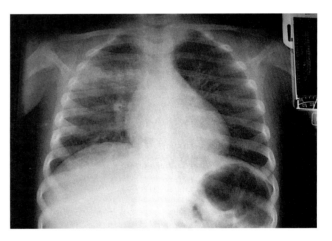

Fig. 13.5 Secondary bacterial bronchopneumonia in measles: this 2-year-old girl developed respiratory distress and high fever as the rash began to stain. The chest X-ray shows extensive nodular pneumonitis as well as a distinct area of consolidation. The patient responded rapidly to intravenous ampicillin plus flucloxacillin and *Staphylococcus aureus* was recovered from sputum cultures.

Mucocutaneous infections occur in debilitated or undernourished children. Impetiginous lesions appear at the angles of the mouth or around the nares. In conditions of poor hygiene necrotizing, synergistic infection may develop. This is called cancrum oris and is nowadays rarely seen except in the poorest rural communities of the world.

Post-measles encephalitis

This complicates about 1 in 1000 infections. Features of encephalitis develop in the second week as the acute illness is resolving. The encephalitis is severe and no specific treatment is available. There is no evidence that corticosteroids or other immunosuppressive drugs influence the course, though dexamathasone may be part of the treatment to lower intracranial pressure. Mortality is about 50% and about 50% of survivors have some permanent neurological sequel.

Subacute sclerosing panencephalitis

This is rare, affecting about 1 in 1 000 000 cases, almost always patients who had measles before the age of 2. Neurological disease begins on average 7–10 years after the acute measles. Clumsiness and poor school performance are followed by progressive spasticity. Myoclonic episodes and salaam-like seizures are common and there is a typical abnormality of the electroencephalogram. The outcome is uniformly fatal.

Measles antigen is plentiful in the brains of SSPE patients, with high antibody titres in cerebrospinal fluid. It appears that virus which lacks surface protein gradually spreads within cerebral cells. Viral antigen can also be demonstrated in the peripheral blood mononuclear cells of sufferers.

Complications of measles
1 Severe, haemorrhagic disease.
2 Measles keratitis.
3 Secondary acute suppurative otitis media.
4 Secondary bacterial bronchopneumonia.
5 Rare cancrum oris.
6 Postinfectious encephalitis.
7 Subacute sclerosing panencephalitis.

Prevention and control

Measles vaccines are produced from live strains of measles virus which have been attenuated by passage in serial cell culture. In most developed countries, measles vaccine is given to all children at 12–15 months of age. Vaccination before this age is not recommended because of a poor immune response, possibly because of interference by maternal antibody. The vaccine is administered by deep subcutaneous or intramuscular injection, usually as part of a combined measles/mumps/rubella (MMR) preparation. It is contraindicated in children with immune deficiency disorders, the only exception being children with human immunodeficiency virus (HIV) infection, in whom the risks from the disease are greater than from the vaccine.

A single injection of measles vaccine induces protective antibody in over 95% of recipients. Protection is usually lifelong, although a mild version of the disease may occur in a vaccinated person when exposed to a case. Minor side-effects occur in 5–10% of vaccine recipients. They include fever, which may be accompanied by loss of appetite and a measles-like rash (mini-measles). These signs usually appear between the sixth and 10th day after vaccination. Occasionally, convulsions occur if the fever is high. Simple measures such as tepid sponging, removal of warm clothing and antipyretic therapy reduce the likelihood of postvaccination febrile convulsions. Very rarely (approximately 1 per 10 million doses) SSPE occurs following vaccination. The risk of neurological complications is 10–100 times greater after the disease than after the vaccine.

Very high vaccination rates are required to prevent the spread of measles. It is estimated that more than 95% of the population must be immune to interrupt transmission. Not all children seroconvert following vaccination. Thus, even countries such as Sweden with vaccination rates close to 100% have so far failed to eliminate the disease completely. For this reason many countries recommend a second dose of vaccine at either 5–6 or 11–12 years of age.

Measles is a notifiable disease. All suspected cases must be notified to the local consultant in communicable disease control so that preventive measures may be taken. Children with measles should be kept out of school until they are no longer infectious (4 days after the appearance of the rash). It is particularly important that contact with immunosuppressed children is avoided.

Unvaccinated children who have been in contact with a case of measles may be protected by vaccination, provided that it is given within 3 days of exposure. Immunosuppressed children, for whom vaccination is contraindicated, may be given temporary passive protection by administration of normal human immunoglobulin, which contains significant quantities of measles antibody.

Mumps

Introduction

Mumps is a systemic viral infection commonly regarded as epidemic parotitis. It has many other clinical presentations capable of causing significant morbidity. Mortality however is extremely low.

Epidemiology

The disease is highly infectious, with a reproduction rate of 10–12. Transmission is through droplet spread and direct contact with saliva of an infected person. The maximum period of communicability is in the 2 days before onset of illness. Virus may however be recovered from saliva from 6 days before the onset of parotitis up to 9 days after onset, and from urine up to 14 days after onset. Very mild or subclinical infections are common, and these can also be infectious. The incubation period is 2–3 weeks (average 18 days). Humans are the only reservoir of infection.

In countries that have not yet implemented mass immunization programmes, epidemics occur at 3-yearly intervals, with the peak incidence during winter and spring. The maximum incidence is in children aged 5–9 years. Deaths from mumps are extremely rare; however, approximately 1500 children were admitted to hospital in the UK each year as a result of mumps complications before vaccination was introduced in 1988. The usual reason for admission was meningitis; mumps was the commonest viral cause of meningitis in children. Immunity following natural mumps infection is generally lifelong.

Virology

Mumps virus is a paramyxovirus of one serological type. It contains a single linear strand of RNA which is associated with an RNA-dependent RNA polymerase to form a helical nucleocapsid. The virus is enveloped and is of variable size, between 120 and 200 nm. It is ether-sensitive, and is destroyed by heating to 56°C for 20 min, and by ultraviolet irradiation. The envelope is approximately 10 nm thick and consists of three layers: the outer layer contains glycoproteins with haemagglutinin, neuraminidase and cell fusion activity. The middle layer is made up of host cell membrane, and the inner layer contains non-glycosylated viral structural proteins. Two complement-fixing antigens are recognized — the V (viral) antigen which is associated with the outer glycoprotein portion of the envelope and the S (soluble) antigen which is associated with the nucleocapsid.

Complement-fixing antibodies to the S antigen appear soon after infection and decline over the next few months. Anti-V antibodies rise more slowly, peaking 2–4 weeks after the beginning of the infection, and persist for years. Neutralizing antibodies develop during convalescence and persist for years.

Clinical features

The features of mumps can appear in any order. Parotitis is the most common, occurring in over 70% of cases. It is usually bilateral but the onset may be asymmetrical and other salivary glands are also sometimes involved. Parotid tenderness and pain on salivation precede swelling by 2–4 days. After increasing for about 3 days the inflammation subsides over 7–10 days.

Orchitis is common in adult men but rare before puberty. It varies greatly in severity, but some men suffer extreme swelling and pain of the testicle, which may take up to a month to resolve completely. Even severe inflammation seldom results in testicular atrophy; bilateral atrophy is even less likely. Mumps orchitis is therefore a rare cause of infertility.

Meningitis and meningoencephalitis are common, but are often so mild as to be overlooked. Clinically significant cases are often admitted to hospital.

Diagnostic puzzles arise when mumps presents as isolated meningitis, pancreatitis (occasionally with acute diabetes) or orchitis. It should always figure in the differential diagnosis of these conditions but not necessarily be first on the list.

Rarer manifestations of mumps include mastitis (which can affect both sexes and all age groups), cochlear infection with hearing impairment, oophoritis in women and arthritis (which often appears in the second week). Myocarditis can occur and may be involved in the rare fatalities in adult cases of mumps.

Clinical features of mumps
1 Parotitis.
2 Meningitis and meningoencephalitis.
3 Orchitis.
4 Pancreatitis.
5 Oophoritis.
6 Cochlear inflammation.
7 Arthritis.
8 Mastitis.
9 Myocarditis.

Differential diagnosis

When parotitis is accompanied by other features of mumps, clinical diagnosis is straightforward. Parotitis alone must be distinguished in children from acute cervical lymphadenitis. In parotid swelling the angle of the jaw is enclosed in the swollen gland, whereas it is superficial to cervical lymph nodes. The serum amylase is often, but not always, raised in parotitis. The white blood cell count is not always a useful feature, as the severe inflammatory effects of mumps can be accompanied by neutrophilia. In cases of doubt there is no harm in giving antibiotics (to cover *Staphylococcus aureus* and *Streptococcus pyogenes*) while awaiting laboratory diagnosis. The other differential diagnosis is pyogenic parotitis, which may also cause a raised amylase. This is usually unilateral; the gland may be fluctuant and any abscess will tend to point below the lobe of the ear, where the cartilage joins the external meatus. Surgical drainage is often required.

Isolated orchitis must be distinguished from testicular torsion or pyogenic epididymo-orchitis. Ultrasound or other imaging may be used in emergency diagnosis. The diagnosis of mumps is usually made clinically, but a laboratory diagnosis may be sought if parotitis is absent or a complication of mumps infection is suspected.

The white cell count and differential are usually normal but a leukopenia and relative lymphocytosis may be present. A leukocytosis may be found in patients with meningitis, orchitis or pancreatitis.

Saliva, cerebrospinal fluid or urine may be collected for culture. Specimens are cultured in primary monkey kidney cell or human embryonic kidney cells. Cultured virus may be identified by haemadsorption, neutralization or fluorescent antibody techniques.

Paired serum samples should be taken for serological investigation. A number of techniques have been described, including haemagglutinin inhibition (HI), virus neutralization, complement fixation (CF) and ELISA. Virus neutralization is the best technique to establish immunity to mumps but it is too cumbersome for routine diagnostic use.

HI and CF are simple to perform but lack sensitivity. A fourfold rise in CF antibodies would confirm a diagnosis of mumps. An elevated titre to S antigen with a low or high titre to V antigen in an acute-phase specimen would indicate recent mumps infection. IgM antibodies may be detected by ELISA and titres reach a peak 1 week after the onset of symptoms, remaining elevated for approximately 1 month. An IgG ELISA may be used to detect local production of antibodies in the cerebrospinal fluid of patients with mumps encephalitis or meningitis.

The usual means of diagnosis is by demonstrating either S antibody by CF or IgM antibody by ELISA.

Treatment

No specific treatment is available. Analgesics and bed rest are helpful in severe cases. A short course of corticosteroids may reduce pain and swelling in severe orchitis.

Prevention and control

Mumps vaccine is a live, attenuated preparation, usually administered as part of combined MMR vaccine. Two mumps vaccine strains (Urabe Am9 and Jeryl Lynn) have been widely used in immunization programmes. Mass vaccination of children aged 12–15 months was introduced in the UK for the first time in 1988 and has greatly reduced the incidence of the disease. A sustained coverage level of 85% or greater is required to prevent transmission of mumps and eliminate the disease.

If coverage levels are low (less then 70%), the total number of cases may decline; however the average age at which infection occurs will increase. This may lead to a net increase in cases among adolescents and adults. Complications occur more frequently in these older age groups, thus a vaccine programme with low coverage may have a negative effect, despite a decline in the total number of cases. It is therefore important to ensure high vaccine coverage levels in young children.

The vaccine is highly effective. More than 95% of recipients develop immunity after a single dose which is usually lifelong. As with other live vaccines, immunodeficiency is a contraindication (see Chapter 25). Minor side-reactions include fever and parotitis (mini-mumps). These occur in up to 5% of recipients, and usually appear in the third week after vaccination. A mild, self-limiting meningoencephalitis occurs after approximately 1 per 11 000 vaccinations with the Urabe Am9 strain, which is not, therefore, used in British immunization programmes. The incidence of meningitis following the Jeryl Lynn strain is not known precisely, but is considerably lower than that for Urabe Am9. These complications must be compared to the risk of meningoencephalitis following natural infection, estimated to occur in 1 per 200 cases.

Mumps is a notifiable disease. Children with the disease should be kept out of school until 10 days after the onset of parotitis. Vaccination of exposed contacts is of no value, although it may be used during outbreaks to protect those who have not previously been vaccinated.

Rubella

Introduction

Rubella is a systemic viral infection with many features, including a rash. Although highly infectious, it often produces subclinical or trivial disease. It is important because even subclinical viraemia can infect the developing fetus, causing severe tissue damage and progressive developmental defects (see Chapter 12).

Epidemiology

The disease is moderately infectious, although less so than measles or varicella. The reproduction rate is 7–8. Transmission is by droplet spread or direct person-to-person contact. The period of communicability lasts from about 1 week before to at least 4 days after the onset of rash. The incubation period from exposure to onset of fever is 2–3 weeks. Humans are the only reservoir of infection.

In the absence of mass immunization, rubella epidemics occur approximately every 6 years. Children are predominantly affected (the average age at infection is 8 years); however, cases may also occur in adolescents and adults. During rubella epidemics, up to 5% of susceptible pregnant women may catch the disease, resulting in subsequent epidemics of congenital rubella syndrome and rubella-associated terminations of pregnancy (Fig. 13.6).

Virology

Rubella virus is a member of the Togaviridae, but unlike other members does not need an arthropod vector for transmission. It is immunologically distinct and differs serologically from the other alphaviruses. It is an icosohedral enveloped virus 60 nm in diameter. The central core containing the nucleocapsid is 30 nm in diameter. It consists of a single-strand RNA and a nucleocapsid protein (protein C) in a helical form. Two viral glycoproteins are associated with the envelope: E1 and E2. Haemagglutinin activity is associated with the viral envelope.

The virus is readily inactivated by ether, trypsin, ultraviolet light, heat and extremes of pH. It will grow in primary monkey cells, or Vero cells, without cytopathic effect.

IgG and IgM antibodies begin to rise as the rash appears, reaching a peak between 7 and 14 days. IgM antibody concentrations fall to low levels within 1 month. HI and CF antibodies rise in the first week and remain elevated for a prolonged period. Passive haemagglutinating antibody begins to rise after 1 month and remains elevated for years.

Clinical features

The average incubation period of 17–18 days is followed by a mild sore throat and mild conjunctivitis, often just a gritty feeling in the eyes. Fever is rarely high and the rash appears on the second or third day. It consists of

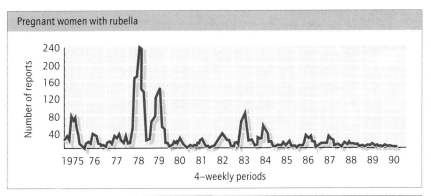

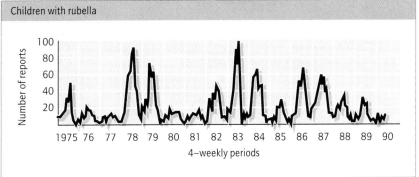

Fig. 13.6 The relationship of rubella epidemics to rubella-affected pregnancies.

fine macules; papules are unusual, petechiae rare. The macules coalesce to a generalized 'blush' in 1 or 2 days, and this fades without desquamation in 3–5 days. Lymphadenopathy commonly affects the neck, and suboccipital nodes may be large and painful.

Arthralgia is common in young adults. It affects the small joints of the hands and feet and occasionally large joints. It can last some weeks, so non-steroidal anti-inflammatory agents may be needed until the discomfort gradually subsides.

Differential diagnosis

Clinical diagnosis is difficult, because many patients lack the rash. Conversely, a rubelliform rash is common in parvovirus infection (in which arthralgia is also common), enterovirus infections, mild allergic rashes and sometimes mild scarlet fever or toxic shock syndrome.

Rubella in pregnancy or exposure of a susceptible pregnant woman can be a disaster. Readiness to suspect rubella and prompt laboratory diagnosis are extremely important in this context. It may also be important to confirm immunity in an exposed pregnant woman.

Laboratory diagnosis

The diagnosis of rubella is usually made by serological techniques. Viral culture should be attempted when strain characterization is required, when vaccine-related infection is suspected, or in complicated neonatal cases. In the absence of CPE, viral growth is detected by challenging infected cells with enterovirus. Control monolayers are destroyed but infected cells resist enteroviral infection and remain intact. Cultured virus is identified by neutralization of virus infectivity with polyclonal rabbit immunoglobulin. Virus shedding from the pharynx may be scanty, but urine is a useful specimen for viral culture.

HI is a widely used technique which detects both IgM and IgG antibodies by their ability to inhibit the agglutination of chick red cells by rubella antigen. Titres of antibody correlate well with the degree of immunity. The diagnosis of acute rubella can be established if a fourfold rise in HI titre is detected, or specific IgM is detected. ELISA and radioimmunoassay are the simplest methods for detecting specific rubella IgM. Congenital rubella can be diagnosed by the presence of IgM antibody or by culture of the virus.

Diagnosis of rubella
1 Immunoglobulin M detection by enzyme-linked immunosorbent assay, radioimmunoassay or particle agglutination.
2 Fourfold rise in haemagglutinin inhibition antibodies in paired sera.
3 Viral culture.

Passive haemagglutination utilizes red cells coated with rubella antigens which are agglutinated in the presence of rubella antibodies. It may successfully be applied for antenatal screening, and the results obtained correlate well with HI. In the single radial haemolysis test the presence of rubella antibody is indicated by complement-mediated lysis of sensitized red cells suspended in an agar gel (Fig. 13.7). It is simple and rapid, facilitating the screening of large numbers of specimens.

Detection of immunity to rubella
1 Single radial haemolysis test.
2 Passive haemagglutination test.

Complications

Immune thrombocytopenic purpura

Rubella is one of the commonest infectious precursors of idiopathic thrombocytopenic purpura. The thrombocytopenia is transient, lasting from 1 to 3 weeks. If mild, it needs no treatment but if necessary it can be treated with intravenous immunoglobulin plus or minus a course of prednisolone.

Encephalitis

This is clinically evident in about 1 in 5000 cases, occurring soon after the rash. It is variable in severity, and can only be treated symptomatically.

Prevention and control

Rubella vaccine is a live, attenuated preparation. In the UK, a policy of selective vaccination of schoolgirls and older susceptible women was adopted in 1970. At that time it was thought that high immunization coverage in women of child-bearing age would prevent cases of congenital rubella syndrome. A vaccination coverage level close to 90% was successfully attained by the mid-1980s and very few women reached child-bearing age non-immune. Rubella epidemics continued to occur

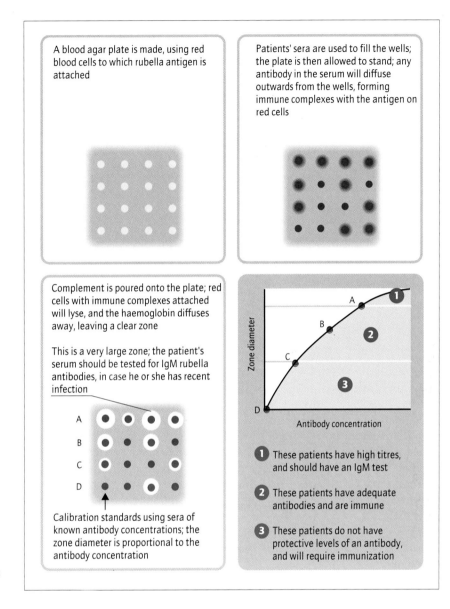

A blood agar plate is made, using red blood cells to which rubella antigen is attached

Patients' sera are used to fill the wells; the plate is then allowed to stand; any antibody in the serum will diffuse outwards from the wells, forming immune complexes with the antigen on red cells

Complement is poured onto the plate; red cells with immune complexes attached will lyse, and the haemoglobin diffuses away, leaving a clear zone

This is a very large zone; the patient's serum should be tested for IgM rubella antibodies, in case he or she has recent infection

Calibration standards using sera of known antibody concentrations; the zone diameter is proportional to the antibody concentration

Zone diameter

Antibody concentration

1 These patients have high titres, and should have an IgM test

2 These patients have adequate antibodies and are immune

3 These patients do not have protective levels of an antibody, and will require immunization

Fig. 13.7 The principle of the radial haemolysis test in screening for immunity to rubella.

among young children of both sexes and adult males. Unfortunately, during these epidemics susceptible pregnant women were still at considerable risk of catching the disease. The risk was greatest among parous women, who became infected mainly by their children; however nulliparous women were also infected, usually by their partners. In addition, some women who had been vaccinated as schoolgirls appeared to lose their immunity. Thus, although selective immunization had reduced the overall number of cases of congenital rubella syndrome, it was apparent that a further reduction in cases could only be achieved by mass vaccination of both sexes in early life. Since 1988, therefore, rubella vaccine (as part of MMR) has been offered to all children at 12–15 months

of age. The aim of this programme is to eliminate rubella, and thereby congenital rubella syndrome. This has now almost been achieved (Fig. 13.8).

As with other live vaccines, rubella vaccine is contraindicated in persons with immunodeficiency. It is also contraindicated in early pregnancy, because of the theoretical risk to the fetus, although vaccination in pregnancy is not an indication for termination. Approximately 95% of vaccine recipients develop immunity following vaccination, which is usually (although not always) lifelong. Side-effects are very mild and include low-grade fever, malaise and rash. In adult vaccine recipients, arthralgia sometimes occurs; very rarely thrombocytopenic purpura may develop.

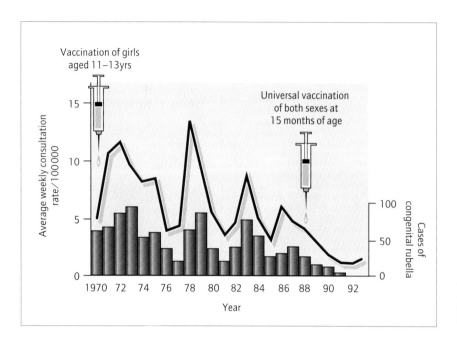

Fig. 13.8 The effect of selective, followed by universal, childhood immunization on the incidence of rubella consultations in general practice and congenital rubella.

Rubella is a notifiable disease. Children should be excluded from school for 7 days after the onset of the rash.

Contact with pregnant women should be avoided. It is particularly important that all health care workers who are likely to be in contact with pregnant women are vaccinated against rubella. Pregnant women who have been in contact with a case, particularly during the first trimester, should be tested serologically for susceptibility or evidence of early infection (IgM antibody) and advised accordingly. Laboratory diagnosis of the case should be sought, as the clinical diagnosis of rubella is unreliable.

Chickenpox (varicella)

Introduction

Chickenpox is a systemic viral infection with a characteristic vesicular rash. Infection is almost always symptomatic but is rarely severe except in adults. Rare cases of fetal injury have occurred after infection in pregnancy (see Chapter 12), and the disease is dangerous in infants aged less than 2 weeks and in the immunosuppressed. Patients on moderate and high doses of corticosteroids are at particular risk of severe illness. Active immunization may become widely available in the near future.

Epidemiology

The disease is highly infectious. The most important sources of infection are cases of chickenpox. Patients with zoster are also infectious, and their susceptible contacts can develop chickenpox. Transmission occurs directly by person-to-person contact, or by air-borne spread of respiratory secretions or vesicular fluid, and indirectly through articles recently contaminated by discharge from vesicles and mucous membranes. The period of communicability is usually from 1–2 days before to 6 days after the first appearance of the first crop of vesicles. This can sometimes be prolonged, particularly in patients with immune deficiency. The incubation period averages 15 days (range 10–25 days). Humans are the only reservoir of infection.

Chickenpox occurs predominantly in young children. Epidemics occur every 1–2 years, usually in winter and early spring. Over 90% of adults have naturally acquired immunity, but in the UK and some other western countries the incidence of chickenpox in individuals over the age of 14 years is steadily increasing (Fig. 13.9). Zoster occurs mainly in older adults, although children, especially those with immune deficiency, may also develop typical lesions (see Chapter 5).

Virology

Varicella-zoster virus (VZV) is a member of the Herpesviridae, and shares morphological and patho-

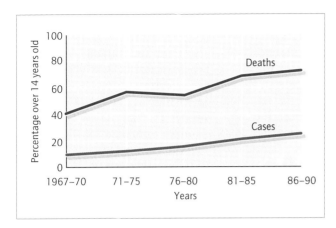

Fig. 13.9 Chickenpox: the increasing incidence in older children and adults in the UK. Courtesy of Dr Elizabeth Miller, Communicable Disease Surveillance Centre.

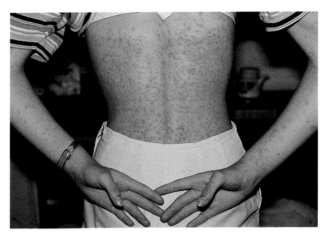

Fig. 13.10 Chickenpox: the very early rash. Many papules are seen, which will all become vesicles in the next few hours.

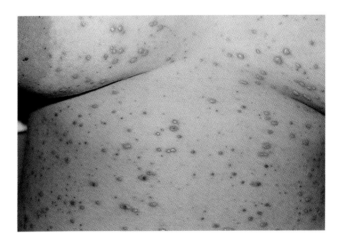

Fig. 13.11 Chickenpox: typical rash showing non-coalescing lesions at all stages of development.

logical characteristics with the other members. Antigenic variation has not been shown, although strain variation can be demonstrated by restriction endonuclease digestion. The virion consists of a central nucleocapsid core 90–95 nm in diameter and an outer membrane envelope 150–220 nm, from which glycoprotein spikes project. The genome consists of double-stranded DNA of mass 80 MDa, coding for 75 protein antigens. There are five major glycoprotein antigens: gp 1–V. Viral infectivity may be neutralized by monoclonal antibodies to gp 1, II and III.

VZV can be isolated in continuous cell culture using many simian and human cell lines, but the virus is strongly cell-associated and therefore difficult to culture from serum and even from cell-free vesicle fluid. The VZV cytopathic effect is characterized by discrete foci of rounded, enlarged cells, and destruction of the monolayer.

Like other herpesviruses, VZV produces lifelong latency, and may reactivate in later life. This reactivation is usually confined to one or two dermatomes served by the dorsal root ganglia, in which the latent virus exists. The mechanism of VZV reactivation remains unknown.

Clinical features

The incubation period is 10–25 days, averaging 15–18 days. Children rarely have a prodromal illness but adults may suffer a few days of fever, headache and myalgia. The appearance of clear vesicles on the trunk is commonly the first sign of disease. They develop from small round papules which are transient and rarely noticed (Fig. 13.10). Many of the vesicles are oval with their long axis along the creases of the skin. These evolve

to opaque pustules which become umbilicated as they dry to crusts. For several days new lesions appear as the older ones evolve (a process called cropping) but successive crops of lesions are smaller and eventually fail to develop (Fig. 13.11). Lesions appear earliest and most densely on the trunk and face. The hands and feet are relatively spared (Fig. 13.12).

Mucosal lesions can affect the conjunctiva, mouth and perineum, where they are sometimes painful or irritating. They are very superficial and usually heal without scarring. Intestinal lesions occasionally cause abdominal pain which may mimic surgical conditions.

A focal pneumonitis occurs in parallel with the rash. It is rarely clinically significant, but occasionally causes

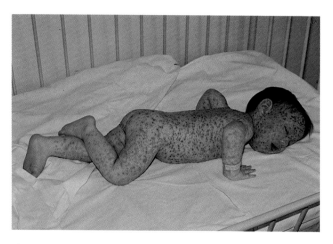

Fig. 13.12 Chickenpox rash: the centripetal distribution spares the hands and feet.

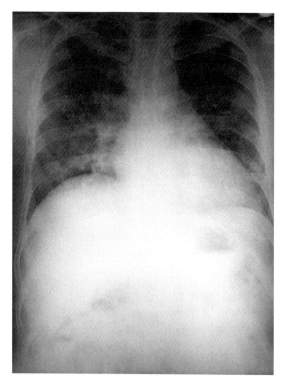

Fig. 13.13 Chickenpox pneumonitis: extensive nodular pneumonitis. Respiratory failure required 5 weeks of assisted ventilation.

severe respiratory disease with blood-stained expectoration and widespread nodular opacities on chest X-ray (Fig. 13.13). The lung lesions tend to calcify on healing, producing a typical X-ray appearance (chickenpox lung).

Differential diagnosis

The diagnosis of chickenpox and shingles is usually made on the basis of the characteristic distribution of the vesicular rash. Diagnostic confusion between atypical varicella infection and smallpox is now irrelevant following the eradication of the latter infection. Disseminated herpes simplex and, occasionally, vesiculating allergic eruptions can cause confusion, but only chickenpox produces typical daily crops of lesions.

Laboratory diagnosis

Specimens which may be collected for laboratory diagnosis include smears of vesicular lesions, vesicular fluid and tissue biopsy or postmortem material. Vesicular fluid can be collected by inserting a small needle into a vesicle and aspirating. Multinucleate giant cells can be found in the cellular debris from the base of vesicles and smears of this material can also be examined by electron microscopy, by immunofluorescence and by culture. Immunofluorescence and electron microscopy are more sensitive than viral culture for the diagnosis of VZV infection. Cultured virus is identified by examination under the electron microscope or by immunofluorescence.

The serological diagnosis of VZV infection is complicated by heterotypic antibody responses to herpes simplex virus in patients previously infected with VZV. A fourfold rise in CF antibody titre is diagnostic of acute VZV infection. The CF test is insufficiently sensitive for the determination of past VZV infection. Techniques used for this purpose include ELISA and fluorescent antibody tests.

> **Diagnosis of chickenpox**
> 1 Electron microscopy of vesicle fluid or scrapings.
> 2 Immunofluorescent staining of vesicle scrapings.
> 3 Culture of vesicle scrapings.
> 4 Fourfold rise in complement-fixing antibodies.

Treatment

Specific treatment is rarely required. Oral aciclovir 10 mg/kg five times daily for 5 days has some effect in reducing the duration of fever and active rash (from about 6.5 to 5.7 days). Pruritis of the rash may be ameliorated by antihistamines. Fewer lesions will develop, and irritation will be less if the skin is kept cool, with light clothing and frequent cool washes. Mild analgesia may be helpful for painful lesions. Aspirin should not be given to children with chickenpox because of the possibility of associated Reye's syndrome.

Problems and complications

Severe forms of chickenpox

Widespread tissue damage occurs, with pneumonitis and sometimes intravascular coagulation, renal damage and disturbed liver function. Smokers are at increased risk of pneumonitis. Danger signs are substernal and epigastric pain, probably indicating many mucosal lesions, and reduced arterial oxygen saturation. By the time that abnormal physical signs appear in the chest, respiratory failure is often already established. In the immunocompromised, pneumonitis may be out of proportion with the rash.

Treatment with aciclovir (10 mg/kg 8-hourly by intravenous infusion) may ameliorate the disease, but must be given early for the best effect, as the advancing lesions are not halted for 24–48 h after commencing therapy. Aciclovir must be given by slow infusion over 1 h to avoid nephrotoxicity, which is related to peak blood levels. The blood urea and creatinine levels should be monitored during therapy.

Falling arterial oxygen saturations may lead to the need for assisted ventilation. Renal failure demands modification of the dose of aciclovir, which is excreted via the kidneys, and must often be treated by haemoperfusion or dialysis. The risk of secondary bronchopneumonia is great, and broad-spectrum antibiotic treatment which includes antistaphylococcal activity is highly advisable.

Secondary bacterial infections

Superinfection of skin lesions by *Staphylococcus aureus* or *Streptococcus pyogenes* is common. These infections can be complicated by erysipelas, scarlet fever or toxic shock syndrome (Fig. 13.14). They should be promptly treated with appropriate antibiotics. If skin lesions become abscess-like or necrotic, swabs should be taken and parenteral antibiotics commenced.

Secondary staphylococcal pneumonia is common, particularly in adults. Any patient with respiratory symptoms should be treated with an antistaphylococcal antibiotic. This applies especially to patients with chickenpox lung who often have mixed viral and staphylococcal pathology. Other secondary bacterial chest infections may occur, and should be treated with amoxycillin or a broad-spectrum cephalosporin.

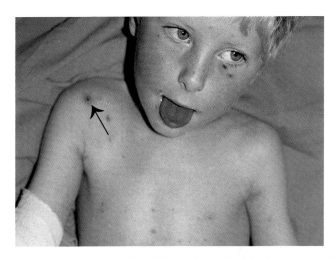

Fig. 13.14 Chickenpox with staphylococcal secondary infection. An abscess has developed in an affected lesion (arrow), and the child has an erythematous rash of toxic shock syndrome.

Treatment of chickenpox
1 Symptomatic — keep the skin cool and give antipruritics.
2 Aciclovir orally 10 mg/kg five times daily (adult 800 mg) for 5 days.
3 Aciclovir i.v. (by infusion over 1 h) 10 mg/kg 8-hourly for 5–7 days.
4 Antibiotic treatment of secondary skin or chest infection — include an antistaphylococcal drug.

Post-chickenpox encephalitis

This is common, but is mild and self-limiting. It is usually a cerebellar disturbance with ataxia and nystagmus which develop as the rash heals. Even cases with other neurological signs or altered consciousness tend to make a prompt and complete recovery. No specific treatment is indicated.

Thrombocytopenia

This is not uncommon. It may make the rash appear haemorrhagic, but the concurrent appearance of dependent purpura and microscopic or macroscopic haematuria will indicate the diagnosis (Fig. 13.15). The condition is transient and can be managed by a brief course of corticosteroids, with or without platelet transfusion, depending on the platelet count. Intravenous immunoglobulin is also effective.

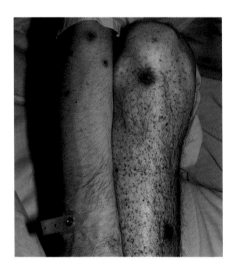

Fig. 13.15 Thrombocytopenia in chickenpox. There has been bleeding into the vesicular lesions and there is a purpuric rash on the leg. The patient had gross haematuria.

Prevention and control

Live attenuated varicella vaccines have been developed and shown to be highly effective. To date these have only been used for immunization of non-immune children with leukaemia, or to protect health care workers who are in regular contact with immunosuppressed children. Mass vaccination in early childhood may be adopted in future, when a combined measles/mumps/rubella/varicella (MMRV) preparation becomes available. Zoster does occur as a complication of vaccination, although less frequently than after the disease.

Varicella-zoster immunoglobulin (VZIG) prepared from plasma containing high titres of specific antibody is available for passive immunization. It is indicated for leukaemic and other immunosuppressed contacts of chickenpox or zoster without a definite history of previous chickenpox, for neonates whose mothers develop chickenpox in the period 7 days before to 7 days after delivery, and for non-immune pregnant contacts. There is no evidence that children with asthma or eczema suffer unusually severe disease or complications.

Children with chickenpox should be excluded from school for 1 week after the appearance of the first crop of vesicles. Patients are no longer infectious when all of the lesions are dry and scabbed. In hospital, cases of chickenpox and zoster should be isolated, because of the risk to immunosuppressed patients.

Human parvovirus B19

Introduction

Human parvovirus B19 (HPV 19) causes a viraemic disease in which the virus particularly attacks rapidly dividing cells. Epidemics of feverish illness with rash and arthralgia are recognized. Infection of red cell precursors occurs and can cause transient aplastic crisis in children with inherited haemolytic anaemias. Infection during the second trimester of pregnancy carries a risk of fetal anaemia and hydrops (see Chapter 12). Persistent infection in the immunocompromised can cause prolonged aplastic anaemia (see Chapter 21).

Epidemiology

The disease appears to be highly infectious. Transmission is person to person, by droplet infection from the respiratory tract. Occasionally the infection may be spread through contaminated blood products. Infection is commonest in children between 5 and 14 years. Outbreaks in schools are common, and usually occur in late winter or spring. The incubation period is 7–22 days (average 14 days).

Virology

Parvoviruses are small DNA viruses which infect a wide range of animal species, including humans. Their role in human disease has only recently been discovered with the association of parvovirus B19 with erythema infectiosum, and aplastic crises in patients with haemolytic anaemias.

Parvovirus is a small, dense icosohedral virus which is not enveloped. The genome is made up of a single-stranded linear DNA which may be of positive or negative polarity. The genome codes for three structural proteins.

The virus may be cultivated in bone marrow, but more conventional techniques are not yet available. The virus is stable to heating at 56°C for more than 1 h. It is resistant to ether and chloroform and survives at room temperature for a prolonged period.

Clinical features

The incubation period of 1–3 weeks is followed by viraemia and often fever. In 2 or 3 days the fever falls and the rash appears. In children the cheeks are often bright red, hence the name slapped cheek syndrome. In all age groups the rash appears on the limbs, and less often on the body. It may be rubelliform but is often reticulate. It fades quickly, recurring transiently if the skin is warm. Bizarre petechial or haemorrhagic rashes are occasionally seen, but the patient is rarely severely ill in spite of the impressive rash. Painful generalized arthralgia can last for several weeks, improving with a fluctuating course. As in rubella, young women are most affected by the joint symptoms.

A pause in erythropoiesis accompanies the rash (and can also occur in the absence of rash). This is caused by infection of red cell precursors in the bone marrow. Reticulocytes become undetectable in the blood film and there may be transient anaemia, often profound in children with inherited haemolytic anaemias. Erythropoiesis resumes as the infection resolves. Immunosuppressed patients may be unable to clear their infection, leading to continued hypoplastic anaemia.

Differential diagnosis

The acute illness must be distinguished from rubella. This is especially important if the patient or a household contact is pregnant. Clinical distinction is poor, so laboratory tests for both rubella and parvovirus should be performed.

Other rash diseases such as scarlet fever and toxic shock syndrome should be suspected if the white cell count is raised. Wide fluctuations in joint symptoms may lead to a suspicion of rheumatic fever.

Laboratory diagnosis

The diagnosis of erythema infectiosum is usually made on the basis of the characteristic clinical features. The difficulties of *in vitro* cultivation of parvovirus mean that serology remains the principal method of diagnosis.

Parvovirus can be visualized by electron microscopy in the serum of infected patients. Antibodies to par-

vovirus can be found in up to 50% of the normal population. Specific IgM and IgG antibody titres rise after the transient viraemia. ELISA for IgG and IgM capture assays have been described. A diagnosis of parvovirus infection can be made by demonstrating IgM antibodies, using ELISA, or parvovirus DNA in blood, using hybridization techniques.

Treatment

There is no specific treatment. Non-steroidal anti-inflammatory agents help the arthralgia. Transfusion may be required for aplastic crises. Normal human immunoglobulin contains antibodies to parvovirus, and intravenous immunoglobulin treatment may terminate or ameliorate bone marrow infection in the immunosuppressed. Anecdotal reports exist of improvement in chronic aplasia after aciclovir treatment.

Prevention and control

There are no specific measures. Exclusion of cases from school is of no value, as most susceptible children will already have been exposed by the time the case is diagnosed.

Human herpesvirus type 6

Human herpesvirus type 6 (HHV 6) is a recently described virus of the herpes group. Originally thought to be a B-lymphotropic virus, it is now known to infect many types of cells. Serosurveys suggest that most people are infected early in childhood, subsequently developing antibodies and harbouring latent virus.

In the late 1980s Japanese workers showed that children with erythema subitum (roseola infantum) excreted HHV 6 and seroconverted to the virus. It seems likely that this disease is the clinical reflection of primary infection. Roseola infantum has long been considered to be a viral infection. It is an illness of infants in which 2 or 3 days of fever are followed by a widespread morbilliform rash which starts on the trunk. As in other viral infections, leukopenia is usual. Small and large outbreaks have been described, with an incubation period of 10–15 days.

Recent reports suggest that HHV 6 may also be a rare cause of severe hepatitis in children.

Kawasaki disease (mucocutaneous lymph-node syndrome)

Introduction

Kawasaki disease is a vasculitic disease of children whose main features are fever, rash, mucocutaneous inflammation and lymphadenopathy. Its cause is unknown, but is thought likely to be an infection because cases sometimes occur in moderate to large epidemics. Although uncommon, the disease has a significant morbidity and mortality, and should therefore be considered in any case of persisting fever and rash.

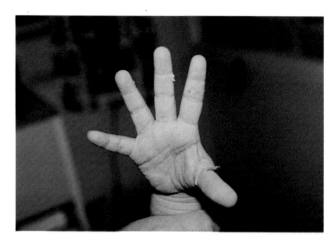

Fig. 13.17 Kawasaki disease: typical desquamation of the finger tips.

Clinical features

The patient is usually a toddler, but rare cases occur in older children and even adults. Illness begins with irregular fever which is often severe. Swelling of the

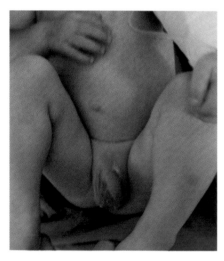

Fig. 13.16 Kawasaki disease: the acute rash affecting the peripheries and the perineum.

hands and feet is common and a red rash soon appears. The rash has different characteristics in different areas of skin; there is usually a 'glove-and-stocking' distribution of intense erythema which is more or less confluent; adjacent areas of the limbs develop roundish slightly raised lesions of various sizes while the rest of the body may be covered with a faint erythema. There is often a shiny or scaly rash on the perineum (Fig. 13.16).

Other early features include oral inflammation, fissuring of the lips and conjunctival injection. There is moderate or gross enlargement of cervical lymph nodes.

After 3–6 days the rash on the hands and feet begins to desquamate. The skin from the ends of the digits often breaks away, characteristically in one piece (Fig. 13.17). Elsewhere the rash may persist for many days.

Even after desquamation of the hands the fever persists, and at this stage systemic features of the disease become increasingly important. Arteritis predominates and, like polyarteritis nodosa of adults, can cause aneurysm formation. Coronary artery aneurysms can be large and multiple, leading to myocardial ischaemia or infarction.

A curious feature of Kawasaki disease is mucocoele of the gallbladder, which is often present, varying in severity from simply an ultrasound finding to an acute surgical emergency.

It is very likely that mild, self-limiting forms of the disease occur. Cardiac events without a preceding illness have not, however been recognized.

Diagnosis

There is no specific diagnostic test, but the evolution of the skin and mucous membrane lesions combined with lymph-node enlargement is quite characteristic. The British Paediatric Surveillance Unit uses a clinical definition.

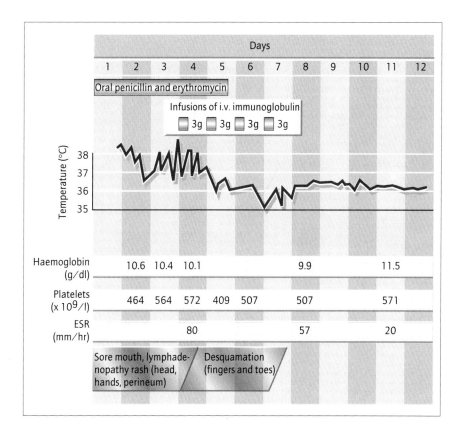

Fig. 13.18 The course of Kawasaki disease and response to intravenous immunoglobulin. ESR, erythrocyte sedimentation rate.

Clinical definition of Kawasaki syndrome
1 Fever, otherwise unexplained, lasting 5 days or more.
2 Bilateral conjunctival congestion.
3 Generalized erythema of buccal and pharyngeal mucosae.
4 Localized cervical lymph-node enlargement.
5 Polymorphous rash with changes in extremities.
6 Desquamation of hands and feet.

As the illness progresses the erythrocyte sedimentation rate and the platelet count both rise dramatically. There is a moderate leukocytosis. Abnormal liver enzyme levels are common — particularly a rising alkaline phosphatase.

Ultrasound imaging often shows distension of the gallbladder. It is essential to perform echocardiography, both to detect any aneurysm existing at presentation and later to check that coronary artery dilatation is not occurring.

Treatment

There is strong evidence that treatment with intravenous immunoglobulin inhibits the development of coronary artery aneurysms. Infusions should be commenced as soon as the diagnosis is evident and should be given daily for 3 or 4 days at a dose of 400 mg/kg. Fever and distress also seem to be reduced by this treatment (Fig. 13.18).

Kawasaki disease is an indication for aspirin treatment, even in children. Full doses of 50 mg/kg daily should be given while the platelet count is raised. Smaller doses, e.g. 10–15 mg/kg daily, may then be used. Most experts would continue aspirin for at least 3 months — longer if the erythrocyte sedimentation rate and platelet count remain raised. Some would add dipyridamole to this regimen, but there is no firm evidence of benefit.

Complications

Myocardial ischaemia or infarction

This is the most important complication. Repeated echocardiography will give warning of developing aneurysms. Large aneurysms of more than 0.9 mm diameter are dangerous, and paediatric cardiologists may even consider surgical intervention if these are seen to form. Myocardial ischaemia is accompanied by pain, as in adults, and electrocardiogram and cardiac enzyme estimations must be performed. Rarely, infarction has occurred after cessation of active treatment. Severe heart failure following infarction may be an indication for heart transplant.

Mucocoele of the gallbladder

This is a rare cause of abdominal emergency in Kawasaki disease. If peritonism or gross pain and enlargement of the gallbladder occur, surgery may be indicated, but the risk of anaesthetic must be taken into account if the heart is compromised.

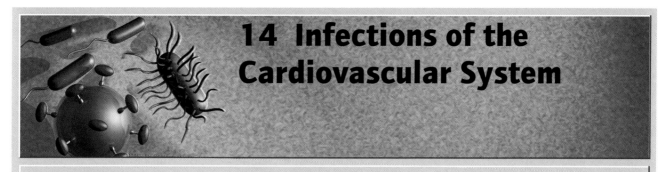

14 Infections of the Cardiovascular System

Introduction

The cardiovascular system has three main structural components:

1 The intimal lining of the blood vessels, or the endocardium in the heart, is composed of endothelium and is in contact with the blood. Damage to the endothelium or endocardium disrupts its smoothness and also initiates the mechanisms of platelet adhesiveness, causing a sticky area of platelet thrombus to develop. This can both trap organisms and protect them from the immunological mechanisms of the blood.

2 The muscular media of the arteries can occasionally be invaded by blood-borne organisms. This can cause aneurysms, leading to altered circulation, thrombosis and even occlusive disease. The myocardium is less susceptible to such direct invasion, though organisms can penetrate from infected heart valves and cause myocardial abscesses. Pathogens with a predilection for muscle tissue may invade the myocardium by the blood-borne route and cause infective myocarditis, in severe cases compromising cardiac function.

3 The pericardium is a mesothelial structure, with the same embryonic origin as the pleura. There is a visceral and a parietal pericardium, with a potential space between. The pericardium can be invaded directly, causing isolated pericarditis, or it can be involved in a pleural or a myocardial inflammatory process. When exudate fills the pericardial space it can compress the heart, reducing its ability to fill and sometimes leading to dangerous tamponade.

Occasionally an infecting organism targets a particular part of the cardiovascular system. Rickettsiae cause an endovasculitis, which predisposes to thrombosis, and haemorrhage from damaged vessels. Late syphilis causes aortitis which damages the elastic layer of the ascending aorta, with aneurysm formation.

Pericarditis

Introduction

Pericarditis is inflammation of the pericardium. While it is often infective in origin, there is a large differential diagnosis, including reactive pericarditis after myocardial infarct, the effect of autoimmune diseases, hypothyroidism and involvement in the pancarditis of rheumatic fever. Malignant invasion of the pericardium will produce signs and symptoms of irritation and effusion, which must be distinguished from infectious disease. Non-infectious pericarditis should therefore be considered in the initial assessment of the patient.

A variety of pathogens can cause pericarditis, either alone or together with myocarditis of varying severity. Acute pericarditis can be a focal complication of bacteraemic disease, such as staphylococcal or streptococcal septicaemia. Contiguous spread of pus from an empyema or from a liver abscess can cause pericarditis with organisms such as pneumococci, enterococci or even *Entamoeba histolytica*. Tuberculosis can cause subacute pericarditis, sometimes with thickening and stiffening of the pericardium (constrictive pericarditis).

Enteroviruses, especially coxsackieviruses
Influenza viruses
Mycoplasma pneumoniae
Streptococcus pneumoniae
Other Gram-positive cocci
Mycobacterium tuberculosis
Coxiella burnetti.

Clinical features

Viral pericarditis

The commonest type of pericarditis is a self-limiting illness with fever, normal or neutropenic white cell count and typical chest pain, accompanied by cardiographic evidence of pericarditis. It is often preceded or accompanied by symptoms of malaise, myalgia or arthralgia, or sore throat, suggesting a viral aetiology. Precordial pain then develops. Usually pleuritic, it often varies with different postures, with swallowing or with the heart beat and sometimes radiates to the neck, shoulders or back. Auscultation may reveal a pericardial rub, which is often transient and variable, disappearing if effusion separates the pericardial layers.

Suppurative pericarditis

This is usually caused by pyogenic bacterial infection. There is swinging fever, neutrophilia in the blood and sometimes other features of infection, such as pneu-monia or pleural effusion. Pain is often severe, and tamponade may occur, with a falling blood pressure and pulse pressure, and a paradoxical rise in the jugular venous pressure on inspiration.

Electrocardiography (ECG) shows upward-curved elevated S-T segments in the anterior chest and sometimes other leads. Echocardiography will often demonstrate pericardial thickening, or effusion if present. On chest X-ray, a pericardial effusion shows as an enlarged, globular heart shadow, which may have a double outline — one for the heart itself and one for the border of the distended pericardium (Fig. 14.1).

Diagnosis

In viral-type pericarditis, nose swab, throat swab, urine and stool should be submitted for virus culture.

An early serum sample should be taken. Immunoglobulin M (IgM) antibodies to enteroviral antigens may be demonstrable in viral pericarditis. Comparison with a later serum sample may allow diagnosis of *Mycoplasma pneumoniae* infection or a rarer condition such as Q-fever. In these disorders, a rising titre of antibodies may be demonstrable.

In suspected pyogenic infections, blood and sputum cultures should be performed. The chest X-ray should be examined for evidence of pneumonia, abscess or tuberculosis. Tapping a pericardial effusion is not without risk; it should be performed as an aseptic technique with ECG or imaging control. Specimens should be submitted for cytology, bacterial culture, acid-fast staining and mycobacterial culture, as indicated.

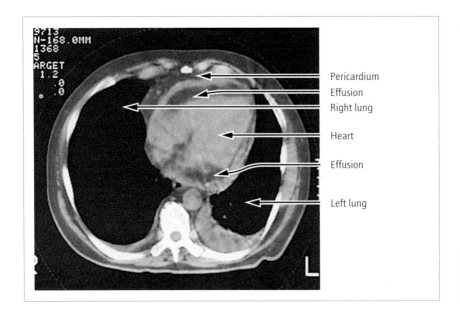

Pericardium
Effusion
Right lung

Heart

Effusion

Left lung

Fig. 14.1 Pericarditis with effusion: computed tomographic scan clearly shows dark fluid between the thickened pericardium and the ventricular muscle.

Management

Viral pericarditis can be treated symptomatically with bed rest and analgesia. Improvement in fever, pain and ECG signs usually occurs in 2 or 3 days and gradual mobilization can then begin. Dysrhythmia or heart failure is rare, as are ECG abnormalities other than S-T elevation, and may warn of accompanying myocarditis.

Pyogenic pericarditis must be treated with immediate intravenous antibiotics appropriate to the situation. If there is localized pneumonia, penicillin must be given; if a lung abscess is present it may be secondary to staphylococcal bacteraemia and cloxacillin or another anti-staphylococcal agent should be included. In a severely ill patient with few clinical signs, *Streptococcus pyogenes* must be considered, and high-dose penicillin immediately commenced.

If tuberculosis is suspected, sputum, urine and gastric aspirate specimens are examined. A tuberculin test should be 'planted' and triple or quadruple therapy then considered. Corticosteroids may also be indicated to limit inflammation and fibrosis of the pericardium (see Chapter 18).

Complications

Pericardial tamponade is caused by sufficient effusion or thickening of the pericardium to interfere with the normal filling of the heart. Warning signs are low systolic or pulse pressure, shortness of breath, first appearing on exertion, and raised jugular venous pressure, often with a paradoxical rise on inspiration. Tamponade can develop suddenly, and occasionally causes severe heart failure, which can be relieved by tapping the effusion. Tapping the pericardium carries a risk of damage to the atrial wall or coronary vessels, and should preferably be carried out by an experienced operator.

In all cases of severe pericarditis, there is a risk of fibrosis of the pericardium, with slow development of tamponade (constrictive pericarditis). Such cases often present with congestive cardiac failure, and signs of tamponade must be carefully sought if the diagnosis is not to be missed. Progressive cases may require surgical decompression.

Myocarditis

Introduction

Myocarditis is inflammation of the myocardium. Most cases are probably of infectious aetiology, and the great majority of these are viral. Many viral cases are purely myocarditis, but myocarditis can also complicate multisystem viral infections such as influenza, mumps or adenovirus infections. The incidence varies from year to year, as would be expected for a viral infection. A few cases occur as part of a systemic disease such as brucellosis or rickettsial infection, or complicate a bacteraemia.

ORGANISM LIST

Coxsackie B (causes about 50% of enteroviral myocarditis)
Coxsackie A
Echovirus
Influenza A and B viruses
Adenovirus (rare)
Mumps (rare)
Rubella
Epstein–Barr virus
Cytomegalovirus
Rarities: rabies, ECM, hepatitis viruses

Coxiella burnetti
Leptospira spp.
Mycoplasma pneumoniae
Neisseria meningitidis and other pyogenic organisms.

Pathology and epidemiology

The pathogenesis of myocarditis is probably different in different types of infection. In infants and young children, and in adults with systemic disease, the myocarditis is concurrent with the acute infection. This is usually the case with bacterial myocarditis.

In many viral infections, particularly coxsackie B infections, the myocarditis is delayed and occurs when viruses can no longer be isolated from the respiratory tract or bowel. In animals this type of myocarditis can be prevented by disabling cell-mediated immunity. Nevertheless, coxsackievirus RNA has been demonstrated by polymerase chain reaction in the myocardium of a high proportion of patients with this type of myocarditis (and also in patients with dilated cardiomyopathy of unknown aetiology).

Clinical features

In adults the disease has a variable presentation. There is usually a history of fever and influenza-like symptoms in the previous 2 weeks, sometimes more recently. Fatigue and exertional dyspnoea are common. Palpitations and precordial pain may be present. Physical examination may reveal fever, tachycardia, dysrhythmia or frank heart failure. Symptoms and signs of pericarditis occasionally coexist.

The ECG shows non-specific changes in the T waves, often inversion. There may be prolongation of the P-R or QRS interval, extrasystoles or heart block. S-T elevation is also sometimes seen, as in pericarditis, which may also be present. Laboratory tests may reveal elevation of the cardiac enzymes, which can persist for many days, but is not always present. The chest X-ray may show cardiomegaly.

Myocarditis is rare in infants, but is often severe or even fulminating, with significant cardiac failure accompanying signs of active viral infection. Older children tend to have relatively mild disease.

In bacterial disease, such as Q-fever or leptospirosis, the other systemic signs of the disease are usually present or predominant (see Chapters 7 and 9).

Diagnosis

The diagnosis will be suggested by the relationship of viral symptoms to the development of cardiological abnormalities. Enteroviruses may be recovered from throat or stool cultures, or respiratory viruses from nasopharyngeal or throat specimens. Endomyocardial biopsy may allow demonstration of virus by culture or immunofluorescence. Diffuse myocardial inflammation can be demonstrated by magnetic resonance scanning.

Management

There is no effective antiviral treatment, though rare cases of Q-fever and other bacterial disease often respond well to appropriate antibiotic treatment. The main treatment is therefore supportive. Bed rest is important, limiting both inflammation and the development of heart failure. If heart failure or severe cardiomyopathy develops, increasing antifailure medication is required, and should be supervised by a cardiologist. In severe and disabling disease, once the acute viral infection is over, cardiac transplant may be indicated.

Endocarditis

Introduction

Endocarditis is infection of the lining of the heart, which particularly damages the cusps of valves. Platelet thrombi form on the infected sites, and these may frag-

ment, producing emboli. The disease is important because it can be difficult to diagnose, requires prolonged and closely supervised treatment and is uniformly fatal if untreated.

Epidemiology

Up to the 1950s, the epidemiology of endocarditis was closely linked to the occurrence of rheumatic heart disease. Spontaneous or native valve disease affected the damaged mitral or sometimes aortic valve. Bacteraemia from the teeth or mouth was almost always the origin of the infecting organism, and this was made more likely by the high prevalence of dental caries and gingival disease, together with the high rate of dental interventions that these demanded.

Both rheumatic heart disease and poor oral health have become less common, but the detectable rate of endocarditis has remained at 1000–1500 cases per year. Predisposing factors are now congenital valve conditions, particularly bicuspid aortic valve and floppy mitral valve. Small ventricular septal defects are at risk, because of the large pressure gradient and intense turbulent flow that they cause; vegetations readily form on the downstream side of the orifice. Elderly patients may have small areas of fibrosis or calcification on valves, or on the myocardial wall, or occasionally a mural thrombus may become infected. While younger patients are at risk from mouth organisms, older patients may have bacteraemias of genital or bowel origin, and enterococci are relatively common in native valve endocarditis of the elderly.

Intravenous drug abusers may suffer repeated bacteraemias, often with skin organisms, but also with pathogens which contaminate their drug preparations. These may include organisms such as *Candida albicans*, derived from lemon juice used as a diluent. Because the source of the contamination is venous, the right side of the heart may be affected. This is otherwise a rare site of endocarditis.

The advent of cardiac surgery and valve replacement has created a new population at risk, either from infection, predominantly with staphylococci from the skin, acquired during surgery, or from infection of the implanted valve itself. Patients whose artificial valves are at risk of thrombus formation receive long-term anticoagulants, which may reduce the risk of vegetations and endocarditis. Surgical patients tend to be either children undergoing treatment for congenital disorders, or the middle-aged and elderly with acquired valvular damage.

Predispositions to endocarditis
1 Congenital valve disease.
2 Septal defects (usually ventricular).
3 Degenerative valve disease.
4 Rheumatic heart disease.
5 Mural thrombus.
6 Intravenous drug abuse (includes right-sided infections).
7 Cardiac surgery, including artificial or biological valve implants.

Pathology

ORGANISM LIST

Native valve infection		Prosthetic valve infection
Young patients	*Elderly patients*	
Viridans streptococci	Enterococci	*Staphylococcus aureus*
Streptococcus sanguis	*Enterococcus faecalis*	*Staphylococcus epidermidis*
Streptococcus mitior	*Streptococcus bovis*	Viridans streptococci
Streptococcus mutans	*Enterococcus faecium*	Enterococci
Streptococcus mitis	*Streptococcus durans*	*Coxiella burnetii*
Streptococcus milleri	Viridans streptococci	
Enterococci	Staphylococci	
Staphylococci	*Coxiella burnetii*	
Coxiella burnetii		

Rare organisms

Small Gram-negative rods (*Cardiobacter*, *Actinobacter*, *Haemophilus* spp.)
Enterobacteriaceae
  Chlamydia psittaci
  Fungi (e.g. *Candida* spp.)
  Mycobacteria (often atypical).

Clinical features

These can be divided into: (i) early manifestations of infection; (ii) embolic events; and (iii) late effects of sepsis and inflammation.

The earliest features are usually fever and heart murmur, with or without associated malaise and fatigue. The onset is often subtle, the fever slight and the murmur easily dismissed as a flow murmur. Charac- teristically, the murmur changes as vegetations develop and valvular patency alters, but this may not occur for days or sometimes weeks. At this stage there is often a mild leukocytosis, and the erythrocyte sedimentation rate and C-reactive protein are both distinctly raised.

Features of embolization may take many days or weeks to occur. Early emboli are seen in more aggressive endocarditis (for instance, *Staphylococcus aureus* endo- carditis), and fungal endocarditis is notorious for pro- ducing frequent and massive emboli. The left side of the heart is affected in the great majority of cases, so emboli are usually systemic. Showers of small emboli may cause eruptions of petechial skin lesions, episodes of haema- turia or splinter haemorrhages in the nails. Large emboli occasionally cause strokes, frank infarcts of the kidneys or acute arterial occlusions. In rare cases of right-sided endocarditis (which may occur in intravenous drug abusers), showers of pulmonary emboli or pulmonary infarcts are typical.

The long-term effects of the infection are those of immunological reaction and tissue damage. The immunological effects include splenomegaly, nephritis and vasculitic lesions of the eyes and skin. The vasculitic lesions occur in the finger pulp or nail margin (Osler's nodes) and in the retina (Roth's spots). Tissue damage affects the valves of the heart, which may rupture or fragment, causing sudden heart failure. Pus may form in the valve rings or cardiac septum, and occasionally ruptures into the pericardial sac.

Clubbing of the fingers (Fig. 14.2) is often an immuno- logically based phenomenon, but its pathology is related to the haemodynamics in the capillary loops of the nail beds. In some cases of endocarditis clubbing occurs early, and responds quickly to effective therapy.

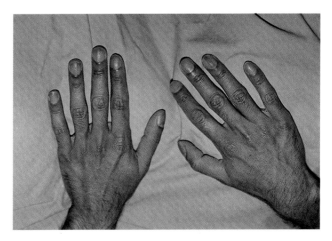

Fig. 14.2 Clubbing of the fingers in endocarditis.

Acute endocarditis

Acute endocarditis occurs when bacteraemia with highly pathogenic organisms involves the heart valves. It behaves differently from the subacute infection caused by less pathogenic organisms. Large vegetations develop quickly; catastrophic valve failure occurs early, and septic emboli may produce necrotic lesions (Janeway lesions), particularly seen on the feet (Fig. 14.3). Infected emboli may also damage arteries, causing marantic aneurysms.

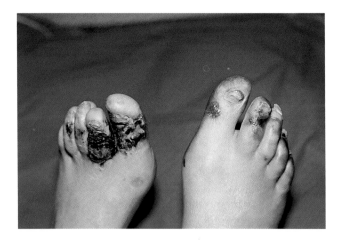

Fig. 14.3 Septic embolic lesions in the feet of a man with acute endocarditis and a huge, friable aortic vegetation.

Diagnosis

The diagnosis must be considered in all patients with fever and a known predisposition to endocarditis. However, apparently spontaneous endocarditis can occur in the elderly, with malaise but very little fever. Changing cardiac function or unexplained murmurs should prompt investigation.

Blood cultures are extremely important. Positive cultures will confirm the diagnosis and provide essential information on the bacterial cause and antibiotic sensitivity. About 10% of patients with endocarditis have negative blood cultures. These should have serological tests for *Coxiella burnetii* and *Chlamydia psittaci*.

Causes of culture-negative endocarditis
1 *Coxiella burnetii*.
2 *Chlamydia psittaci*.
3 Fastidious streptococci or Gram-negative rods.
4 Mycobacterial endocarditis.
5 Fungal endocarditis (*Aspergillus* spp. are virtually never recovered from blood cultures).

Echocardiography is useful in demonstrating vegetations on affected valves, and sometimes intra-cardiac abscesses. Transoesophageal echocardiography is useful for defining some aortic valve lesions not visible on standard views. Negative results, however, do not exclude the diagnosis. Other imaging techniques, such as computed tomography or magnetic resonance scans, can demonstrate intracardiac abscesses. Contrast ventriculography and angiography may be necessary to define connections between abscesses and the blood stream, or to check on the patency of the coronary ostia in aortic valve disease.

When surgery is performed, tissue specimens become available for culture and microscopy. Organisms concealed in vegetations may then be recovered, or rarities such as mycobacteria demonstrated by histological staining.

Management

The mainstay of management is adequate antibiotic treatment. Many viridans streptococci are sensitive to benzylpenicillin, while a few, including enterococci and *Streptococcus 'milleri'*, respond much better if gentamicin is added to a penicillin. Other organisms may need different regimens, depending on the results of sensitivity testing. Q-fever or ornithosis should be treated with tetracycline, with erythromycin as the drug of second choice.

The duration of treatment should be at least 4 weeks. While fully sensitive viridans streptococci can be well-treated in this time, less sensitive organisms usually require 6 weeks of parenteral treatment. Examples of typical regimens are:
1 For sensitive viridans streptococci: intravenous benzylpenicillin 2.4 g 6-hourly plus low-dose gentamicin (60–80 mg twice daily) for 2 weeks, followed by either benzylpenicillin alone for 2 weeks or oral amoxycillin 500 mg 8-hourly for 2 weeks.
2 For streptococci less sensitive to penicillin: benzylpenicillin plus low-dose gentamicin for 4–6 weeks.
3 For staphylococcal endocarditis: intravenous flucloxacillin up to 1.5 g 6-hourly plus either fusidic acid 500 mg 8-hourly or rifampicin 300–600 mg twice daily (both of which may be given orally) for 4–6 weeks. For staphylococci resistant to flucloxacillin, vancomycin or teicoplanin may be given (blood levels must be monitored if vancomycin is chosen).
4 For penicillin-allergic patients: vancomycin can be substituted for benzylpenicillin, and can be given alone for the treatment of staphylococcal endocarditis (blood levels must be monitored to avoid nephrotoxicity and ototoxicity). Teicoplanin is also an effective treatment.

5 For children: the doses of commonly used antibiotics are:

(a) Benzylpenicillin i.v., 150–300 mg/kg daily in four to six divided doses.

(b) Gentamicin 2 mg/kg 8-hourly.

(c) Amoxycillin orally 250 mg 8-hourly (may be increased to 750 mg 12-hourly below age 5 years, and 1.5 g 12-hourly over age 5 years).

(d) Vancomycin i.v. infusion, 10 mg/kg 6-hourly (with plasma concentration monitoring).

(e) Teicoplanin i.v., 10 mg/kg 12-hourly (may be reduced to 10 mg/kg daily after a good response).

Use of vancomycin or teicoplanin for the treatment of endocarditis

1 Vancomycin i.v. infusion, either: 500 mg over 60–90 min, 6-hourly or 1.0 g over at least 100 min, 12-hourly (peak level 1 h after infusion should not exceed 30 mg/l, trough should not exceed 10 mg/l).

2 Teicoplanin i.v. 400 mg 12-hourly (may be reduced to 400 mg daily after a good response).

A resolving fever and stabilization of cardiac function are signs that infection is resolving. The C-reactive protein level is also a useful monitor of progress, falling to normal as infection is controlled.

Complications

Continuing fever

Continuing fever and elevated C-reactive protein are rarely due to inappropriate antibiotic treatment. The usual cause is inaccessibility of the infecting organisms, because they are replicating in necrotic tissue or abscesses. In these circumstances, surgery is often needed to remove pus or devitalized tissue. Accurate preoperative imaging of loculated infection greatly assists the surgeon in operating effectively and safely.

Persisting production of emboli

Persisting production of emboli can lead to disabling strokes, myocardial infarction or limb ischaemia. Routine anticoagulation is considered unwise in uncomplicated endocarditis, because of the risk of bleeding from small (or sometimes large) sites of intra-arterial infection. However, when embolization threatens life or function, anticoagulation is indicated to limit the size and friability of vegetations.

Control of the infection is also important in limiting embolization. In some cases, especially of fungal endo-

carditis, the best chance of arresting the problem is surgery to remove the affected valve and vegetations.

Severe value dysfunction

Severe valve dysfunction is an unpredicatable event. The changing status of vegetations and loss of devitalized tissue can cause sudden haemodynamic changes. Occasionally there is complete valve failure. In left-sided endocarditis this usually causes acute heart failure, with signs of aortic or mitral regurgitation. Emergency surgery and valve replacement is the only reasonable treatment.

Prevention and control

About two-thirds of endocarditis cases affect patients with an identifiable cardiac abnormality. Most of these will have a positive medical history or physical signs, allowing identification of their risk. Antibiotic prophylaxis should be offered to at-risk patients undergoing procedures likely to cause bacteraemia. Although it has never been possible to show by prospective or retrospective studies that prophylaxis prevents cases, the costs of prophylaxis are low, and the benefit of saving even one case is relatively enormous.

The British Society for Antimicrobial Chemotherapy recommendations are as follows for standard-risk patients.

1 For dental extractions, scaling, periodontal surgery without general anaesthesia; for surgery or instrumentation of the upper respiratory tract; for urogenital examination or instrumentation:

(a) amoxycillin 3 g orally 1 h before; *or*

(b) clindamycin 600 mg orally 1 h before; *or*

(c) erythromycin stearate 1.5 g 1–2 h before *plus* 0.5 g 6 h later (not recommended for urogenital procedures).

Note: for urogenital procedures in the presence of colonized or infected urine, an antibiotic effective against the urinary organism must be chosen. Trimethoprim 300 mg orally 1 h before may be useful in this situation.

2 For the same procedures under general anaesthesia:

(a) amoxycillin 1 g intramuscularly 1 h before induction and 0.5 g orally 6 h later; *or*

(b) amoxycillin 3 g orally 4 h before and 3 g orally postoperatively; *or*

(c) amoxycillin 3 g orally plus probenecid 1 g orally 4 h before induction.

3 For obstetric and gynaecological procedures; for gastrointestinal procedures:

(a) only patients with prosthetic heart valves require prophylaxis; others are at negligible risk.

4 For patients requiring general anaesthesia who have prosthetic heart valves or are allergic to penicillins:

(a) if not allergic to penicillin, amoxycillin 1 g plus gentamicin 120 mg i.m. at induction *plus* amoxycillin 0.5 g orally 6 h later; *or*

(b) if allergic to penicillin, vancomycin 1 g infused over 1 h *plus* gentamicin 120 mg intravenously at induction, or 15 min before the procedure.

Infective endarteritis

Infective endarteritis can arise by haematogenous spread in any bacteraemic condition, though it is assumed that some insult to the endothelium must have occurred to allow adherence of organisms.

The atheromatous lower aorta is particularly at risk, because of endothelial ulceration and because aneurysms form, and often contains thrombi. In the affected age groups, bacteraemias are often of bowel or urinary tract origin, so *Escherichia coli* or enterococci are common pathogens.

Pre-existing aneurysms in other vessels, such as the popliteal or femoral arteries, may also be infected. These are often traumatic or autoimmune in origin, affecting younger people. They may be infected with staphylococci, endocarditis organisms or rarities such as salmonellae.

Infected emboli from endocarditis itself may damage or occlude arteries, causing a metastatic or marantic arteritis which can become aneurysmal.

Syphilitic aortitis (see Chapter 11) is a special case in which late infection of the ascending aorta destroys the elastic tissue, causing the development of a potentially massive and fragile aneurysm. This must be treated with care, as the Jarisch–Herxheimer reaction can increase inflammation and friability of the infected tissue.

15 Bacteraemic Infections

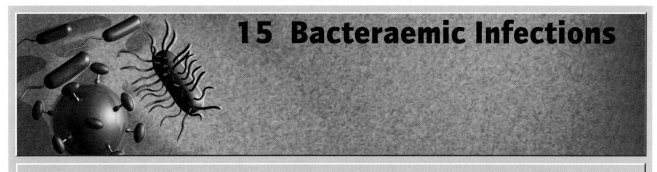

Introduction

Bacteraemia is the condition in which bacteria circulate in the blood stream. Surprisingly, it is not always associated with illness or even with a feverish reaction. Repeated cultures of blood show that bacteria are detectable for 12–48 h after mild tissue trauma, such as dental extractions, and endoscopic examination of the bladder or biliary tree. Self-limiting bacteraemia is also fairly common in salmonella and other bowel infections.

Conditions where transient bacteraemia is common
1 Dental treatment.
2 Endoscopic procedures.
3 Urinary tract infections.
4 Severe bowel infections.
It does not usually cause disease or require treatment.

These bacteraemias are transient and resolve without treatment because of the powerful bactericidal properties of the blood (see below). Several mechanisms of bacterial killing work in parallel to defend the body tissues from circulating pathogens.

Epidemiology

Bacteraemia is common. Approximately 30 000 blood isolates are reported from laboratories in the UK each year. This probably represents only a small fraction of the true incidence, as many cases are not diagnosed and not all laboratories report their isolates.

The infections reported are biased towards more seriously ill patients and may not be representative. Nevertheless, it is clear that a high proportion of bacteraemias are acquired by people in hospital, already ill, who are unable to tolerate infecting organisms. Approximately 60% of reported bacteraemias fall into this category. Neonates and the elderly are at greatest risk.

A wide range of pathogens cause bacteraemia. The distribution of the most important organisms is shown in Fig. 15.1. They may be considered under four general categories: (i) staphylococci and streptococci; (ii) Enterobacteriaceae; (iii) anaerobic and aerobic opportunists; and (iv) community-acquired bacteraemias.

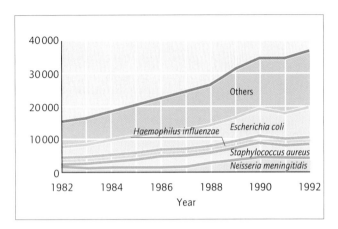

Fig. 15.1 Trends in the occurrence of bacteraemias in the UK.

Stapyhlococci and streptococci

These are both community- and hospital-acquired. The epidemiology of staphylococcal bacteraemia is described later in this chapter (p. 295). Over 7000 streptococcal bacteraemias are reported each year, of which half are due to *Streptococcus pneumoniae*. Pneumococcal bacteraemia occurs mainly in the elderly and is often accompanied by pneumonia. It also affects patients of all ages with underlying risk factors such as sickle-cell disease, asplenia, chronic renal, cardiac, liver or lung disease and diabetes mellitus. Eighty-four capsular types have been characterized, of which 8–10 cause most of the bacteraemic infections.

Enterobacteriaceae

Enterobacteriaceae include *Escherichia coli*, *Klebsiella*, *Citrobacter*, *Enterobacter*, *Proteus* and *Salmonella* species. These gastrointestinal organisms are usually hospital-acquired. The great majority (between 7000 and 8000 per year) are due to *E. coli* and occur in elderly, often surgical, patients. *Klebsiella* infection is commonly associated with antibiotic treatment.

Anaerobic and aerobic opportunists

Anaerobic opportunists include *Bacteroides*, *Clostridium* and anaerobic streptococci, and aerobic opportunists include *Acinetobacter*, *Aeromonas*, *Pseudomonas* and *Serratia*. These are also mainly hospital-acquired, affecting elderly, postoperative, debilitated or immuno-suppressed patients.

Community-acquired bacteraemias

These include *Neisseria meningitidis*, *Haemophilus* spp. and *Listeria monocytogenes*. Meningitis is often an accompanying feature. Meningococcal and *Haemophilus* bacteraemias occur mainly in children under the age of 4. A second, smaller peak of meningococcal disease occurs in young teenagers (see Chapter 16). Asplenic patients and those with complement deficiencies are at increased risk of meningococcal disease. The incidence of invasive *H. influenzae* disease is now declining as a result of childhood immunization. Listerial bacteraemia particularly affects adult immunocompromised patients and pregnant women. Infection in pregnancy often results in stillbirth or neonatal bacteraemia (see Chapter 12).

Defences of the blood

Phagocytes

The phagocytes are mobile cells which ingest particulate matter, including bacteria. The main phagocytes of the blood are the neutrophils, but cells of the monocyte–macrophage line are also phagocytic. The pathogens are ingested into small vesicles called phagosomes. Within the neutrophil these fuse with lysosomes, forming phagolysosomes into which are liberated proteolytic enzymes and highly oxidative agents, including free radicals, which poison and destroy the bacteria. Phagocytes are particularly protective against staphylococci and pseudomonads, which are common pathogens in people with agranulocytosis, or defective phagocyte oxidative pathways (as in chronic granulomatous disease).

Neutrophils are active in both blood and tissues. They leave the blood stream by rolling along the endothelial capillary wall, then adhering to endothelial cells, and finally passing between the cells into the tissues (Fig. 15.2). Neutrophil-associated substances such as CD18 and integrin are important in adhesion to endothelium. Many neutrophils are destroyed in the inflammatory process; others emerge on the surfaces of epithelia and are shed from the body.

Alternative complement pathway

The alternative complement pathway is a soluble defence mechanism. The third component of complement, C3, adheres to bacterial surfaces, where it is slowly broken down to C3a and C3b. In the presence of factor B, active C3bBb is formed, and is stable in the

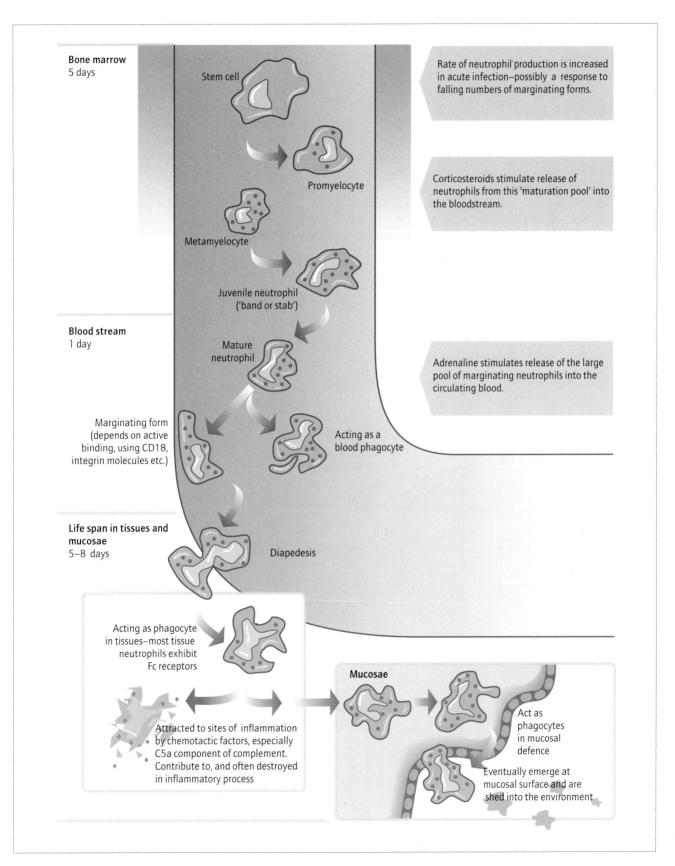

Bone marrow
5 days

Stem cell

Promyelocyte

Metamyelocyte

Juvenile neutrophil
('band or stab')

Blood stream
1 day

Mature
neutrophil

Marginating form
(depends on active
binding, using CD18,
integrin molecules etc.)

Acting as a
blood phagocyte

**Life span in tissues and
mucosae**
5–8 days

Diapedesis

Rate of neutrophil production is increased
in acute infection–possibly a response to
falling numbers of marginating forms.

Corticosteroids stimulate release of
neutrophils from this 'maturation pool' into
the bloodstream.

Adrenaline stimulates release of the large
pool of marginating neutrophils into the
circulating blood.

Acting as phagocyte
in tissues–most tissue
neutrophils exhibit
Fc receptors

Attracted to sites of inflammation
by chemotactic factors, especially
C5a component of complement.
Contribute to, and often destroyed
in inflammatory process

Mucosae

Act as
phagocytes
in mucosal
defence

Eventually emerge at
mucosal surface and are
shed into the environment

Fig. 15.2 The life cycle of the neutrophil.

presence of properdin. The 'membrane attack' complex can then be formed at the cell surface, disrupting the membrane and destroying the bacteria (Fig. 15.3).

The alternative complement pathway does not depend on the presence of antibody, and therefore provides a non-specific means of destroying bacteria. It is particularly important in defending against Gram-negative cocci, and people with defects in this pathway are at increased risk of gonococcal and meningococcal bacteraemia. These bacteraemias are not more severe in complement-deficient patients, but in rare individuals who lack properdin they are aggressive and fulminating.

Iron binding

Iron binding is a prominent property of blood, depending on both specific and non-specific iron-binding proteins. Bacteria replicate inefficiently, and have reduced capacity to produce toxins when they lack iron. Iron-binding proteins such as ferritin are among the fast-reacting proteins of the blood; a large increase in their concentration may have an important antibacterial function.

Spleen

The spleen plays an important part in removing bacteria from the blood. It not only provides conditions for

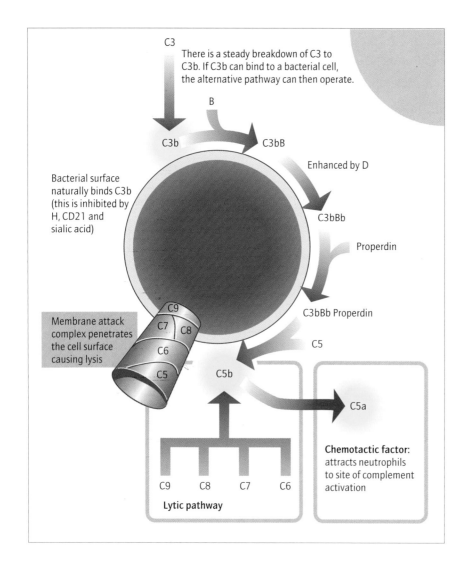

C3

There is a steady breakdown of C3 to C3b. If C3b can bind to a bacterial cell, the alternative pathway can then operate.

B

C3b   C3bB

Enhanced by D

Bacterial surface naturally binds C3b (this is inhibited by H, CD21 and sialic acid)

C3bBb

Properdin

C3bBb Properdin

C5

Membrane attack complex penetrates the cell surface causing lysis

C9
C7   C8
C6
C5

C5b

C5a

Chemotactic factor: attracts neutrophils to site of complement activation

C9   C8   C7   C6

Lytic pathway

Fig. 15.3 Action of the alternative complement pathway.

phagocytosis in its sinusoids, but it removes engorged phagocytes from the blood stream and promotes their destruction by other cells. People who lack a functioning spleen are at greatly increased risk of pneumococcal bacteraemic diseases.

Antibodies

Antibodies circulate in the blood and can adhere to or agglutinate bacteria. In the presence of attached antibody, the classical complement pathway can be activated (Fig. 15.4). This is much faster than the alternative pathway, rapidly destroying bacteria and generating large amounts of chemotactic factors to summon phagocytes and cytotoxic cells. Phagocytes bear receptors which will attach to antibody on bacteria. This process is called opsonization, and makes subsequent phagocytosis of the organism much faster. As well as directly disabling organisms, therefore, antibodies also enhance or recruit other defensive mechanisms of the blood. The effects of deficiencies of alternative complement pathway components are negated if the individual has antibodies to an organism, as the classical complement cascade can be rapidly activated.

The disadvantage of antibodies is that they must be developed following exposure to the particular organism. Unless the patient is already immune, the nonspecific bactericidal mechanisms must 'buy time' while an antibody response is mounted.

Bactericidal properties of the blood
1 Phagocytes.
2 Alternative complement pathway activity.
3 Iron binding (deprives bacteria of iron).
4 Specific antibody.
5 Classical complement pathway activity.
6 Removal of capsulated bacteria by the spleen.

Pathogenesis of bacteraemia

The natural defences of the blood are overcome when bacteria enter the circulation faster than they are removed, or when the bacteria replicate in the blood. When this happens, or when bacteraemia is associated with illness, the resulting disease is often called a septicaemia.

Septicaemia is the term used for an illness in which bacteria enter the blood stream faster than they can be removed.

There are three ways in which bacteria may enter the blood in large numbers:

1 Escape from a site of natural occurrence is a common means of entry. Typical sites of origin include the bowel, urogenital system or skin. When the integrity of such tissues is damaged by trauma, inflammation or malignancy, natural barriers to the passage of bacteria are disrupted. Manipulation, examination under anaesthesia or surgery all increase the likelihood that bacteria will be released into the blood stream.

Some pathogens cause bacteraemia by colonizing a surface such as the respiratory tract, invading the epithelium and then escaping into the blood. This is the probable pathogenesis of pneumococcal, meningococcal and *H. influenzae* bacteraemic diseases.

2 Release from a site of deep sepsis is also common. Abscess cavities are lined with granulation tissue, which is full of tiny, fragile blood vessels. These are easily invaded and entered by pathogens. The same is true of tissue surrounding a devitalized or necrotic area.

3 Inoculation of bacteria can occur by bite, scratch, trauma or iatrogenic injury with a needle or surgical instrument. Some bacteria, e.g. *Streptococcus pyogenes*, are so pathogenic, and successful at evading the antibacterial actions of blood and tissues, that a trivial injury can lead to overwhelming infection. Animal bites may inoculate organisms such as *Pasteurella multocida*, flea bites transmit plague, and inoculation accidents in hunters are an important means of transmission of tularaemia.

Bacterial numbers may be amplified by rapid replication at the site of the inoculum or in a draining lymph node, from where blood stream invasion proceeds.

Pathological accompaniments of bacteraemia

Pathology at the site of origin

Pathology at the site of origin may seem to be an obvious accompaniment, but the effects of the bacteraemia itself can obscure the origin. Such problems as an asymptomatic gallstone or stricture of a branch of the biliary tree can cause overwhelming Gram-negative sepsis which will not be permanently cured until the causative local infection is removed. Renal or hepatic abscesses, collecting system infection behind a ureteric stricture, a small undrained empyema or an infected intracranial sinus are all capable of maintaining a bacteraemia, unless the loculated infection is drained or removed. These predisposing conditions are easily overlooked unless actively sought.

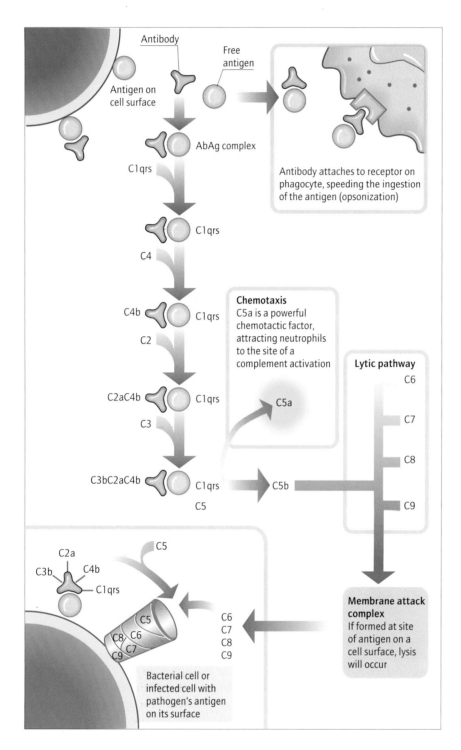

Fig. 15.4 Action of the classical complement pathway.

The heart must always be examined to exclude endocarditis. Apparent cure of the bacteraemic disease after 1–2 weeks' antibiotic therapy can be followed by recrudescence and cardiac damage because of inadequately treated endocarditis (Fig. 15.5).

Effects of exotoxins

Effects of exotoxins are widespread. Staphylococcal and streptococcal exotoxins can both cause rashes. Streptococcal toxins include leukocidins, haemolysins and

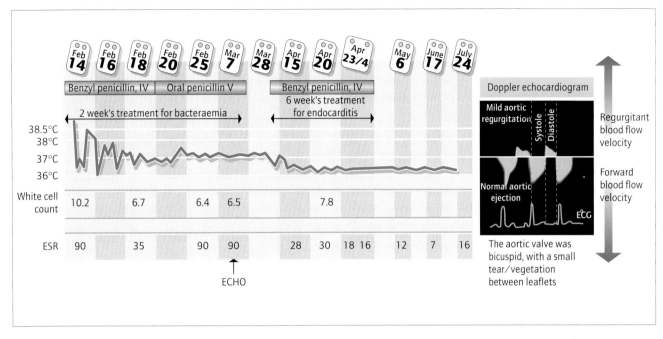

Fig. 15.5 Endocarditis complicating bacteraemic disease: this 27-year-old presented with septic arthritis of the ankle and was found to have *Streptococcus pyogenes* bacteraemia; after completing treatment at 2 weeks, the erythrocyte sedimentation rate (ESR) rose and a systolic murmur led to the diagnosis and treatment of endocarditis. ECG, electrocardiogram.

hyaluronidase. Both Gram-positive and Gram-negative bacteria are capable of producing toxins which cause tissue necrosis. *Clostridium perfringens* bacteraemia is sometimes associated with severe, toxin-mediated haemolysis.

Effects of inflammatory responses

Effects of inflammatory responses probably contribute to fever and rigors. The effects of massive complement activation, kinin activation and release of toxic agents from phagocytes are highly damaging, and add to the classical pathways of fever production. They promote endothelial damage, platelet activation, vascular shunting and poor ventilation–perfusion matching.

Effects of endotoxin

Endotoxin is a complex lipopolysaccharide which is a major component of the cell walls of Gram-negative organisms. Small amounts are naturally released from the gut into the portal circulation and are detoxified in the liver. Large amounts are highly toxic, probably acting by causing the release of tumour necrosis factor from leukocytes. The main effects are on the circulatory

system, with variable degrees of vasodilatation or constriction (depending on the concentration of endotoxin) and loss of endothelial integrity. Hypotension and loss of fluid from the intravascular space result in tissue ischaemia and renal dysfunction. These circulatory changes contribute to redistribution of fluid in the lungs, predisposing to pulmonary oedema or adult respiratory distress syndrome.

Metastatic infections

Metastatic infections occur when tissues are seeded with bacteria from the blood stream. Common sites affected include the lungs, the bones, the kidney and the susceptible endocardium. In some bacteraemias, e.g. *Streptococcus 'milleri'*, the brain is also at risk. Meningitis, arthritis and empyema are relatively frequent complications of bacteraemias caused by Gram-positive cocci.

Some bacteraemias are trivial or silent, but present with complications. *Salmonella* bacteraemias may not even be accompanied by bowel symptoms, but result in osteomyelitis in sickle-positive individuals, or soft-tissue abscess in others. Staphylococcal joint infection is probably the result of silent bacteraemia, as is streptococcal pericarditis or pneumococcal peritonitis.

Diagnosis of bacteraemia

Clinical diagnosis

Clinical diagnosis of a bacteraemia can sometimes be assisted by the presence of typical physical signs. Typical rashes may accompany streptococcal, staphylococcal, meningococcal and gonococcal bacteraemias. Large-joint arthritis commonly accompanies gonococcal bacteraemia. Lobar pneumonia is often present in pneumococcal bacteraemia. Nodular opacities or frank lung abscesses may be seen in staphylococcal bacteraemia. Disease or obstruction of the urinary tract, biliary tree or bowel often leads to Gram-negative and/or enterococcal bacteraemia, often with a contribution from the anaerobic *Bacteroides fragilis*. Recent instrumentation or surgery makes bacteraemia more likely.

In contrast, early hypotension is much more common in Gram-negative bacteraemias, particularly those caused by Enterobacteriaceae. Shock is usually absent until the terminal stages of Gram-positive bacteraemias. An important exception to this is the early presence of shock in *Clostridium perfringens* bacteraemia.

Laboratory diagnosis

Laboratory diagnosis depends on obtaining positive results from blood cultures. A minimum of two sets of blood cultures should be obtained; more than three are usually unnecessary, and do not increase the likelihood of a positive diagnosis. Other specimens which should be cultured include urine, and sputum if obtainable. Specimens such as pus, urinary catheter urine, wound swabs, drain aspirate, throat swabs, joint aspirate, cerebrospinal fluid and diarrhoea stool may be cultured in appropriate circumstances.

Blood specimens should be collected when bacteraemia is most likely, usually when the fever is rising. This consideration is less relevant in infections where continuous bacteraemia is the rule, such as endocarditis or cannula-related sepsis. The yield from blood culture increases with increasing quantity of sample obtained. However, with increasing sample volume the dilutional effect of the blood culture medium is reduced, and this means that the inhibitory effect of the blood (found in serum and white cells) may prevent a positive culture being obtained. A 1 in 10 dilution is usually required and the sample size should be adjusted appropriately. In neonates and small children a positive culture can be obtained with a much smaller volume as the degree of bacteraemia is usually higher.

The media should be nutritious and able to support the growth of aerobic and anaerobic pathogens. More than one medium is required and microbiology laboratories provide blood culture sets. These vary from laboratory to laboratory but usually consist of one bottle suitable for the growth of aerobic, capnophilic and facultative anaerobic organisms and a second culture to which reducing agents have been added, which is suitable for the isolation of anaerobic species such as *Bacteroides*. Blood culture bottles can be subcultured within 6 h for a rapid result and the supernatant examined by Gram stain to yield a rapid presumptive diagnosis. The supernatant can also be examined for the presence of specific bacterial antigens such as pneumococcal capsular polysaccharides and streptococcal group antigens. Many laboratories now use automated blood culture systems which detect the presence of bacterial growth. The methods employed include radiometric, infrared or colorimetric detection of carbon dioxide production or changes in electrical impedance of the medium caused by bacterial growth. These allow rapid detection of positive cultures without the need for routine subculture, saving considerable laboratory time and materials, and optimizing positive diagnosis.

Management

Antibiotic treatment

Effective antibiotic treatment is the surest way to abolish bacteraemia and terminate its effects. A rational choice of antibiotics may be possible if the history and examination point to a particular pathogen or group of pathogens, as follows:

1 Probable coccal bacteraemia (excluding enterococci) can be treated with benzylpenicillin or a broad-spectrum cephalosporin, plus an antistaphylococcal drug such as flucloxacillin, fusidic acid or rifampicin (Table 15.1).

2 Probable coliform bacteraemia, as in urinary pathology, can be treated with broad-spectrum cephalosporin, aminoglycoside or (if hospital-acquired, and resistance is likely), a mixture of the two. In community-acquired infections it is rarely justified to start with a ureidopenicillin, imipenem or other very broad-spectrum agent. In hospital-acquired bacteraemia, locally prevalent antibiotic-resistant patterns may necessitate such initial treatment, dictated by local knowledge of the sensitivities of likely organisms (Table 15.2).

3 Probable mixed bacteraemia, as with bowel, biliary or genital tract origin, often requires a multidrug approach in the initial stages. Treatment for coliforms should be

Organism	May originate from	Antimicrobial treatment
Staphylococcus aureus	Skin, nasopharynx (50% of all cases). Intravenous devices or pacemaker systems (recently implanted) (25% of all cases). Bone and joint disease or surgery or prosthesis (10% of all cases). Genitourinary disease or surgery (2% of all cases)	Cloxacillin or flucloxacillin *Alternatives or additions*: fusidic acid,* rifampicin,* teicoplanin, vancomycin, clindamycin,*† ciprofloxacin
Streptococcus pneumoniae	Lung infection (50% of all cases). Intracranial or meningeal infection (10% of all cases). Patients with altered immunity, splenectomy or alcoholism (up to 10% of all cases). Rarely, intrapartum infection or peritonitis	Benzylpenicillin or erythromycin *Alternatives and for penicillin-resistant organisms*: third-generation cephalosporins, e.g. cefotaxime or ceftriaxone *For multiply resistant organisms*: teicoplanin or vancomycin
Coagulase-negative staphylococci	Intravascular devices including pacing systems, haemodialysis and parenteral nutrition systems (over 50% of all cases). Peritoneal dialysis systems. Intracerebral shunts and valves connected with the right atrium. Intracardiac prostheses	Depending on results of laboratory testing, but start with cloxacillin or flucloxacillin plus one alternative, as for *S. aureus* *Other possibilities*: erythromycin, trimethoprim, ciprofloxacin
Group A streptococci	Skin and soft tissues (most cases). Rarely, postpartum infections, genitourinary disease or surgery, bone and joint infection, pharyngitis	Benzylpenicillin, third-generation cephalosporin or erythromycin *Alternative*: clindamycin
Group B streptococci	Neonatal infection (over 50% of all cases). Genitourinary infection or surgery, including termination of pregnancy	Benzylpenicillin *plus* gentamicin *Alternatives*: third-generation cephalosporins
Group C and G streptococci	Skin and soft tissue infection	Benzylpenicillin or third-generation cephalosporin
Streptococci milleri	Meningitis, ventriculitis, brain or liver abscess	As for group B streptococci

* May be given orally, but beware of emerging resistance.
† Beware of pseudomembranous colitis.

Table 15.1 Sources of coccal bacteraemias, and suggested empirical treatments

combined with metronidazole to cover the possibility of anaerobic bacteraemia (Table 15.3).

4 Enterococci are among the most difficult organisms to treat, as they are moderately resistant to many drugs, including the broad-spectrum cephalosporins. Ampicillin plus an aminoglycoside is a synergistic combination against enterococci, and is the treatment of choice except for rare, hospital-derived, gentamicin-resistant organisms. This mixture is adequate for many community-acquired coliforms also. Vancomycin plus gentamicin is also synergistic against enterococci, but cannot be used in mixtures with beta-lactams, as vancomycin is antagonistic to their actions (Table 15.4).

Some reports of vancomycin-resistant enterococci are now appearing. Most affected are intensive care units, particularly those with many surgical cases. Imipenem/cilastatin or meropenem may be effective (but *E. faecium* is resistant to meropenem).

General management of bacteraemic patients: systems and life support

However effective the chosen antibiotic therapy, the bacteraemic patient needs support until it has time to act. The effects of bacteraemia can be extremely damaging, and some patients have circulatory and organ failure at presentation.

Supporting the circulation

Supporting the circulation is usually the first priority. Shock occurs relatively early in Gram-negative bacteraemias, because of the high concentrations of endotoxin produced by many Gram-negative organisms. In Gram-positive bacteraemias the blood pressure is usually maintained until a late or preterminal stage, but

Organism	May originate from	Antimicrobial treatment
Escherichia coli (the cause of over 50% of all Gram-negative bacteraemias and about 25% of all bacteraemias)	Urinary tract colonization or infection, especially after instrumentation. Intestinal disease or surgery. Pancreaticobiliary disease, instrumentation or surgery	Ampicillin, amoxycillin or third-generation cephalosporin, e.g. cefotaxime or ceftriaxone *Alternatives*: gentamicin or other aminoglycoside (20–30% risk of resistance to ampicillin) Plasmid-mediated resistance to antibiotics is easily acquired in hospital, and has also (rarely) been associated with community-acquired infections
Klebsiella sp.: K. pneumoniae subsp. *pneumoniae* subsp. *aerogenes* subsp. *ozaenae* K. oxytoca	*K. pneumoniae* subsp. *pneumoniae* causes about 50% of all *Klebsiella* bacteraemias. Origins are as for *E. coli* plus rare cases of suppurative lobar pneumonia	Usually resistant to ampicillin Hospital-acquired strains often resistant to first- and second-generation cephalosporins and gentamicin *May be sensitive to*: third-generation cephalosporins, ureidopenicillins, e.g. piperacillin, carbapenems, e.g. imipenem/cilastatin or meropenem, tebramycin or amikacin
Enterobacter sp. and *Serratia* sp.	As for *E. coli*. Increasingly common in intensive care units and immunosuppressed patients	Third-generation cephalosporins Gentamicin and other aminoglycosides Ureidopenicillins Carbapenems
Proteus sp. (a member of the family Proteaceae which also includes *Morganella* and *Providencia*)	Genitourinary and pelvic disease, surgery and instrumentation. Renal or urinary tract stones (to which *Proteus* predisposes by metabolizing urea and forming alkaline ammonia)	As for *Enterobacter*
Salmonella sp.: including *S. typhi* and *S. paratyphi* sp.	Food- and water-borne intestinal infection	Ciprofloxacin *Alternatives*: chloramphenicol, ampicillin (if sensitive) (see also Chapter 8)

Table 15.2 Sources of Gram-negative bacteraemias and suggested empirical treatments

when shock develops it is indistinguishable from that of Gram-negative disease and demands urgent treatment.

The initial step is to obtain an adequate intravascular fluid volume. There is some controversy as to whether crystalloid fluids (such as saline solutions) or colloids (such as albumin or polygels) are most effective. Crystalloids are quite widely distributed in the interstitial fluid as well as intravascularly; they provide filterable solute for the renal tubules and can replenish lost intracellular fluid, but they are also quickly excreted. Colloids tend to remain in the vascular space; they improve blood pressure and organ perfusion but cannot pass through glomeruli. Different colloid substances are broken down in the circulation at different rates, and the

longer-lasting ones may be hard to recover if the patient becomes overhydrated or develops pulmonary oedema.

Current practice is to give crystalloids first for an immediate effect, and then to follow up with colloid. The three most useful monitors of circulatory function are the blood pressure, the central venous pressures and the urine output. The blood pressure need not be completely normalized, provided that cerebral function, urine output and tissue perfusion are adequate. A right atrial pressure of 5–10 mmHg is usually adequate. Higher pressures are not often helpful and may contribute to congestive cardiac failure and poor tissue perfusion. The pulmonary capillary wedge pressure may be measured, using a flotation balloon catheter. If it is substantially

Organism	May originate from	Antimicrobial treatment
Pseudomonas sp. and *Burkholderia* sp.	Immunocompromised patients (25% of all cases). Intensive care unit cases. Biliary tract disease, surgery or instrumentation	Gentamicin, tobramycin or amikacin. Azlocillin or piperacillin. Cefotaxime or ceftazidime. Aztreonam. Imipenem or mecropenem. (Often a combination of aminoglycoside with another drug is used, as resistance is common in hospital-acquired infection)
Acinetobacter sp.	Immunocompromised patients (33% of all cases). Intravenous devices. Cardiac prostheses. Rarely, neurosurgical procedures	Third-generation cephalosporins, e.g. cefotaxime, ceftriaxone. Imipenem or meropenem *Alternatives*: gentamicin or other aminoglycoside if sensitive. Piperacillin if sensitive
Bacteroides sp. (especially *B. fragilis*)	Abdominopelvic disease or surgery. Liver abscess. Rarely, postpartum	Metronidazole *Alternative*: clindamycin, meropenem
Clostridium sp. (including *C. perfringens*)	As for *Bacteroides*, but also biliary tract sepsis, perineal or lower limb trauma, soil-contaminated or necrotic wounds	Metronidazole *Alternatives*: benzylpenicillin
Anaerobic cocci (including *Peptococcus* and *Peptostreptococcus*)	Postpartum infections. Abdominopelvic disease or sepsis. Rarely, neonatal bacteraemia	Metronidazole, benzylpenicillin or ampicillin *Alternatives*: clindamycin
Enterococci (including *Enterococcus faecalis*, *E. faecium* and *Streptococcus durans*)	Intravascular cannulae, especially in intensive care unit patients (25% of all cases). Pancreaticobiliary disease, surgery or instrumentation. Abdominopelvic disease or surgery	Ampicillim plus gentamicin *Alternatives*: vancomycin plus or minus gentamicin. Imipenem/cilastatin, meropenem (not *E. faecium*)

Table 15.3 Sources of 'hospital' bacteraemias and suggested empirical treatments

higher than the right atrial pressure, the left ventricle is not adequately moving blood from the lungs, which may be oedematous; in these circumstances there is often poor systemic perfusion and/or a high vascular resistance.

The difference between the body's core temperature and skin temperature gives an idea of skin, and therefore tissue, perfusion. If the skin temperature (usually measured at the foot) is more than 2°C lower than the core (measured rectally or at the eardrum), this suggests inadequate tissue perfusion. If the temperatures are nearly equal, there may be pathological vasodilatation and increased cardiac output, indicating possible endotoxaemia or uncontrolled sepsis.

Drugs used to support the circulation

These are only effective if there is sufficient intravascular fluid volume, indicated by adequate central venous pressure. Dopamine is routinely used in infusions of up to 4 μg/kg per min, as this has an inotropic effect on the heart and a vasodilator effect on the kidney and general circulation. Higher doses cause vasoconstriction and tachycardia, and may contribute to heart failure.

Dobutamine may be added in infusions of 2.5–10 μg/kg per min for extra inotropic effect.

Poor tissue perfusion can be exacerbated by persistent vasoconstriction, and inappropriate shunting of blood. This can affect the pulmonary circulation as well as the periphery. In intractable pulmonary oedema, reducing cardiac afterload by inducing vasodilatation can produce clinical improvement. Various vasodilator drugs are available, including infusions of glyceryl trinitrate, isosorbide dinitrate and sodium nitroprusside. Prostacyclin is a natural vasodilator which reduces platelet aggregation. Its potential in bacteraemic shock has yet to be fully assessed, but it is increasingly used, especially when its antiplatelet action is desirable. It potentiates the action of anticoagulants.

Managing hypoxia

Tissue oxygenation depends on both adequate lung function and good tissue perfusion. Bacteraemic patients may have a defect of pulmonary gas transfer caused by both interstitial oedema and ventilation–perfusion mismatch. Increasing the percentage of inspired oxygen will increase the arterial oxygen saturation, and this can be

Antimicrobial agent	Adverse reactions and problems	Action to avoid adverse reactions and problems
Benzylpenicillin Flucloxacillin Ampicillin	Skin rashes	Avoid penicillins; cephalosporins may be given cautiously
	Cholestasis	Not usually intolerable; resolves on discontinuing drug
	Anaphylaxis (rare)	Avoid all penicillins. Avoid other beta-lactams where possible
	Agranulocytosis (rare)	Check white cell count during prolonged, high-dose treatment. Will occur with all beta-lactams — avoid
Erythromycin	Nausea	Substitute another drug (clarithromycin or non-macrolide drug)
Cephalosporins	Skin rashes	Avoid cephalosporins
	Thrombocytopenia (rare) Defective coagulation (rare)	Check platelet count during high-dose treatment. Oral cephalosporins may be given cautiously in future
Aminoglycosides	Impaired renal function Ototoxicity	Renally excreted; reduce dose in renal impairment; *always* monitor peak and trough blood levels. Avoid co-administration of frusemide (also ototoxic)
	Exacerbation of myaesthenia gravis	Avoid
Clindamycin (a lincoside)	Antibiotic-associated diarrhoea and pseudomembranous colitis	Discontinue drug if diarrhoea occurs. Persisting diarrhoea with fever and abdominal pain, may be treated with oral vancomycin (see p. 173)
Vancomycin (a glycopeptide)	Hypersensitivity reaction with vasodilatation, collapse and possible renal failure	*Never give by rapid injection.* Always infuse dose over at least 60 min for each 500 mg
	Ototoxicity	Reduce dose in renal impairment, monitor peak and trough blood levels. Use with *caution* if combined with aminoglycoside
	Nephrotoxicity	
Teicoplanin (a glycopeptide)	As for vancomycin, but does not cause hypersensitivity reaction. Less toxic	*May* be given by intravenous or intramuscular injection. *No* requirement for blood-level monitoring
Ciprofloxacin (a 4-quinolone)	Skin rashes	Discontinue or substitute an alternative drug
	Diarrhoea	Avoid
	Precipitation or exacerbation of epilepsy	
	Enhances effect of warfarin, aminophyllined sulphonyl ureas	Avoid or use with caution and frequent monitoring

Table 15.4 Adverse effects of antimicrobial agents used in treating bacteraemias

monitored by pulse oximetry or arterial blood-gas estimations. Removal of carbon dioxide is not increased, however, and care must be taken not to allow the patient to become severely hypercapnic as this impairs cardiac function, increases acidosis and raises intracranial pressure.

Positive-pressure ventilation will overcome decreased lung compliance and may also expel fluid from the oedematous lungs. It can be beneficial for both oxygen and carbon dioxide exchange. Positive end-expiratory pressure or continuous positive airways pressure may afford a better improvement. They have the disadvantage of reducing venous return and cardiac output, so often cause a requirement for increased cardiovascular support. Dopamine, dobutamine and even isoprenaline are sometimes given for this purpose in intensive care settings.

Combating toxaemia

The idea of removing toxins from the circulation by blood or plasma exchange is attractive, and has been trialled on several occasions in both Gram-positive and Gram-negative infections. Perhaps because of the difficulty of comparing gravely ill patients with multiple metabolic problems, the results have not been conclusive and benefit has not been demonstrated. High-dose corticosteroids have also been tried for their tissue-protective effects of inhibiting inflammation, but it is now generally accepted that they have no demonstrable benefit. Prostacyclin is being considered for its anti-inflammatory, vasodilator and antiplatelet properties but is, as yet, unproven.

Direct inhibition of endotoxin effects is theoretically possible, using monoclonal antiendotoxin antibodies. Two large trials have been criticized for their methodology. While there is slight evidence that the treatment offers some advantage in patients who have Gram-negative organisms in their blood, this is outweighed by a decrease in survival in non-bacteraemic patients receiving antibody treatment. Antibody preparations are not therefore currently available for clinical use.

Increasing knowledge of pathogenetic mechanisms in sepsis suggests that inhibition of granulocyte action may reduce the production of inflammatory mediators and damaging enzymes. Similarly, inhibition of the action of tumour necrosis factor may be beneficial. Antitumour necrosis factor, anti-CD18 and integrin antagonists are all under consideration as treatments for septic shock. The balance of therapeutic benefit versus the cost of inhibiting natural immune responses is currently unmeasured.

Nutrition

Patients with bacteraemic diseases have very high calorie requirements, and rapid turnover of macro- and micronutrients. Nowadays it is considered important to support nutrition early in intensive management. Intragastric feeding is physiological and prevents atrophy of the intestinal mucosa; well-designed enteral diets are available for this purpose. Nasogastric intubation is unpleasant and increases management requirements in intubated patients, so endoscopically placed gastrostomy catheters are increasingly used when long-term enteral nutrition is needed.

Patients with reduced bowel function cannot absorb enteral nutrients and must be fed parenterally. This is usually done via a dedicated lumen of a multilumen right atrial catheter. A gradual change is made to enteral feeding as soon as improving bowel function allows.

General management of bacteraemic patients
1 Optimize intravascular and tissue fluid volumes, using crystalloid and colloid infusions and measure arterial and central venous pressures.
2 Support circulatory function, using inotropic and/or vasodilator agents.
3 Optimize oxygen delivery to the tissues by giving oxygen with or without positive-pressure ventilation.
4 Combat toxaemia (theoretical treatment) with anti-tumour necrosis factor antibodies or other antagonists of toxic mediators.
5 Maintain adequate nutrition, using enteral or parenteral feeding techniques.

Staphylococcal septicaemia

Introduction and epidemiology

Staphylococcus aureus is the commonest cause of Gram-positive septicaemia. Although it can complicate hospital treatments or trauma (intravenous cannulae, temporary and permanent pacing catheters, surgical and traumatic wounds are all important portals of entry), half of all cases are community-derived and affect previously healthy people. It is an important disease because it affects all age groups, has an insidious onset, and the diagnosis is often overlooked or missed because sufferers do not initially appear gravely ill. It carries a high mortality in the elderly.

Pathology

It is easy to imagine the replication of staphylococci within an intravenous device, or in the track which it makes from the skin. In patients with no such predisposing factor, the means of establishment of bacteraemia is not understood. There appears to be no tendency for a particular strain of *Staphylococcus* to predominate.

Phagocytosis is important in defence against staphylococci. Children with cystic fibrosis have poor phagocyte function, and tend to suffer severe staphylococcal chest infections. It is known that patients whose phagocytes cannot mount a bactericidal respiratory burst, as in chronic granulomatous disease, are at risk of repeated staphylococcal infections.

Clinical features

The onset of illness is often slow, with increasing fever and malaise eventually causing the patient to become bed-bound. In some cases a large joint may be painful, often without effusion or surrounding inflammation. The underlying disease may be hinted at by severe periarticular tenderness of all joints, by groups of small pustules on the skin, or by pleurisy or cough.

By the time of admission to hospital patients usually have high, swinging fever, but are haemodynamically normal. Very few patients have an obvious skin infection, abscess or toxic rash, though rare cases have coexisting toxic shock syndrome (see Chapter 5).

The white cell count is often misleadingly normal, but the proportion of neutrophils is usually near 90%. After some days of illness a conventional leukocytosis develops. The platelet count may be slightly reduced. Renal function is moderately impaired; proteinuria and microscopic haematuria are common. In half or more of cases the chest X-ray is abnormal, showing nodular opacities or abscesses, an area of consolidation, effusion or pleural abscess.

If the condition is untreated, progressive renal failure tends to occur (probably because of numerous foci of infection in the kidneys). Disseminated intravascular coagulation is common and can cause loss of digits or limbs. Metastatic infections are a real danger and include acute endocarditis, pneumonia, suppurative arthritis, soft-tissue abscesses and sometimes abscesses of the kidney, liver or brain.

Diagnosis

Even in patients who have received oral antibiotics, blood cultures are usually positive in all bottles within 18–24 h.

Management

As soon as cultures have been obtained, treatment should begin with intravenous cloxacillin or flucloxacillin, in divided doses totalling at least 6 g/day. A second drug is usually added, as in some tissue sites flucloxacillin does not reach bactericidal levels. Either fusidic acid or rifampicin can be used. Both are well-distributed in the body, but fusidic acid penetrates the cerebrospinal fluid less readily than rifampicin. Rifampicin may be preferable in the presence of meningitis or endocarditis. Fusidic acid is difficult to give via peripheral veins as it is very irritant, but both drugs are well-absorbed orally or intragastrically. Neither fusidic acid nor rifampicin should be given alone, because bacteria can make a one-step mutation to become completely resistant to them. A population of resistant organisms can emerge within 4 or 5 days.

Most *S. aureus* organisms are sensitive to aminoglycosides on laboratory testing. These may be useful additional drugs. Possibly because of relatively poor penetration into abscesses, they sometimes produce disappointing results when used as antistaphylococcal monotherapy.

In patients who have skin allergies to penicillins, cephradine or cefuroxime may be substituted, but should not be given to patients who have anaphylactic reactions to penicillin. In such difficult situations, clindamycin, teicoplanin or ciprofloxacin may be useful.

Vancomycin is the treatment of choice for organisms resistant to cloxacillin. This drug must be given as an infusion over 90 min. This avoids the severe hypersensitivity reaction of vasodilatation (red man syndrome) and acute hypotension. It also avoids high peak levels, which predispose to nephrotoxicity and ototoxicity. Peak and trough levels should be monitored at the end of infusion and immediately before the next dose. They should not be greater than 30 and 10 mg/l respectively. The dose should be reduced in renal impairment. Aminoglycosides and loop diuretics enhance vancomycin toxicity. Teicoplanin may be an effective alternative, but some staphylococci have increased minimum inhibitory concentration (MIC) and minimum bacteriocidal concentration (MBC) values for this drug.

Important antistaphylococcal drugs

Flucloxacillin i.v., 1–2 g 6-hourly (child under 2 years, 250–500 mg 6-hourly; 2–10 years, 500 mg to 1 g 6-hourly); *or*

Cloxacillin i.v., 500 mg to 1 g 4–6-hourly (child under 2 years, 125–250 mg 6-hourly; 2–10 years, 250–500 mg 6-hourly); *plus*

Fusidic acid orally 750 mg 8-hourly (child under 1 year, 50 mg/kg daily; 1–5 years, 750 mg daily; 5–12 years, 1.5 g daily, all in three divided doses) or i.v. 580 mg 8-hourly; *or*

Rifampicin orally or i.v., 300–600 mg 12-hourly (child under 3 months, 5 mg/kg 12-hourly; 3 months to 12 years, 10 mg/kg 12-hourly to maximum 600 mg/day); *or*

Gentamicin by slow i.v. injection, 2–5 mg/kg daily in three divided doses (child under 2 weeks, 3 mg/kg 12-hourly; 2 weeks to 12 years, 2 mg/kg 8-hourly); plasma levels should peak (1 h after dose) not above 10 mg/l, trough not above 2 mg/l.

Alternative drugs

1 Cephradine i.v. 1–2 g 6-hourly (child 50–100 mg/kg daily in four divided doses).

2 Cefuroxime i.v. 750 mg to 1.5 g 6–8-hourly (child 60–100 mg/kg daily in three divided doses).

3 Trimethoprim by slow i.v. injection or infusion, 150–250 mg 12-hourly (child 6–9 mg/kg daily in two or three divided doses).

4 Vancomycin i.v. infusion over 90 min, 500 mg 6-hourly (neonate up to 1 week, 15 mg/kg followed by 10 mg/kg 12-hourly; 1–4 weeks, 15 mg/kg followed by 10 mg/kg 8-hourly; child over 1 month, 10 mg/kg 6-hourly) plasma levels should peak (1 h after dose) not above 30 mg/l, trough not above 10 mg/l.
5 Teicoplanin i.v. 400 mg 12-hourly for three doses, then 400 mg daily — may be reduced to 200 mg daily after good response (child over 2 months, 10 mg/kg daily — may be reduced to 5 mg/kg daily after good response).
6 Clindamycin orally 300–600 mg 6-hourly — may be increased to 900 mg 6-hourly in life-threatening disease (child over 1 month, 30–40 mg/kg daily — *minimum* 300 mg daily at any age); discontinue immediately if diarrhoea or colitis develops.

Coagulase-negative staphylococci

Coagulase-negative staphylococci are common causes of bacteraemia in neonatal intensive care. They are particularly associated with the use of indwelling intravenous devices, and are a hazard of cardiac surgery. Many are resistant to flucloxacillin and cloxacillin. They must therefore be treated as methicillin-resistant staphylococci, with teicoplanin, vancomycin, gentamicin, fusidic acid, clindamycin or trimethoprim, depending ultimately on the results of sensitivity testing.

The duration of treatment will depend on response. Uncomplicated cases can be adequately treated with 7–10 days' antibiotics. Cases with multiple abscesses or loculated infections need longer courses. Formal drainage may be required for conditions such as empyema, large lung abscess or secondary bone infection. Complicating endocarditis needs long-term treatment and follow-up (see Chapter 14).

Streptococcal septicaemia

Introduction and epidemiology

Streptococcus pyogenes is a common commensal of the skin and upper respiratory tract. It can also colonize the female genital tract following examination or manipulation during pregnancy and delivery. It causes infections of the tonsils (see Chapter 6) and the skin (see Chapter 5).

Many cases of streptococcal septicaemia appear to originate in the skin or throat. The originating infection may, however, be trivial. Examples include small cuts or abrasions, which may have healed by the time bacteraemia is recognized. A minority of cases are streptococcal puerperal fever, which may follow normal or assisted delivery, Caesarean section or other gynaecological procedures (see Chapter 12).

Although a rarer cause of bacteraemia than *Staphylococcus aureus*, the meningococcus or the pneumococcus, *Streptococcus pyogenes* is a dangerous organism; the mortality of treated streptococcal septicaemia is 25–30% in most western countries.

Pathology

No specific predisposition to streptococcal bacteraemia is recognized. There are many strains of *S. pyogenes*, and it is well-recognized that some are more virulent than others. Different strains predominate for several years at a time in slow epidemic fluctuations. M1 types have produced serious disease in the UK in the 1990s. These strains have shown a significant incidence of resistance to erythromycin.

Clinical features

The presenting complaint is usually of severe feverish illness with a short history of 1 or 2 days. If a preceding event is recognized, this has an onset 3–5 days before the development of bacteraemia. Small skin lesions may have healed in this time, even though colonized by the streptococci. A sinister warning feature is severe pain and induration of regional lymph nodes draining the original site. This may be seen in the axilla if a hand or arm lesion is implicated, in the inguinal region following erysipelas or injury of the leg, or in the tonsillar nodes in the case of tonsillitis. The affected nodes are often surrounded by extensive oedema, and sometimes by spreading erythema. Sloughing of the nodes is occasionally seen.

There is not usually any other physical finding, unless areas of erysipelas, cellulitis or a scarlet fever-like rash develop. The appearance of erysipelas, other than in the typical sites on the face or leg, is strongly suggestive of bacteraemia. Occasionally the fever is accompanied by a septic arthritis or abscess of a lymph node or parotid gland. Puerperal fever may be marked by pelvic pain and offensive lochia.

Non-specific features of severe illness may be prominent. These include watery diarrhoea, persistent vomiting, meningism or pain in the back or thighs.

The white cell count shows a modest leukocytosis of 12 or $13 \times 10^9/l$. Renal and liver function is usually maintained, as is the blood pressure, until the preterminal stages. As illness progresses, an ill-defined pneumonia or a pleural effusion may occur. In untreated cases, shock and profound hypoxia can develop very quickly and are extremely difficult to reverse.

Diagnosis

Initial suspicion must often be based on clinical clues. Appropriate specimens from throat, skin or other lesions may produce a growth of beta-haemolytic streptococci within 24 h. Blood cultures are not reliably positive for up to 3 days in some cases, as *S. pyogenes* has a slow initial growth curve.

Management

The most urgent requirement is high-dose intravenous antimicrobial therapy. *S. pyogenes* is very sensitive to benzylpenicillin on laboratory testing, and this is the treatment of choice. A suitable dose is 1.2 g 2-hourly. It is notoriously difficult to eradicate streptococcal bacteraemia, so the dose should not be reduced too soon after an apparently good response. High dosage for 4–5 days may be needed before intermittent recurrences of fever and toxaemia are controlled. A further 7 days or more of conventional dosage are then advisable.

Even though normotensive and well-oxygenated on presentation, a significant proportion of patients will need respiratory and circulatory support and monitoring as their treatment continues. Tissue damage caused by the streptococcal toxins tends to progress for many hours after the start of treatment. Erythemas may appear; inspired oxygen requirements may increase; inotropic support may be indicated and a few patients need a period of positive-pressure ventilation.

It may be tempting to alter the treatment if an intermittent or slow response to therapy occurs. This is not always wise, as few drugs are as effective as penicillin. Broad-spectrum cephalosporins are not reliable alternatives, nor is ciprofloxacin. Erythromycin is ineffective against a minority of virulent strains. A change of therapy should therefore be made only for compelling reasons, or when it is impossible to maintain high-dose penicillin treatment. Failure to respond or cessation of progress after a response may be better managed by increased penicillin dosage (limited only by nausea, drowsiness or other penicillin toxicity) than a change of drug.

Additional drugs such as clindamycin or an aminoglycoside do not always confer benefit, but could be tried in the face of deterioration in the patient's condition.

Complications

A common complication of treatment is an unpredictable intermittent fever caused by mild hypersensitivity to the high penicillin dosage. So long as the patient's physical condition is improving, this is not an indication to change the treatment.

The classic poststreptococcal conditions of rheumatic fever, erythema nodosum and erythema multiforme are rarely seen, but scarlet fever may occur. When it does, it is often severe, with pleural effusion, ascites, renal impairment and hypotension.

Tissue necrosis occasionally occurs, even when the bacteraemia is relatively easily controlled. The commonest example is suppuration of affected lymph nodes. Rare cases are reported of necrosis of lymph nodes or infected tissues.

Gram-negative septicaemia

Introduction and epidemiology

Gram-negative septicaemia almost always originates from the organs of the abdomen or pelvis. In young age groups appendicitis, trauma or gastroduodenal surgery are the commonest predispositions. In middle age, gallbladder or biliary disease and bowel surgery are more common. In the elderly, or those such as multiple sclerosis sufferers, bladder emptying is inefficient and the urine is often colonized with organisms; the urinary tract then becomes an important source of bacteraemia.

Escherichia coli is by far the commonest cause of Gram-negative bacteraemias.

Clinical features

While many Gram-negative bacteraemias are continuous, some are intermittent, with bacteria being released into the blood on one or two occasions in any day or week (Fig. 15.6). In either case, the bacteraemia is accompanied by fever, usually severe rigors, tachycardia and a lowered blood pressure. In continuous bacteraemias the blood pressure can be sufficiently low to compromise cerebral and renal perfusion, while in the intermittent type, it usually normalizes when the bacteraemia ceases after 30–90 min.

Significant abnormality of the prothrombin time tends to occur early in Gram-negative bacteraemias, and elevation of fibrin degradation products may indicate consumptive coagulopathy. The white cell count usually

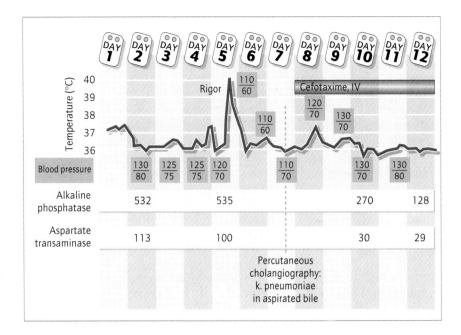

Fig. 15.6 Intermittent Gram-negative bacteraemia: this patient's gallbladder was colonized with *Klebsiella pneumoniae*; his fevers were accompanied by rigors and hypotension; the fever and liver function improved with antibiotic treatment.

shows a neutrophilia, but in overwhelming sepsis there may be a low white cell count.

Diagnosis

Apart from the task of identifying the organisms in the blood, early management should include detecting their origin and treating any underlying condition. Imaging of the pancreaticobiliary system or renal drainage system is particularly worthwhile in intermittent bacteraemias. Disease of the bowel will often reveal itself by causing pain or bowel dysfunction. This is helpful when ulcer disease, malignancy or diverticulitis are the origin of the infection. Patients with colonized urine, however, often have clinical features of bacteraemia but without urinary symptoms.

It is often impossible to guess clinically whether a patient has an *E. coli* septicaemia or one of the less common enterobacterial, enterococcal or anaerobic infections. Only the results of blood culture can confirm this.

Management

General supportive measures are often required. The choice of antimicrobial chemotherapy usually needs to include initial cover for Enterobacteriaceae, enterococci and anaerobes. Combinations of drugs are recommended in this setting. Ampicillin or amoxycillin plus an aminoglycoside is effective against *E. coli* and enterococci. A broad-spectrum cephalosporin is effective against many coliforms, but may not be adequate for enterococci, and an aminoglycoside may be added. Imipenem/cilastatin or meropenem is often effective against both, and is useful in intensive care units where gentamicin-resistant enterococci may exist. Metronidazole is reliable additional treatment to cover anaerobic organisms.

Typical regimens for treating Gram-negative bacteraemia

Ampicillin i.v. 500 mg to 1 g 4–6-hourly (child under 10 years, 50–100 mg/kg daily in four to six divided doses); *or*

Cefotaxime i.v. 1–2 g 8-hourly (neonate 100–200 mg/kg daily; child 150–200 mg/kg daily, both in two to four divided doses); *plus*

Gentamicin by slow i.v. injection, 2–5 mg/kg daily in three divided doses (child under 2 weeks, 3 mg/kg 12-hourly; 2 weeks to 12 years, 2 mg/kg 8-hourly). Plasma concentrations should peak (1 h after dose) not above 10 mg/l, trough not above 2 mg/l; *plus*

Metronidazole rectally, 1 g 8-hourly or i.v. 500 mg 8-hourly (child, any route, 7.5 mg/kg 8-hourly).

Alternatives

Imipenem (with cilastatin) i.v., 2–4 g daily in three or four divided doses (child over 3 months, 60 mg/kg daily in four divided doses — maximum 2 g/day).

Meropenem i.v. 1 g 8-hourly (2 g 8-hourly for meningitis) (child 3 months to 12 years, 10–20 mg/kg 8-hourly).

For pseudomonal infections
Gentamicin or another aminoglycoside may be given with (but not mixed in the same syringe or infusion) azlocillin i.v. 2–5 g 8-hourly (neonate 100 mg/kg 12-hourly; 7 days to 1 year, 100 mg/kg 8-hourly; 1–14 years, 75 mg/kg 8-hourly); *or*
Piperacillin i.v., all ages, 200–300 mg/kg daily in four to six divided doses.

The antibiotic spectrum may be narrowed, or the least toxic drugs selected, when the results of culture are available.

Complications

The most important complication is failure of the fever, hypotension and clotting abnormalities to resolve on appropriate antibiotic treatment. The usual reason for this is loculated infection, in which the organisms are relatively inaccessible to the antibiotic.

If the kidney or pancreaticobiliary system is the suspected source of the bacteraemia, the drainage of these systems must be examined. Ureteric stricture, or obstruction by inspissated pus, may prevent resolution of infection in the ipsilateral kidney. Biliary stricture will prevent healing of gallbladder disease.

If the bowel is suspected, radiography, ultrasound or isotope imaging may reveal an abscess as the source of infection. Appropriate drainage will often permit resolution of the local infection and abolish bacteraemia.

Follow-up of patients with bacteraemia

In patients responding to treatment of their bacteraemia, it is tempting to cease follow-up when the temperature has resolved and chemotherapy has been terminated. Patients should be reviewed, however, as recurrence sometimes occurs. A particular danger is that of persisting undetected predisposition (such as a carcinoma of the colon or a biliary stricture) or unrecognized complicating endocarditis. Examination should always be performed to detect abdominal tenderness, an enlarged liver or gallbladder or developing heart murmurs. It is also useful to review the erythrocyte sedimentation rate or C-reactive protein measurement, as a rise in either can give early warning of continuing infection.

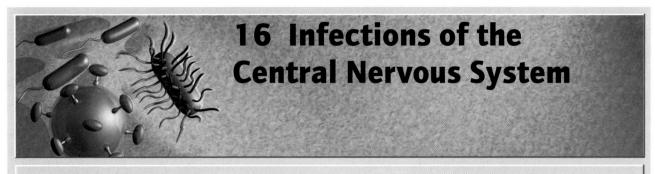

16 Infections of the Central Nervous System

Introduction

Structural and functional considerations

The structure of the nervous system is such that the brain and spinal cord form a special compartment of the body. The cerebrospinal fluid (CSF) is different from other body fluids, in particular having a low protein content, including very low immunoglobulin levels. The central nervous system (CNS) has no lymphatics, but depends on migration of lymphocytes to and from the blood circulation.

The layers of the meninges support and protect the brain and spinal cord, and contain the CSF. Together with their blood vessels, choroid plexuses and arachnoid processes, the meninges constitute a structural and functional barrier between the blood and the CSF. This is called the blood–brain barrier. It permits the brain to maintain its own homeostatic environment, with its own acid–base equilibrium. It inhibits the entry of organisms, and of many drugs and toxins.

During an inflammatory process, fast-reacting proteins appear in the CSF, mostly by diffusion from the blood, with the low-molecular-weight, more diffusible proteins appearing in highest concentrations. Immunoglobulins diffuse into the CSF but can also be locally manufactured once lymphocytes have migrated from the circulation. Both lymphocytes and neutrophils are able to enter the CSF during infection and inflammation.

It is possible to deduce that a specific antibody is being manufactured locally, and not just diffusing into the CSF, by comparing the ratio of its CSF : blood concentrations with the ratio for an antibody unlikely to be involved with acute CNS disease. For instance, if herpes simplex antibody is manufactured locally in a case of herpes simplex encephalitis, its CSF : blood concentration ratio will be higher than that of, say, rubella antibodies. Most virology departments will estimate these types of ratios in suspected viral infections. The relationship between the ratios is an antibody index.

An antibody index

$$\frac{\text{CSF : serum ratio of the antibody in question}}{\text{CSF : serum ratio of reference (e.g. rubella) antibody}}$$

If this index is greater than 2, local production of the antibody in question may be assumed.

The more the blood–brain barrier is disrupted by inflammation, the more protein and cells appear in the CSF. This may have advantages in permitting more effective immune responses, and also in allowing the rapid entry of therapeutic drugs such as penicillins or vancomycin which penetrate the intact blood–brain barrier rather poorly. The immediate disadvantages of inflammation and exudation are the elevation of intracranial pressure, with consequent reduction in cerebral perfusion pressure (the difference between blood pressure and CSF pressure) and reduced cerebral blood flow. Intense inflammation causes protein accumulation and fibrin deposition. This can obstruct the aqueduct, or the foramina of the brain, causing local or general hydrocephalus.

Inflammatory changes can be inhibited by the use of corticosteroids and by some non-steroidal anti-inflammatory drugs, especially if these are given early, but it is not clear whether this improves the outlook in many diseases.

Rising CSF pressure is also related to changes in the water content of the brain. It is now recognized that increased brain water is not necessarily equivalent to cerebral oedema, as the water may be in other compartments than the interstitium. In meningitis, particularly, it is no longer the custom to limit fluid intake as, rather than preventing a rise in intracranial pressure, it reduces blood volume and impairs cerebral perfusion. In encephalitis there may be true cerebral oedema, often demonstrable by computed tomographic (CT) or magnetic resonance (MR) scanning. It may then be possible to reduce oedema with dexamethasone treatment.

Effects of meningeal inflammation
1 Increasing cerebrospinal fluid (CSF) protein and cell count.
2 Increased entry of water-soluble antibiotics.
3 Increased brain water.
4 Increased CSF (= intracranial) pressure.
5 Reduced cerebral perfusion pressure.
6 Risk of CSF obstruction leading to hydrocephalus.

The incidence of deafness following some types of acute meningitis is reduced by early dexamethasone treatment. The reason for this is uncertain; it may be reduction of oedema or inflammation, or possibly protection of the cochlear hair cells from the action of endotoxin.

Pathogenesis of CNS infections

Many infections of the brain and spinal cord are blood-borne. This is suggested by the fact that the causative organism colonizes or infects other sites of the body before causing CNS disease. Thus, the viruses of meningitis are often found in the throat and bowel as well as in the CSF; a neonate with cutaneous herpes simplex lesions is at risk of developing encephalitis; in bacterial meningitis, the causative organisms appear first in the nasopharynx, then in the blood and lastly in the CSF.

It is relatively uncommon for the CNS to be infected by the spread of organisms from adjacent structures. However, pneumococcal infection may arise from chronic infection in the paranasal sinuses or the middle ear. This is much more likely if there is a defect in the meninges, usually a tear in the dura mater following head injury, surgery or other damage (in this situation recurrent meningitis may occur). It is thought that amoebic meningitis arises by migration by amoebae through the cribriform plate.

There are rare examples of spread of pathogens along nerve trunks or between segments of the spinal cord. Rabies viruses enter peripheral nerves and migrate to the CNS where they then cause infection. The incubation period is proportional to the length of nerve which must be traversed. Transection of the nerve trunk or amputation of the injured limb will prevent rabies in animals. Herpes zoster viruses can enter the spinal cord via a dorsal root and spread segment by segment, causing an ascending myelo-encephalitis.

Modes of pathogenesis of central nervous system infections
1 Infection during viraemic phase of viral infections.
2 Blood-borne spread from local or bacteraemic bacterial infection.
3 Contiguous spread from intracranial infective focus.
4 Entry of bacteria through a defect in the dura.
5 Rare spread through cribriform plate.
6 Rare spread along nerve fibres and connections.

Meningitis and meningism

Introduction

Meningitis is inflammation of the meninges. Meningism is the group of symptoms and signs which accompanies the inflammation. The symptoms are headache, neck stiffness, nausea or vomiting and photophobia. The headache is global and usually described as the worst ever experienced. Photophobia is the most variable of the symptoms; in severe cases it may be very marked, but it can occur in a number of other conditions such as tension headache and migraine.

Main features of meningism
1 Headache.
2 Neck and back stiffness.
3 Nausea and vomiting.
4 Photophobia.

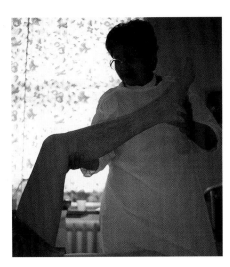

Fig. 16.1 Kernig's sign of meningism: the patient's leg cannot be straightened because of hamstring spasm.

Typical signs of meningism are uncommon in infants and small children, who rarely exhibit the features of neck and back stiffness. They usually simply appear flaccid, though in late disease they may develop opisthotonus. A bulging fontanelle is a useful sign of raised intracranial pressure in an infant. Fever and persistent vomiting are important warnings of meningitis in the under-2s, in whom meningism may also be absent.

Warning signs of meningism in infants
1 Bulging fontanelle.
2 Vomiting.
3 Strange cry.
4 Convulsions.
5 Opisthotonus.

Meningism can occur without meningitis. Quite distinct meningism can accompany upper lobe pneumonia, urinary tract infection and high fevers such as the prodromal fever of dysentery. In these conditions CSF examination is normal, and the subsequent investigation and evolution of the disease make the true diagnosis obvious. The mechanism of meningism without meningitis is unknown.

True meningism can also occur without significant fever in non-infectious conditions. The most important of these is subarachnoid haemorrhage, in which headache and nausea have a very abrupt onset and may be accompanied by collapse, loss of consciousness and/or abnormal neurological signs. Malignant infiltration of the meninges can also present with meningism. Leukaemic meningitis and metastatic melanoma are the commonest causes of this. Meningism is a rare adverse reaction to non-steroidal anti-inflammatory drugs, described most often after ibuprofen.

Conditions where meningism can occur without meningitis
1 Small children with high fevers.
2 Upper lobe pneumonias.
3 Acute urinary tract infections.
4 Subarachnoid haemorrhage.
5 Meningeal malignancies.

Physical signs of meningism

The two traditional tests for meningism are: (i) to attempt to flex the neck and touch the chin to the chest; and (ii) to elicit Kernig's sign (Fig. 16.1). These will easily demonstrate moderate-to-severe meningism, but mild meningism is sometimes missed. More subtle signs are the tripod sign, elicited when the patient is unable to sit up from a supine position without making a tripod with the hands resting on the bed behind him or her; and the inability to curl forwards enough to touch the nose to the knees (Fig. 16.2).

The detection of minimal meningism can be extremely important, first because it permits early clinical suspicion in developing meningitis, and second because diseases such as tuberculous meningitis may cause only the mildest meningism before major neurological deficit occurs.

Lumbar puncture

This is the most rapid diagnostic test for meningitis. It permits the distinction of bacterial meningitis from viral meningitis or meningoencephalitis. It often allows a rapid aetiological diagnosis of bacterial infection by Gram stain or slide agglutination test on CSF.

Nevertheless, lumbar puncture is not without risk; many fear that raised intracranial pressure will cause herniation of the brain through the foramen magnum if fluid is removed from the spinal theca. In fact, many thousands of lumbar punctures are performed without adverse incident. This is probably because the duration of raised intracranial pressure before presentation to medical care is short, and fibrosis has not yet interfered with normal CSF flow. Even if a degree of hydrocephalus is present, it is communicating, so that removing CSF from the lumbar theca will simply reduce intracranial pressure. Since fluid is incompressible, only a tiny amount need be removed to improve intracranial pressure and decrease the resistance to cerebral blood

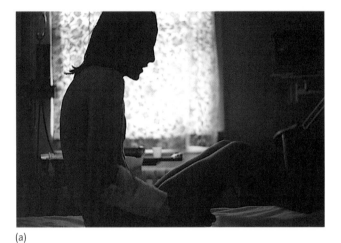
(a)

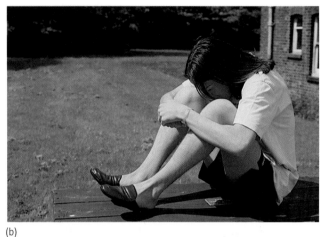
(b)

Fig. 16.2 Meningism can be easily demonstrated: this patient with meningococcal meningitis could not oppose his nose and knees (a), but after recovery (b), the manoeuvre was easily performed.

flow. Patients with moderate meningism often feel better and have reduced headache after lumbar puncture (Fig. 16.3).

The risk of herniation is greater, however, when the history of headache is longer than 3 or 4 days, when there are neurological signs of a space-occupying lesion or when it is known or suspected that a patient might have a history of tonsillar herniation. The presence of papilloedema also indicates increased risk. The absence of papilloedema means little, however, as it develops slowly, and is not always present when the CSF pressure

is high. If lumbar puncture may be dangerous, then a judgement must be made whether there is time to obtain an emergency CT scan. Where there are on-site facilities this can usually be carried out. In most cases, lumbar puncture can be performed after the scan has shown no contraindication. Otherwise, ventricular puncture may be required.

In rare situations it is possible to deduce the diagnosis and give emergency treatment without performing a lumbar puncture. This is so with childhood meningitis, particularly in the presence of a meningococcal rash. Problems may arise with this in the uncommon cases of streptococcal or staphylococcal meningitis with a purpuric rash. *Haemophilus influenzae* bacteraemia also occasionally causes a rash, but emergency treatment will usually cover for this disease, which is becoming less common since the introduction of immunization.

CSF examination

This is important as it provides not only diagnostic but prognostic information. It is essential that a simultaneous specimen of blood be obtained for glucose estimation so that the result of CSF glucose may be interpreted. Other important investigations include blood cultures, throat swabs and stool specimens (for viral culture).

Three specimens of CSF are collected into numbered universal containers, and one is collected into a blood sugar estimation bottle. From infants, only 10–12 drops of fluid should be taken for each specimen, while from older children and adults 1–2 ml can be collected.

The CSF cell count is performed by examining an unspun, unstained specimen in a counting chamber. The

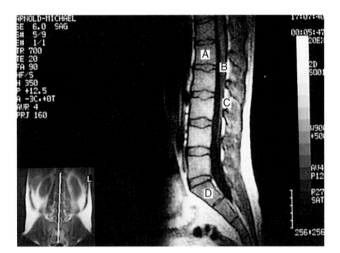

Fig. 16.3 Lateral magnetic resonance image of normal lumbar spine, showing the termination of the spinal cord at the L1/L2 level, leaving a space below filled with CSF and nerve roots; the optimum track for lumbar puncture is shown by the dotted line. A, body of 1st lumbar vertebra; B, lower extreme of the spinal cord; C, track of the lumbar puncture between spines of the 3rd and 4th lumbar vertebra; D, the sacrum.

cell types are identified by examination of a Giemsa-stained centrifuged deposit. The presence of neutrophils is associated with bacterial infections such as *Neisseria meningitidis*, *H. influenzae* or *Streptococcus pneumoniae*. The presence of lymphocytes is associated with infection with viruses, mycobacteria or *Leptospira*. A lymphocytic or mixed pleiocytosis may be seen in cases of partially treated pyogenic infection or in brain abscess.

Further information can be obtained from biochemical tests. The CSF protein level reflects the degree of meningeal inflammation. It is often two or three times normal in viral infections of the CNS, and up to five or 10 times normal in bacterial infections. In abscesses and chronic infections, such as tuberculous meningitis, it may reach very high levels. The CSF glucose level is usually normal in viral infections, significantly low in bacterial meningitis, and negligible in advanced tuberculous meningitis. As acute intracranial disorders can raise the blood glucose (often to 8–12 mmol/l), it is essential to compare the CSF glucose with a simultaneous blood glucose estimation.

Normal CSF composition includes:

1 Cells: <6 white blood cells, all lymphocytes; no red blood cells (in an atraumatic tap).

2 Protein: 0.1–0.4 g/l (lumbar theca); 0.07–0.25 g/l (ventricular).

3 Glucose: up to 1.7 mmol/l below blood glucose.

The centrifuged deposit should be stained by Gram's method to demonstrate pyogenic organisms. The sensitivity of Gram's stain is about 10^4 cfu/ml. This can be improved upon by using acridine orange. Ziehl–Nielsen stain should be employed if tuberculosis is suspected, or

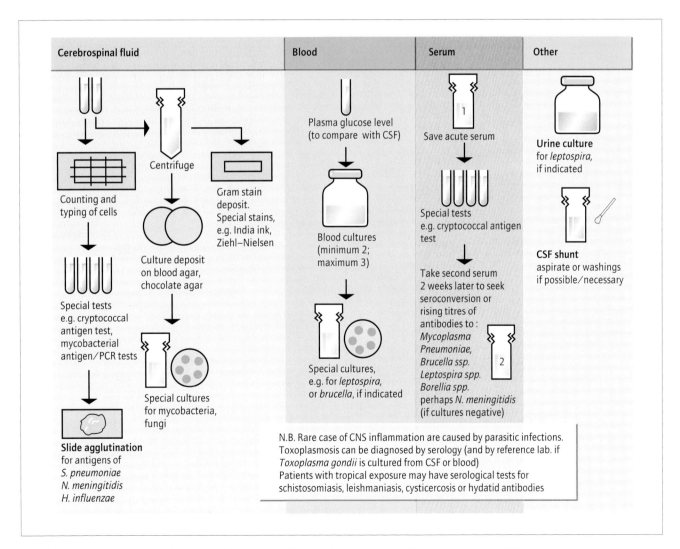

Fig. 16.4 Scheme for the investigation of bacterial meningitis. CNS, central nervous system; CSF, cerebrospinal fluid; PCR, polymerase chain reaction.

indicated by the cell count or biochemical examination. If cryptococcosis is suspected in an immunosuppressed patient, the CSF should be examined by an India ink method which outlines the fungal capsule in sharp relief.

Specimens from the centrifuged deposit are inoculated on to a range of media capable of growing the main pathogens. This usually includes blood and chocolate agar, together with an enrichment broth (such as tryptose broth, intended to amplify the sometimes scanty organisms). All colonies growing after 24 h are identified and sensitivity testing performed. If there is no bacterial growth after 24 h the enrichment broth is subcultured. It is important that all isolates are sent to reference laboratories for confirmation and typing (Fig. 16.4). In England and Wales they should also be reported to the Communicable Disease Surveillance Centre (CDSC; see Chapter 25), to update national records of current types and antimicrobial sensitivities of important pathogens.

The aetiological diagnosis of viral meningitis by CSF culture is often unrewarding. A better diagnostic yield, in enteroviral infections, is obtained from stool culture. Mumps or measles virus may be recovered from urine cultures. In suspected herpetic encephalitis, anti-herpes simplex virus antibody can be measured in the CSF, and the CSF : serum antibody ratio compared with that of rubella or measles (Fig. 16.5). Positive identification of viral agents in CNS disease should also be reported to CDSC .

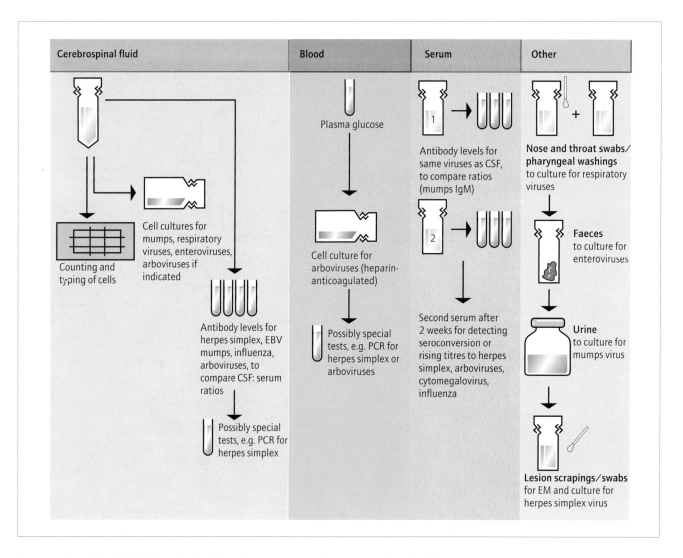

Fig. 16.5 Scheme for virological investigation of central nervous system disease. CSF, cerebrospinal fluid; EBV, Epstein–Barr virus; EM, electron microscopy; IgM, immunoglobulin M; PCR, polymerase chain reaction.

Rapid diagnostic techniques

The importance of pyogenic meningitis as a medical emergency has focused research on rapid diagnostic techniques. Some attempted to distinguish bacterial from viral infections, based on the detection of lactate or C-reactive protein. Unfortunately, CSF lactate was difficult to measure reliably, and was not clinically useful. C-reactive protein levels were found to indicate the intensity of inflammation rather than its aetiology.

The common bacteria causing pyogenic meningitis possess polysaccharide capsules, whose antigens can be detected by rapid methods. These methods include latex agglutination, coagglutination, counterimmunoelectrophoresis and enzyme immunoassay (EIA). Positive results can be obtained after antibiotics have been commenced and cultures become negative. Effective tests are available for *S. pneumoniae*, *H. influenzae* and *N. meningitidis* serogroup A, C and W135. Satisfactory results are more difficult to obtain with the less immunogenic *N. meningitidis* serogroup B.

The concentration of antigen indicates prognosis in *S. pneumoniae* infection, but studies for other pathogens are awaited. The impact of polymerase chain reaction (PCR)-based detection methods on rapid diagnosis in pyogenic meningitis is likely to be slight, because of the delay imposed by the amplification and detection stages. PCR may prove useful in diseases where CSF microscopy and culture are relatively slow or insensitive. Tuberculous meningitis and herpes simplex encephalitis are examples where useful PCR methods are becoming available.

Rapid diagnostic techniques which can be performed on cerebrospinal fluid
1 Gram stain of centrifuged deposit.
2 Special stains:
  (a) Ziehl–Nielsen (for acid-fast organisms).
  (b) India ink (for capsulated yeasts).
3 Slide agglutination tests:
  (a) *Neisseria meningitidis* A, C, W135, Y.
  (b) *Streptococcus pneumoniae*.
  (c) *Haemophilus influenzae*.
4 Antigen test: *Cryptococcus neoformans*.
5 Polymerase chain reaction DNA detection tests:
  (a) *Mycobacterium tuberculosis*.
  (b) Herpes simplex.

Examination for other pathogens

CSF examination contributes to the investigation of other infective conditions such as syphilis, Lyme disease and trypanosomiasis. In syphilis and Lyme disease serological investigations are important. In supected cerebral trypanosomiasis CSF should only be examined after the blood has been cleared of parasites with suramin. Trypanosomes can be concentrated by an anion exchange chromatography. The presence of parasites or of morula cells indicates CSF infection and the need for treatment with arsenical preparations.

Viral meningitis

Introduction

Viral meningitis is common worldwide. Approximately 1000 laboratory-confirmed cases are reported each year in the UK, but this is only a fraction of the total incidence as most infections are mild or inapparent. The illness is usually self-limiting, rarely lasting for more than a week. Its importance lies in the differential diagnosis from tuberculous (see Chapter 18) and acute bacterial meningitis, and from rare diseases such as listeriosis, borreliosis and cryptococcosis. In some places where immunization is still rare, viral meningitis can be caused by poliovirus, and may be followed by paralysis.

ORGANISM LIST

Echovirus
Coxsackievirus
Poliovirus
Mumpsvirus
Herpes simplex type 2
Herpes zoster
Influenza virus type A or B
Arboviruses (usually meningoencephalitis)
A rare effect of many virus infections, such as rubella and Epstein–Barr virus infection.

Enterovirus meningitis

Introduction and epidemiology

Young children are the usual source of enterovirus infection. Faecal virus shedding may persist for several weeks and spread usually occurs as a result of environmental contamination, particularly under conditions of crowding and poor hygiene. Enterovirus meningitis is commonest in children aged 5–14 years, but also occurs in other age groups. Intrafamilial spread is common, and outbreaks have been described in hospital nurseries, boarding schools and other residential institutions.

By far the commonest cause of enteroviral meningitis is echovirus infection. The predominant serotypes are 6, 9, 11, 19 and 30. There are annual epidemics of echovirus infections in the late summer (Fig. 16.6). They cause the so-called summer flu, with fever, sore throat and often headache. A proportion of infected individuals develop

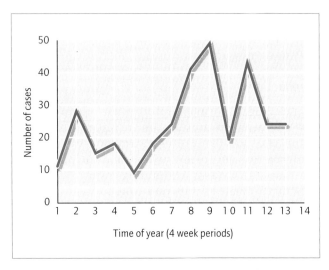

Fig. 16.6 Echovirus epidemic curve: this common infection dominates the epidemic curve for all viral meningitis notifications.

meningitis, with or without a preceding or accompanying sore throat. Enteroviruses types 70 and 71 are also important causes of outbreaks.

Coxsackievirus meningitis is caused predominantly by serotypes A9, B4 and B5. Coxsackie A infections affect all age groups; type B disease occurs mainly in infants and preschool children.

Enteroviruses can cause a rare, generalized chronic brain infection in individuals with agammaglobulinaemia.

Clinical features

There may be a personal or family history of sore throat in the preceding 5–7 days. The patient then develops increasing headache over 12–36 h, usually with nausea and vomiting. Although the headache is severe, there is no alteration in consciousness or neurological function. There is usually meningism, but this varies from minimal to severe and is not always in proportion to the severity of the headache.

Other clinical features are few. There may be cervical lymphadenopathy; rarely there is clinical pharyngitis. The white cell count and differential are almost always normal, as is blood biochemistry.

Lumbar puncture and CSF examination should be carried out in patients with other than mild meningism. This is to exclude bacterial meningitis or other diagnoses such as subarachnoid haemorrhage. Cases with minimal meningism may be observed overnight before a decision on lumbar puncture is made, and the investigation often turns out to be unnecessary.

Typical CSF changes in viral meningitis are as follows:
1 Cells: 40–250, all lymphocytes.
2 Protein: 0.45–0.9 g/l.
3 Glucose: 1.0–1.7 mmol/l below blood glucose.

There may be a proportion of neutrophils in the CSF cell count if the lumbar puncture is performed early in acute disease. The presence of 50% or more of lymphocytes, however, is reassuring evidence against acute bacterial meningitis.

A lymphocytosis, or predominantly lymphocytic pleiocytosis, can occur in the CSF in:
1 Tuberculous meningitis.
2 Partly treated bacterial meningitis.
3 Intracranial abscess.
4 Leptospirosis.
5 Lyme borreliosis.
6 Viral encephalitides.
7 Lymphocytic leukaemias.
These conditions should be considered, however briefly, if there is anything atypical about the presentation or course of viral meningitis. CSF glucose levels are usually depressed in tuberculous meningitis, an important feature in the differential diagnosis (see Chapter 18).

The blood glucose is elevated in diabetic patients, and can be raised in acute brain insult (though viral meningitis is rarely sufficient to do this). It should always be checked at the time of lumbar puncture.

Diagnosis

The typical clinical and CSF findings during the epidemic period of the year are sufficient to make the diagnosis. All of the differential diagnoses are rarities; they include tuberculous meningitis, neuroborreliosis and, when the CSF cell count includes neutrophils, intracerebral abscess and partly treated bacterial meningitis. On rare occasions an exacerbation of multiple sclerosis or an autoimmune transverse myelitis causes CSF pleiocytosis, but this is often accompanied by typical neurological abnormalities.

Enteroviruses are transiently present in the pharynx and the CSF. They are excreted for several days or weeks in the faeces. Enteroviruses and their detection are discussed more fully in Chapter 6.

Serological diagnosis is unreliable. Test systems exist for detecting immunoglobulin M (IgM) antibodies to coxsackieviruses, but they have variable sensitivity and specificity.

Management

This is symptomatic. As with many acute viral infections, bed rest produces non-specific improvement in malaise. Analgesics and antiemetics are helpful. Lumbar puncture is often followed by improvement in the headache. Fever and headache are often much improved within 48–72 h. Occasionally severe tension headache or cervical spondylosis delays recovery. The use of a non-steroidal anti-inflammatory analgesic will often help, as will a small dose of promethazine for its mild sedative and muscle-relaxing effect.

If there is no improvement in a week, the differential diagnosis should be reconsidered.

Poliomyelitis

Introduction

Poliomyelitis is unique among enteroviral meningitides in causing infection and death of anterior horn cells. This is exceptionally rare in other enteroviral infections. Polio remains endemic in some areas where vaccination is not readily available, and still causes rare outbreaks in western countries. It remains the commonest worldwide cause of paralysis and limb-wasting in young age groups.

Epidemiology

Humans are the only known reservoir of infection. In acute infection, virus excretion lasts for up to a week in oropharyngeal secretions and for up to 6 weeks in faeces. Faecal–oral transmission is the major method of spread in conditions of poor hygiene. Where sanitation is good, pharyngeal spread is more important.

There are three distinctive patterns of disease: endemic, epidemic and sporadic. Endemic disease occurred in the prevaccine era and is still seen in some parts of the world with poor vaccine coverage. Virus circulated extensively among infants and young children and most individuals had been infected by 3 years of age. Because a large proportion (over 99%) of polio infections in young children are asymptomatic, the incidence of neurological disease is relatively low when the disease is endemic.

During the 20th century, many temperate countries experienced a shift from endemic to epidemic disease. This occurred as living conditions improved and virus circulation among young children diminished. The effect was to increase the average age at which infection occurred to teenagers and young adults, in whom neurological disease is much commoner; 10% of infections at this age are paralytic. Large outbreaks of paralytic polio occurred in the UK, USA and many other countries during the 1940s and 1950s. These outbreaks were usually due to type 1 poliovirus.

Following the introduction of vaccination in the 1950s, polio was rapidly brought under control. The last outbreak in UK was in 1977 and occurred in unvaccinated itinerant gypsies. Since then there have been only sporadic cases, in unvaccinated travellers to countries where the disease is still common. Some developed countries, e.g. Holland, have continued to experience occasional outbreaks in groups that refuse vaccination on religious grounds. In other countries, outbreaks in highly vaccinated populations have occurred due to vaccine failure. This may occur when reduced-potency vaccine has been used, or due to competitive inhibition of oral poliovaccine in the intestine by other enteric viruses. An unusual outbreak occurred in Finland in 1984 due to an antigenically altered type 3 poliovirus, against which vaccination with inactivated vaccine (routinely used in Finland) was ineffective.

Live polio vaccines carry a minute, but definite, risk that the vaccine virus will mutate to a virulent form. Half of the resulting clinical cases have occurred in vaccine recipients; the remainder affect contacts of recipients.

Pathogenesis

Poliovirus enters the body through the alimentary tract and the oropharynx. This is followed by a viraemic phase, during which the virus enters the spinal cord. The virus infects and kills anterior horn cells, leading to lower motor neurone degeneration.

Clinical features

The incubation of poliomyelitis varies from 3 to 35 days, but is usually between 1 and 3 weeks. Probably over 90% of cases are inapparent or mild. Sometimes an influenza-like illness, an acute pharyngitis or a mild diarrhoeal disease may be recognized as caused by poliovirus. Otherwise the disease may be divided into non-paralytic and paralytic, depending on the outcome.

Non-paralytic poliomyelitis

Non-paralytic poliomyelitis is simply viral meningitis caused by poliovirus. It is indistinguishable from other enteroviral meningitides, except for the results of viral culture and serology, and it has an identical self-limiting course.

Paralytic poliomyelitis

Paralytic poliomyelitis begins as a feverish illness, often with myalgia and/or meningism, but is followed after 2–5 days by the development of lower motor neurone lesions. The muscles affected are often painful in the day or two before paralysis is evident. Trauma, such as vigorous exercise, injection, vaccination or tonsillectomy, makes paralysis of the local muscles more likely. Paralysis is also more likely and more extensive in older age groups, so that a toddler may have a weak leg while an adult may develop a quadriparesis.

Paralysis develops over about 48 h. Fasciculation is common at the onset, then reflexes and movement are lost. The muscle groups affected are asymmetrical, and there is a complete absence of upper motor neuron or sensory features. If the upper arms are affected, the diaphragm is at risk; if bulbar weakness occurs, the airway must be guarded.

Clinical spectrum of poliovirus infection
1 Inapparent seroconversion.
2 Non-neurological (usually pharyngeal or diarrhoeal).
3 Non-paralytic (viral meningitis only).
4 Paralytic (anterior horn cell death).

Examination of the CSF reveals a lymphocytic pleiocytosis of up to 500 cells/mm^3, with other changes consistent with viral meningitis. The peripheral white cell count may be raised during the myalgic early stages, but is otherwise normal.

Diagnosis

The diagnosis is usually clinically evident. However, culture of throat swabs, CSF and faeces should permit identification and typing of the causative virus. Virus persists in the faeces for up to 6 weeks after the onset of paralysis. In later cases, rising titres of antibodies may be detectable in serum, and local synthesis of antibody may be demonstrable by comparing serum and CSF titres.

Typing of the virus may be important in identifying a community outbreak or in defining a vaccine-associated case. Poliovirus can be serologically typed into types 1, 2 and 3, and further typed when necessary by RNA studies. Three corresponding attenuated vaccine viruses also exist, which can be distinguished from wild virus by their different RNA structure.

Diagnosis of poliomyelitis
1 Cell culture of stool, throat swab or cerebrospinal fluid (CSF).
2 Serotyping of virus isolates by neutralization tests.
3 RNA studies if vaccine-associated polio is suspected.
4 Demonstration of local antibody production in CSF.
5 Demonstration of rising titres of serum antibodies.

Management

There is no specific treatment but bed rest is recommended until the fever has resolved, as this may limit the severity of paralysis.

Once the patient is afebrile and stable, physiotherapy should be commenced. The rate and extent of recovery of power are variable, but improvement can continue for up to 2 years. Children are more likely to have a good or apparently complete recovery than are adults.

Complications

Secondary bacterial infection is common; in the chest if the intercostal muscles, glottis or diaphragm are weak, and in the bladder if catheterization is necessary. Appropriate cultures and antibiotic treatment are important in maintaining the patient's health during recovery.

Persisting muscle paralysis may lead to contracture or deformity, especially in growing limbs. Expert orthopaedic advice may be needed to optimize posture and give the best functional result.

Prevention and control

Inactivated poliovaccine (IPV) was introduced in 1956 and was followed by live oral poliovaccine (OPV) in 1962. Since 1967, only OPV has been used in the UK, although IPV is still recommended for immunization of pregnant women, immunosuppressed patients and their household contacts. The standard UK OPV schedule is three doses at monthly intervals starting at 2 months of age, with booster doses before entry to school and at 15 years of age (see Chapter 25).

Both OPV and IPV protect against poliovirus types 1, 2 and 3. OPV has the benefit of being orally administered and provides intestinal as well as humoral immunity, whereas the immunity from IPV is largely humoral. For this reason OPV is the vaccine of choice for control of epidemics, where the aim is to interrupt transmission of circulating virus. Following vaccination with OPV, vaccine virus is excreted in the faeces for up to 6 weeks. OPV can thus spread to, and immunize, close contacts of recently vaccinated individuals. This means that good population immunity can be achieved even where up-take of the vaccine is low.

The main disadvantage of OPV is that it causes paralysis in approximately 1 per 2 million recipients, with a similar risk for non-immune contacts. An average of two vaccine-associated cases of polio are reported per year in the UK. Nevertheless, OPV remains the most widely used vaccine in national immunization pro-grammes. A novel approach used in some countries is a combined OPV/IPV schedule.

Advantages of oral poliovaccine
1 Can be administered orally.
2 Confers mucosal as well as systemic immunity.
3 The vaccine infects and immunizes close contacts.
Disadvantages of oral poliovaccine
1 Vaccine must be kept refrigerated.
2 Three doses are needed.
3 There is a small risk of mutation to virulence, and paralytic disease.

Although polio remains endemic in many Asian coun-tries, it has been virtually eradicated in some developing countries, notably in South America. The World Health Organization aims to eliminate polio globally by the year 2000.

Polio is a notifiable disease. Cases should be isolated in hospital. In an outbreak, extensive virus circulation usually precedes the first case; a single case of indigenously acquired polio requires vaccination of a wide network of contacts.

Herpes simplex type 2 meningitis

This is almost always associated with primary genital herpes simplex, of which it is an uncommon com-plication. Occasional cases occur in the absence of detectable genital lesions. The meningitis is benign, behaving like an enteroviral infection.

It is sometimes accompanied by sacral myelo-radiculitis with pain in the perineum, buttock or leg, associated paraesthesiae, and occasionally difficulty of micturition or defecation. Although the condition is usually self-limiting, it can persist for weeks. It is there-fore reasonable to offer treatment with aciclovir, which

should be given intravenously in a dose of 10 mg/kg 8-hourly (see Chapter 11).

Bacterial meningitis

Introduction

This section deals with diseases of children and adults but not of neonates, who have particular types of bac-terial meningitis associated with the birth process and early bacterial colonization. Neonatal meningitis is discussed in Chapter 12.

Bacterial meningitis is always a medical emergency because of the high mortality of untreated or late-treated cases. The importance of meningitis is the preventable morbidity which different types cause in various age groups. Prompt treatment can minimize the mortality to 4–8% in childhood types, and to 8–25% in adults. Many cases recovering after early treatment have little or no neurological deficit.

ORGANISM LIST

Haemophilus influenzae
Neisseria meningitidis
Streptococcus pneumoniae
Listeria monocytogenes
Mycobacterium tuberculosis

Streptococcus 'milleri'
Other Gram-positive cocci
Escherichia coli.

Between 15 and 25% of cases of bacterial meningitis have negative blood and CSF cultures. This is more often because of sampling problems or previous anti-biotic treatment than because of an unusual bacterial aetiology.

Rare cases of bacterial meningitis after neurosurgery may be caused by Gram-negative rods such as *Acinetobacter* spp.

Lumbar puncture and CSF changes in purulent meningitis

With the exception of tuberculosis and leptospirosis, bac-terial meningitis causes neutrophil pleiocytosis in the CSF. All bacterial meningitis causes a raised protein level and low glucose. Some laboratories also estimate CSF lactate levels. Endotoxin accumulates in the CSF of patients with Gram-negative bacterial meningitis, but this is usually only measured for research purposes.

The range of changes seen in any type of bacterial meningitis is extremely wide. Any number of neutrophils in the CSF is abnormal; some patients have fewer than 10/mm^3; others may have 2000 or more. The protein level is usually more elevated in bacterial than viral meningitis; levels greater than 1.0 g/l are common. A low glucose level is rarely found in viral meningitis, but is usual in bacterial infections.

In bacterial meningitis, the degree of abnormality in the CSF is closely related to the prognosis. In particular, high neutrophil counts, high protein, high lactate and high endotoxin levels are associated with a poor prognosis. Since these levels tend to rise in parallel, the protein level and neutrophil count often give a reasonable indication of prognosis.

Haemophilus influenzae meningitis

Introduction and epidemiology

Haemophilus influenzae meningitis is almost exclusively a disease of small children, appearing with the loss of maternal antibodies at about 6 months of age and becoming increasingly rare after the age of 5. It is caused by an encapsulated *H. influenzae* of capsular type b (Hib), which is asymptomatically carried in the nasopharynx of many infants and toddlers, but rarely colonizes adults. Antibodies to the organism are naturally acquired in unimmunized populations, and appear to inhibit colonization as well as to prevent infection.

Other important childhood bacteraemic diseases are also caused by Hib. These include pneumonia, acute epiglottitis, facial cellulitis and some bone and joint infections. Different children in the same family or nursery may therefore be affected by different diseases when infected with Hib.

A few cases of *H. influenzae* meningitis are caused by capsular types a, c–f or non-capsulate strains. This is particularly true in those rare cases of adult *H. influenzae* meningitis, which are usually a complication of chronic CSF fistulae, and which are rarely type b infections (Fig. 16.7).

Before the introduction of routine immunization, Hib was the second commonest cause of bacterial meningitis in the UK after *N. meningitidis*. One in 600 children developed invasive disease before the age of 5. The case fatality ratio was 4–5% and up to 30% of survivors had permanent neurological sequelae (see below). The disease is now disappearing in most western countries.

Older children and adults rarely contract *Haemophilus* meningitis. Cases occasionally occur in patients with chronic CSF fistulae; over half of these are caused by non-encapsulated *H. influenzae*.

Microbiology

H. influenzae is a small Gram-negative coccobacillus which is catalase- and oxidase-positive. As it requires nicotinamide adenine dinucleotide phosphate (NADP) and haematin for active growth, it produces little or no growth on unsupplemented blood agar, but it grows well on chocolate blood agar. The organism is aerobic but isolation and growth are favoured by an atmosphere with enhanced carbon dioxide.

Pathogenesis

The main pathogenicity determinant of *H. influenzae* is the capsule. Although the organism is capable of producing one of six different capsular polysaccharides (or none), almost all isolates from clinical disease are serotype b. Susceptibility to Hib infection correlates with the absence of antibodies to the type b capsule. Recent data from molecular studies have confirmed the importance of the polyribitol ribosyl phosphate (PRRP) capsule in experimental meningitis. Other pathogenicity determinants include the lipopolysaccharide, outer membrane protein, pilus proteins and the IgA protease.

Pathogenicity factors of *Haemophilus influenzae*
1 Polyribitol ribosyl phosphate (PRP) capsule, especially capsular type b.
2 Cell-wall lipopolysaccharide.
3 Outer membrane protein.
4 Pilus proteins.
5 Immunoglobulin A protease.

In respiratory infections the capsule is not a vital pathogenicity requirement. Infection tends to occur in individuals with bronchiectasis or chronic obstructive airways disease. In this environment the organisms are partly protected from the activities of the host immune system. In addition it appears that bacterial antigens and the host's inflammatory response to them sets up a cycle of damage, colonization and damage, with progressive loss of respiratory function.

Clinical features

Hib meningitis often has a slow onset over 3 or 4 days, beginning as an apparent cold or respiratory infection. The development of drowsiness, vomiting, convulsions

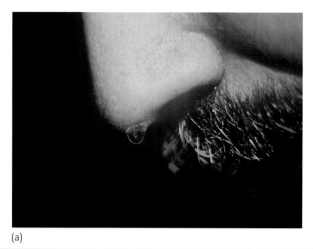

(a)

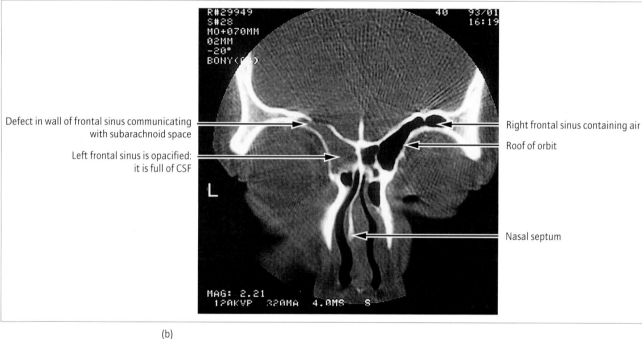

Defect in wall of frontal sinus communicating with subarachnoid space

Left frontal sinus is opacified: it is full of CSF

Right frontal sinus containing air

Roof of orbit

Nasal septum

(b)

Fig. 16.7 Cerebrospinal fluid (CSF) rhinorrhoea in a man who developed *Haemophilus influenzae* type b meningitis many years after a head injury. (a) Clear CSF dripping from the nose; (b) contrast computed tomographic scan showing CSF leaking via a skull defect into the frontal sinus (arrow). The sinus is opaque compared with the air-filled sinus on the right. (Courtesy of Dr W.R.C. Weir and the *Journal of Infection*.)

(not always during periods of fever) and a strange cry in infants, is the usual sign of more severe illness. Toddlers will usually complain of headache or photophobia. The condition may fluctuate initially, improving when the temperature is lower, or reduced by paracetamol medication, and worsening with feverish episodes.

Examination shows a feverish, irritable or hypotonic child, often drowsy and intermittently vomiting. Infants may have a bulging fontanelle; older children have frank meningism and occasionally opisthotonus.

The white cell count is usually high — $15–20 \times 10^9/l$ with a neutrophilia. The blood sugar may also be raised to 8–10 mmol/l in the face of acute cerebral insult, but this will resolve without specific treatment in 36–48 h.

Diagnosis

Lumbar puncture reveals changes typical of bacterial meningitis. Gram stain will often demonstrate small, Gram-negative rods in the CSF, but these are not easy to identify and are rarely seen if significant antibiotic treatment has already been given.

In a child below the age of 6, purulent meningitis without a rash may be caused by Hib. However, rare cases occur of Hib meningitis with a purpuric rash, and not all cases of meningococcal meningitis (which is now much commoner than Hib meningitis) have the typical rash.

If Gram stain and culture are negative, serological evidence of Hib infection may be obtained by performing a latex agglutination test on the CSF, using the Hib PRP antigen. Failing this, blood cultures may prove positive 24–36 h after admission.

Diagnosis of *Haemophilus influenzae* type b (Hib) meningitis
1 Demonstration of small, Gram-negative rods in cerebrospinal fluid (CSF) deposit.
2 Demonstration of Hib antigen in CSF by latex agglutination.
3 Positive CSF culture.
4 Positive blood culture.

Management

The first priority is immediate and adequate intravenous antibiotic treatment. This should be commenced at the start of resuscitation, as soon as specimens have been obtained for culture. The treatment of choice is a broad-spectrum cephalosporin, such as cefotaxime or ceftriaxone, which penetrates excellently into the CSF and is highly bactericidal to Hib. Cefuroxime does not reach such good CSF concentrations and carries a slight risk of late relapse. Chloramphenicol is the drug of second choice but with this, and more with ampicillin, there is an increasing risk of resistance. About 12% of Hib may be ampicillin-resistant, and 4–6% chloramphenicol-resistant. Antibiotic treatment should be continued for at least 1 week, and probably for 10 days in severe cases. In rare cases another Hib-related condition such as pneumonia coexists with meningitis, and may require prolonged treatment.

Dexamethasone has been studied for its possible beneficial effect in Hib meningitis. While it makes only a few hours' difference to the duration of fever, and does not alter mortality, it reduces the incidence of deafness after recovery in some trials. The dose is 8 mg twice daily during the first 3 days of antibiotic treatment. However, if antibiotic treatment is in any way suboptimal, dexamethasone treatment may increase the late relapse rate (probably by inhibiting the entry of antibiotics such as cefuroxime or ampicillin into the CSF).

Treatment of *Haemophillus influenzae* type b meningitis
1 Cefotaxime, i.v. 150–200 mg/kg daily in three or four divided doses; alternative, ceftriaxone, i.v. or i.m. 50 mg/kg daily in a single dose (up to 80 mg/kg can be given i.v.); both for 7 days.
2 Second choice: chloramphenicol, i.v. or orally 50–100 mg/kg daily in four divided doses for 10–14 days; *plus* dexamethasone, orally, i.m. or i.v. 8 mg twice daily for the first 3 days only.

Other priorities include adequate rehydration and haemodynamic support, control of convulsions and, on rare occasions, specific measures to control raised intracranial pressure.

A single dose of diazepam, intravenously (250 μg/kg) or rectally (500 μg/kg), may be sufficient to control convulsions occurring during the acute fever at presentation. As fever and inflammation are controlled, fits often cease. If fits persist, phenytoin may be given by slow intravenous infusion to a total of 5–15 mg/kg. This can often be followed by oral administration of phenytoin or sodium valproate until the acute illness is controlled, when weaning from the anticonvulsant may be attempted.

Lumbar puncture rarely produces coning and may be of value in reducing intracranial pressure. It is hazardous in some cases with very high CSF pressure caused by gross cerebral oedema. Warning signs of this include sluggish pupillary reactions, decerebrate posturing and bradycardia. Unrelieved pressure will 'incarcerate' the brain inside the skull, occluding the cerebral circulation and leading to cerebral vein thrombosis or cerebral ischaemia. Anaesthesia, artificial hyperventilation or insertion of a CSF drain may occasionally be needed to avoid this.

Complications

Apart from the immediate problems of treatment, late problems can occur after the initial resolution of fever.

Recurrence of fever

Recurrence of fever is occasionally seen, sometimes with a neurological complication. It probably represents a small subdural area of infection, or cerebral vein thrombosis with persisting inflammation, which may be demonstrable on CT or MR scan. It usually responds to continued or increased antibiotic treatment. Tapping of subdural collections is occasionally indicated.

Convulsions

Convulsions may develop during the course of healing. They are rarely caused by frank abscess formation, but a cerebral vein thrombosis, subdural collection, rising intracranial pressure or small area of gliotic scarring may be responsible. A CT or MR scan is indicated to detect these.

Hydrocephalus

Hydrocephalus is rare but can develop at any time after treatment commences. It may present as increasing fits or deteriorating cerebral function with neurological deficit, drowsiness or coma. Imaging is required to make the diagnosis, and neurosurgical advice on temporary or permanent CSF drainage may be necessary.

Neurological impairment

Neurological impairment is rarely gross in those who survive the infection. The commonest problem is reduced hearing, which occurs in 9–15% of survivors. It should always be sought, as it affects subsequent schooling and social development if untreated. Other cranial nerve defects may occur, including squint, ptosis, reduced visual field or acuity and impaired balance. These may improve considerably with time, but residual defects do occur.

More global neurological problems are rare, but monoparesis, spasticity, learning difficulties and epilepsy are all recognized sequelae of severe childhood meningitis. Intensive follow-up and rehabilitation under the care of a developmental paediatrician is indicated in these cases.

Complications of *Haemophilus influenzae* type b meningitis

1 Impaired hearing in 9–15% of survivors.
2 Convulsions (rarely, persisting epilepsy).
3 Subdural collections of fluid (rarely, subdural empyema).
4 Cerebral vein thrombosis.
5 Rare visual, motor or sensory deficit.
6 Very rare hydrocephalus.

Prevention and control

Polysaccharide Hib vaccines were first produced in the 1970s. These were very effective in older children, but were much less effective in children under 2 years of age, the group most at risk from disease. In addition they did not prime the immune system for subsequent boosting, as the immunity was mainly B-cell-mediated.

The immunogenicity of Hib vaccines has now been greatly improved by conjugating the polysaccharide moeity to T-cell-dependent proteins, such as tetanus toxoid or CRM_{197}, a non-toxic derivative of diphtheria toxin. Conjugate vaccines are effective in infants from 2 months of age and elicit an immune response which primes for subsequent boost with natural polysaccharide.

Hib vaccine was introduced in the UK immunization schedule in 1992. Three doses are given at 2, 3 and 4 months of age (see Chapter 25). Booster doses are not recommended. Unvaccinated children over 1 year of age are protected by a single dose; however immunization is not worthwhile in children above age 4. There are no specific contraindications to Hib vaccine. A mild-to-moderate local reaction occurs in up to 10% of vaccine recipients.

Household contacts of patients with Hib should be given chemoprophylaxis (and vaccine, if unvaccinated) if there is a child under 4 years in the household. The case should also receive prophylaxis before discharge from hospital. Recurrent infections are rare, but have been documented, thus the index case should also receive vaccine. Nursery contacts should be given chemoprophylaxis (and vaccine, if unvaccinated) where two or more cases occur within 120 days of each other.

The regimen for chemoprophylaxis is rifampicin 20 mg/kg daily for 4 days, up to a maximum of 600 mg daily. Patients must be informed of the possible adverse effects, which include interference with oral contraception, red coloration of urine, sputum and tears, staining of contact lenses, skin rashes and gastrointestinal reactions.

Prophylaxis of *Haemophilus influenzae* type b (Hib) meningitis

Rifampicin, orally 20 mg/kg daily (maximum 600 mg daily) for 4 days, to *all* household or nursery contacts, when other children below age 4 are present; *plus*
(In unvaccinated children) Hib vaccine 0.5 ml i.m. or deep s.c. as a single dose (infants below 13 months require three injections at intervals of 1 month; the vaccine is not indicated above age 4 years).

Haemophilus meningitis is a notifiable disease in the UK (see Chapter 25).

Meningococcal meningitis

Introduction

This disease, caused by *Neisseria meningitidis*, is an important cause of morbidity and mortality in children and young adults. It is a bacteraemic disease with a rapid and acute onset. About 85% of cases have signs of meningitis, which often leads to a prompt diagnosis. The minority with bacteraemia alone tend to present with more advanced disease, and have approximately twice the mortality of those with meningitis.

Epidemiology

N. meningitidis is the commonest cause of bacterial meningitis in the UK (Fig. 16.8). Approximately 1000 laboratory-confirmed cases are reported annually, 40% of these occurring between January and March. Two-thirds of the cases are due to serogroup B infections. In recent years group B, type 15, subtype P1.16/P1.7 has predominated. This is in contrast to the 'meningitis belt' of sub-Saharan Africa, where the predominant strains are group A, and sometimes group C, which cause explosive epidemics during the dry season from December to March.

The peak incidence of meningococcal meningitis is at 6 months of age, coinciding with loss of maternal antibody. A second, smaller peak occurs in teenagers and young adults. Many infections are sporadic, but outbreaks sometimes occur in households, schools and military establishments. Group C strains cause outbreaks more frequently than others. During outbreaks, the age distribution shifts towards older children.

Certain conditions predispose to meningococcal infection, notably functional or anatomical asplenia and complement deficiency. There is also some evidence that recent upper respiratory infection (especially influenza) temporarily increases the risk of meningococcal disease.

Pathogenesis

N. meningitidis are small Gram-negative cocci. They are carried in the nasopharynx, and cause septicaemia and meningitis in a minority of hosts. They are aerobic, catalase- and oxidase-positive, non-motile and possess a polysaccharide capsule, which is the main antigen and determines the serotype of the species. The main serogroups of pathogenic organisms are A, B, C and W135 and their prevalence varies with time and geographic location. Up to 50% of the bacterial outer membrane is a lipo-oligosaccharide (LOS), analogous to the lipopolysaccharide of Gram-negative bacteria, in that it contains a lipid A subcomponent. This antigen causes activation of macrophages and release of tumour necrosis factor, a mediator of shock in serious meningococcal septicaemia. The LOS may also assist in invasion of the CNS, by altering the permeability of the blood–brain barrier.

Meningococcal serogroups can be subdivided by serotyping, based on the outer membrane protein (OMP) 2 antigen. This is one of three OMPs which act as porins, controlling the influx of water-soluble molecules through the lipophilic outer membrane. Some OMP types are associated with more serious infections.

Neisseria express either one of two types of pili, which are important in adherence to host epithelium. Class I pili are similar to those produced by *N. gonorrhoeae*. Pilus production can be switched on and off and this may give the organism advantages in colonization and transmission.

Pathogenicity factors in *Neisseria meningitidis*
1 Capsular polysaccharide.
2 Outer membrane lipo-oligosaccharide (endotoxin-like).
3 Outer membrane proteins.
4 Pili.
5 Immunoglobulin A protease.

Antibodies to the capsular polysaccharide are bactericidal and protective, but the response to serogroup B antigen is weak because it cross-reacts with host tissues.

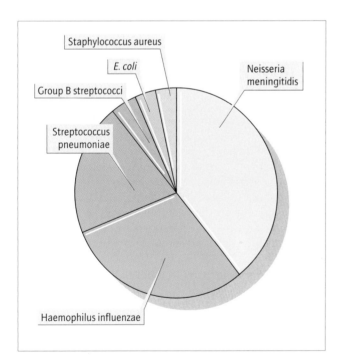

Fig. 16.8 Pie chart of the commonest causes of bacterial meningitis in 1992 in the UK. The proportion of cases due to *Haemophilus influenzae* fell in 1993 and 1994 following the introduction of vaccines against *H. influenzae* type b.

There is a strong immune response to meningococcal iron regulation proteins, which may assist in controlling infection by denying the organism iron. Like many other upper respiratory tract colonists, *N. meningitidis* produces an IgA protease which cleaves secretory IgA. This may block the bactericidal activity of IgG and paradoxically enhance the invasiveness of the organism.

Complement is important in protection against meningococcal disease. Defects of the alternative complement pathway cause enhanced susceptibility to infection. Rare defects in properdin predispose to catastrophic infection. Immunization permits recruitment of the classical complement pathway and abolishes this predisposition.

Clinical features

The disease has a short incubation period, evidenced by the rapid appearance of those secondary cases which occur. Most are seen 2–5 days after the primary case, although some occur up to 4 weeks later. In most cases the illness develops rapidly, over less than 24 h, but a slower onset sometimes occurs and causes diagnostic uncertainty. Fever, malaise and increasing headache are accompanied by nausea and often vomiting. Photophobia may be extreme.

A typical petechial and purpuric rash appears in the majority of patients (Fig. 16.9) sometimes preceded by a measles-like rash or generalized erythema which lasts for only a few hours. The rash, a feature of disseminated intravascular coagulation (DIC), is an important clue to diagnosis, but varies widely in its severity and extent. Some cases present with only one or two lesions (Fig. 16.10),

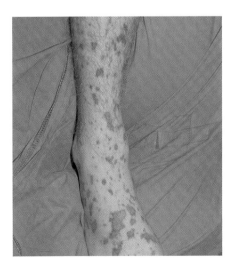

Fig. 16.9 Meningococcal meningitis: acute rash in a teenage boy; the legs, buttocks and elbows are often most affected.

and a few have petechiae only in the conjunctiva or other mucosal surface. A careful search for petechiae is warranted, as their presence makes the diagnosis very likely. A few cases present with vasculitic lesions (Fig. 16.11), or extensive, necrotic lesions (purpura fulminans; Fig. 16.12).

Patients with rapidly advancing disease may present with, or quickly develop, features of endotoxaemia such as hypotension, sluggish peripheral circulation and pulmonary oedema. As the disease progresses, drowsiness and confusion are common and coma sometimes develops.

The white cell count is usually raised to $15–20 \times 10^9/l$. The erythrocyte sedimentation rate is low, consistent with DIC, and fibrin degradation products are present in elevated amounts. The prothrombin time or international normalized ratio (INR) is often slightly prolonged, but serious bleeding or very low platelet counts are unusual.

Lumbar puncture reveals purulent CSF with a neutrophilia, raised protein and low sugar levels. Gram-negative diplococci may be seen inside and outside the neutrophils (Fig. 16.13), though they may not be detectable after antibiotic treatment. Blood and CSF cultures are usually positive.

Meningitis in an infant sometimes has a fluctuating onset, with intermittent fever accompanied by lassitude, high-pitched crying and perhaps vomiting, separated by periods of apparent normality. A bulging fontanelle or altered responsiveness eventually prompts the performance of diagnostic tests.

Older children and adults may have chronic meningococcal bacteraemia, which starts as an influenza-like illness with fever and arthralgias. The flat rash of DIC becomes progressively more papular and autoimmune-like (Fig. 16.14), and is then difficult to distinguish from Henoch–Schönlein disease, which is a common misdiagnosis. Joint swelling and small effusions may appear in the hands, knees or ankles. The condition can persist for weeks with a fluctuating course, but there is significant risk of progression to acute meningitis or bacteraemia.

The white cell count is usually elevated. The erythrocyte sedimentation rate rises as the condition persists, increasing the chance of misdiagnosis of autoimmune or collagen disease. Blood cultures are positive during feverish episodes, though several may need to be taken before the true diagnosis is confirmed.

Diagnosis

The clinical picture and evolution of the disease are often unmistakable, allowing the physician to treat promptly

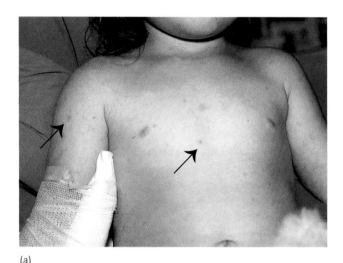

(a)

Fig. 16.10 Acute meningococcal meningitis:(a) this 3-year-old girl had only a handful of odd-shaped spots on the trunk and shoulders (arrows); (b) this 20-year-old woman had a conjunctival lesion.

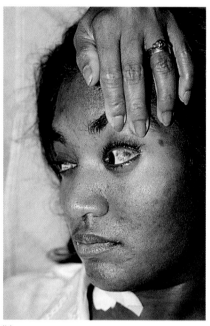

(b)

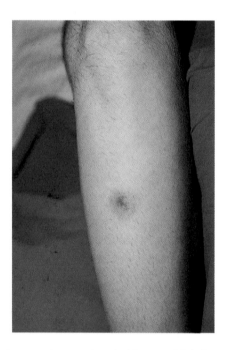

Fig. 16.11 Acute meningococcal meningitis: a vasculitic lesion on the shin; there were three others on the hand and arms.

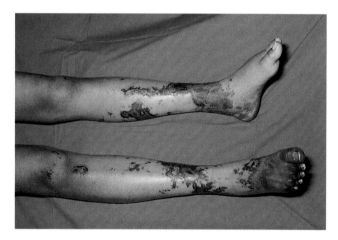

Fig. 16.12 Acute meningococcal meningitis: purpura fulminans.

without performing a confirmatory lumbar puncture. Occasionally, the typical rash is associated with staphylococcal, streptococcal or Hib infection, and some meningococcal cases have no rash. Where there is doubt, therefore, lumbar puncture offers the advantage of rapid diagnosis. Blood cultures should always be carried out.

Management

Meningococci are extremely sensitive to benzylpenicillin, which inhibits their replication within hours of the first dose. Intravenous penicillin treatment is therefore an urgent priority, and attending general practitioners should give a first dose pending hospital referral. This policy almost certainly saves lives, as the disease can progress alarmingly in the time it takes to reach hospital. For the first 24–48 h, most specialists would give 1.2 g 2-hourly. This is because penicillin is very rapidly excreted, so frequent dosage is required to maintain blood and CSF penicillin levels. Once the fever has resolved,

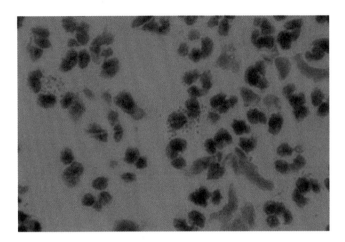

Fig. 16.13 Rapid diagnosis of meningococcal meningitis. Cerebrospinal fluid smear shows neutrophils, and intracellular and extracellular Gramnegative diplococci.

1.2 g 4-hourly or 2.4 g 6-hourly can be given to complete 5 days' treatment.

Many patients claim to be allergic to penicillin, often meaning that it causes diarrhoea or gastric irritation. The treatment of meningococcal disease is so urgent that only a history of anaphylaxis or angioneurotic oedema should be taken as a contraindication to penicillin. In such truly allergic patients there is significant risk of cross-allergy to cephalosporins, so the drug of second choice is chloramphenicol 2 or 3 g/day in divided doses for an adult or 50 mg/kg day in a child.

Treatment of meningococcal meningitis
1 General practitioner treatment: benzylpenicillin i.v.; infant below 1 year, 300 mg; child 1–6 years, 600 mg; older child or adult, 1.2 g, given immediately.

---

2 Hospital treatment: benzylpenicillin i.v. 1.2 g 2-hourly for 24–48 h (child 1–12 years, 200 mg/kg daily), reducing to 1.2 g 6-hourly to complete 5 days' course (child reduced to 100 mg/kg daily).
3 Alternative: cefotaxime i.v. 2.0 g 8-hourly (child 150–200 mg/kg daily) for 5 days; or ceftriaxone i.v. 2–4 g daily (child 50–80 mg/kg daily) as a single dose.
4 In severe penicillin allergy: chloramphenicol i.v. or orally, 2–3 g daily in three or four divided doses (child 50–100 mg/kg daily).

Uncomplicated cases become afebrile within 6–12 h of commencing treatment. The headache progressively resolves, skin lesons fade, or heal by scabbing and re-epithelialization, depending on their size. Neurological sequelae are rare.

More seriously ill patients with reduced blood pressure and impaired cerebral function will also lose their fever in the first day or two. However, the pathology of the DIC and haemodynamic disturbance resolves more slowly. There are platelet plugs containing trapped organisms in many small blood vessels. The activated platelets promote inflammation, complement activation and coagulation. There is often little improvement in haemodynamics or cerebral function in the first 24–36 h in such patients. During this time support measures as for Gram-negative bacteraemia and endotoxaemia are often needed (see Chapter 15).

Patients with established pulmonary oedema and severe purpura are gravely ill and require vigorous support. There is no evidence that heparin benefits the DIC once penicillin treatment has been commenced. Corticosteroids do not appear to improve the prognosis. Even with the best intensive care, 40% of these patients fail to recover.

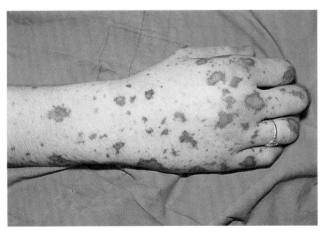

(a)

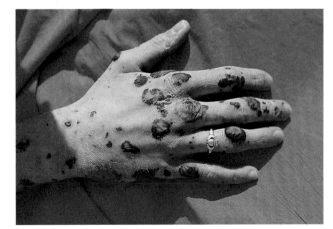

(b)

Fig. 16.14 (a) Early meningococcal rash; (b) the same rash after 1 week's evolution.

Many who die have bilateral haemorrhagic necrosis of the adrenal glands (Waterhouse–Friderichsen syndrome).

Plasmapheresis or exchange transfusion has not proved effective in treating severe disease, probably because they cannot remove the infected platelet thrombi from the circulation.

Complications

Other manifestations of meningococcal infection

Other manifestations of meningococcal infection may precede or complicate the meningitis. This is uncommon, but can cause diagnostic confusion. Many meningococcal infections are fairly trivial, for instance conjunctivitis, pharyngitis or otitis media. Others may be severe, including pericarditis, endocarditis, myocarditis and, rarely, septic arthritis. Most will respond to standard antimeningitis treatment, but endocarditis requires 4–6 weeks' treatment.

Necrosis

Necrosis of purpuric and ecchymotic lesions can cause severe pain. Adequate analgesia is important. Some lesions ulcerate and a few leave full-thickness skin defects which later require grafting. Large lesions of fingers or toes can cause loss of digits by gangrene. Nevertheless, secondary infection of these lesions is rare, and healing is often better then expected.

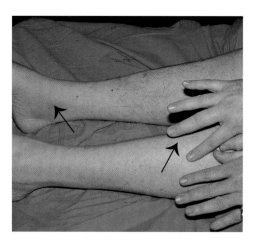

Fig. 16.15 Postmeningococcal synovitis affecting the finger and ankle (arrows).

Reactive arthritis

Reactive arthritis is a common late complication, affecting more than 50% of adolescents and young adults after 5–7 days. The fingers or knees are most often affected, usually asymmetrically (Fig. 16.15). Aspiration reveals neutrophils but no organisms. Immune complexes containing meningococcal antigen are demonstrable in the synovium. The condition resolves spontaneously and good symptomatic relief is afforded by non-steroidal anti-inflammatory agents.

Serositis

Serositis with effusion is much rarer than arthritis, but is probably also an immune-complex disorder. A pleural or pericardial effusion may be detected on X-ray, and occasionally requires aspiration. A rapidly reducing course of prednisolone will often terminate recurrent effusions.

Neurological sequelae

Neurological sequelae are rare except in the severest cases. Deafness or other cranial nerve lesions are the most likely. Occasionally an apparently recovering patient will collapse with respiratory arrest. This is usually due to acute basilar artery pathology secondary to meningeal or intracerebral purpuric lesions. It is often fatal.

Abscess formation

Abscess formation is rare but may occur at the original site of sepsis, such as the middle ear or a paranasal sinus. While this may respond to the treatment of the meningitis, surgical decompression and drainage are often indicated, both to remove the persisting infection and to prevent recurrence of the meningitis.

Prevention and control

Meningococcal vaccines are available against group A, C, Y and W135 strains. Unfortunately, no group B vaccine is available at the present. Vaccines are prepared from purified polysaccharide capsular antigen, and like the early Hib vaccines (see p. 315), they are less effective in young children and provide only temporary T-cell-independent immunity. Vaccination is indicated for those at particular risk from meningococcal disease. These include military recruits, household contacts of cases due to vaccine-preventable strains, asplenic patients and those with certain complement deficiencies. Vaccination has been successfully used to control outbreaks of group C disease in schools and military training camps. Travellers to the African meningitis belt and Haj pilgrims visiting Mecca (where an outbreak occurred in 1987) should also be vaccinated.

Chemoprophylaxis should be given to household and mouth-kissing contacts of cases in the 10 days preceding admission. During outbreaks chemoprophylaxis may be more widely extended to include classroom, nursery or other institutional contacts. The regimen is rifampicin 10 mg/kg every 12 h for 2 days, up to a maximum of 600 mg per dose. This differs from the regimen for Hib prophylaxis (see p. 315). Compliance may be poor due to gastrointestinal side-effects. Ciprofloxacin as a single oral dose of 500 mg is a good alternative but is not licensed for this use. Ceftriaxone 1 g intramuscularly may be used in pregnancy. The index case should receive chemoprophylaxis before discharge from hospital to prevent reintroduction of the infecting strain into the household. This is important, but often overlooked.

> **Prophylaxis of meningococcal disease**
> 1 Rifampicin orally, 600 mg 12-hourly for 2 days (infant 6–12 months, 5 mg/kg 12-hourly; child 1–12 years, 10 mg/kg 12-hourly).
> 2 Alternative: ciprofloxacin orally, 500 mg, single dose.
> 3 In pregnancy: ceftriaxone i.m. 1 g, single dose.
> 4 Meningococcus types A plus C polysaccharide vaccine, for school and military outbreaks with these types, 0.5 ml i.m. or deep s.c. (not effective below age 18 months).

Complications

Swabbing of contacts and cases after chemoprophylaxis is not essential.

A case of meningococcal meningitis, particularly in a school, often causes alarm and may attract media attention. Good communication and public education can minimize this. It is advisable to inform parents when a case occurs in a school, nursery or college. Meningococcal meningitis and septicaemia are both notifiable diseases (see Chapter 25).

Pneumococcal meningitis

Introduction and epidemiology

Pneumococcal meningitis is the commonest bacterial meningitis in the middle-aged and elderly, but can affect all age groups. While it can be apparently spontaneous it also has an increased incidence in certain susceptible patients:
1 Those with defects of the dura mater, for instance after head injury or surgery (see Fig. 16.7).
2 Those with chronic infections in the skull, for instance chronic suppurative otitis media or sinusitis. Patients with large nasal polyps are susceptible, especially after polypectomy.
3 Individuals who lack a spleen for any reason, for instance in haemolytic diseases, after abdominal trauma or after splenectomy for lymphoma or other malignancies.
4 Alcoholics are at increased risk of all types of pneumococcal disease.

Pneumococcal meningitis is an important disease because of these increased susceptibilities. It also has the highest mortality of the common bacterial meningitides. Many studies show that mortality increases with increasing age.

Clinical features

The incubation period is uncertain, as most cases are intrinsically derived. The onset is often rapid, over 1 or 2 days, but a few cases have a gradual onset, with meningism evolving during the course of an ear or sinus infection.

Most patients have marked meningism by the time of presentation, and impairment of consciousness is common. A significant proportion of cases present with spurious or non-specific complaints such as diarrhoea or vomiting, and are often too confused to complain spontaneously of headache. Signs of meningism must be actively sought if such cases are not to be missed.

Other features of severe pneumococcal disease, such as pneumonia or peritonitis, are occasionally present.

The white cell count is usually high; $15-25 \times 10^9/l$ is common. A low count indicates a poor prognosis. The plasma creatinine is often slightly elevated. Lumbar puncture shows a marked neutrophil pleiocytosis, and Gram-positive diplococci are relatively easy to demonstrate in most cases. Blood cultures are positive within 18–24 h.

Management

Specific treatment is with high-dose intravenous benzylpenicillin. However, penicillin tolerance is beginning to appear in indigenous pneumococci. It is important to give high enough doses to inhibit or kill tolerant bacteria while awaiting the results of culture sensitivity testing. A dose of 1.2 g 2-hourly produces adequate, sustained blood penicillin levels. Treatment should be continued for 10–14 days, to avoid the risk of recrudescence.

If the organism is found to be penicillin-tolerant, high-dose cefotaxime or ceftriaxone is a better treatment. Although slightly less effective than benzylpenicillin against fully sensitive streptococci, these drugs continue to penetrate the blood–brain barrier even when healing has restored its function. Penicillin penetrates less well through the intact blood–brain barrier, so produces initial improvement but tends to fail after 2 or 3 days.

Pneumococci completely resistant to penicillin are rare in the UK, but are common in Spain, Portugal, South Africa and parts of the Pacific. These organisms are often resistant to cephalosporins, chloramphenicol and erythromycin. The drug of choice in such circumstances is teicoplanin or vancomycin.

> **Treatment of pneumococcal meningitis**
> 1 Benzylpenicillin i.v. 1.2 g 2-hourly, then 2.4 g 4–6-hourly for 10–14 days.
> 2 Alternative and *for penicillin-tolerant pneumococci*: cefotaxime 2 g 8-hourly for 10–14 days; *or* ceftriaxone i.v. 2–4 g daily, single dose for 10–14 days.
> 3 For penicillin-resistant pneumococci: teicoplanin i.v., 400 mg 12-hourly for three doses, then 400 mg daily; *or* vancomycin i.v. 500 mg 6-hourly initially, but then to maintain plasma levels at peak not more than 30 mg/l and trough not more than 10 mg/l.

Patients with severe pneumococcal sepsis can develop renal failure, shock and pulmonary oedema. These problems should be treated vigorously, just as they would be in a patient with endotoxic shock (see Chapter 15).

Recurrence

Recurrence is a real possibility after pneumococcal meningitis in a susceptible patient. It is particularly likely in those with dural tears, who may have many attacks. CSF rhinorrhoea or otorrhoea can be confirmed by the presence of tau protein in the fluid, and the dural defect may be demonstrable by contrast injection and CT scan (see p. 312 and Fig. 16.7). Attempts should be made to prevent recurrence by repair of the predisposing condition, by immunization and prophylaxis. Occasionally an attack of meningitis in such patients is caused by an alternative organism, such as *Haemophilus influenzae*.

Other complications

Other complications are similar to those of meningitis in general. They include cranial nerve lesions, early or late hydrocephalus, visual defects or paresis of varying severity. Metastatic pneumococcal sepsis may occur.

Prevention and control

Pneumococcal polysaccharide vaccine contains antigen from 23 capsular types of pneumococci, which account for 90% of the invasive infections in the UK. The efficacy is approximately 70%, but is reduced in children under 2 and in those with immunological impairment. Vaccination is indicated for those at increased risk (see p. 321). Revaccination is not generally recommended because of the risk of severe systemic reactions. Asplenic patients and those with nephrotic syndrome, whose antibody levels are likely to decline more rapidly, should however be reimmunized after 5–10 years.

Splenectomized patients should be advised that they are at increased risk of pneumococcal disease. In addition to vaccine they should receive long-term penicillin prophylaxis (see Chapter 21).

Listerial meningitis

Introduction

Listeriosis is best known as an infection of pregnant women and neonates (see Chapter 12). However, 35–40% of recognized cases occur in older children and adults. Approximately half of non-neonatal infections attack patients who are immunosuppressed; the rest affect apparently immunocompetent individuals. Among the immunosuppressed, those at most risk are those on corticosteroid therapy, anticancer therapy, and those with chronic uraemia or immunosuppression following organ transplant. Listeriosis rarely affects patients with acquired immunodeficiency syndrome (AIDS).

Listeria monocytogenes is a small, Gram-positive rod which is common in nature. It is found in human and animal faeces, sewage slurry and land on which it is spread, vegetables, soft cheeses, pâtés, and some pre-prepared meat meals which have been kept chilled. The organism is robust, able to grow between 4 and 40°C, and able to survive temperatures of up to 60°C. Minor failures of pasteurization have been followed by large, milk-borne outbreaks. Its ability to replicate at refrigeration temperatures allows it to contaminate chilled food while other bacteria are inhibited.

The organism grows well on blood agar and exhibits a narrow band of beta-haemolysis. It is catalase-positive. It is motile by virtue of its flagella, and exhibits a characteristic, end-over-end 'tumbling' motion at 22°C. *Listeria* are able to survive inside macrophages and have frequently been used as a model of intracellular parasitism. Increasing interest is being shown in listeri-olysin as the major pathogenicity determinant. This is one of the family of cysteine-based toxins homologous to streptolysin O and pneumolysin (see p. 137).

Clinical features

The commonest manifestation of non-neonatal listeriosis is purulent meningitis. In the immunocompetent it often presents as acute meningitis, and must be differentiated from the commoner types. In about a third of patients it causes either bacteraemia alone or an unusual type of meningoencephalitis with a predominance of brainstem abnormalities.

In the immunosuppressed it may cause meningitis, bacteraemia or occasionally peritonitis; it rarely causes brainstem encephalitis.

In a pregnant woman the infection is often a trivial feverish illness, or merely a colonization of the bowel or genital tract. The only sign of maternal infection may be the birth of an affected infant.

Manifestations of listeriosis
1 In the immunocompetent: acute meningitis; rarely, brainstem encephalitis.
2 In the immunosuppressed: acute or subacute meningitis; bacteraemia; peritonitis.
3 In pregnant women: mild feverish illness; asymptomatic colonization of bowel or genital tract.

Diagnosis

Diagnosis depends on the results of blood and CSF culture. The disease must be suspected in cases of brainstem encephalitis, who may have minimal or no meningism, and are often immunocompetent. CT or MR scanning may suggest brainstem and/or meningeal inflammation. On occasions the CSF microscopy and culture are positive while blood cultures remain negative, even without prior antibiotic treatment. It is therefore important to obtain a CSF culture if CNS listeriosis is suspected.

Management

Management is with intravenous antibiotics. The choice is not easy, as *L. monocytogenes* is sensitive to penicillin, tetracycline and many other agents on laboratory testing but less so, apparently, in clinical use. High-dose ampicillin may be effective. Some would advocate addi-tional gentamicin, but it is uncertain whether this offers extra benefit. Chloramphenicol is effective, and readily enters the inflamed brain. It is probably the treatment of choice in encephalitis. Cephalosporins are poorly active and unreliable in listeriosis.

Treatment of listeriosis
1 Ampicillin i.v., 500 mg 4-hourly or 1 g 6-hourly for 10–14 days; *plus or minus* gentamicin 2–5 mg/kg daily in divided doses (avoid peak concentration above 10 mg/l, and trough above 2 mg/l).
2 Alternative: chloramphenicol i.v. or oral, 2–3 g, daily in three or four divided doses.

Prevention and control

Prevention and control depend largely on food hygiene. Adequate reheating of hospital cook–chill and cook–freeze meals substantially reduces the risk of infection among immunocompromised patients. High-risk foods (especially pâté and soft cheeses) should not be served to such patients. Pregnant women should also avoid these foods.

Streptococcus 'milleri' meningitis and ventriculitis

S. 'milleri' is the name used for a group of related streptococci, an uncommon cause of bacteraemia and meningitis. It tends to cause widespread infection with collections of thick pus. It is one of the few causes of simultaneous abscess formation in the brain and the liver. When it causes meningitis, it often leads to purulent and inflammatory obstruction of the foramina of the brain. The resulting loculated infections produce ventriculitis as well as severe meningitis.

The organisms are streptococci which may be alpha-, beta- or non-haemolytic, and of Lancefield group A, C, F or G. The commonest type is beta-haemolytic group F. Group A forms typically produce microcolonies on culture. Diagnosis depends on careful assessment of streptococci isolated from blood, CSF or pus cultures.

The importance of the organism is its reduced sensitivity to penicillin, which is, however, more effective than ampicillin. The treatment of choice is high-dose benzylpenicillin plus standard doses of gentamicin. A search should be made for distant infection and abscesses, particularly in the liver, as drainage may remove an additional source of sepsis.

Encephalitis and meningoencephalitis

Introduction

Encephalitis is inflammation of the brain. It can occur entirely independently of meningitis or the two can coexist, when the condition is called meningo-encephalitis.

The clinical features of encephalitis are those of cerebral irritation and dysfunction. The irritation often appears first, initially resembling bad temper or extreme restlessness. Fits may occur at this stage. The personality may change, giving an appearance of distraction or mild confusion. Some patients complain of ataxia or generalized weakness. If the temporal lobes are affected there may be aphasia or loss of short-term memory. On examination the reflexes are often over-brisk and the plantars may be upgoing. Brain swelling may trap cranial nerves, causing focal signs such as ophthalmoplegia or ptosis.

As cerebral dysfunction increases, fits become more likely and drowsiness or coma develops. In extreme cases bulbar function is impaired, the pupil reactions are sluggish or absent, intermittent breathing patterns develop and the outlook is grave.

General features of encephalitis
1 Irritability.
2 Altered personality.
3 Drowsiness.
4 Ataxia.
5 Excessively brisk tendon reflexes.
6 Upgoing plantar responses.
7 Signs of cerebral or brainstem failure (sluggish or absent pupil reflexes, intermittent breathing patterns).
8 Signs of brain swelling (focal neurological signs, papilloedema).
Signs of meningitis may coexist.

There are non-infectious causes of cerebral dysfunction, which can sometimes mimic encephalitis. Acute confusional states can complicate fever, especially in the old and the very young. Certain infections are likely to cause confusion or encephalopathy; legionnaire's disease, typhoid fever and typhus are examples. A non-cerebral source of infection should therefore be excluded in cases of global cerebral disturbance. Drugs may also cause encephalopathy. Opiate analgesics, high doses of phenytoin, indomethacin and some antidepressants are common examples.

ORGANISM LIST

Herpes simplex virus type 1
Tick-borne encephalitis virus
Japanese B encephalitis virus
Many mosquito-borne arboviruses
Rabies virus.

Encephalitis of varying severity can follow a number of viral infections. Its onset is 10–14 days after the onset of acute infection, so it is often assumed to be an immunopathological event and is called postinfectious encephalitis. A severe form can follow natural measles infection, and a benign form with cerebellar abnormalities is seen after chickenpox (see Chapter 13). Acute viral infections can be complicated by simultaneous encephalitis. This is quite common and transient in mumps, and is well-recognized and more severe in influenza A and B. These types of encephalitis are mentioned under their specific disease headings and will not be further discussed here.

Other infections causing fever and encephalopathy
1 Legionnaire's disease.
2 Typhoid and paratyphoid fever.
3 Typhus fevers.
4 Rare neurobrucellosis.
5 Rare neuroborreliosis.

Herpes simplex encephalitis

Introduction

Herpes simplex is a common infection of humans, usually affecting body surfaces, but herpes simplex encephalitis is rare. It is important because it attacks previously well individuals, causing a high mortality and much prolonged disability. If recognized early it can be treated with antiherpes medication, much improving the prognosis.

Epidemiology

Fewer than 50 laboratory-confirmed cases are reported in the UK each year. Encephalitis is usually caused by type 1 virus, whereas meningitis is usually due to type 2 virus. The disease arises sporadically and affects mainly young and middle-aged adults. Infection in children is rare. Both sexes are equally affected. The case fatality ratio may be as high as 70% in untreated cases.

Clinical features

The incubation period is uncertain, as the disease is almost always intrinsic. The onset varies from a rapid onset of fever and neurological abnormalities, fits and coma, to several days of slowly declining cerebral function. In many cases the temporal or frontotemporal regions of the cerebral cortex are affected earlier and more severely than the rest. Focal signs may reflect this, with memory loss, dysphasia and unsteady gait in a drowsy or irritable patient. Headache is not a common complaint, though cold- or flu-like symptoms may be present.

A careful search may reveal a herpes simplex lesion of the lip, skin or eye but this is absent in more than half of cases. There is rarely any other physical sign. The white cell count is normal, except when cerebral necrosis occurs, when there may be a neutrophilia. If there is significant cerebral destruction the aspartate transaminase levels may be raised.

The CSF almost always contains an excess of lymphocytes, though this varies from a few dozen to more than 200. Red blood cells may also be present in the absence of a traumatic tap. The protein level is moderately elevated, and the glucose is normal.

Diagnosis

When focal neurological signs are present, these help to distinguish encephalitis from a confusional state. Imaging is helpful in showing cerebral inflammation and often in demonstrating localization in the temporal lobes. MR is probably most helpful, but CT is also useful. There are typical electroencephalographic abnormalities in many cases. However, not all herpes simplex encephalitis shows localization, and temporal lobe involvement is not pathognomonic of herpes simplex.

Lumbar puncture is carried out after imaging. It is unusual to isolate herpes simplex virus from the CSF. A wide variety of antigen detection systems have been tried, but none are reliable. PCR DNA detection techniques may demonstrate herpes simplex virus DNA in CSF samples. Differential herpes simplex and rubella antibody levels may be estimated in blood and CSF, and may suggest intrathecal production of herpes simplex antibodies. It is rarely justifiable to perform brain biopsy, as neither a positive nor a negative result would influence the necessity to attempt specific antiviral therapy.

Diagnosis of herpes simplex encephalitis
1 Demonstration of temporal lobe oedema on brain imaging.
2 Demonstration of encephalitic electroencephalographic changes in the temporal cortex.
3 Demonstration of intrathecal anti-herpes simplex virus (HSV) antibody production.
4 Demonstration of HSV DNA in cerebrospinal fluid by polymerase chain reaction.
5 Demonstration of HSV immunoglobulin M, seroconversion, or rising immunoglobulin G titres in serum.

Management

Since herpes simplex is the commonest cause of infective encephalitis in Europe, and since antiviral therapy is effective, it is reasonable to offer all cases of acute encephalitis treatment with an antiherpes drug. The treatment of choice is intravenous aciclovir 10 mg/kg 8-hourly. There is no evidence that the addition of other antiviral agents or of corticosteroids offers any benefit, though it is reasonable to give dexamethasone if generalized cerebral oedema is demonstrated on imaging.

The response to treatment is not rapid. Fever will often subside in 2 or 3 days, but cerebral abnormalities improve slowly, and recovery is often incomplete. Treatment is continued for 2 weeks, sometimes longer, but improvement can continue for many weeks after cessation of therapy. Physiotherapy and speech therapy may help the patient regain social and motor skills as quickly and completely as possible.

Arbovirus encephalitides

Although none affecting humans are endemic in the UK, arboviruses are a common cause of encephalitis in both the new and the old world. The arboviruses are a heterogeneous group of organisms found in the Togaviridae, Flaviviridae and Bunyaviridae. They replicate in the cells of vertebrate and invertebrate hosts and cause encephalitic diseases, amongst others. They are transmitted by many different vectors, including mosquitoes, ticks and sandflies (Table 16.1).

In the forests of Germany, Austria, Scandinavia and Eastern Europe, tick-borne encephalitis is endemic. It is transmitted to humans from its natural rodent hosts in the summer months when ticks are active.

In north India, Pakistan, parts of Indonesia and the Far East, including Japan, Japanese B encephalitis is transmitted by mosquitoes, and causes outbreaks and epidemics with high morbidity.

Name	Vector	Distribution
Alphaviruses		
Eastern equine encephalitis	Mosquito	Americas
Venezuelan equine encephalomyelitis	Mosquito	Americas
Western equine encephalomyelitis	Mosquito	Americas
Flaviviruses		
Japanese encephalitis	Mosquito	Asia, Pacific islands
Kyanasur forest disease	Tick	India
Louping ill	Tick	UK
Murray Valley encephalitis	Mosquito	Australia, New Guinea
Powassan virus encephalitis	Tick	North America, Russia
St Louis encephalitis	Mosquito	Americas
Tick-borne encephalitis	Tick	Europe, Asia
Bunyaviruses		
Rift Valley fever	Mosquito	Africa
California encephalitis	Mosquito	USA

Table 16.1 Principal human neurological diseases caused by arboviruses

In the USA there are four main types of encephalitis. The commonest is St Louis encephalitis, but eastern equine, western equine and Californian encephalitis also cause significant human disease. All are transmitted from birds and rodents by mosquitoes to horses and humans.

In Australia, Murray Valley encephalitis is transmitted by mosquitoes.

Like most arboviral infections, these have incubation periods of a week or less. The onset of illness is rapid, with features of viral-type meningitis. Cerebral disturbance develops over the next 1–2 days. The diseases vary in severity and there are many inapparent infections. However, Japanese B encephalitis can have a mortality rate of 7–20%, with up to 30% incidence of intellectual or psychological problems in survivors. There is no specific treatment, and trials of prednisolone and dexamethasone have failed to show benefit.

Arbovirus infections can be diagnosed by culture or serology. Culture diagnosis requires specialized high-containment laboratory facilities and is rarely attempted in clinical practice. Immunofluorescence, EIA and PCR may be used to diagnose specific viral infections. The detection of virus-specific IgM is useful in many instances.

Mosquito control is an important factor in prevention of the mosquito-borne encephalitides. Safe and effective vaccines exist for tick-borne encephalitis (for which an immune globulin is also available for postexposure prophylaxis) and for Japanese B encephalitis.

Rabies

Rabies is caused by a rhabdovirus, transmitted from animals to humans by salivary contamination of a bite or open skin lesion. Many animals and birds are capable of infection by rabies virus. Human infections can result from contact with dogs, wolves, cats, bats, squirrels, skunks and occasionally horses or other animals. Rare cases of iatrogenic transmission have occurred in recipients of corneal grafts harvested from patients who have died from 'ascending polyneuropathy'.

The virus is neurotropic. It enters the peripheral nerves in the infecting lesion and migrates towards the CNS, where it eventually causes an encephalomyelitis. The incubation period varies with the length of nerve which the virus must traverse. It is often 3 or 4 weeks for a bite on the face or head, and a year or more for a bite on the foot.

No tests are available to diagnose rabies before the onset of clinical disease. Clinical rabies can be diagnosed by detecting serum neutralizing antibodies which appear as early as the sixth day of clinical illness. Rabies virus can be isolated from human tissues, including saliva, brain, CSF and urine. The virus may also be demonstrated by immunofluorescent antibody staining of impression smears of skin, cornea or other patient material. Histological examination of brain tissue shows perivascular inflammation and the characteristic cytoplasmic inclusion bodies known as Negri bodies. These are absent in up to a third of patients, particularly in persons who have received vaccination.

Illness is often heralded by irritation or paraesthesia at the site of the originating lesion. There is then a feverish illness, sometimes with ascending paralysis which may be the only manifestation of the disease. Encephalitis, with altered personality, agitation and altered consciousness often follows. Stimulation of the face and mouth, by attempts to drink, or by draughts of air, can precipitate painful and terrifying spasms of the face and neck — the typical picture of hydrophobia. If the history of exposure is not identified, the agitation of the encephalitis can be mistaken for hysteria or 'rabies phobia'.

Rabies is uniformly fatal, whether it presents as the paralytic or hydrophobic form. An individual decision must therefore be made in each case on the expediency and humanity of extended intensive care.

Pre-exposure immunization is available for those occupationally exposed. Postexposure prophylaxis is highly effective, and has three main components:
1 Washing the wound with any disinfectant will reduce the viral load and greatly reduce the risk of infection.
2 Human rabies immunoglobulin (HRIG) should be given as soon as possible; half of the dose of 20 U/kg is given as an intramuscular injection; the other half is infiltrated into the site of the infecting wound.
3 Immunization with diploid-cell vaccine is commenced immediately in a different intramuscular site, with doses on days 0, 3, 7 and 14, and after 1 and 3 months.

Neuroborreliosis

Among the postprimary manifestations of Lyme disease is a meningoradiculitis which can occur 2–6 months after the initial infection. A history of tick bite and/or erythema chronicum migrans, facial or other nerve palsy (see Chapter 20) is helpful in suspecting the condition.

The usual clinical features are headache, fever, varying degrees of neck and back stiffness, with localized pain and dysfunction of the affected spinal nerve roots, often the lumbosacral ones.

The CSF contains excess lymphocytes, and often a few red cells. The protein is raised and the sugar may be normal or slightly low.

IgM antibodies to *Borrelia burgdorferi* may have disappeared, but IgG antibodies should be present both in serum and CSF. Attempts may be made to recover spirochaetes from CSF culture, but negative results do not exclude the diagnosis.

Treatment is with intravenous cefotaxime or ceftriaxone. However, the optimum duration is unknown; a significant proportion of patients are not cured by 2 weeks' therapy. The addition of tetracycline, doxycycline or high-dose ampicillin for 6–10 weeks may be more successful.

Chronic encephalitis

Creutzfeldt–Jakob disease (CJD) is a spongiform encephalopathy related to scrapie of sheep, bovine spongiform encephalopathy (BSE) and kuru of the New Guinean islanders. The pathogenic agents of the diseases are not fully understood, but no nucleic acid is demonstrable in infectious material. Instead, infectivity seems to be associated with an abnormal form of a fibrillar protein called prion protein. The agent is extremely resistant to heat and chemical agents, including formalin disinfection; it requires prolonged autoclaving to sterilize contaminated materials.

Genes for prion protein can be found in the animals affected by the respective spongiform encephalopathies, and susceptibility to infection seems to have a strong genetic basis. It is suspected that spongiform encephalopathies may be caused by infectious proteins which perpetuate their own production from the host's genome.

The natural route of infection is probably via the diet. Iatrogenic transmission has followed the use of reusable stereotactic instruments for neurosurgery, human dura mater grafts, biologically derived human growth hormone and gonadotrophin (manufactured from pituitary glands harvested postmortem). The incubation period for natural infection is probably in the region of a decade or more.

The clinical disease is a presenile dementia. Rare before the age of 40, its peak onset is in the 60s. Illness begins with clumsiness, ataxia and tremor, and progresses to intellectual and motor impairment, leading to death in 18–24 months. No treatment alters this course.

Great care is required in disinfection of any reusable item which has come into contact with infected nervous tissue. For instance, 1 h of autoclaving at 134°C (or three periods of 20 min) is recommended for adequate sterilization.

Cerebral and intracranial abscesses

There are many ways in which space-occupying infections of the CNS can occur. Most are derived from bacteraemia which may be transient or never clinically evident. Some are complications of septicaemia. Others follow CNS invasion by contiguous spread from adjacent bone or intracranial sinus. Extradural or subdural collections of pus may compress the brain or spinal cord, or occlude an important blood supply, producing both local and long tract signs without actual CNS invasion.

Infectious lesions of this type often produce fever, but are otherwise difficult to distinguish clinically from tumours. Imaging is important in making an early diagnosis, or allowing biopsy or aspiration under imaging control. A CT scan will define lesions and their position, and will demonstrate enhancement of the inflamed, oedematous area surrounding inflammatory lesions. An MR scan will readily demonstrate oedema, and define fluid in an abscess cavity; enhancement can be used to suggest a rim of immunologically active cells in the abscess wall.

The importance of early suspicion and diagnosis is paramount as the prognosis is relatively good before impaired consciousness and severe neurological deficit occur, but the prognosis is definitely bad once these changes are established.

Cerebral abscess

Epidemiology

Traditionally, brain abscess has been associated with suppurative disease of the middle ear and mastoid cavity, and less often with ethmoid or frontal sinus disease. These are still important but, in children, an almost equal number of abscesses are of bacteraemic origin, associated with cyanotic congenital heart disease.

Rarer sources of brain abscesses are bacteraemias in patients with bronchiectasis, or with necrotic and ischaemic bowel lesions. Several reports exist of brain abscess as a rare complication of injection sclerotherapy for oesophageal varices. Bacteraemic disease may be complicated by brain abscess, and listeriosis is occasionally accompanied by brainstem abscess.

ORGANISM LIST

Anaerobic Gram-positive cocci
Prevotella melaninogenicus
B. fragilis
Fusobacterium spp.
Actinomyces spp.
Aerobic staphylococci and streptococci
Haemophilus aphrophilus
Other *Haemophilus* spp.

Listeria monocytogenes
Facultative Gram-negative rods.

The bacteriology of abscesses is often mixed, with more than one anaerobe identified, or a mixture of aerobes and anaerobes.

Clinical features

These are a mixture of headache, reduced consciousness, features of raised intracranial pressure, localizing signs and, rarely, fits. Up to half of patients have papilloedema at presentation, and a similar number have vomiting and altered consciousness. Only about half of patients have a significant fever. The headache may develop against the background of pain in the ear or the sinus, and should always be taken seriously in these circumstances, as it offers the chance to make an early diagnosis. If the abscess affects the meninges, or ruptures into the CSF, the headache becomes one of meningism, with nausea, vomiting, neck and back stiffness and photophobia.

The localizing signs depend on the site of the abscess. Frontal abscesses cause subtle signs of altered personality, paucity of conversation and apparent depression; parietal lesions cause classic features of hemiparesis and sometimes dysphasia; temporal lesions cause memory defects, sometimes aphasia and altered personality; visual field defects may be a sign of occipital lesions, or ataxia and tremor of cerebellar abscess.

Approximately equal numbers affect the frontal, parietal or temporal lobe. Occipital lobe abscesses occur less often and brainstem abscesses are also occasionally seen. Multiple lesions are uncommon but may complicate bacteraemic disease, actinomycosis and nocardiosis. Subdural empyema occurs less often than intracerebral abscess, but the organisms involved and the clinical presentations are similar.

The symptoms of raised intracranial pressure are global headache (worse on lying down and often waking the patient at night), increasing somnolence, rising blood pressure and falling pulse.

Fits are more common when the abscess is subdural or cortical.

Diagnosis

The two main aims of diagnosis are to demonstrate and localize the lesion, and to identify the pathogenic organisms.

Early imaging is essential to make the diagnosis (Fig. 16.16). In the presence of evolving localizing signs, it is

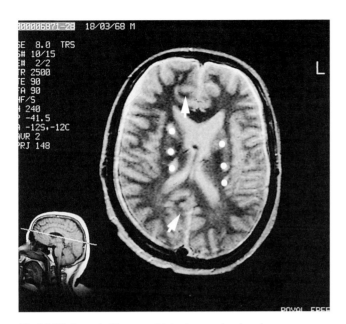

Fig. 16.16 Computed tomographic brain scan, showing abscesses surrounded by oedema (arrows) and several areas of enhancing tissue (circles).

unsafe to perform lumbar puncture because deformity of the brain may block the flow of CSF and cause herniation of the cerebellum or brainstem if the theca is opened. Lumbar puncture should be deferred until after imaging, even when meningism is present.

Blood cultures should always be set up to identify any coexisting bacteraemia.

When the abscess has been demonstrated, it is a neurosurgical choice whether it should be drained or aspirated at craniotomy, whether needle drainage alone is possible and whether indwelling drainage is required. Pus should be obtained for aerobic and anaerobic culture when drainage is performed.

Management

Broad-spectrum antibiotics should be given at diagnosis, to cover the likely range of pathogens. Agents which penetrate the brain well and are effective include chloramphenicol, cefotaxime, ceftriaxone and metronidazole. High doses of the cephalosporin should be given to achieve the best possible tissue levels as early as possible. Some specialists still use penicillin, chloramphenicol and metronidazole, a mixture which has also stood the test of time. However, penicillin penetrates the blood–brain barrier less well than the broad-spectrum cephalosporins. Treatment can be modified if

necessary when the results of blood and pus culture are known.

Neurosurgery is an important part of treatment. Single abscesses can be aspirated or drained via burr holes or at craniotomy. In a few cases the cavity may require excision. Small abscesses, especially if multiple, may be treatable with antibiotics alone, but require close follow-up by imaging to ensure adequate resolution.

Treatment of cerebral abscess
1 Cefotaxime i.v. 2–4 g, 8–hourly; *or* ceftriaxone i.v. 2–4 g, daily; *plus* metronidazole i.v. or rectal, 500 mg 8-hourly.
2 Alternative: benzylpenicillin, i.v. 2.4 g 4–6-hourly; *plus* chloramphenicol i.v. or oral, 2–3 g daily in three or four divided doses; *plus* metronidazole i.v. or rectal, 500 mg 8-hourly.
Drainage by needle or burr-hole approach is often indicated.

It is important to examine the patient clinically, by X-ray and, if necessary by further imaging, to detect any precipitating lesion. Sinusutis, otitis or, in the spinal column, osteomyelitis are all common and easy to miss if not deliberately sought.

There is the possibility of a distant, complicating abscess or septic focus. The liver and the lung should be particularly examined for evidence of this.

Other space-occupying lesions of the CNS

Apart from tumours, tuberculomata and cysticercal lesions can cause chronic space-occupying lesions in the brain.

Tuberculomata have a rather typical appearance, similar to abscesses, on CT and MR scanning. They may be associated with tuberculosis of the meninges, or of another body system. A positive tuberculin test can be helpful in suggesting the diagnosis. Treatment is with triple or quadruple antituberculosis therapy. Corticosteroids are often needed to avoid early increases in inflammation (see Chapter 18).

Cysticercosis is the condition in which tissue cysts of *Taenia solium* develop in the brain and/or other tissues. It is not endemic in western countries where tapeworm infestation is extremely rare, but is the commonest cause of epilepsy in individuals from endemic areas. Imaging of the brain shows round cystic lesions, often with surrounding oedema (Fig. 16.17). Cysts with surrounding oedema will often die as a result of the inflammatory immune reaction; calcified cysts are usually dead. Scolices are sometimes visible in living cysts.

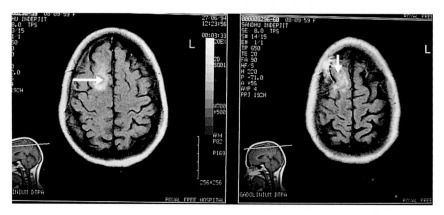

Fig. 16.17 Cerebral cysticercosis: this 44-year-old woman from Kenya had recent-onset epilepsy. The computed tomographic brain scan shows a cystic lesion with enhancing halo in the right frontal lobe (arrows). Serology was positive.

The commonest manifestation is epilepsy, but raised intracranial pressure, nausea or vomiting is also often seen. Single cysts may block the flow of CSF, or affect the spinal cord, behaving like space-occupying lesions. Cysticercal antibody tests are available. Stool examination for eggs and proglottides is advisable, but is often negative. Treatment with albendazole or praziquantel can ameliorate symptoms and greatly reduce the frequency of seizures.

Treatment of cerebral cysticercosis
1 Albendazole orally, 400 mg 12-hourly for 8–10 days.
2 Alternative: praziquantel orally, 20 mg/kg 8-hourly for 1 day (consider simultanous prednisolone 40–60 mg, continued for 3–5 days).

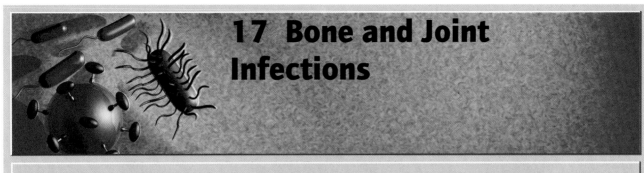

17 Bone and Joint Infections

Introduction: structural considerations

Structure of bone

Bone is a complex connective tissue formed of osteoid material which is hardened by the calcium salt hydroxyapatite. Its structure is best seen in the hard, or cortical, parts of the long bones.

The basic structure is comprised of concentric lamellae of bone surrounding a small blood vessel which runs in a central canal, or Haversian canal. The bone is laid down by cells called osteoblasts, which surround the blood vessel and also form a layer beneath the highly vascular periosteum. The osteoblasts separate the perivascular tissue fluid from the bone tissue fluid, which fills the Haversian system and the Volkmann's system, which forms transverse connections across the bone lamellae. Each Haversian system is bounded by a 'cement line', which separates each set of lamellae, and across which blood vessels do not pass (Fig. 17.1).

If the blood supply of a Haversian system is lost or damaged, the bone lamellae within that cement line will die. The dead tissue may demineralize, fibrose or occasionally be replaced by cartilage. Healing and remodelling can take place if the disease process is controlled.

As bone grows it is remodelled. This is achieved by small, advancing points of bone resorption, performed by groups of cells called osteoclasts or osteocytes. The resorption is followed by ingress of osteoblasts which build a new Haversian system, usually in a different orientation to the first, fragments of which are left supporting the new system (Fig. 17.2).

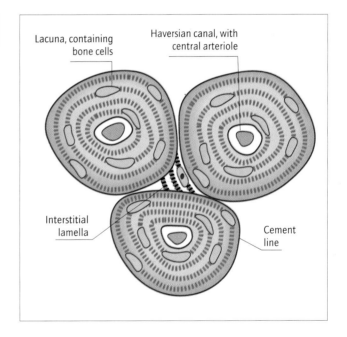

Fig. 17.1 The Haversian system of bone structure.

Each bone is surrounded by a tough, vascular membrane or periosteum. The periosteum is rich in sensory nerves, and has a lymphatic supply both of which are absent from the interior of the bone.

Bone growth in childhood

Bone growth in childhood takes place by the extension of the central, or diaphyseal, part of a bone at a car-

331

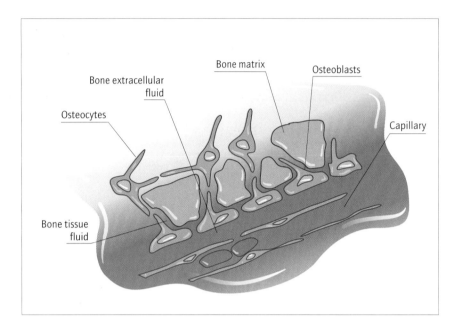

Fig. 17.2 The cells and fluid compartments of bone; antibiotics must enter the bone tissue fluid to treat intraosseous infection effectively.

tilaginous plate, the epiphyseal plate. The growing part of the bone is called the metaphysis (Fig. 17.3). On the other side of the epiphyseal plate is the epiphysis, which is initially composed entirely of cartilage but develops a centre of ossification as the child develops. When the rate of ossification overtakes that of cartilage growth, the epiphysis becomes fully ossified.

Blood vessels do not cross the epiphyseal plate; the epiphysis has its own blood supply, usually derived from a single afferent vessel. In most bones the epiphyseal artery can enter the epiphysis directly, but in the head of the femur it must traverse the joint capsule, as the epiphysis is entirely intracapsular. This artery is more at risk of damage than others, due to pressure or deformity affecting the joint.

In the epiphyseal plate there is a proliferative layer, in which osteoid is manufactured, and a deeper maturation layer. Finally, in the deepest layer, next to bone, is the level at which mineralization, or ossification, occurs. These areas are served by many capillary loops, in which blood flow slows significantly as it passes from the arterial to the venous side. It is thought that this rather stagnant flow may predispose to the deposition of bacteria, and may explain the predisposition of the growing metaphysis to haematogenous osteomyelitis.

Structure of joints

Most large joints are synovial joints. The ends of the bones which move over one another are covered with articular cartilage. The bones are held together by a tough, fibrous joint capsule. The capsule is lined with vascular synovial membrane which secretes synovial fluid, and where the capsule joins with the articular cartilage there is a fibrocartilaginous zone overlapped by the vascular edge of the synovial membrane.

The articular cartilage does not grow once adulthood has been reached. It is not bound to the underlying bone by fibrous tissue, and it receives no blood vessels from the bone. It is attached merely by the irregular-shaped, interlocked surfaces of bone and cartilage. The cartilage receives its nutrition by diffusion from the synovial fluid, and since the cartilage has an open, water-saturated structure, this process of diffusion is increased by joint movement. If the cartilage is damaged, it is not replaced, but may repair by a sort of fibrous scar.

Sometimes the joint capsule is attached very near to the end of the articulating bone. The metaphysis is then extracapsular. In the femur, by contrast, the capsule of the hip joint is attached far down the neck, and the femoral neck is therefore intracapsular. This means that infection of the neck of the femur can extend directly into the joint space, or that joint infection may invade directly into the bone.

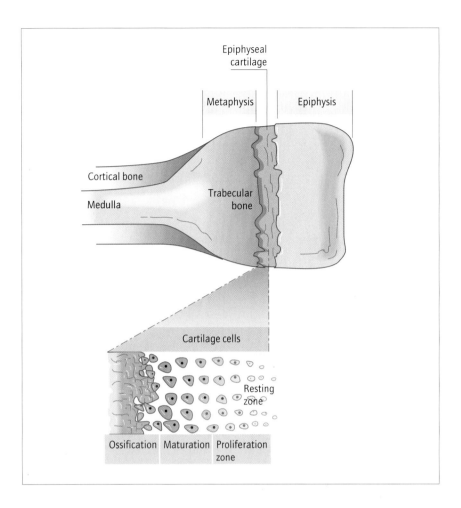

Fig. 17.3 General structure of a growing bone.

Osteomyelitis

Introduction

Osteomyelitis is infection of bone. It can arise by haematogenous spread, by extension from an infected joint, by direct invasion as a result of trauma, or by iatrogenic infection following surgery or instrumentation. This chapter is concerned with acute haematogenous osteomyelitis.

Epidemiology

The commonest type of acute haematogenous osteomyelitis is a disease of children, affecting growing bones. The source of infection is probably a transient bacteraemia, arising from the skin, mouth or respiratory system. The infection usually affects a single long bone (Fig. 17.4), and arises in the metaphysis, possibly because of the rich blood supply and the vulnerable capillary loops (see above).

Adults and elderly people can be affected by a different type of haematogenous osteomyelitis, which develops as a result of a predisposition. An example of this is the ability of bacteria to pass up the valveless venous plexus of the pelvis to the lower spine. Infection, instrumentation or invasive tumour of the lower bowel or urogenital tract can release bacteria into this plexus and cause 'metastatic' Gram-negative spinal ostomyelitis.

Occasionally a haematogenous infection occurs in a bone already damaged by degenerative or malignant disease. This is often an axial bone such as a vertebra or part of the pelvis.

Some intravenous drug users develop pseudomonal osteomyelitis of the spine or pelvis, possibly after injecting into inguinal veins.

Coliform bacteria or salmonellae may escape from an infected bowel and cause distant osteomyelitis, usually of the axial skeleton (Fig. 17.5). Salmonellae are said to

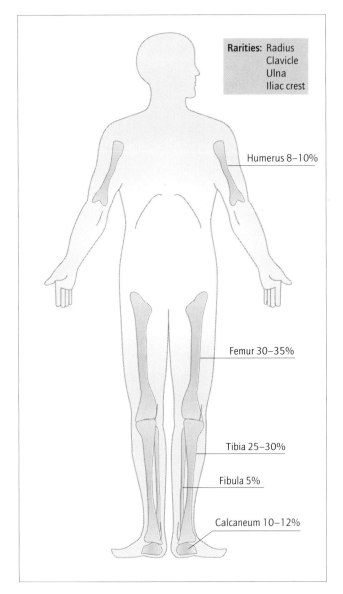

Fig. 17.4 Bones most often affected by childhood osteomyelitis. The spine is rarely affected in children, but is more commonly involved in adults.

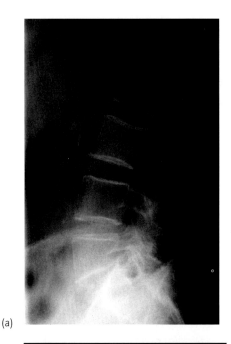

(a)

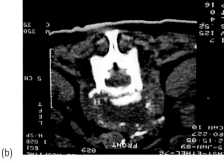

(b)

Fig. 17.5 Osteomyelitis of the lumbar spine complicating *Salmonella enteritidis* colitis. (a) X-ray; (b) computed tomographic scan showing destruction of the body of the second lumbar vertebra.

have a predilection for the bones of individuals with sickle-cell disease, possibly because of stagnant bone circulation following sickling crises (Fig. 17.6).

Finally, bone may be infected by extension from an overlying site of soft-tissue infection. An example of this is osteomyelitis underlying a deep pressure sore, or a diabetic foot ulcer (Fig. 17.7).

Pathology

Osteomyelitis is caused by pyogenic organisms. Inflammatory oedema and pus therefore form in the infected

bone and track through the Haversian and Volkmann's canals. At the site of infection, bone ischaemia and necrosis occur. When the exudate reaches the periosteal surface of the bone, the periosteum is elevated by the fluid. The osteoblasts underlying the periosteum then begin to generate new bone.

Formation of sequestra and involucra

While the infected area of bone suffers progressive necrosis, it is gradually surrounded by an accumulation of new bone, which encloses it. The old, dead bone is called a sequestrum, and the surrounding live bone is termed an involucrum. These have typical X-ray appearances, with a sclerotic sequestrum surrounded by the more normal-appearing involucrum, from which it is

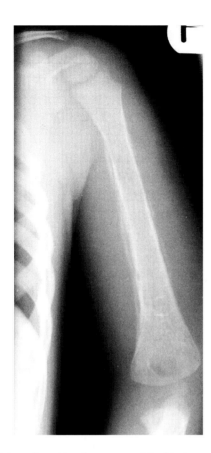

Fig. 17.6 *Salmonella typhimurium* osteomyelitis of the humerus in a child with sickle-cell disease. Note the elevated periosteum.

separated by a lucent area (Fig. 17.8). The sequestrum has no blood supply, and so is inaccessible to antibiotics and most immunological processes. It is therefore often a

site of persisting infection which prevents the healing of the osteomyelitis.

Brodie's abscess

Sometimes the infected part of a bone not only dies, but is completely replaced by pus. This intraosseous abscess is enclosed in a sclerotic membrane, and becomes surrounded by a sclerotic bony reaction. The infection may become quiescent when it is contained in this way, but there is a high risk of recrudescence and new extension in the future.

If pus continues to accumulate, it may track through the tissues, causing a local abscess or reaching the skin surface to produce a draining sinus. If the infection is near the joint surface of an intracapsular bone, it may track through the synovial membrane and cause a pyogenic arthritis.

ORGANISM LIST

Staphylococcus aureus (90%)
Streptococcus pyogenes (4%)
Haemophilus influenzae (4%)
Escherichia coli
Proteus spp.
Klebsiella spp.
Pseudomonas spp.
Neisseria meningitidis
Salmonella spp.
Brucella spp.
Mycobacteria
Anaerobic bacteria (anaerobic streptococci, *Bacteroides* spp., *Fusobacterium* spp., etc.).

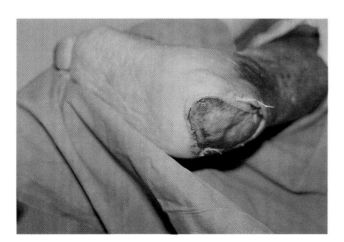

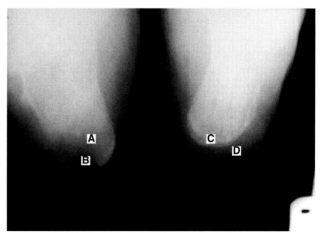

Fig. 17.7 Osteomyelitis of the calcaneum: this immobile, elderly man had a deep heel ulcer colonized with methicillin-resistant *Staphylococcus aureus*; this infection extended to the underlying periosteum and bone. (a) The ulcer; (b) X-ray showing loss of structure of the calcaneum. A, defect in both cortical layer and bone structure; B, absence of soft tissue; C, normal outline of continuous layer of bone cortex; D, soft tissue of the heel.

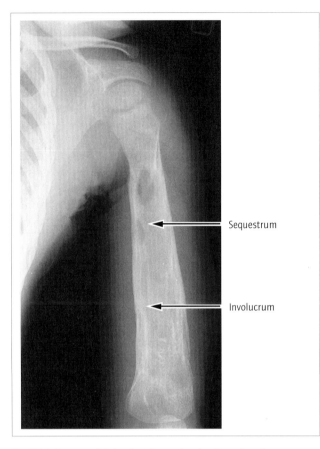

Fig. 17.8 Osteomyelitis in a long bone, showing formation of a sequestrum and involucrum.

Clinical features

The onset of osteomyelitis is insidious in most cases. In children a common presentation is with a feverish illness and poorly localized pain. While infection is confined within the bone, there may be little change in the white cell count, and the illness and pain may be passed off as 'flu-like'. Infants and toddlers may not be able to describe the pain, but instead they stop using the affected limb, displaying a 'pseudoparalysis'.

As infection progresses, the affected bone site becomes surrounded by soft-tissue swelling. Later changes, such as the development of draining sinuses, of deformity of bones or of pathological fractures, are the unfortunate consequences of delayed diagnosis.

Diagnosis

X-ray changes are slow to develop, except for soft-tissue shadows. They are not usually helpful in early diagnosis. Later on, areas of lucency appear where bone is demineralized or destroyed, and the elevation of perios-

teum and formation of subperiosteal bone are typical X-ray findings in established disease.

Isotope scans of the skeleton, using technetium or gallium, will show early signs of vascularity or inflammation respectively. They do not always distinguish between the changes of rheumatic inflammation, infection or tumour circulation.

Magnetic resonance scanning shows extremely early changes of oedema and altered blood flow. Although expensive, it can be an important early diagnostic investigation if others are unhelpful (Fig. 17.9).

Bacteriological diagnosis

Bacteriological diagnosis is not always easily obtained. Blood cultures are often negative, and pus is not always obtainable for examination, especially in early disease. Needle aspiration of subperiosteal fluid or pus is sometimes possible. Imaging-directed needle aspiration may yield pus from abnormal bone, or from within or outside the periosteum.

An operative approach can be used to obtain pus, infected bone or adjacent tissue. If a large collection of pus, a sequestrum or a Brodie's abscess is already present, drainage may well contribute to treatment, and a bacteriological diagnosis can help the choice of antibiotic management.

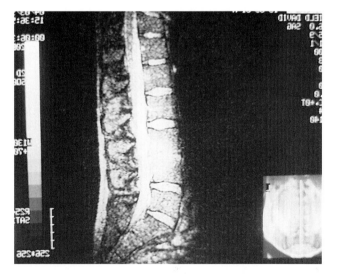

Fig. 17.9 Magnetic resonance scan showing infection of an intervertebral disc (discitis): the patient 'strained' his back while suffering from a severe sore throat. Persisting back pain and fever led to imaging and needle aspiration, revealing a *Fusobacterium necrophorum* infection (see Chapter 7).

Management

Confirming the diagnosis

Confirming the diagnosis is an important part of management. Blood cultures should be taken, and a careful examination made for skin, chest, throat or ear sepsis, which may provide clues as to the infecting agent. Urine should be cultured, especially in elderly patients.

Imaging studies may show evidence of bone inflammation at a suspicious site. This allows follow-up by clinical and further imaging examination, to confirm healing or to detect the development of pus.

Antimicrobial treatment

Antimicrobial treatment should be commenced as soon as specimens have been obtained. In all age groups an antistaphylococcal agent should be included. Agents which penetrate bone well include fusidic acid, flucloxacillin or cloxacillin. In all but the mildest cases, it is advisable to begin with intravenous treatment.

In unvaccinated children up to age 5, it is advisable to treat empirically for *Haemophilus influenzae* as well as *Staphylococcus aureus*. Cefuroxime is effective against both organisms.

Clindamycin is particularly useful in osteomyelitis, being effective against staphylococci and some other Gram-positive cocci, as well as against anaerobes. It penetrates bone very well. The possibility of pseudomembranous colitis should be borne in mine when using this drug.

In the elderly, especially those with infected urine or urinary tract obstruction, cefotaxime may be given to cover for Gram-negative rods. It is also useful in osteomyelitis of the diabetic foot, where Gram-negative rods may be involved.

Most cases of acute osteomyelitis should be treated for a minimum of 6 weeks, and for longer if any evidence of inflammation remains.

Antibiotic treatment of osteomyelitis
1 First choice:
  (a) Flucloxacillin i.v. 1–2 g 6-hourly (child under 2 years, 250–500 mg 6-hourly; 2–10 years, 500 mg to 1 g 6-hourly *or* cloxacillin i.v. 1 g 6-hourly (child proportionately as for flucloxacillin); *plus*
  Fusidic acid orally 750 mg 8-hourly (child up to 1 year, 50 mg/kg daily in three divided doses; 1–5 years, 250 mg 8-hourly; 5–12 years, 500 mg 8-hourly) *or* fusidic acid i.v., adult over 50 kg, 580 mg 8-hourly; adult under 50 kg and child, 6–7 mg/kg 8-hourly.

  (b) Clindamycin orally, 150–300 mg 6-hourly (child 3–6 mg/kg 6-hourly).
2 For child under 5 years, consider cefuroxime i.v. 60–100 mg/kg daily in three or four divided doses.
3 For elderly people, consider cefuroxime i.v. 750 mg 1.5 g 8-hourly *or* cefotaxime i.v. 2 g 8-hourly plus an antistaphylococcal drug.
4 For methicillin-resistant *Staphylococcus aureus* or enterococci, teicoplanin i.v. 400 mg 12-hourly for three doses, then 400 mg daily (child 10 mg/kg daily, reducing to 6 mg/kg daily after first 2–5 days).

Treatment may be modified in the light of bacteriological information, when it becomes available. Difficult infections such as those with enterococci may be treated with teicoplanin. Treatment should be continued until the fever has subsided, the erythrocyte sedimentation rate or C-reactive protein has fallen to the normal range and healing of the bone is established.

Patients with 'difficult' organisms, such as methicillin-resistant *Staphylococcus aureus*, enterococci or mixed facultative and anaerobic infections, are often also difficult patients to treat. They may be long-term patients, frail, demented or otherwise debilitated. It is sometimes impossible to maintain continued parenteral treatment in such patients. As long as a steady response is obtained, treatment with combinations of oral drugs such as fusidic acid, rifampicin, trimethoprim and/or metronidazole can be successful.

Surgical treatment

Surgical treatment is usually reserved for those cases requiring release of clinically or radiologically apparent pus. It is rarely productive to operate on a suspected site, as it may not be the exact site of infection. Exceptions are the calcaneum and the sacroiliac area, which are accessible to aspiration. Otherwise a fruitless anaesthetic and a scar are the only likely result of early, 'blind' operative intervention.

Evidence of pus formation should be sought by daily examination for fluctuance or localization of inflammation. The erythrocyte sedimentation rate or C-reactive protein can be used to monitor the continuation or diminution of inflammatory reaction during treatment. When pus is present, drainage will alleviate the infection, producing improvement in the patient's fever and general condition, and allowing healing of the bone.

Surgery may also be indicated when a sequestrum has formed. The orthopaedic specialist will decide whether or when there is adequate new bone formation to compensate for the defect caused by sequestrum removal.

Problems and complications

Failure to respond

Failure to obtain a response to treatment is the commonest problem. This may be because the causative organism is unusual (for instance, *Brucella* sp.), and not covered by the chosen antibiotic regimen. It can also be because the organism has an unexpected resistance, such as a methicillin-resistant *S. aureus*. Care should be taken that an adequate antibiotic dosage is being used, and that the route of administration is optimal.

Problems of prolonged antibiotic treatment

Problems of prolonged antibiotic treatment may result from the need to use antibiotics for several months in severe infections. Many patients tolerate this surprisingly well. Candidal infections of mucosae or skin folds may be troublesome if broad-spectrum agents must be used; intermittent or concurrent anti-*Candida* medication will often help, if necessary using itraconazole or fluconazole (though fluconazole resistance can occur, especially in hospital environments).

Prolonged ciprofloxacin treatment can cause otherwise unexplained anorexia and weight loss. Long-term metronidazole can cause peripheral neuropathy. Prolonged high-dose beta-lactam medication can cause sudden, idiosyncratic agranulocytosis, which quickly resolves if treatment is stopped, but which precludes further use of any beta-lactam because of complete cross-reactogenicity.

Mistaken diagnosis

A mistaken diagnosis is always a possibility in bone disease. Bone tumours and cysts, or the effects of trauma, can all cause a painful, warm and immobile limb. Failure to respond to antibiotics should prompt a reconsideration of the diagnosis and a review of imaging studies.

Damage to epiphyseal cartilage

Damage to epiphyseal cartilage occasionally follows extensive osteomyelitis. It is an irreversible situation. This causes progressive distortion and failure to elongate at the affected site. The least favourable sites for this to occur are the lower end of the femur and the upper tibia,

as gait, stature and knee function are all severely affected.

Invasion and suppurative arthritis

Invasion and suppurative arthritis of a neighbouring joint can occur if a bone metaphysis is intracapsular, or partly so. The hip and the shoulder are therefore the joints affected by this problem.

Chronic osteomyelitis

Epidemiology

The epidemiology of chronic osteomyelits has changed with the development of powerful antibiotics. Only half of cases, or fewer, are nowadays the result of persisting infection after acute blood-borne osteomyelitis. The remainder of cases follow fractures (sometimes associated with non-union), or complicate surgery.

Bones

The bones involved are mainly the femur and the tibia, which together account for over 70% of cases in many series. Any other bone may be involved, however, including vertebrae, the bones of the foot (especially in diabetics) or the skull (complicating severe otitis externa, for instance).

Bacteria

The bacteria are similar to those of acute disease. Over half of cases are caused by *S. aureus*. Gram-negative infections are slightly less common, and are more often caused by *Pseudomonas* spp. or *Proteus* spp. than by *Escherichia coli*. Mixed Gram-positive and Gram-negative infections occur. Between 10 and 20% of cases are due to anaerobic infection.

Causes of chronic osteomyelitis
1 *Staphylococcus aureus* (>50%).
2 Anaerobic infections (10–20%).
3 *Pseudomonas* spp.
4 *Proteus* spp.
5 *Escherichia coli*.
6 Mixed Gram-positive and -negative infections.

Clinical features

Clinical features include pain, swelling, deformity and, in the case of fracture or surgery, defective healing.

Some cases have intermittently or continuously discharging sinuses.

Diagnosis

Diagnosis is made on clinical and radiological grounds, and by identifying a causative organism. Pus or swabs from sinuses are often contaminated by skin commensals or saprophytes, so specimens obtained directly from infected bone or periosteum are preferred.

Management

Management may be simply a prolonged course of appropriate chemotherapy, but surgery may also have an important role. Surgical intervention may include removal of sequestra and other devitalized tissue, plastic surgery and vascular surgery to fill tissue defects and optimize blood supply, and bone grafting to restore anatomy and function when infection has been controlled.

Complications

Complications are rare, except for the inconvenience of the lesion and the systemic effects of chronic infection. The only important complication is the occasional occurrence of squamous cell carcinoma in the infected tissue. This is associated with increased pain, progressive bone destruction and metastasis to regional lymph nodes.

Suppurative arthritis

Introduction and epidemiology

Suppurative arthritis is usually a blood-borne infection, arising either from an inapparent bacteraemia or as a complication of a bacteraemic disease. The natural history of the disease is slightly different in children and adults. In children the joint infection often arises apparently spontaneously, while in adults pre-existing disease such as rheumatoid arthritis, gout or pseudogout may predispose to septic joint disease, and complicate its diagnosis. In children, but rarely in adults, arthritis of the hip can be an extension from osteomyelitis of the upper femur.

ORGANISM LIST

In children
  Staphylococcus aureus (50%)
  Haemophilus influenzae (20%)*
  Streptococcus pyogenes (16%)
  Gram-negative rods (7%)
  Anaerobes
  Staphylococcus epidermidis

In adults
  Staphylococcus aureus (70%)
  Gram-negative rods (15%)
  Streptococcus pyogenes (7%)
  Neisseria gonorrhoeae (3%)
  Staphylococcus epidermidis
  Mixed organisms
  Anaerobes

*Becoming less common since commencement of immunization programme.

Rarities
  Borrelia burgdorferi
  Salmonella spp.
  Brucella spp.
  Pasteurella spp.

Clinical features

The joints most commonly affected are similar in children and adults. The knee is involved approximately twice as commonly as any other joint. The hip, ankle, elbow and wrist are progressively less often affected. In adults the shoulder rivals the hip or ankle in frequency; in children it is about as commonly affected as the wrist.

In children the onset of suppurative arthritis is often abrupt, with fever, pain and swelling of the joint. The main exception occurs when the hip is affected in a small child or infant. The swelling may not be apparent, and the child often complains of abdominal pain. Constipation or abdominal distension may further confuse the diagnosis.

Misleading clinical signs in childhood hip infections
1 Pseudoparalysis of the leg.
2 Abdominal pain.
3 Abdominal distension.
4 Constipation.

A small child may have been exposed to a case or an outbreak of *Haemophilus influenzae* disease, such as meningitis or pneumonia, raising the possibility of a *Haemophilus* arthritis. This will become much less likely as the *H. influenzae* type b (Hib) vaccination programme becomes established.

In adults the onset may also be rapid, but is not always so. Especially in individuals with pre-existing joint disease, there may be a gradual swelling and slow accumulation of effusion.

There may be a clue in the recent medical history, suggesting a source of infection. Recent salmonella gastroenteritis or an episode of urinary retention or urinary tract manipulation may suggest a Gram-negative aetiology.

When the joint infection is part of a bacteraemic disease, there may be other manifestations of the infection on general examination. In staphylococcal septicaemia there may be a cellulitic skin rash, or nodular pneumonitis, with a tendency to abscess formation. In streptococcal infections there may be an erysipelas-like rash on the trunk or arm, a scarlet fever-like rash or a follicular tonsillitis. Painful lymphadenitis tends to accompany severe streptococcal infections.

There may be a typical rash in gonococcal bacteraemia (see Chapter 11).

Diagnosis

In children the diagnosis is often clinically obvious, but in adults there is a wide range of differential diagnoses, some of which can coexist with infection. The differential diagnoses include rheumatoid arthritis, acute osteoarthritis, acute gout or pseudogout.

Examination of effusion

Examination of effusion is the best rapid diagnostic test. In acute infective arthritis the protein level is high, the glucose level low and there is a neutrophilic pleiocytosis. This picture can also occur in exacerbation of inflammatory joint disease, however, so bacteriological examination is critical.

Gram-stained preparations will often show typical Gram-positive cocci in staphylococcal and streptococcal infections, and their grouping in masses or chains may indicate the type of bacteria involved. Gram-negative organisms such as *H. influenzae* or coliforms may also be demonstrable, but the small *Haemophilus* organisms in particular are more difficult to see. Most pyogenic organisms will be detectable in culture in 24–36 h, though speciation and sensitivity testing may take a further day. Previous treatment with antibiotics may make culture difficult, slow or impossible.

Cultures from other sites

Cultures from other sites, such as blood cultures, should also be obtained, as should urine cultures and specimens from skin, throat and sputum, when indicated. In patients at risk through known exposure or overseas residence, cultures for mycobacteria should be set up. It is worth remembering that about 80% of patients with tuberculous arthritis have a strongly positive tuberculin test. Brucellosis is a recognized cause of infective arthritis in Middle Eastern and East European countries. It often affects the knee or the spine.

Differential diagnosis

Exclusion of differential diagnoses is helpful, and can include examination of joint aspirate for crystals, as well as serological tests for rheumatoid factors and other autoantibodies. On rare occasions arthroscopy and synovial biopsy may be useful in diagnosing typical rheumatoid changes, or in obtaining tissue specimens for culture.

Management

Early eradication of infection minimizes damage to the joint, particularly to the articular cartilage, which is eroded by proteolytic enzymes and other inflammatory mediators. There is general agreement that intravenous antibiotic treatment is justified, to obtain high levels of agent in the synovial fluid and adjacent tissues.

Adults

For adults an antistaphylococcal drug is essential. This may be flucloxacillin or cloxacillin. Fusidic acid (or sometimes rifampicin) may be added, as it penetrates bones and joints well. Teicoplanin is useful for methicillin-resistant *Staphylococcus aureus*, and may be used for other staphylococci. Ciprofloxacin is well-distributed even when given orally, but is less effective against streptococci than staphylococci, even at high doses. Clindamycin is an option, especially if anaerobic infection is present. Antibiotic treatment is usually continued for 3–4 weeks. Oral continuation treatment is possible with ciprofloxacin, fusidic acid or rifampicin, but neither of the latter two drugs should be given alone, because of the risk of one-step mutation to resistance by the infecting organism.

Adults with urinary or bowel sepsis

For adults with urinary or bowel sepsis it is advisable to consider the possibility of Gram-negative infection. A broad-spectrum cephalosporin such as cefotaxime is useful in this setting, and can be given with an antistaphylococcal drug.

Children

For children the possibility of *H. influenzae* infection still exists. A broad-spectrum cephalosporin is the antibiotic of choice in this setting, and an additional antistaphylococcal drug can safely be added. Cefuroxime is effective against both *S. aureus* and *H. influenzae*.

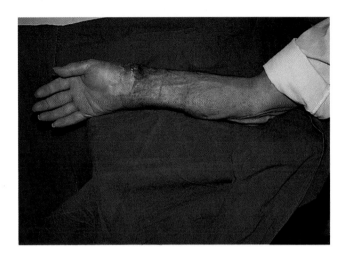

Fig. 17.10 Destructive tuberculous infection of the wrist, with draining sinus. Concurrent pulmonary tuberculosis responded well to triple therapy, but the wrist only healed after debridement and arthrodesis.

Surgical intervention

Surgical intervention is not often needed. When the joint is distended by pus, rather than just serous fluid containing neutrophils, then adequate aspiration protects the cartilage from inflammatory damage. Aspiration and irrigation may be performed. In severe cases, persistent effusion can be drained by an indwelling suction drain.

In the rare case of extensive joint destruction, it may be possible to carry out arthroplasty or arthrodesis when the infection has been fully controlled (Fig. 17.10).

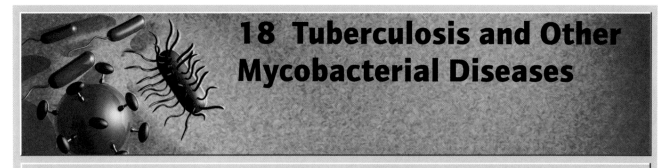

18 Tuberculosis and Other Mycobacterial Diseases

Introduction

Tuberculosis is a granulomatous disease caused by infection with some species of mycobacteria. Depending on the portal of entry of the infection, and on the degree of haematogenous spread, many organs and systems of the body can be affected. The commonest sites of infection are the lungs or the lymph nodes. Other important sites are the bowel, the peritoneum, the meninges, the kidneys and the bones and joints. Even the skin can occasionally be involved.

The disease is important because it is common in many countries (Fig. 18.1), because its commonest, pulmonary form is highly infectious and because it can cause severe morbidity and high mortality in people of all ages.

Epidemiology

Tuberculosis is one of the commonest infections of humans. It is estimated that 1.7 billion persons are infected and that there are 20 million active cases and 3.3 million deaths a year. Most of these cases are in the developing world, although the incidence in many developed countries is now starting to rise after almost a century of steady decline (Table 18.1). There are a number of possible reasons for this recent increase: a deterioration in living conditions, particularly in inner cities and among refugees, spread of the human immunodeficiency virus (HIV), intravenous drug abuse and worsening standards of health care. In developed countries, the disease mainly affects two group: elderly, predominantly male, 'skid row' populations, and recent

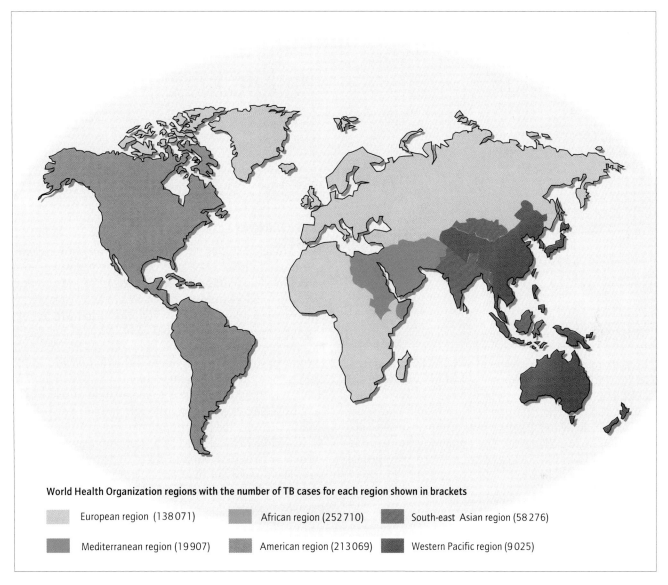

World Health Organization regions with the number of TB cases for each region shown in brackets

European region (138 071)   African region (252 710)   South-east Asian region (58 276)

Mediterranean region (19 907)   American region (213 069)   Western Pacific region (9 025)

Fig. 18.1 Incidence of tuberculosis (TB) reported in different regions of the world in 1993. Courtesy of the World Health Organization.

immigrants from developing countries. Health care workers, teachers and veterinary workers also have an increased risk of disease compared to the general population. Outbreaks occur in conditions of crowding, such as shelters for the homeless, hospitals and prisons. In 1990, the incidence in the UK was 10.3 per 100 000 population, slightly lower than the average for western Europe (14.0 per 100 000).

The prevalence of infection detected by tuberculin testing rises with age. In the UK, tuberculin sensitivity among school children aged 10–13 years, who are routinely tested prior to bacillus Calmette–Guérin (BCG) administration, is between 1 and 2%.

Most infections in developed countries are caused by *Mycobacterium tuberculosis*. Infection due to *M. bovis* is, however, still a problem in countries where the disease has not been controlled in cattle, and milk is consumed raw.

The rise of tuberculosis among HIV-infected individuals is often due to reactivation rather than primary infection. This phenomenon has mainly been observed in areas where the prevalence of HIV infection is high, such as parts of Africa and some US cities. Another problem in these areas is the emergence of strains of *M. tuberculosis* resistant to several antituberculosis drugs.

Country	Incidence per 100 000	Current trend
Austria	18.3	Up
Belgium	14.8	Down
Denmark	6.5	Up
Finland	15.5	Down
France	15.0	Down
Germany	18.4	Down
Ireland	17.9	Up
Italy	7.3	Up
Netherlands	9.2	Up
Norway	8.5	Up
Spain	23.1	Down
Sweden	6.5	Stable
Switzerland	16.5	Up
United Kingdom	10.5	Stable

Table 18.1 Tuberculosis: recent trends in western Europe (from Raviglione, M.C. *et al.* (1993) *Bulletin of the World Health Organization*, 71, 297–306, with permission)

Microbiology

There are more than 85 species of mycobacteria, and new species continue to be proposed. Most mycobacteria are environmental organisms which rarely, if ever, cause human disease. Their natural habitat is soil, and fresh and estuarine water. Only a minority of species are obligate human pathogens. The remaining human diseases arise when host defences are reduced by physical or immunological defect.

Classification

Obligate pathogens

This group includes those organisms whose isolation or detection implies that a disease is present. It includes the organisms of the *M. tuberculosis* complex: *M. tuberculosis*, *M. africanum*, *M. bovis*, BCG and also *M. leprae*, which is in a group of its own. This is important since the identification of any of these organisms in a patient specimen implies the presence of disease, and the need for specific chemotherapy.

Pulmonary opportunists

M. kansasii and *M. xenopi* infection are found most commonly in patients who have anatomical abnormalities of the lower respiratory tract. Chronic obstructive airways disease and bronchiectasis are common predisposing conditions. Surprisingly, these species have not often been isolated from patients with acquired

immunodeficiency syndrome (AIDS). Infection is usually pulmonary, resembling indolent progressive pulmonary tuberculosis.

The most commonly isolated mycobacteria in the UK
1 *Mycobacterium tuberculosis*.
2 *M. kansasii*.
3 *M. avium-intercellulare*.
4 *M. bovis*.
5 *M. xenopi*.
6 *M. chelonei*.
7 *M. fortuitum*.

Skin pathogens

This group includes *M. marinum*, a cause of chronic granulomatous infection and ulceration of the skin, and sometimes subcutaneous tissue. It is found in old, concrete-lined swimming pools, rivers and fishtanks or aquaria. Infection occurs when the organism enters through broken or macerated skin. *M. ulcerans* is the causative organism of buruli (tropical) ulcers. This is a chronic destructive ulcer, often of the foot or leg, which erodes the skin and the subcutaneous tissues, including bone. It is thought to be due to inoculation of the organism by sharp vegetation, though it has never been isolated from the environment in endemic areas. *M. tuberculosis* can also act as a skin pathogen, causing a chronic scarring infection of the skin, principally on the face. The disease is called lupus vulgaris because of the wolf-like facies of sufferers in the pre-antibiotic period.

Opportunist pathogens

In the past, opportunist infections with mycobacteria were uncommon. Now, due to the appearance of AIDS, opportunist infections are quite common in these severely immunocompromised patients.

AIDS-related opportunists

Organisms of the *M. avium-intracellulare* (MAI) complex have been associated with AIDS patients in the latter part of the disease process. The infection is acquired through the gastrointestinal tract but as immunity fades, invasion occurs and the organism may be isolated from the blood and other tissues. Infection often takes the form of cervical adenopathy. Infection with *M. avium-intracellulare* is rare in immune-competent patients but has been associated with outbreaks of pulmonary infection in a hospital environment.

Rapid growers

These organisms include *M. fortuitum* and the *M. chelonei* complex, and differ from other mycobacteria in the speed of their growth. Isolates grow on Löwenstein–Jensen and other selective media in 2–48 h. The organisms have low virulence but can be associated with significant infections in some circumstances. *M. chelonei* has caused systemic infections in neutropenic patients. In contrast, both *M. chelonei* and *M. fortuitum* can cause abscesses in patients who have been injected with 'sterile' fluids contaminated by this organism (for example, at sites of injection of insulin in diabetics whose needles or multidose insulin containers have become contaminated).

Pathogenesis

This is an extremely complex subject which has proved difficult to research; however, a number of important pathogenic attributes of mycobacteria can be identified. The mechanisms of mycobacterial pathogenicity are gradually being elucidated by the use of molecular cytology and immunology techniques.

In contrast to many bacteria, the cell wall of the mycobacteria is very lipid-rich. Up to 40% of the dry weight of the organism is made up of lipid, and several lipid antigens have been identified as potential pathogenicity determinants.

Handling of mycobacterial antigens by the immune system

Once ingested by antigen-presenting cells, mycobacterial antigens are processed and presented in the classic way, in association with human leukocyte antigen (HLA) class II molecules. T-lymphocytes bearing receptors which can recognize this complex bind to the macrophage, causing the release of interleukin 2 (IL-2), and the activation of T-helper cells. IL-2 stimulates both antigen-specific T cells and antigen non-specific N cells. All of these cell types are capable of producing gamma-interferon, which has an important role in activating bactericidal mechanisms in macrophages.

Basis of the wasting effect of mycobacterial infections

The macrophage releases several cytokines while reacting to mycobacteria. These include tumour necrosis factor (TNF), IL-3 and granulocyte–macrophage colony-stimulating factor (GM-CSF), which probably have an important role in inducing symptoms such as fever and wasting. Mycobacterial lipoarabinomannan is a strong inducer of TNF.

Inhibition of cell-mediated immune responses

Macrophage activation may be inhibited by mycobacterial lipid antigens such as lipoarabinomannan, and capsule-like materials such as the phenolic glycolipid of *M. leprae*. These are thought to act by scavenging reactive oxygen intermediates and interfering with the efficiency of the microbicidal oxidative system. Protein antigens of mycobacteria, such as catalase and superoxide dismutase, may also act in this way.

Mycobacterial antigens may interfere with the activation of T-cell responses. Lipoarabinomannan has been implicated in blocking the stimulatory effect of gamma-interferon by inhibiting its interaction with macrophage surface molecules such as protein kinase C. Lymphocytes and macrophages which are recruited to the site of infection, but cannot destroy the mycobacteria, contribute to the progressive formation of granulomatous infiltration.

Mechanisms of survival within macrophages

A key characteristic of the pathogenic mycobacteria is the ability to survive inside macrophages. Mycobacterial ingestion is mediated via the CR1 and CR3 receptors which do not stimulate microbicidal oxidative responses. Mycobacteria are able to survive inside macrophages by inhibiting phagosomal-lysosomal fusion or by escaping from the phagosome into the cytoplasm, in both cases avoiding the effects of lysozymes.

Heat-shock proteins are produced by phagocytosed mycobacteria, and this may also be an adaptive mechanism to survival inside the macrophage.

> **Possible pathogenicity factors of *Mycobacterium tuberculosis***
> 1 Lipoarabinomannan (induces tumour necrosis factor and scavenges oxidizing molecules).
> 2 Catalase (scavenges oxidizing molecules).
> 3 Superoxide dismutase (scavenges oxidizing molecules).
> 4 Inhibitors of phagosomal-lysosomal fusion.
> 5 Heat-shock proteins.

Primary tuberculosis

This is an acute or subacute illness which follows primary infection in a non-immune host. There is usually a small focus of inflammation, with a few mycobacteria surrounded by a dense granuloma. When this occurs in the lung it is called a Ghon focus. Regional lymph nodes are often enlarged, and the combination of primary granuloma and enlarged nodes is called a primary complex.

Primary tuberculosis is not always associated with clinical illness; indeed, naturally acquired immunity to tuberculosis often follows healing of an inapparent primary complex. When tuberculous lesions heal they often calcify, leaving an irregular, X-ray-dense shadow which is easily identified.

Postprimary tuberculosis

This is the type of disease caused by reinfection or reactivation of infection in a person previously sensitized to mycobacterial antigens. It can follow primary infection or immunization after a variable period of time, up to many years. The resulting vigorous tissue reaction causes the formation of exuberant granulomata, often with central, cheesy necrosis, called caseation. In pulmonary infection, necrotic tissue is coughed away, leaving cavities within the granulomata. In solid organs or soft tissues, the caseous material resembles pus, and may discharge via the body surface. The abscess-like lesion is indurated rather than hot and inflamed, and is therefore called a cold abscess.

The reaction does not destroy the mycobacteria, however, as the immune system is suppressed and mycobacteria survive within macrophages. Lesions contain large numbers of organisms, which are released from caseating tissues. Postprimary, cavitating pulmonary tuberculosis is highly infectious to susceptible individuals because of the large numbers of mycobacteria released during coughing.

Miliary or disseminated tuberculosis

This type of disease occurs when local defences are overwhelmed and large numbers of mycobacteria enter the blood stream. It may also follow rupture of an active granuloma into a blood vessel. Many organs are affected by the resulting infection, which varies in the severity of presentation from mild fever and malaise to severe, debilitating illness.

When the tissue granulomata are large enough to be macroscopically detectable they are visible in the organs as small white nodules rather like millet seeds. This is the origin of the expression miliary tuberculosis, used to describe the condition.

Other types of mycobacterial infection

There are many species of mycobacteria in nature, of which only a few cause typical types of tuberculosis in humans. Other organisms, called environmental mycobacteria, are occasionally pathogenic. They tend to enter the soft tissues via small skin lesions or injection sites, and the usual result is a granuloma of the skin or a subcutaneous cold abscess.

ORGANISM LIST

Human organisms
  Mycobacterium tuberculosis
  M. africanum
  M. bovis
  BCG.

Other mycobacteria capable of causing typical tuberculosis
  M. kansasii
  M. avium-intracellulare complex
  M. xenopi.

Mycobacteria which can cause cold abscesses
  M. fortuitum
  M. chelonei
  M. scrofulaceum
  BCG (if mistakenly injected subcutaneously).

Mycobacteria associated with skin lesions
  M. marinum
  M. ulcerans.

Organism of leprosy
  M. leprae.

Primary tuberculosis

Introduction

Primary tuberculosis characteristically affects certain organs and systems. The commonest affected organ is the lung, but the pleura, lymph nodes, peritoneum, pericardium and meninges are other sites where primary disease occurs.

Clinical features

The clinical presentation is a combination of general features of tuberculosis and of signs and symptoms related to the affected site.

The general features are common to all kinds of tuberculosis. These are fever, night sweats, anorexia and weight loss. There is no predictable change in the blood count, the liver function tests or other blood biochemistry. The erythrocyte sedimentation rate or C-reactive protein may be raised, but often remains within the normal range.

Erythema nodosum

Erythema nodosum sometimes accompanies primary tuberculosis, and is occasionally the first sign of the disease. As tuberculosis has become less common, other associations with erythema nodosum, such as sarcoidosis or streptococcal infections, are important differential diagnoses (see Chapter 5). Nevertheless, tuberculosis should always be carefully excluded in patients first presenting with the condition.

In rare cases, erythema nodosum develops early in the treatment of tuberculosis. This is similar to the situation in leprosy, where the condition is well-recognized as a complication of treatment, occurring with a surge of cell-mediated immune reactivity.

Affected site

The clinical features relating to the affected site are often helpful in suggesting the diagnosis, both because of the typical site but also because of the typical type of lesion produced.

Primary pulmonary tuberculosis

Primary pulmonary tuberculosis, when it is clinically evident, often causes a persistent, dry cough in addition to general features. The site of the infection is usually the periphery of the mid-zone of one lung. The lesion, or Ghon focus, is too small to produce abnormal signs on physical examination, but is visible on chest X-ray as a fluffy, approximately round opacity with a diameter of 1–2 cm. The mediastinal lymph nodes on the affected side may be enlarged and, together with the Ghon focus, this is the primary complex (Fig. 18.2).

Endobronchial tuberculosis

Endobronchial tuberculosis sometimes occurs as a primary infection, particularly in children. Granulomata develop in the bronchial mucosa of one of the larger airways, causing partial obstruction. There is a persistent, wheezy cough and often a fixed wheeze on auscultation over the affected airway. The narrowed section of bronchus may be visible on chest X-ray.

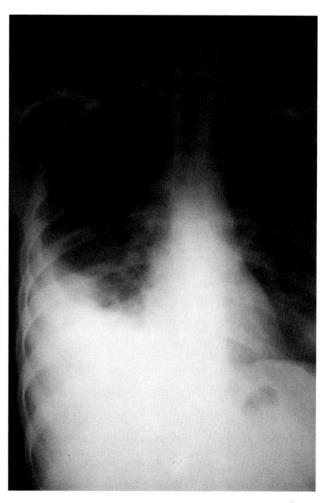

Fig. 18.3 Primary tuberculosis: pleural effusion in an Indian teenager with malaise, night sweats, weight loss and low-grade fever.

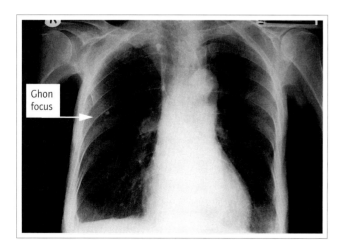

Fig. 18.2 Primary tuberculosis: Ghon focus on chest X-ray. The density of the lesion suggests healing and calcification.

Pleural tuberculosis

Pleural tuberculosis occurs when granulomata affect the pleura. Pleuritic pain is the characteristic clinical feature, and a pleural rub is occasionally heard on auscultation of the chest. As with other inflamed serous surfaces, exudate tends to produce an effusion. Effusion may cause shortness of breath; the typical physical signs are detectable on chest examination, and any pre-existing pleural rub disappears as the pleural surfaces are separated. The chest X-ray shows the characteristic opacity with an upcurved surface (Figs 18.3 & 18.4).

Tuberculous pericarditis

Tuberculous pericarditis is similar to pleural infection, but the granulomata affect the pericardium. The features of tuberculosis are combined with those of pericarditis (see Chapter 14; Fig. 18.5). In very slowly developing cases the patient may present with heart failure due to tamponade caused by giant effusion or constrictive pericarditis.

Lymph-node tuberculosis

Lymph-node tuberculosis usually affects the cervical or mediastinal nodes. In children, caseating or suppurating

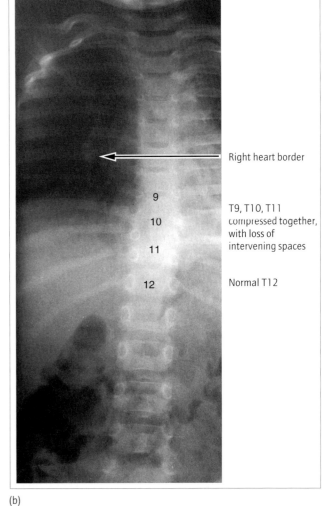

Right heart border

T9, T10, T11 compressed together, with loss of intervening spaces

Normal T12

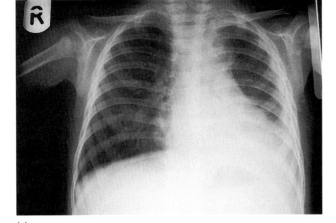

(a)   (b)

Fig. 18.4 This Bosnian refugee was born in internment and did not receive bacillus Calmette–Guérin (BCG). At age 18 months she had persistent cough, fever and back pain, with evidence of (a) left-sided pleural disease on chest X-ray and (b) spinal osteomyelitis, with loss of two disc spaces and vertebral volume in the lower thoracic spine.

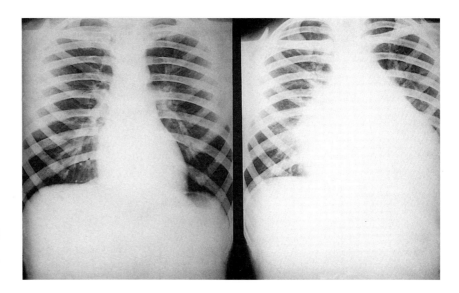

Fig. 18.5 Tuberculous pericarditis in a 57-year-old Pakistani businessman: he presented with several days' increasing chest pain, anorexia and fever. Echocardiography revealed the small pericardial effusion, which rapidly enlarged over the next 10 days.

lymphadenitis may be due to *M. scrofulaceum.* Swollen cervical nodes are easily detectable. The swelling develops at a varying rate from very slowly to alarmingly suddenly, when lymphoma must be urgently excluded. Cold abscess formation is nowadays rare, as early diagnosis and treatment usually prevent it (Fig. 18.6).

Mediastinal lymph-node swelling may cause cough, due to extrinsic tracheal irritation. A dull, central chest pain is also a fairly common symptom. Physical signs are few, unless compression of an airway produces a fixed wheeze. The chest X-ray often shows a nodular shadow

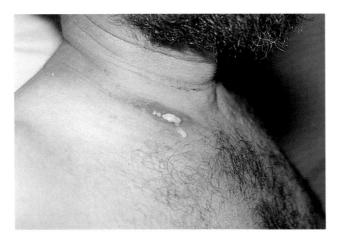

Fig. 18.6 Tuberculous lymphadenitis: this 42-year old man had typical symptoms and a swollen cervical lymph node for 4 months. Chemotherapy did not prevent the formation of a draining sinus.

widening the mediastinum, with or without narrowing of a central airway (Fig. 18.7).

On rare occasions a swollen lymph node ruptures an airway, protruding into it and obstructing it. Complete tracheal obstruction may be fatal, but urgent bronchoscopy with bypass or resection is sometimes possible.

Tuberculous peritonitis

Tuberculous peritonitis is most common in Asians. It presents with the usual general features, accompanied by abdominal discomfort and distension. Minor amounts of ascites are common, showing as separation of bowel loops on X-ray or as collection in the pelvis or peritoneal reflections on imaging. Massive ascites is extremely rare.

Diagnosis of tuberculosis

The diagnosis of tuberculosis is suggested by the typical quartet of clinical features, and the site may be indicated by localizing symptoms and signs.

Confirmation of the diagnosis is not always easy, as there are relatively few mycobacteria in the primary lesion, and they are encased in a dense granuloma. Very few cases of primary pulmonary tuberculosis have a positive sputum examination. Pleural, pericardial or ascitic fluids rarely yield positive smears or cultures. Only about 1 in 5 cases of tuberculous meningitis have positive cere-

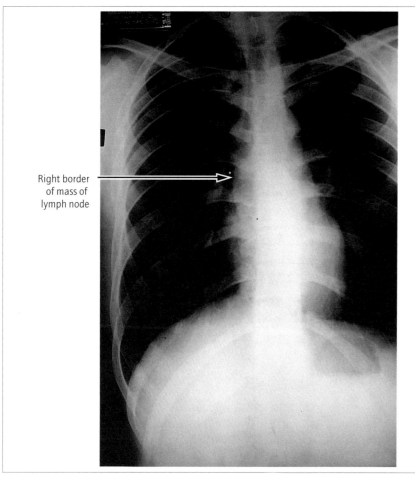

Right border
of mass of
lymph node

Fig. 18.7 Tuberculous lymphadenitis: this teenager presented with typical symptoms of tuberculosis, plus a cough and substernal chest pain. The swollen gland was compressing the trachea.

brospinal fluid bacteriology. Although bacteriological examination should always be performed, as it is diagnostic when positive, it is not reliable in excluding tuberculosis.

Tuberculin tests

The tuberculin test is an intradermal test for cell-mediated hypersensitivity to tuberculoprotein. Three methods of tuberculin testing are available: (i) the Heaf test, which is widely used for screening large numbers of individuals, for instance before BGC immunization; (ii) the tine test, which is similar to the Heaf test; and (iii) the Mantoux test, which is particularly applicable to individual cases, and can be performed in different dilutions. The Heaf test is the most widely used (Fig. 18.8). Concentrated purified protein derivative (PPD) is inoculated into the skin, using an automated, six pointed instrument (Heaf gun).

The tuberculin test is negative in those who have never been exposed to infection with tuberculosis. It becomes positive 3–5 weeks after infection. A strongly positive tuberculin test is good evidence of active tuberculosis unless the diagnosis is disproved. A grade three or four Heaf or tine test, a strongly positive (greater than 15 mm) 1 : 1000 (10 tuberculin unit) Mantoux test, or a positive (greater than 6 mm induration) 1 : 10 000 (1 tuberculin unit) Mantoux test can all be taken as indicating tuberculosis (Fig. 18.9).

Strongly positive tuberculin tests, not necessarily indicating current disease, can be found in individuals repeatedly exposed to tuberculoprotein or mycobacteria. Nurses and doctors in chest or infectious diseases departments, overseas aid workers or previously immunized individuals recently exposed to a case of tuberculosis may present this problem. If the positive individual is well and has a normal chest X-ray, treatment is probably not indicated, unless the positivity is related to a recent family contact (see section on prevention and control, below).

The tuberculin test may be misleadingly negative if performed too soon in the course of the disease, as it may not have had time to convert to a positive response. This is a particular problem in erythema nodosum and sometimes in tuberculous meningitis, which can both occur very soon after exposure to infection. It is worth repeating the test after 1 or 2 more weeks in cases where the disease is strongly suspected.

A debilitated patient or one with overwhelming tuberculous infection may have a falsely negative tuberculin test because of suppression of cell-mediated responses. This is not such a common problem in primary tuberculosis, which is rarely severely debilitating, as in postprimary disease (see below). Improvement in the patient's general condition, or 7–10 days' antituberculosis treatment, is often followed by the ability to mount a strong positive response.

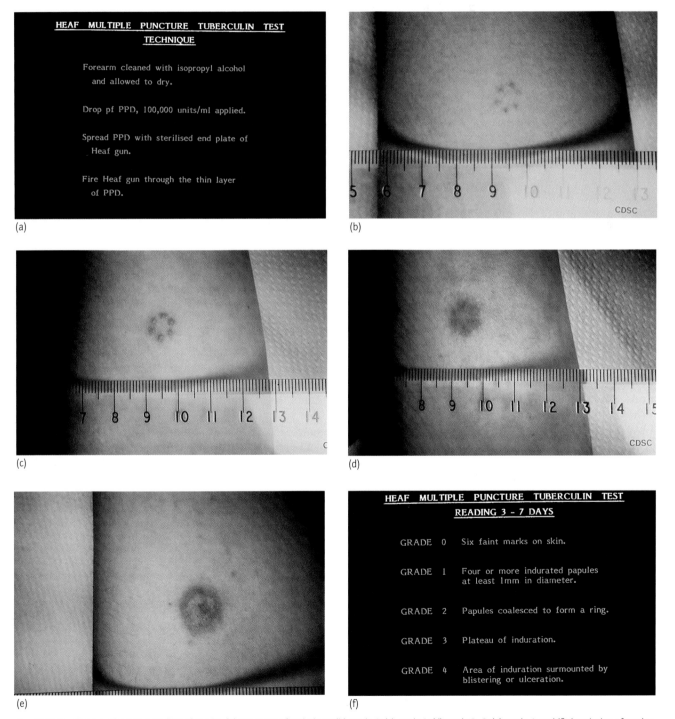

Fig. 18.8 Heaf test method and grading of results. (a) Summary of technique; (b) grade 0; (c) grade 1; (d) grade 2–3; (e) grade 4; and (f) description of grades.

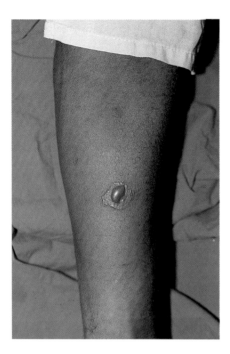

Fig. 18.9 Strongly positive Mantoux test: this patient had a short history and high fever; the main reaction is 18 mm in diameter. (0.1 ml of fluid containing 10 or 1 units of PPD is injected intradermally: the diameter of the resulting induration is measured 48–72 hours later.)

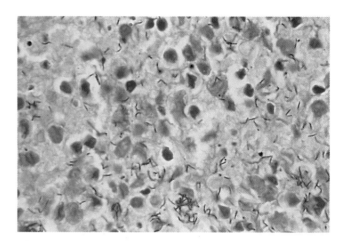

Fig. 18.10 Ziehl–Nielsen-stained material obtained from a caseating mediastinal lymph node. Many acid-alcohol-fast bacteria are seen, with the typical 'cording' or clustering appearance of *Mycobacterium tuberculosis*.

Histology and cytology as diagnostic tools

In some cases, infected tissue such as pleura or lymph node is accessible to biopsy or fine-needle aspiration. When pleural effusion exists, needle biopsy of the pleura is usually possible. Excision biopsy of cervical lymph nodes is a straightforward procedure, which contributes to cure. Fine-needle aspiration of affected lymph nodes can also be performed, and the aspirate can be examined for acid-fast bacilli (Fig. 18.10).

Histological examination of biopsy material shows granulomata, which are often caseating. In the absence of caseation, a firm diagnosis of tuberculosis cannot be made, and sarcoidosis or other granulomatous conditions must be excluded by other means. Tissue sections can be stained to demonstrate acid-alcohol-fast bacilli, which are diagnostic if present. Culture of the tissue should always be carried out, as this increases the chance of making a diagnosis by about 50%. It is important not to place all of the tissue obtained into formalin or other fixative, as this prevents its use for culture. Some tissue should be sent unfixed to the laboratory.

Microbiological diagnosis

Specimens

Sputum is the most important specimen for the diagnosis of pulmonary tuberculosis. Early-morning specimens are preferable. In some patients excretion of bacilli may be intermittent or scanty; other patients find it impossible to produce a satisfactory specimen. In these circumstances morning aspiration of the gastric contents (to recover swallowed organisms) may yield a positive diagnosis. Unfortunately, microscopic examination of gastric aspirate can give false-positive results, so these specimens are only suitable for culture.

Cerebrospinal fluid is required for the diagnosis of meningitis. Other naturally sterile fluids may be examined, but the diagnostic yield is often disappointing: culture and histological examination of a pleural biopsy increase this yield. Early-morning urine specimens can be used for the diagnosis of renal tuberculosis. Twenty-four-hour collections are less useful because of frequent contamination with other bacteria. Pus may be submitted for microscopy and culture if tuberculosis is suspected. Blood culture has become more important in the diagnosis of mycobacterial infections following the HIV epidemic. *Mycobacterium avium-intracellulare* infection can readily be demonstrated in blood culture. In these patients faecal smear and culture can yield a positive diagnosis, as intestinal infection is present before dissemination takes place.

In the laboratory, specimens which are normally sterile can be processed without decontamination on non-selective media, while those which possess a normal bacterial flora require decontamination before inoculation. Cerebrospinal fluid, pus and blood do not require decontamination but sputum and faeces do. Urine, which may sometimes be contaminated, should be examined by Gram's stain and, if non-mycobacterial organisms are seen, is subject to a decontamination procedure (see below).

Specimens which may be examined for mycobacterial infection

Body fluids
1 Sputum (D,S,C).
2 Gastric aspirate (C).
3 Effusion fluids (S,C).
4 Early-morning urine specimens (S,C).
5 Cerebrospinal fluid (S,C).
6 Pus (D,S,C).
7 Blood (C).
8 Faeces (D,S,C).
9 Fine-needle lymph-node aspirate (S,C).

Tissues
1 Lymph-node biopsy (H,S,C).
2 Liver biopsy (H,S,C).
3 Pleural biopsy (H,S,C).
4 Uterine curettings (H,S,C).
5 Biopsy of affected skin (H,S,C).
6 Bone marrow (H, S, C).

(Key: C, culture; D, decontamination; H, histology; S, smear and acid-fast staining.)

Microscopy

The examination of sputum smears is central to the diagnosis of pulmonary tuberculosis. Early-morning samples are collected, and if there is delay in processing these should be refrigerated to prevent overgrowth of other bacteria. Since sputum is contaminated with mouth flora, it must be decontaminated before it can be used for culture. Several specimens from the same patient can be pooled and decontaminated using 4% sodium hydroxide. This acts by killing the other bacteria present in the specimen. This effect is not absolutely specific, so care is necessary if false-negatives are not to result.

The treated specimen is centrifuged, and the deposit used for microscopic examination and inoculation of culture medium (see below). Slides can be stained in two ways: by a modification of the Ziehl–Nielsen method, in which hot carbol-fuchsin is used to stain the mycobacteria; or the phenol auramine technique, which uses a fluorescent dye easily visible under ultraviolet illumination. Auramine staining enables large numbers of specimens to be screened more quickly. All positive slides are then overstained by the Ziehl–Nielsen method so that the identity of the fluorescent objects can be checked. This technique is particularly suited to laboratories with a large throughput. In smaller laboratories, or where an ultraviolet microscope is not available, Ziehl–Nielsen is the method of choice.

The lower limit of detection by stained smear is approximately 10^4 cfu/ml. Excretion of bacilli can be intermittent and, thus, a negative result does not exclude the diagnosis. The importance of microscopic diagnosis of tuberculosis cannot be overemphasized. Not only does it provide a rapid and relatively sensitive diagnostic technique, but is also identifies patients who are excreting large numbers of organisms and are therefore infectious.

Culture of mycobacteria

All but a few species of mycobacteria are slow-growing. This means that other bacteria present in the specimen would rapidly overgrow if not adequately suppressed. Specimens from sterile sites can be inoculated directly on to isolation medium but those from sites with a normal bacterial flora (e.g. sputum) require decontamination. Growth of contaminating species is further inhibited by the incorporation of dyes, for instance malachite green in Löwenstein–Jensen medium, or antibiotics, as in Kirchner's selective medium. Culture must be performed in screwcapped containers to prevent the release of infectious organisms, and to prevent desiccation (Fig. 18.11).

Many different media are used in the isolation of mycobacteria. All contain a source of fatty acids; fresh eggs in Löwenstein–Jensen, or purified oleic acid in Middlebrook's medium. Liquid media increase the diagnostic yield because they permit inoculation of a larger amount of specimen. A positive diagnosis is made when colonies grow on solid medium, or liquid medium becomes cloudy. Colonies of *Mycobacterium tuberculosis* (MTB) on solid media are usually rough and a buff colour, and the smear often shows cording (see below), but these characteristics are not sufficiently typical to allow a presumptive diagnosis.

Automated methods

More recently, the diagnosis of mycobacterial infection has been improved by the introduction of radiometric

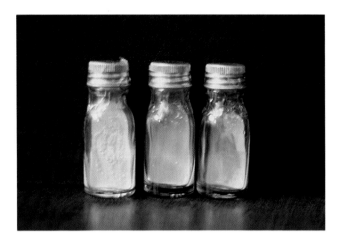

Fig. 18.11 Culture of mycobacteria on Löwenstein–Jensen medium. Results at 3 weeks show the typical, breadcrumb-like growth of *Mycobacterium tuberculosis* in the middle bottle (left is *M. fortuitum*, right is *M. kansasii*).

detection of mycobacterial growth. This technique utilizes a Middlebrook broth which incorporates ^{14}C palmitate. This is metabolized by the organism to produce $^{14}CO_2$, which is detected by the machine. This has reduced the time taken to detect a positive isolate from about 21 days to approximately 10 days.

Identification

Organisms isolated in this way must be shown to be mycobacteria on the basis of acid-fast staining by Ziehl–Nielsen's method. Acid-fast bacteria are reported as '*Mycobacterium* sp. isolated'. The organisms are then subcultured on to identification and sensitivity media. Identification is often performed in two stages — screening and definitive. The first stage uses screening tests which will identify different members of the *M. tubercu-*

losis group by their microscopic morphology (cording), ability to grow on medium incorporating paranitro-benzoic acid and their pyrazinamide sensitivity or resistance.

Definitive diagnosis is based on biochemical tests, ability to grow at various temperatures and ability to produce coloured pigments in the presence or absence of light (Table 18.2).

Sensitivity testing

From the first days of antituberculosis chemotherapy the problem of rapid development of resistance has been apparent: patients treated with streptomycin mono-therapy produced organisms resistant to therapy after a few months. A single-step mutation caused methylation of the target site on the bacterial ribosome.

Resistant mutants arise to all antimycobacterial agents to varying degrees. Mutation to rifampicin resistance occurs once in 10^8 cell divisions. In a patient with pulmonary tuberculosis there are approximately 10^{13} MTB, making resistance inevitable. In combination chemotherapy the likelihood of resistance developing to all of the agents in a combination is multiplied (i.e. 10^8 rifampicin $\times$ 10^6 ethambutol and 10^6 pyrazinamide = 10^{20}, i.e. the risk is once in 10^{20} divisions). Generally, if 1–10% of a patient's mycobacterial population is resistant to an antimicrobial, laboratory tests will indicate resistance to that drug.

In countries where antituberculosis therapy is closely controlled, wild strains are usually sensitive to all agents. Where there is little or no control, patients may take only one drug (or one effective drug) for long periods of time, and resistance is more common. A high cost of medical care, poor advice and the choice of inadequate regimens contribute to this. Extreme poverty may deny treatment to many. Also patients must understand the need to continue therapy after they return to

	Cording	Growth on pNB	Rapid growth	Pigment	Growth at 37°C	Growth at 25°C
Mycobacterium tuberculosis	+	–	–	–	+	–
M. bovis	+	–	–	–	+	–
M. avium-intracellulare	–	+	–	–	+	+
M. kansasii	–	+/–	–	+	+	+
M. fortuitum	–	+	+	–	+	+

pNB, paranitrobenzoic acid.

Table 18.2 Some laboratory characteristics of commonly identified mycobacteria.

apparently normal health. Where drugs are provided free by government schemes, they may be sold by patients to supplement inadequate incomes.

Testing for antimicrobial resistance

There are several different ways of testing for resistance in mycobacteria, including new and rapid sensitivity methods depending on radioactive growth detection.

The resistance ratio method

This is the method most commonly employed in UK reference centres. It uses Löwenstein–Jensen medium into which are incorporated antituberculosis drugs in differing dilutions. Essentially, a minimum inhibitory concentration (MIC) is obtained of the isolate, and of a range of simultaneously tested control strains. An organism with an MIC below that of the controls, by a factor of a least 4, is considered sensitive.

The proportion method

In the proportion method a culture of MTB is inoculated on to plates containing test antibiotic or no antibiotic. A strain is considered resistant to a test antibiotic if the proportion of bacteria growing, compared to the non-drug control, is greater than 1%.

Radiometric growth detection methods

Radiometric detection of growth in liquid media incorporating different concentrations of antibiotic allows determination of MICs within 7–14 days.

Molecular techniques

Mycobacterial DNA can be detected in clinical specimens, using the polymerase chain reaction (PCR), and a commercial kit is now available offering sensitivity similar or superior to that of culture. Great care is required in the application of PCR techniques if false-positive results from contamination are not to occur. Detection of antimicrobial resistance genes may also become possible using these methods.

Typing mycobacteria

New typing techniques using analysis of restriction fragment length polymorphisms show promise in elucidating the epidemiology of tuberculosis.

Postprimary tuberculosis

Introduction

Postprimary tuberculosis produces expanding granulomata which readily caseate and release large numbers of mycobacteria. In contrast to primary tuberculosis, spontaneous remission is uncommon. Progressive tissue destruction is common, and is an important cause of morbidity and mortality worldwide.

The tissues affected by postprimary tuberculosis are different from those involved in primary disease. The commonest site affected is the apex of the lung. Less common are kidneys, bones and joints, the male and female genital tracts and the bowel.

Pulmonary tuberculosis

Introduction and epidemiology

Pulmonary tuberculosis is one of the most important epidemic respiratory infections worldwide. Approximately 75% of all infections due to *M. tuberculosis* present as pulmonary tuberculosis.

Pathology

The usual cause is *M. tuberculosis*, but as discussed above, other mycobacteria can cause pulmonary disease often in people with debility or immunosuppression. Pulmonary tuberculosis may exist alone or coexist with postprimary tuberculosis in other sites.

Clinical features

The typical quartet of fever, night sweats, anorexia and weight loss is usually prominent. Cough is usual and there is often sputum, which may appear purulent but is rarely copious. Nowadays haemoptysis is rarely seen, but a few patients have episodes of blood-streaking in the sputum and the occasional case expectorates fresh blood or blood clot.

A few patients have no sputum, and children rarely expectorate their sputum, as it is immediately swallowed.

Physical examination may be surprisingly uninformative. Most patients with pulmonary tuberculosis have few, if any, definite abnormal signs. Crepitations over the affected apex or dullness to percussion and perhaps bronchial breathing are the commonest findings. Classic signs such as whispering pectoriloquy and aegophony are extremely rare.

The chest X-ray often shows typical changes which are virtually diagnostic. A ragged-edged opacity is seen in

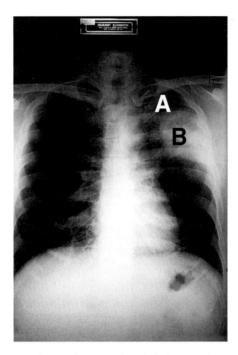

Fig. 18.12 Postprimary pulmonary tuberculosis. Sputum microscopy and culture were both positive. A, apical opacity; B, large thick-walled cavity.

the apex of the lung, occasionally of both lungs. The opacity is not homogeneous, but contains small and large lucencies which represent cavities. Often one or two particularly large and thick-walled cavities are present (Fig. 18.12).

Laboratory findings are variable. The erythrocyte sedimentation rate and C-reactive protein may be elevated, but are not always abnormal. As debility and weight loss progress, the blood albumin level falls and anaemia often develops. On rare occasions bizarre haematological abnormalities occur, including thrombocythaemia, leukaemoid reactions or pancytopenia. The pathogenesis of these abnormalities is poorly understood.

Even when the sputum is scanty it usually contains many acid-alcohol-fast bacilli and yields a growth of mycobacteria, allowing speciation and antimicrobial sensitivity testing. In children and others from whom sputum cannot be obtained, the gastric fluid is an alternative source of respiratory secretions. These accumulate in the stomach during recumbency overnight. Early-morning gastric aspirate can be cultured for mycobacteria in the same way as sputum.

The tuberculin test yields variable results. In early disease and in non-debilitated patients it is often strongly positive. However, in debilitated or hypo-albuminaemic patients and those with advanced disease, cell-mediated responses are depressed and the test is negative. In these patients the test usually becomes strongly positive within a week of commencing effective therapy.

Diagnosis

The diagnosis is usually evident from the history and the chest X-ray appearances. Confirmation is obtainable from examination of sputum or early-morning gastric aspirate. It is rarely necessary to perform a tuberculin test, which has a sensitivity of only 50–60% (i.e. is positive in 50–60% of cases) in untreated postprimary pulmonary disease.

While 70–75% of all reported tuberculosis cases have pulmonary disease, there is a broad overlap between pulmonary and non-pulmonary tuberculosis. Of those with non-pulmonary disease in various sites, about 30% also have lung lesions. Thus, approximately 10% of pulmonary tuberculosis cases have coexisting non-pulmonary disease.

Pulmonary tuberculosis often responds readily to appropriate chemotherapy, but disease in other sites may be much slower to improve. It is not uncommon, for instance, to find that a patient with pulmonary and articular disease will have an improving chest X-ray and a deteriorating joint (see Fig. 17.10). Similarly, a patient with pulmonary and renal involvement may have completely healed lung lesions, but persisting low-grade infection in a kidney. It is therefore important to examine cases of pulmonary tuberculosis for evidence of extra-pulmonary and disseminated disease. At the least a series of urine examinations and a full physical examination should be carried out.

Complications

Before treatment

Before the start of treatment and for a short time afterwards, the important complications are caused by locally extending lesions or dissemination of disease. Local extension erodes lung tissue and can reduce lung function significantly, especially in patients who already have chronic bronchitis or other pre-existing lung disease.

Infected caseous material or sputum may overflow into other parts of the bronchial tree, causing tuberculous bronchopneumonia. This causes multinodular segmental or lobar opacities on chest X-ray. If several areas of lung are involved, significant impairment of ventilatory function may occur.

Occasionally a cavity will erode a pulmonary blood vessel, causing haemoptysis. The appearance of blood-streaked sputum or fresh blood clots is alarming. Bed rest, lying on the side of the lesion to minimize drainage into the opposite lung, and a check of the platelet count are advisable. Many cases resolve, especially if antituberculosis treatment is in progress. A few cases have severe bleeding, requiring transfusion, or even emergency lobectomy, but catastrophic and fatal haemorrhage is very rare.

Patients with severe, extensive pulmonary disease sometimes develop tuberculous laryngitis, with persisting harsh cough and hoarseness of the voice. Such patients are extremely infectious. However, they usually respond rapidly to antimicrobial chemotherapy, though some scarring and hoarseness may remain after healing.

After treatment

After the start of treatment, there is a sudden release of immune function from the suppressive effect of the disease. This is most intense in patients who are severely debilitated or cachectic when treatment begins. The resulting surge of inflammation can make the patient severely ill, with a high, swinging fever, anaemia, an erythrocyte sedimentation rate rising towards 100 mm/h and a rapidly falling albumin, leading to hypotension and peripheral oedema.

Such patients often need circulatory support; whole blood or albumin is better is such cases than plasma substitutes. Corticosteroids in the form of oral prednisolone or intravenous hydrocortisone will suppress some of the inflammatory responses. The dose should be tailored to achieve stability of blood pressure and body weight, and then gradually tailed off as the patient gains condition. Attention to nutrition, with adequate protein, vitamin and mineral intake, assists in recovery.

In patients with both pulmonary and extrapulmonary disease, care should be taken to ensure that both have been adequately treated before chemotherapy is discontinued. This is because infection at different sites tends to respond at different speeds (see above).

Tuberculous meningitis

Introduction

Tuberculosis is an unusual cause of bacterial meningitis. Nevertheless, there are more than 200 cases per year in the UK. Meningitis is a relatively common manifestation of primary tuberculosis in children and young adults, in whom it can develop within 3–4 weeks of exposure. It also

occurs in adults and the elderly, in whom it is more often associated with extensive tuberculosis elsewhere in the body. It is a diagnostic opportunistic condition in AIDS, and is particularly seen in cases originating in Africa.

The disease is important because the diagnosis is often difficult, and early cerebrospinal fluid changes are similar to those of viral meningitis. Delayed diagnosis or treatment can lead to severe complications which may be irreversible.

Clinical features

The disease often has an insidious onset. It can present as fever of unknown origin, personality disorder, meningitis of slow onset, or with a neurological complication. Headache may not be prominent, but mild or minimal meningism is often demonstrable by careful examination.

There may be few other physical signs except for fever, which is almost always significant. Older patients may have signs of pulmonary tuberculosis, or of disease elsewhere. Not all patients complain of the classic quartet of fever, night sweats, anorexia and weight loss, commonly seen in pulmonary tuberculosis.

Haematological and biochemical examination of the blood is often normal, though tuberculosis can produce unpredictable changes in the white cell count. If the meningitis is part of miliary or systemic disease, the liver function tests may be mildly abnormal. The erythrocyte sedimentation rate is not predictably altered.

The cerebrospinal fluid appears clear in tuberculous meningitis, even though it contains excess white cells. Depending on the stage and severity of the disease, from 10 to 500 lymphocytes per cubic millimetre may be found, and sometimes more. The cerebrospinal fluid protein is elevated, sometimes so much that it forms a 'spidery' white clot if the fluid is allowed to stand. The glucose is low, and may even be undetectable in advanced cases.

Diagnosis

The most important factor in diagnosis is suspicion. Examination of the cerebrospinal fluid is mandatory. In many cases it will be advisable to perform imaging of the brain before lumbar puncture. This may show oedema or hyperaemia of the meninges, but is often normal in early cases.

Mild changes in the cerebrospinal fluid, with slightly raised protein, a few excess lymphocytes and a minimally low sugar, are difficult to distinguish from the changes of viral meningitis. A careful search should therefore be made for acid-fast bacilli, and cultures for mycobacteria should be set up immediately. However, only 20–25% of cases have organisms identified in the cerebrospinal fluid. Polymerase chain amplification of mycobacterial DNA in cerebrospinal fluid samples may greatly increase the chance of early diagnosis.

A strongly positive tuberculin test is good evidence of the diagnosis. A negative test is unhelpful, as false negativity is common in debilitated patients or those with advanced disease. Furthermore, the rapid onset of childhood tuberculous meningitis sometimes means that the disease presents before the tuberculin test has converted to positivity. It is always worthwhile repeating the test after 1–2 weeks, or after a few days' trial of therapy when suppression of cell-mediated immunity has ceased.

Management

Treatment should be commenced without delay, and without awaiting bacteriological confirmation. It is usual to give quadruple therapy, including isoniazid, rifampicin, pyrazinamide and ethambutol. The ethambutol and pyrazinamide are discontinued after 2 or 3 months. Streptomycin does not cross the blood–brain barrier, and is not a first-line drug in tuberculous meningitis.

The granulomatous inflammation of tuberculosis easily causes vascular and neurological lesions, especially if fibrosis occurs. It is therefore usual to give corticosteroids such as prednisolone for the first 2–4 weeks of treatment. A typical dose would be 40 mg daily for the first 7–10 days, diminishing to 20–25 mg after this, and then tailing off as fever resolves. Corticosteroids may also improve the chance of resolution if neurological damage is present when treatment is started. As long as effective antituberculosis treatment is given concurrently they have no adverse effect on the tuberculosis.

Trials of short-course chemotherapy have not been completed for tuberculous meningitis. Treatment is usually continued for at least a year, depending on the speed and completeness of response.

Complications

Tuberculomata

Granulomatous, space-occupying lesions may already be present when the patient presents. As treatment reduces the suppression of cell-mediated immunity, they may enlarge and cause signs of cerebral space-occupying lesions. Treatment with dexamethasone or prednisolone often reduces inflammation and swelling, and should be given until the tuberculomata have responded to chemotherapy. On rare occasions they remain a threat to cerebral function, and require neurosurgical intervention.

Focal lesions

Focal spinal cord or brain lesions can be caused directly by granulomata or by granulomatous compression of blood vessels. Cranial nerve lesions, paraparesis and cauda equina syndromes are the commonest problems. Cauda equina lesions are often due to multiple granulomata, and tend to present with a mixture of leg weakness and bladder dysfunction.

Hydrocephalus

Hydrocephalus may occur as a result of extensive fibrosis or as part of a poorly controlled granulomatous process. In either case, corticosteroids offer hope of prevention and improvement. Temporary or permanent cerebrospinal fluid drainage may be needed, depending on the response to further therapy.

Renal tuberculosis

Introduction

Tuberculosis of the renal tract is assumed to be primarily blood-borne in origin. The kidney is almost always involved; granulomatous lesions of the collecting system, the ureters, the vas deferens and epididymis are assumed to occur when mycobacteria descend from the kidney.

The renal lesion starts as a destructive granuloma of the medulla, usually affecting one or more pyramids. Swelling deforms the adjacent renal calyx, and destruction of the pyramid may cause a bulbous enlargement of the cavity of the calyx. If the disease is untreated, the kidney is slowly replaced by a tuberculous abscess. The process of renal damage is speeded up if the ureter becomes blocked by seedling granulomata, as back-pressure and hydronephrosis then complicate the infectious process.

Tuberculous epididymitis presents as a slowly enlarging, low-grade inflammatory lesion. The affected epididymis is indurated, dull-red and mildly tender. Late or untreated cases may progress to a discharging, cold abscess.

Clinical features

The clinical features of renal tuberculosis are variable. Probably a significant proportion of cases have minimal symptoms for a considerable time. Dull pain in the flank on the affected side is common in established disease. Low-grade or swinging fever is also common. Many cases have classic symptoms of urinary tract infection and some have superimposed bacterial infections, probably because deformity and partial ureteric obstruction predispose to bacterial colonization. Some cases come to light because they present with a complicating epididymitis.

A significant proportion of patients with renal tuberculosis have coexisting pulmonary disease. At least a chest X-ray should therefore be carried out, and sputum or gastric aspirates examined if an opacity is present. If there is cough and sputum, examination for acid-alcohol-fast bacilli is mandatory.

Diagnosis

The diagnosis of renal tuberculosis is based on the demonstration of acid-fast bacilli or culture of mycobacteria from urine. The specimen of choice is the whole of an early-morning voiding of urine, in which acid-fast bacilli will have collected overnight in relatively concentrated urine.

Imaging of the kidneys may show typical distortion of the calyces, expansion of a kidney by the inflammatory and granulomatous process, or areas of calcification related to partial healing. It is advisable to perform imaging or renal scanning which can show ureteric obstruction, as hydronephrosis and insidious loss of renal function occurs when a granuloma blocks a ureter. Early relief of obstruction will avoid effective loss of a kidney.

Tuberculous epididymitis

This presents as a progressive, indurated swelling of the affected epididymis. The inflammation is subacute, with dusky red swelling and relatively little pain. Both sides may be affected, often asymmetrically.

Usually a complication of renal tract tuberculosis, the diagnosis is made by demonstrating the renal infection. If this proves difficult, biopsy with histology and culture will confirm the aetiology and exclude malignancy.

Tuberculosis of the female pelvis

Tuberculosis of the female genital tract usually causes subacute or chronic salpingitis. The mucosa of the tube is affected, and granulomata develop in the endometrium,

many of them being shed during the menses. Progressive distortion and eventual occlusion of the tubes lead to infertility, which is often the only manifestation of the disease.

Clinical features are few and relatively minor in most cases. They include minimal vaginal discharge, mild to moderate suprapubic discomfort, or dyspareunia in the presence of a large cold abscess. Occasionally the condition presents subacutely with suprapubic pain and a moderate fever.

The diagnosis may be suggested by an ultrasound appearance of tubal swelling. Laparoscopy permits inspection of the tubes, and biopsy material may then be obtained. Dilatation and curettage are the traditional means of obtaining premenstrual endometrium for histological and microbiological examination. Typical granulomata may be seen in the tissue. Acid-fast bacilli may be demonstrable, and mycobacteria can often be recovered by appropriate cultural methods.

Tuberculosis of bones and joints

Introduction

Tuberculosis of bones and joints originates via blood-borne infection. The joints most often affected are the spine and the hip. The knee and the wrist are less common sites, and involvement of other joints is uncommon. Synovitis without joint involvement is occasionally seen, especially affecting the extensor tendons of the wrist and hand.

The granulomatous process begins in the cartilage of the joint, and spreads by a process of caseation and destruction into adjacent bone. The capsule of a joint may rupture, allowing a cold abscess to track and extend, sometimes erupting at the skin as a sinus. Destruction of bone surfaces and cortex can lead to severe deformity of the joint. The classic example of this is Pott's disease of the spine, in which infection originates in a disc and spreads to the two adjacent vertebrae (see Fig. 18.4b). Collapse of the vertebral bodies produces an angular kyphosis at the level of the infection.

Clinical presentation

The clinical presentation is often with fever and pain. Soft-tissue swelling of the synovium and capsule follows, and effusion develops. Clinical examination will reveal these signs in limb joints, but in the spine and sometimes the hip, imaging may be required to demonstrate soft-tissue changes and features of inflammation. This is important, as bone changes occur late, and considerable disease must exist before X-ray changes are detectable. The bone changes are indistinguishable on X-ray from those of pyogenic chronic osteomyelitis.

On occasion the joint infection is revealed by the appearance of an abscess where pus has tracked to a distant site. The classic example of this is the appearance of an abcess in the groin at the insertion of the psoas muscle. This is the result of infection in the lumbar spine, with pus tracking along the psoas from its spinal origin (see Fig. 22.6).

Diagnosis

Diagnosis depends on suspecting and recognizing the tuberculous nature of the joint or bone disease. Joint effusions usually have a high protein content and a predominantly lymphocytic pleiocytosis. Synovial swellings may produce an exudate containing soft masses of inflammatory material, which look similar to melon seeds.

Demonstration of acid-fast bacilli or culture of mycobacteria may be possible from aspirated effusion or from synovial biopsy. In advanced disease, bone biopsy may yield positive results. In early disease culture may be negative and synovial biopsy inconclusive; a strongly positive tuberculin test is then helpful if present.

Problems in treatment

Problems in treatment of bony tuberculosis can arise because there is often a considerable delay between the start of treatment and the resolution of inflammation and pain. Sinus formation and bone destruction may progress for some weeks after treatment is commenced.

Surgical drainage and debridement of devitalized bone may contribute to cure if there is extensive disease (see Fig. 17.10). There is little evidence that prolonged bed rest or long-term splinting of joints affects the rate of healing or degree of final deformity. However, both may be useful in limiting pain in the early stages of treatment.

Miliary or disseminated tuberculosis

In some circumstances local defences against tuberculous infection are overcome and many mycobacteria enter the blood stream, causing widespread infection. In miliary tuberculosis small granulomata develop in many organs. They are visible radiographically in the chest X-ray and pathologically on the surfaces and cut sections of the solid organs. Here they look similar to millet seeds, which is the origin of the term miliary. In rare cases they can be seen in the retina on fundoscopy.

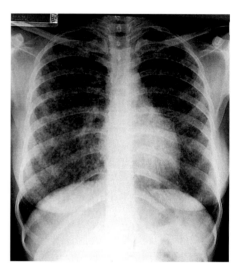

Fig. 18.13 Miliary tuberculosis. Both lung fields contain numerous small, ill-defined, round opacities (the solid organs are similarly affected).

The diagnosis of miliary tuberculosis may be suggested by the chest X-ray appearances (Fig. 18.13). There is rarely significant sputum production, and sputum examination is usually negative. There is often a modest elevation of liver alkaline phosphatase levels in the blood, because of the many space-occupying granulomata in the liver. The white cell count and erythrocyte sedimentation rate are not predictably abnormal.

Liver biopsy material may show small granulomata. These are not always caseating, and acid-fast bacilli are not always demonstrable on Ziehl–Nielsen or auramine staining. Some of the material should be saved unfixed for culture, as this may yield a diagnostic growth of mycobacteria, allowing speciation and sensitivity testing.

Disseminated tuberculosis is not always miliary. The disease may present simply as a fever, often with weight loss, with or without an elevated erythrocyte sedimentation rate, abnormal white cell counts or liver function tests. Biopsy of reticuloendothelial tissue does not reveal granulomata. The tuberculin test may be strongly positive, but is negative in about 40% of cases. This condition, known as cryptogenic miliary tuberculosis, must be suspected on epidemiological grounds or by exclusion.

Treatment of tuberculosis

Introduction

The mainstay of treatment in tuberculosis is effective antimicrobial chemotherapy. In the great majority of cases this will produce cure of the disease with a negligible chance of relapse.

There are two phases in the treatment of tuberculosis. In the initial phase, lasting for 8 weeks, three or four drugs are given, of which two are usually rifampicin and isoniazid. This ensures that at least two or three are effective while the sensitivities of the organism are tested, if possible. It also greatly reduces the load of organisms by using drugs with a range of actions to attack rapidly replicating intracellular and extracellular mycobacteria, as well as commencing therapy against more slowly metabolizing organisms. This is followed by the continuation phase, during which rifampicin and isoniazid are continued for a further 4–7 months. If toxicity prevents the use of one or both of these, then other drugs must be substituted, and the duration of therapy adjusted. If rifampicin cannot be given, treatment must usually be continued for 12–18 months.

Mycobactericidal drugs used in tuberculosis

Rifampicin

This is the single most important drug in the treatment of tuberculosis, as it continues to kill even slowly replicating mycobacteria throughout the course of treatment. Its inclusion in a treatment regimen therefore permits short-course chemotherapy of 6–9 months' duration. It is extremely well-absorbed by mouth and widely distributed in the body. It penetrates moderately well into the cerebrospinal fluid.

The unwanted effects of rifampicin include gastro-intestinal distress and a red-orange discoloration of urine, tears and other body fluids. Soft contact lenses will also become discoloured.

The most important side-effect is hepatocellular liver damage. There is always a temporary elevation of transaminases in the blood when antituberculosis treatment is commenced, but this should peak by 3–4 weeks, and slowly subside thereafter. Levels should not climb to more than three or four times the upper limit of normal. In patients with hepatic impairment the rifampicin dose should not exceed 8 mg/kg daily.

In some cases of miliary tuberculosis, granulomata in the liver expand at the beginning of treatment, producing early liver enzyme abnormalities which are not the effect of drug toxicity. It is worth temporarily withdrawing liver-toxic drugs while continuing the other drugs and giving a course of prednisolone. When liver function tests have returned to normal, rifampicin and isoniazid may be cautiously reintroduced.

A rare effect of rifampicin is the production of a viral-like syndrome of fever, myalgia and anorexia, particularly in patients on intermittent or interrupted therapy. This does not improve as therapy continues, and the drug must usually be withdrawn.

Rifampicin is a powerful inducer of hepatic enzymes. It increases the metabolism of the components of the contraceptive pill, making this method of contraception less reliable. Patients using oral contraception may be advised to take two pills daily instead of one, but barrier methods are probably more reliable during rifampicin therapy.

Rifabutin is a closely related drug, useful in some infections due to 'atypical' mycobacteria.

Isoniazid

This drug is highly effective in killing rapidly replicating mycobacteria. It is responsible for the early dramatic reduction in bacterial load in patients who receive it. It is given with rifampicin for the whole duration of chemotherapy, and contributes to the effectiveness of short-course treatments. It penetrates well into the cerebrospinal fluid.

The unwanted effects of isoniazid include nausea and vomiting, hypersensitivity rashes and occasional cerebral disturbance or convulsions.

It can produce hepatocellular damage, especially in middle-aged and elderly patients.

Peripheral neuritis is an important side-effect which occurs in slow acetylators of the drug. The neuritis is painful and disabling, improving only slowly and often incompletely on withdrawal of isoniazid. This side-effect can be completely avoided by giving pyridoxine supplements to patients taking isoniazid. The usual pyridoxine dosage is 10 mg/day.

Ethambutol

This is a slightly less powerful drug than rifampicin and isoniazid. It is useful in combination with the two main drugs for the initial phase of therapy. It can also be used as one of two drugs for continuation therapy, but the duration of treatment must be longer than with rifampicin and isoniazid continuation therapy.

Ethambutol can cause optic neuritis, loss of red-green colour discrimination and visual impairment. These are particularly likely in the elderly and in patients with renal impairment. Prolonged or high dosage also carries the risk of ocular effects. The patient notices loss of acuity and colour appreciation, both of which are reversible if the drug is promptly discontinued. Regular enquiry for visual symptoms and testing of colour vision before and during treatment are advisable. The drug should not be given to preschool children or others who cannot effectively report visual defects.

Pyrazinamide

This is a bactericidal drug which is well-absorbed and enters the cerebrospinal fluid particularly well. It is highly effective against replicating intracellular organisms, but not against slowly metabolizing organisms later in the course of treatment. It is a useful addition to initial therapy, especially in the treatment of tuberculous meningitis, but is less useful after the first 2–3 months.

Pyrazinamide can be hepatotoxic, and also produces rashes, including urticaria. On occasions it can precipitate acute gout.

M. bovis is resistant to pyrazinamide.

Streptomycin

This is an effective drug whose usefulness is limited by ototoxicity, vertigo and nephrotoxicity, as well as the necessity for intramuscular administration. The usual dose of 1 g daily should be reduced in those over age 40, in small patients and in those with renal impairment. It is highly advisable to check pre- and postdose streptomycin levels at intervals.

The total dose given should not exceed 100 g, above which toxicity becomes much more likely. Streptomycin is most useful as part of the initial phase of treatment.

Additional and second-line drugs

Amikacin

This aminoglycoside may be effective when streptomycin is not. It must be given intramuscularly, and has the same side-effects as other aminoglycosides, so should not be given in combination with them. Like streptomycin, it can be given in a daily or a twice-weekly regimen.

Capreomycin

This aminoglycoside is only used in tuberculosis. The principles of its use are the same as for amikacin. As well as ototoxicity and vertigo, it can cause renal impairment, hepatotoxicity and skin reactions.

Prothionamide

This is a bacteriostatic drug, which is useful in resistant *M. tuberculosis* infections. It penetrates well into the cerebrospinal fluid. Side-effects are mainly those of

gastrointestinal distress, but there is a long list of rare side-effects, including rashes, blood dyscrasias and liver dysfunction.

Clarithromycin

This macrolide drug is particularly useful in treating *M. avium-intracellulare* infections, but may also be effective against *M. tuberculosis*. It is a broad-spectrum antibiotic, which can predispose to *Candida* infections. Its use is limited by nausea in some patients.

Ciprofloxacin

This broad-spectrum antibiotic has proved effective against several types of mycobacteria. Its use in maintenance therapy is somewhat limited by anorexia and weight loss, which may worsen with increasing duration of treatment. It is also more likely than other drugs to lead to candidal overgrowth, frank candidiasis and antibiotic-associated diarrhoea.

Cycloserine

This is a rather toxic mycobacteriostatic drug, which can be used in combination with other antimycobacterial agents. It has unpleasant side-effects, including headache, dizziness, depression, convulsions and allergic rashes. It tends to be a drug of last choice.

Non-tuberculous mycobacterioses

Introduction

While classic mycobacteria and some other species are capable of causing systemic granulomatous disease, other mycobacteria can cause local disease. These *Mycobacterium* species are usually environmental organisms, and the commonest diseases caused are skin infections or inoculation abscesses. They can all cause more extensive disease, or mycobacteraemic disease, in immunosuppressed individuals (see Chapter 21).

Mycobacterium chelonei

This organism is often found in water, and can inhabit hydrotherapy pools if they are not regularly cleaned and adequately chlorinated. It is most commonly seen in cold abscesses at injection sites, particularly in insulin-dependent diabetics, who have many injections. After fruitless treatment with conventional antibiotics, drainage or aspiration is often undertaken, and the true aetiology of the infection may then be discovered.

The infection can be treated with amikacin. Attempts at excision or drainage often result in extension or recurrence. Possible alternative drugs include clarithromycin, cefoxitin, doxycycline and clofazimine.

Mycobacterium fortuitum

This organism also causes inoculation abscesses. It is a rare cause of bone and joint disease, especially in the diabetic foot. It is often sensitive to a wide range of antimicrobial agents, including amikacin, cotrimoxazole, clarithromycin, cefoxitin and ciprofloxacin.

Mycobacterium marinum

This organism is found in river and pond water, and also affects domestic fishtanks. It typically causes 'swimming pool granuloma', an indolent, granulomatous lesion on the dorsum of the hand or the finger. This is probably because it enters epidermal abrasions. Untreated lesions sometimes spread to involve subcutaneous tissue, including fascia and tendons.

It is sensitive to a number of drugs, including co-trimoxazole, rifampicin, ethambutol, ciprofloxacin, streptomycin and doxycycline.

Mycobacterium ulcerans

This is the causative organism of tropical ulcer. It is an environmental organism, which is probably inoculated into the skin of the leg or foot by spiky vegetation. The resulting lesion is an expanding, undermining ulcer whose true extent is much larger than the visibly broken skin. Most cases respond rapidly to treatment with rifampicin or rifabutin.

Prevention and control of tuberculosis

Introduction

The most effective interventions for the control of tuberculosis are those that improve living conditions. The decline in tuberculosis that occurred during the latter half of the 19th century and the early part of the 20th century preceded other control measures and is attributed to improvements in housing conditions, nutrition and social deprivation (see Chapter 25).

Reductions in infection due to M. bovis have been achieved in many countries by a combination of testing and treating cattle and pasteurization of milk.

Bacillus Calmette–Guérin vaccine

BCG vaccine contains a live attenuated strain derived from M. bovis. It is given as a single intradermal dose. The vaccine is contraindicated in patients with immunosuppression, including asymptomatic HIV-positive individuals. A local reaction develops at the immunization site within 2–6 weeks, beginning as a small papule which increases in size; it may ulcerate and gradually heals, leaving a small scar.

Estimates of protection by BCG have varied in different field trials, from zero in one study in India, to 90%. Many studies, including those in the UK, have shown protection of approximately 70%, lasting for at least 20 years. Policies for the use of BCG vary considerably between countries. In developing countries, where infection in young children is common, the vaccine is routinely administered at birth. Many developed countries only offer the vaccine to groups at particular risk of tuberculosis. These high-risk groups may include contacts of cases with respiratory tuberculosis, health care workers, teachers and immigrants from developing countries. In the USA, the number of groups recommended for BCG is very limited and control rests on case detection and contact tracing (see below). In the UK BCG is given routinely to all tuberculin-negative school children at 10–13 years of age.

Tuberculin testing

BCG vaccine can safely be given without prior tuberculin sensitivity testing to infants up to 3 months of age. In older infants, children and adults, a tuberculin test should be performed first.

A negative tuberculin test indicates that the individual has not previously been infected or received BCG vaccination; such individuals can be given BCG. A weakly positive test indicates past infection or previous vaccination and BCG is not required. A strongly positive reaction may indicate active disease; such individuals should be referred for further investigation.

Management of the case and close contacts

Most patients with pulmonary tuberculosis can be treated at home and need not be separated from other household members, provided chemoprophylaxis is given to young children in the household (see below). Where hospital admission is required because of severe disease or for social reasons, the patient should be nursed in a single room until no longer infectious. With modern antimicrobial therapy this is usually achieved within 2 weeks, even though some bacilli may still be seen in sputum smears. Patients who are sputum-negative or with non-pulmonary disease can be nursed in a general ward.

Close contacts of sputum-positive cases should be tuberculin-tested and have a chest X-ray. Close contacts are defined as household members, and classroom contacts (if the index case is a teacher or a school child). Where the tuberculin test is negative, it should be repeated 2–3 months after the last exposure to determine whether tuberculin conversion has occurred. Chemoprophylaxis is indicated for the following contacts:
1 Children under 16 with a strongly positive tuberculin test, irrespective of BCG vaccination status.
2 Adults with a strongly positive tuberculin test and no previous BCG vaccination.
3 Adults who have tuberculin-converted.
4 Young (< 35 years) Asian adults with a strongly positive tuberculin test.

Isoniazid is the drug of choice for chemoprophylaxis. It is usually given for 6 months, although longer chemoprophylaxis may be indicated for HIV-positive contacts.

BCG vaccine should be given to unvaccinated contacts under 35 years of age who remain tuberculin-negative.

Drug-resistant tuberculosis

Mycobacterium tuberculosis has tended to remain sensitive to first-line anti-tuberculosis drugs, mainly because of the policy of using multiple-drug therapy of adequate duration. In the UK, less than 5% of isolates are resistant to one drug (usually INAH), and less than 2% to two drugs. In recent years, multiple-resistant organisms have become increasingly recognized. Poor social conditions, failure to take multiple drugs and failure to complete adequate treatment have contributed. There have been large outbreaks of drug-resistant tuberculosis in refugees, and 'down and outs', and some smaller hospital outbreaks among immunosuppressed patients.

Control of the situation is gained by energetic carefinding, adequate isolation of cases in hospital (see Chapter 23), close supervision of drug taking (directly observed therapy in the patient's own environment) and diligent contact-tracing and follow-up. Treatment with three or four effective drugs should be continued for at least 9 months after sputum clearance and clinical cure. There is no evidence that drug-resistant tuberculosis is more infectious than tuberculosis caused by sensitive organisms.

Screening of immigrants

Screening is indicated for all immigrants from countries where tuberculosis is common, such as the Indian sub-

continent. The aims are to detect active disease, identify infected individuals who may require chemoprophylaxis, and identify unvaccinated individuals who may require BCG.

Leprosy

Introduction

Leprosy is an indolent disease, mainly affecting the skin, nerves and mucosa, but also capable of infecting the eye, muscles and testicles. It is caused by *M. leprae*, which has low infectivity and is extremely slow-growing, with approximately one replication per fortnight. It has never been cultured in artificial media, but will grow slowly in some animals.

Spread is by close contact, usually among families and particularly from individuals with extensive mucosal lesions.

Its importance is that it produces peripheral nerve lesions, leading to paralysis and anaesthesia of limbs, trophic ulcers and Charcot joints. In untreated cases there is no means of preventing these effects, which produce devastating deformities, including autoamputation.

Clinical features and grading of disease

The clinical features of leprosy, as with tuberculosis, depend on whether the sufferer is sensitized to the organism. However, the first presentation is often rather mild, and is called indeterminate leprosy. It consists of an ill-defined area of skin which gradually loses some of its pigmentation, and becomes hypoaesthetic. The face or hand is often affected, and the patient more often presents because of a cut or burn of the site, precipitated by diminished sensation, than because of the cosmetic appearance.

Tuberculoid disease

Tuberculoid (TT) disease occurs in those who mount a strong cell-mediated response to the infection. It is characterized by one or two areas of hypopigmented skin, and localized, asymmetrical inflammation and thickening of peripheral nerves. Nerve thickening may be visible or palpable in the ulnar nerve at the elbow, the accessory nerve in the posterior triangle of the neck or the peroneal nerve at the knee. Biopsy of affected skin shows typical granulomata, with palisades of epithelioid cells, surrounding collections of Langhans-type giant cells and active lymphocytes. Bacteria are rarely, if ever, seen in these lesions.

Lepromatous disease

Lepromatous (LL) disease is associated with an absent cell-mediated response. There is intense oedema of the affected tissues, which contain no granulomata and no lymphocytes. Only undifferentiated macrophages are seen, and these are packed with acid-fast bacilli. There is mycobacteraemia, with spread to distant areas of the skin, nerves, nasal and pharyngeal mucosa, eye, muscles, testicles and reticuloendothelial tissues such as the spleen, liver and bone marrow (especially that of the phalanges).

Disease is expressed as multiple lesions which are often symmetrical. Skin lesions are nodular, and not hypoaesthetic because the small nerves are oedematous rather than inflamed. The nasal mucosa is affected early, and the discharge from it is highly infectious. Facial and lip swelling, often with a collapsed bridge of the nose, causes a typical (leonine) facies. Nerve trunks are swollen, the Schwann cells become packed with bacilli and proliferate, adding to physiological and anatomical disruption. There is gradual loss of sensation, starting with small-fibre functions and eventually affecting all modalities. Involvement of the eye can cause conjunctivitis or keratitis; muscle involvement causes weakness of small muscles, including the smooth muscles of the skin and superficial blood vessels; bone involvement leads to loss of alveolar bone from the jaw, of the nasal septum and of phalangeal joint surfaces.

Borderline leprosy

Borderline (BB) leprosy is an intermediate form in which lesions contain a lymphocytic infiltrate, and macrophages evolve to epithelioid cells, but no giant cells are seen and bacilli survive within the epithelioid cells. There is a continuous spectrum of intermediate forms between tuberculoid, the intermediate borderline and the extreme lepromatous disease. These are distinguished by histological features, by the degree of localization of skin, nerve and other lesions, and by the number of bacilli (on a scale of 1–6) detectable in lesions.

Borderline disease is unstable, and a small fluctuation in immune response or bacterial activity can cause a shift either way along the spectrum.

Diagnosis

The three aspects of diagnosis comprise:
1 Physical examination for typical skin lesions, anaesthesia in lesions or nerve distributions and nerve thickening.

2 Biopsy of atypical or indeterminate skin lesions (this is also helpful for staging the disease).
3 Examination of split-skin smears for acid-fast bacilli (a small cut is made through the epidermis, without drawing blood, and the blade is then used to scrape a little tissue fluid from the exposed dermal tissue and transfer it to a microscope slide, where it is allowed to dry before staining).

Treatment

Multiple drug treatment is now recommended worldwide. The first-line drugs are rifampicin, dapsone and clofazimine. Rifampicin reduces the bacillary load in a few days, while dapsone kills residual organisms. Clofazimine is as effective as dapsone, and also has an intrinsic anti-inflammatory effect, which lessens the likelihood of reactive conditions complicating treatment.

These are given in a regimen which depends on the bacillary load, and for this purpose, leprosy cases are divided into paucibacillary (indeterminate, TT and BT cases), and multibacillary (BB, BL and LL cases, cases with multiple skin or nerve lesions, and those with bacilli in their split-skin smears).

Paucibacillary cases are given rifampicin 600 mg monthly plus dapsone 100 mg daily for 6 months.

Multibacillary cases are given rifampicin 600 mg and clofazimine 300 mg monthly plus dapsone 100 mg and clofazimine 50 mg daily. All drug dosages are continued for 2 years. Clofazimine has the disadvantage that it causes first reddening of the skin, viscera and body fluids, and eventually a grey skin colour. The three-drug regimen is adequate, even for dapsone-resistant organisms, and prevents the emergence of further resistance. Prothionamide is a useful second-line drug, used if clofazimine is refused or if adverse reactions occur to other drugs.

Patients are followed up 6-monthly after completing treatment. Paucibacillary patients are examined for new lesions until disease-free for 2 years. Multibacillary patients also have split-skin smears, and treatment is continued if these are positive. Follow-up of these patients continues for 5 years without disease.

Complications

Several types of immunological change can occur in leprosy; all are more common after the start of treatment:
1 Changes in the staging of the disease, either downgrading towards the lepromatous end of the spectrum or upgrading towards the tuberculoid end.

2 Type 1 reactions, which represent increasing sensitivity to bacterial antigens, are associated with marked swelling of both skin and nerve lesions, with a risk of rapidly developing paralysis or anaesthesia (especially in the relatively unstable BB stage).

3 Type 2 reactions, affecting many LL and some BL stages, with the development of nodular, inflamed lesions of erythema nodosum leprosum on the face and limbs, and sometimes inflammation of the uveal tract, fingers, peripheral nerves and testicles.

In all cases multiple drug treatment should be continued. Mild type 1 reactions which do not threaten nerve function will often respond to standard doses of aspirin, or to chloroquine 150 mg three times daily. These drugs can be combined for their additive effect. Type 2 reactions respond well to thalidomide in diminishing doses from 400 mg daily to 50 mg daily (but great care must be taken to avoid using this in a pregnant woman). The lowest dose can be given for some months if necessary. Severe reactions of either type may threaten nerve or eye function, or cause severe inflammation and fever. These are treated with prednisolone 40–80 mg daily, with a slow reduction in the dose and gradual replacement by milder treatments.

Many patients need physiotherapy, orthopaedic shoes or supportive limb braces to overcome established nerve lesions. In some, tendon transplants may improve hand or wrist function. Emergency surgery to open nerve sheaths or surrounding fascia can limit damage caused by severe inflammatory swelling.

Prevention and control

This is based on case-finding, often by local health workers; on treating infectious cases, who are the reservoir of infection; and on educating the public about the curability of the disease and the needlessness of suffering nerve lesions and disfigurement.

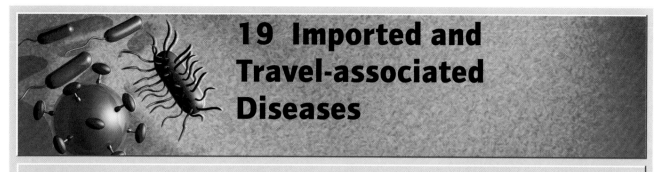

19 Imported and Travel-associated Diseases

Introduction

Worldwide travel has increased enormously since the 1950s, as it has become easier, quicker and more affordable (Fig. 19.1). Slower international sea travel has largely been replaced by air travel, allowing movement around the world in a shorter time than the incubation period of almost any disease. Only the most hostile areas are inaccessible to tourism, but even these may be entered by geologists and other researchers. Overland travel is popular, as is the experience of sharing unfamiliar living conditions with local people.

Travellers are vulnerable to infections unfamiliar to their home-based medical services, presenting diagnostic problems, difficulties in management and unexpected complications. Contagious diseases are also hazardous to contacts and can be serious public health problems.

Unfamiliar features of imported diseases
1 Presenting features.
2 Diagnostic methods.
3 Management requirements.
4 Unexpected complications.
5 Unexpected infectiousness.

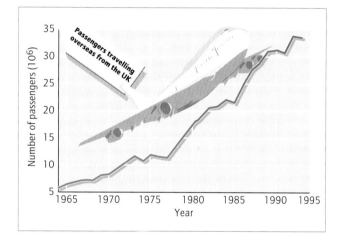

Fig. 19.1 Recent trends in air passenger travel from the UK from the International Passenger Survey, with permission.

Other factors which increase the vulnerability of travellers include:
1 The temptation to take risks with food, water, animals and sexual contacts when relaxing away from the conventions of home.
2 The different epidemiology of some diseases in different environments (e.g. heterosexual versus homo-

367

sexual transmission of human immunodeficiency virus (HIV), prevalence of open pulmonary tuberculosis or existence of epidemic diseases such as polio and diphtheria).

3 The incomplete understanding of health hazards and protective measures with which travellers often arrive at a destination.

4 The stress that accompanies long journeys across time zones may make travellers unusually susceptible to some diseases.

5 In the case of refugees, privation, malnutrition and pre-existing disease or injury may widen the range of infections to which they are vulnerable.

DISEASE LIST

(Rather than listing organisms, diseases of travel can conveniently be considered in aetiological or epidemiological groups.)

Diseases which are common worldwide
Influenza
Community-acquired pneumonias
Meningococcal disease
Sexually transmitted diseases.

Diseases related to climate and environment
Sunburn
Heat exhaustion and heatstroke
Dermatophyte infections
Folliculitis
Cold injury
Altitude sickness.

Diseases controllable by public health measures
Sanitation, food hygiene and safe drinking water
Hepatitis A
Hepatitis E
Viral gastroenteritis

Traveller's diarrhoea
Bacterial food poisoning
Bacillary dysentery
Enteric fevers
Cholera

Giardiasis
Amoebiasis
Cryptosporidiosis

Helminth infections.

Immunization
Poliomyelitis
Diphtheria.

Education
HIV infection.

Risks of contact with mud and water
Leptospirosis
Hookworms
Strongyloidiasis
Guinea worms (increasingly rare)
Schistosomiasis
Liver flukes.

Diseases with arthropod vectors
Dengue fevers
Arboviral encephalitides
Other arboviral infections, e.g. phlebotomus fever

Rickettsial infections
Plague
Lyme disease

Malaria
Leishmaniasis
Trypanosomiasis
Filariasis
Onchocerciasis.

Some important zoonoses
Brucellosis
Rabies
Tularaemia
Anthrax.

Viral haemorrhagic fevers
Yellow fever
Dengue haemorrhagic fever
Hantavirus infections (including Korean haemorrhagic fever)
Lassa fever and other arenavirus infections
Marburg fever
Ebola fever
Crimean-Congo haemorrhagic fever.

Many of these diseases are discussed in some detail in other chapters. Important or common diseases not mentioned elsewhere will be described in detail in this chapter. Brief information on presentation, diagnosis and management will be given for the remainder.

Diseases which are common worldwide

Introduction

However exotic a traveller's destination, the most common infection risks will be those of 'cosmopolitan' diseases. Travellers are not exempt from urinary tract infections, common respiratory infections and epidemic diseases. Indeed, crowding, stress, fatigue and altered patterns of hydration may predispose to clinical expression of common infections.

Some epidemic diseases may be active at the destination while in abeyance at home. Influenza and meningococcal disease are good examples; their epidemics wax and wane around the world from time to time.

Influenza prophylaxis

Pandemics of influenza A begin in eastern Asia and spread westwards across the world, following the winter season, first southwards to Australasia and then northwards to Europe and North America. World Health Organization 'spotter' laboratories maintain surveillance of virus types, to warn of the emergence of new epidemic strains. Appropriate vaccines can quickly be constructed. Local outbreaks of influenza A and B can also be defined and combated in this way.

Immunization is useful for travellers who will enter areas of influenza activity, and should be offered to individuals with special susceptibilities who would be given the vaccine routinely in the UK. It affords about 75% protection to healthy recipients. Debilitated and elderly recipients are not so well-protected, but the severity of illness and the risk of death are significantly reduced.

Prophylaxis of meningococcal disease

Group B meningococci remain the prevalent epidemic organisms of Europe and North America, but in the Middle East, Africa and South America most epidemics are of group A. In the late 1980s a large epidemic of group A disease affected many Muslim pilgrims travelling through Mecca and the Middle East. Local outbreaks of group A and C meningococci also occur in many countries, and immunization is available against both of these.

Meningococcus vaccine, containing polysaccharide antigens of group A and C, affords good protection to adults and older children for at least 3 years after a single dose. Like other polysaccharide vaccines, it is poorly immunogenic in children aged less than 18–24

months. A polyvalent A/C/Y/W135 vaccine is also available in some countries.

Diseases related to climate and environment

Health problems in hot climates

Sunburn

Sunburn is skin damage caused by radiant heat from the sun. Most cases are superficial and heal completely by desquamation without scarring, A few are severe, and cause blistering. Prolonged exposure to sunlight causes ageing and wrinkling of the skin, while both chronic and repeated severe exposure predispose to malignant skin conditions, including melanoma.

Sunburn is prevented by avoiding direct strong sunlight or covering the skin, but this precludes the development of a fashionable tan. Barriers to damaging ultraviolet B (UVB) radiation can be applied as suntan creams, whose protection number indicates the recommended duration of exposure for untanned European skin. UVA radiation is less damaging, but is not excluded by most creams; those containing a partly opaque suspension of titanium oxide are the simplest protection against UVA. Tanning protects from sunburn, but must be accomplished gradually. It does not prevent the ageing or carcinogenic effects of prolonged exposure.

Heat exhaustion

Heat exhaustion is caused by excessive sodium and water loss in sweat. People unacclimatized to hot environments secrete large amounts of sweat with a high sodium content, which falls slowly during the first month of acclimatization. This process cannot be speeded by exercise or medication, so most brief holidays do not allow acclimatization.

The symptoms of heat exhaustion are malaise, nausea, headache and collapse. Replacement of sodium and water results in rapid improvement. It can be achieved with oral rehydration solutions, as for acute diarrhoea, or simply by giving plentiful dilute squash or fruit drinks to which salt has been added (about 1.5 teaspoons per pint, or 3 per litre).

Exercise in hot conditions may cause sweating of up to 4 l/h, so travellers should take plentiful fluids and add salt to their meals. Salt tablets may be of benefit if strenuous sport is played. It is sensible to rest in the midday heat, as local people usually do.

Sunstroke

Sunstroke is a condition of hyperpyrexia and shock. It is most often induced by excessive exercise, associated with too much clothing or failure of sweating due to dehydration. It is a medical emergency which can lead to liver damage, haemolysis, shock, renal failure and death.

The collapsed patient should be moved into the shade and excess clothing removed. The temperature should be reduced by tepid sponging or by wrapping in moist sheets. Fanning is helpful at this stage. When the core or rectal temperature is below 40°C the damage to tissue ceases, and slower cooling may be allowed to continue naturally. The patient requires frequent observation in case the temperature rises again, and haematological and biochemical assessment should be carried out without delay.

Skin infections in hot climates

In hot climates the skin is constantly moist and easily becomes macerated, or traumatized by the friction of moist clothing. The openings of hair follicles or sweat glands may be blocked by soft keratin plugs, causing an uncomfortable condition of hyperaemia and papular swelling, often called a sweat rash. In these circumstances dermatophyte infections easily occur. Staphylococcal folliculitis is also common. A healthy skin can be maintained by avoiding insect attack and wearing loose, light clothes, preferably made of absorbent natural fibres. Both the clothes and the skin should be regularly washed. Antiperspirants are not as effective in hot climates as in temperate ones.

Prevention of insect bites

Insect bites are common in hot climates and are easily infected by staphylococci or streptococci (such streptococcal infections make nephritis a common paediatric problem in tropical countries). Insect repellents are effective in reducing bites. Loose clothing is also a useful barrier; the arms and legs should be covered at dusk when mosquitoes are highly active. Window and door screens keep insects out of buildings; those few which enter can be killed with 'knock-down' sprays. In malarious areas mosquito-proof bed-nets offer important additional protection; they may also be impregnated with permethrin, which much increases protection against nocturnal bites.

Rarer skin infections are also worthy of note. *Acinetobacter* infections will not respond to the usual narrow-spectrum antibiotics used for skin infections. Cuts and abrasions from coral may become infected by marine vibrios and are similarly resistant to treatment. Both will often respond to oral tetracycline.

In areas where diphtheria exists, skin ulcers and abrasions may be colonized or infected with *Corynebacterium diphtheriae*. Infected lesions often have a greyish membrane at the base, and a slight serosanguineous discharge. In local child populations the small dose of toxin produced in the lesion often induces natural immunity. Troublesome lesions respond rapidly to treatment with penicillins or erythromycin, but it should be remembered that such lesions are infectious and could transmit classic diphtheria to susceptible contacts. Immunity declines slowly after childhood immunization, so a significant number of adults may be susceptible. Older travellers and arrivals from overseas may never have been immunized.

Skin infections in hot climates
1 Staphylococcal folliculitis.
2 Staphylococcal and streptococcal infections of insect bites.
3 Infections with *Acinetobacter*, pseudomonads or marine vibrios.
4 Colonization or infection with *Corynebacterium diphtheriae*.
5 Dermatophyte infections.

Effects of cold and altitude

Frostbite

Frostbite occurs when the skin is sufficiently frozen to cause tissue damage. As thawing takes place, fluid leaks from affected blood vessels and painful blisters appear. Deeper injury can cause necrotic and anaesthetic lesions which are very prone to secondary infection. Temporary superficial freezing (frostnip) may be completely reversible if rapidly thawed by applying a warm hand or clothing.

Altitude sickness

Altitude sickness is the result of excessive accumulation of interstitial fluid. It occurs when rapid ascent is made without time for physiological acclimatization. Individuals vary widely in their susceptibility. There is evidence that mild diuretic medication can lessen the severity of altitude sickness.

Warning signs of headache or persistent cough should not be ignored, as severe cerebral and/or pulmonary oedema can quickly follow. Prompt descent to a lower altitude is the treatment of choice. In neglected cases there is a risk of convulsions and death from cerebral oedema. Pulmonary oedema is also dangerous and may be complicated by secondary pneumonia.

Diseases controllable by public health measures

Traveller's diarrhoea

Introduction

This is an important disease of travellers, most often caused by enterotoxigenic *Escherichia coli* (ETEC; see Chapter 8). It affects from 8 to 50% of travellers, depending on the local sanitary standards. Up to half of cases are obliged to rest or remain in bed for at least 1 day.

Clinical features

Symptoms usually begin a few days after reaching the destination, most often on the third day. Malaise and watery diarrhoea quickly develop, sometimes accompanied by low-grade fever or a brief episode of vomiting. The illness lasts an average of 4 days and few patients have more than five or six diarrhoea stools per day. An attack caused by ETEC is followed by immunity to the local type of ETEC.

Management

Most cases are brief and are unlikely to be significantly shortened by treatment with antibiotics.

In endemic areas 40–60% of ETEC are susceptible to agents such as amoxycillin, trimethoprim or co-trimoxazole. Ciprofloxacin is currently effective against nearly 90% of ETEC. Elderly and debilitated patients, who tend to suffer prolonged or complicated illness, may be advised to take a 2- to 3-day course of oral ciprofloxacin at the first sign of diarrhoea.

Prevention

Although several antibiotics and also bismuth preparations can reduce the incidence of diarrhoea in travellers, resistant ETEC soon become prevalent in locations where antibiotics are frequently used. Few experts therefore recommend chemoprophylaxis of traveller's diarrhoea unless the necessity is exceptional.

Adherence to certain dietary rules can contribute to prevention, especially in the short term. Travellers who suffer from diarrhoea have more often taken chopped fresh fruit, sandwiches with mixed fillings, raw or lightly cooked seafood and untreated water (including ice cubes).

Research is proceeding into the development of conjugate vaccines containing enterotoxin antigens. These are primarily intended for the prevention of gastroenteritis in children, but they may become a useful safety measure for travellers.

Water safety

It is safest to avoid untreated water, including fruits and salads washed in it and ice cubes made from it. Commercial brands of mineral water are usually safe. Tap water may be purified by boiling. Alternatively it can be filtered in a portable filter, and purifying tablets then used to destroy viruses.

Typhoid and paratyphoid fevers

Introduction

These diseases, caused by *Salmonella typhi* and *S. paratyphi* type A or B, are uncommon but often severe infections of travellers. They can be contracted in many countries where sanitation is poor or drinking water is insufficiently safe. Even with modern treatment, morbidity is considerable, and an increasing tendency to antibiotic resistance means that some cases are difficult to treat.

Pathology of enteric fever

For a few days after infection, salmonellae are replicating in the gut, and may be recovered from the faeces. This is followed by the primary bacteraemia which is usually asymptomatic. During the remainder of the incubation period, the organism is located in reticuloendothelial cells, and cannot be cultured from blood, faeces or urine. A secondary bacteraemia heralds the reinvasion of the gut, particularly of the Peyer's patches, and the onset of symptoms. During this period salmonellae can be isolated from the urine in some patients. Treatment of the infection may render the blood sterile, but bone marrow cultures may remain positive until late in the course of antimicrobial treatment.

Clinical features

Typhoid fever is the typical enteric fever. The incubation period varies widely, from 6 or 7 days to 4 weeks, but

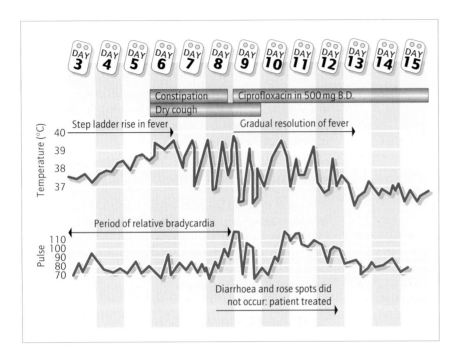

Fig. 19.2 Clinical chart of the course of typhoid fever.

averages 2 weeks. The insidious onset is often mistaken for flu. Symptoms include fever, which increases daily, headache, abdominal discomfort, constipation and often a dry cough. The pulse rate often fails to rise in step with the temperature, producing the effect of a relative bradycardia (Fig. 19.2). There may be a neutrophilia at this early stage. Confusion is common, varying from taciturnity or bad dreams to frank delirium or apparent psychosis. Confused patients are often very restless and may hurt themselves while attempting to escape from hospital.

After 7–10 days the fever reaches its peak; a handful of rose spots often appear on the flanks, buttocks or costal margins (Fig. 19.3), and diarrhoea begins. At this stage tachycardia reaches the expected level for a feverish patient and the white blood cell count usually shows a neutropenia.

In untreated cases complications can be expected from the second week of illness. The commonest are intestinal bleeding or perforation, usually from deeply ulcerated Peyer's patches. Bleeding may be slight, and mixed with greenish diarrhoea stools, but can also be catastrophic. Similarly, small perforations can become walled off by omentum, causing temporary local signs of peritonism which resolve with continued treatment. Large or multiple perforations require emergency surgery. Bleeding and perforation are the main causes of fatalities from enteric fevers.

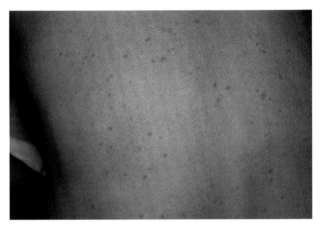

Fig. 19.3 Rose spots on the ninth day of typhoid fever.

Late features and complications of typhoid fever
1 Bowel haemorrhage.
2 Bowel perforation.
3 Acute cholecystitis.
4 Osteomyelitis (especially spinal).
5 Other, rare metastatic infections.
6 Relapse.
7 Prolonged *Salmonella typhi* excretion.

Relapse is an important feature of typhoid, with an incidence of 10–15%. It can occur after either treatment or spontaneous resolution, often being less severe than the original illness, but occasionally it is severe or fatal. It is more likely after inadequate treatment.

Less common presentations

Less common presentations of enteric fevers are important to recognize. Paratyphoid A resembles typhoid almost exactly, except that rose spots are rarely seen. Paratyphoid B may have an incubation period of 4–5 days. It is usually a diarrhoeal disease from its onset, the greenish watery stools becoming bloody as the feverish illness progresses. In this disease a widespread rash of rose spots often develops.

Typhoid fever is often atypical in children. The fever does not follow the classic evolution but is often high, swinging and persistent. Bowel signs and symptoms are minimal in many cases; signs of pneumonia may predominate. Splenomegaly is common, particularly after the first week or 10 days. Although untreated disease may last for weeks, fatalities are relatively few.

Possible presentations of typhoid fever in infants and children
1 Complications of high fever.
2 Apparent acute pneumonia.
3 Fever with splenomegaly.

Respiratory features are common in all age groups. Cough is a frequent symptom and the chest X-ray sometimes shows a frank segmental or nodular pneumonitis; *S. typhi* may be isolated from sputum. In infants typhoid may be mistaken for acute pneumonia.

Rare features of typhoid include acute cholecystitis, and osteomyelitis which particularly affects the lumbar spine.

Clinical diagnosis

Laboratory diagnosis of enteric fever is not always quick or easy, especially if speculative antibiotic treatment has been given before blood culture is performed. The evolution of clinical features often permits diagnosis, which can be made with near-certainty if typical rose spots appear.

Laboratory diagnosis

In common with other Enterobacteriaceae, salmonellae can be readily cultured on simple nutrient-selective media.

In cases of suspected enteric fever blood, urine and faeces should be submitted for bacteriological culture. In difficult cases, or those recently treated with antibiotics,

bone marrow culture can yield positive results. Blood culture has a sensitivity of approximately 60%, and bone marrow 80%. Using conventional culture systems detection of positive isolates may be delayed, but in automated systems, positives can be detected within 24 h and subculture commenced. Isolation of *S. typhi* in faeces alone must be interpreted with caution, as it may indicate asymptomatic carriage rather than true infection.

Laboratory diagnosis of typhoid fever
1 Blood culture.
2 Bone marrow culture.
3 (Urine or faeces culture in appropriate clinical illness.)
4 Widal agglutination test (carefully interpreted).

The Widal test is an agglutination test, nowadays rarely performed, as cultural techniques provide more certain diagnosis. However, it may be valuable in cases already treated with antibiotics.

The somatic O antigen or the flagellar H antigen of the salmonellae is added to tubes containing dilutions of the patient's serum. In the presence of specific antibodies, the bacterial antigen is agglutinated, forming a delicate mat at the bottom of the tube. If no specific antibody is present a button is formed at the bottom of the tube. The titre is recorded as the lowest dilution in which agglutination is detected.

In natural infection the anti-O titre is first to rise, remaining elevated for approximately 6 months after recovery. The anti-H titre rises later in the course of infection, remaining elevated for a prolonged period. A similar pattern of responses is found following vaccination. The background titre in populations varies; in developing countries a background titre of 320 could be expected, in comparison to 80 in developed countries. A single titre greater than these may be useful evidence for an enteric fever. A fourfold rise in titre is only likely to occur in time to make a retrospective diagnosis. Previous vaccination can cloud the picture, but if it was more then 6 months previously, rises in the O antibody titres can be observed.

Antigen detection

S. typhi lipopolysaccharide antigen can be detected in the serum and the urine of patients with typhoid. Techniques reported include counterimmunoelectrophoresis and enzyme-linked immunosorbent assay (ELISA). Results can be obtained more rapidly than from bacterial culture, and remain positive after chemotherapy has been initiated.

Management

Typhoid fever

The choice of antibiotic for typhoid fever lies between ciprofloxacin, chloramphenicol, co-trimoxazole and high-dose amoxycillin. Except in the case of amoxycillin, standard doses are adequate but ciprofloxacin should be continued for at least 10 days and the other drugs must be given for 2 weeks to minimize the risk of relapse. The dose of amoxycillin should be 500 mg to 1.0 g 8-hourly (100 mg/kg daily in divided doses for a child). All of these agents can be given by mouth if the patient is able to take them.

Ciprofloxacin and chloramphenicol act most quickly, the fever usually falling in 2–5 days (average 3.5 days). They are also the most likely to be effective, though clinically significant chloramphenicol resistance occurred in an outbreak of typhoid in Pakistan and north India in early 1991; this organism was sensitive to ciprofloxacin. Co-trimoxazole and amoxycillin are often recommended for typhoid in children and in natives of endemic areas. Adverse reactions to chloramphenicol are rare in the treatment of typhoid. While a small dose-related fall in the white cell count may occur, the opposite often happens as typhoid-related neutropenia resolves. Two weeks' treatment is rarely enough to precipitate sudden agranulocytosis.

Antibiotic treatment of typhoid fever
1 Oral ciprofloxacin 500 mg twice daily for 10 days (child 7.5 mg/kg twice daily).
2 Intravenous ciprofloxacin may be given in a dose of 200 mg twice daily (child 5 mg/kg twice daily) until oral therapy is possible.
3 Alternatives:
  (a) Chloramphenicol, orally or i.v., 2–3 g daily in divided doses (child 50–100 mg/kg daily) for 2 weeks.
  (b) Co-trimoxazole orally, 960–1440 mg twice daily (child 6–12 years, 480 mg; 6 months to 5 years, 240 mg; 6 weeks to 5 months, 120 mg; all 12-hourly for 2 weeks).
  (c) Amoxycillin orally 500 mg to 1g, 8-hourly for 2 weeks (child up to 10 years, 250 mg 8-hourly).

Severely ill patients may suffer exacerbation of fever and prostration at the start of specific treatment, with falling serum albumin and the appearance of hypotension. This will often respond to treatment with intravenous hydrocortisone 100 mg three times daily. The dose can be rapidly reduced according to the patient's response.

Paratyphoid fevers

Paratyphoid A and B are less predictable than typhoid in their response to antibiotics. Chloramphenicol or ciprofloxacin are the drugs of choice and are usually effective, though ciprofloxacin-resistant paratyphoid B has been seen in our practice.

Prevention and control

Avoiding high-risk food and drinking water can much reduce the chance of exposure to enteric fevers.

Immunization is available against typhoid fever:
1 Killed whole-cell vaccine is given in two 0.5 ml doses, 4–6 weeks apart, and provides 65–75% protection for approximately 3 years, after which a booster dose is recommended. This vaccine causes a high rate of feverish reactions, which can be minimized by giving second and booster doses as a 0.1 ml dose, intradermally.
2 Vi-polysaccharide vaccine (Typhim Vi), given in a single 0.5 ml dose, provides protection equivalent to whole-cell vaccine, with fewer febrile side-effects, but sometimes irritation at the injection site. A booster is recommended after 3 years.
3 Oral Ty21a live vaccine (Vivotif), given in three doses of one capsule each on alternative days. The capsules must be kept refrigerated, and taken before food, with warm water. Booster doses are recommended at yearly intervals.

Cholera

Introduction

In spite of its rarity in developed countries, cholera is still an important infection worldwide. It may occur as part of an epidemic or arise sporadically in the developing world. It is occasionally found in travellers returning from endemic countries.

Epidemiology

Cholera is spread mainly through drinking faecally contaminated water. Food, especially shellfish, may also be a vehicle of infection. Large epidemics occur in countries with inadequate facilities for the disposal of sewage and safe drinking water. Cholera is a pandemic infection, capable of causing epidemics that affect many countries around the globe simultaneously. Smaller epidemics and outbreaks have been reported in Mediterranean and East European countries.

During the 19th century, several cholera pandemics spread from India throughout Asia, Europe and the Americas. During the first half of the 20th century, the disease was largely confined to Asia. The seventh cholera pandemic spread from Indonesia in 1961, and has now reached all continents, including South America, where the disease has reappeared for the first time this century (Fig. 19.4). In most countries, infection is due to the E1 Tor biotype, although the classic biotype has re-emerged in Bangaladesh. More recently the new serotype, 0139, has appeared as a cause of epidemic illness in Bangladesh and India. It is now recognized as the eighth pandemic.

Cholera is rare in developed countries. There is a small focus of infection in Texas and Louisiana due to a unique strain of *Vibrio cholerae* 01. There has been no indigenous cholera infection in the UK this century. Travellers to endemic areas are only occasionally affected. Since 1981 only 45 cases of cholera have been imported into England and Wales. It has been estimated that the risk of infection in a traveller is about 1 in 500 000.

Pathogenesis

Cholera is a toxin-mediated disease caused by the 01 and 0139 serotypes of *V. cholerae*. Cholera toxin is very closely

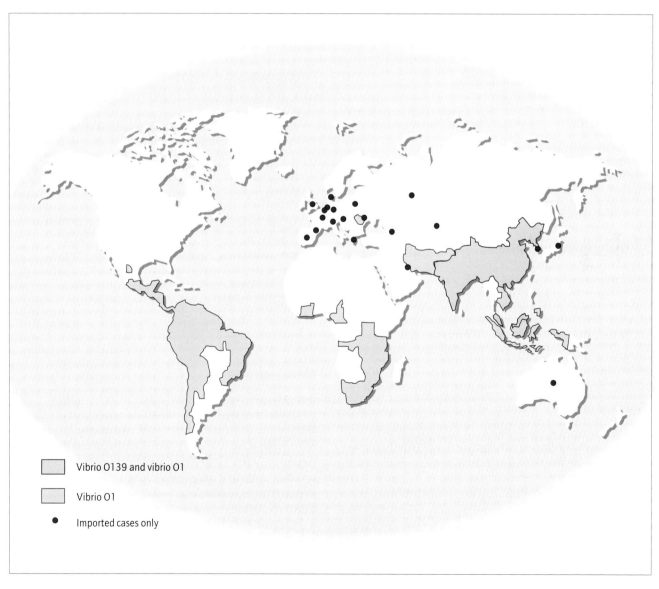

Fig. 19.4 Progress of the seventh (01) and eighth (0139) cholera pandemics across the world: the situation in 1993.

related to the heat-labile toxin of *Escherichia coli* (see Chapter 8). In the future, the same vaccine may be effective against both heat-labile *E. coli* and cholera toxin.

Clinical features

The usual incubation period is 3 or 4 days. The severity of illness is extremely variable, many patients simply having a gastroenteritis-type disease. In classic cholera there is an abrupt onset of severe diarrhoea, at first watery and brown, but quickly changing to pale fluid stools containing only a little mucus and cell debris — the so-called rice-water stools. Fever is not prominent. Continuous fluid loss quickly leads to dehydration and collapse. The diarrhoea contains many organisms and is highly infectious. This, coupled with the difficulty of maintaining personal and domestic hygiene, contributes to the rapid spread of the disease.

Diagnosis

Clinical suspicion will be alert in an epidemic or outbreak situation. There are few diseases which cause such sudden dehydration in adults, though child cases in particular may be hard to distinguish from other gastroenteritides. Examination of the diarrhoea stools will give an early result but, even so, treatment should not be delayed pending diagnosis.

Laboratory diagnosis

Microscopy

Vibrio cholerae have characteristic darting motility, and can be seen in freshly passed stool specimens from patients with acute disease. This rapid diagnosis can be confirmed by demonstrating inhibition with specific antiserum.

Isolation

Specimens should be transported to the laboratory with minimum delay but, if this cannot be avoided, specialized transport media such as that of Cary-Blair can be employed.

Media for the isolation of pathogenic vibrios have a high pH (8.6) and incorporate bile salts which together inhibit the growth of other enteric bacteria. The most commonly used medium is thiosulphate citrate bile sucrose (TCBS) agar. *V. cholerae* ferments sucrose after 24 h incubation. This organism produces yellow colonies due to a colour change of bromothymol blue

indicator with the falling pH. Other vibrios, including food-poisoning species such as *V. parahaemolyticus*, will grow well on this medium. Most, including *V. parahaemolyticus*, are non-sucrose-fermenters whose colonies appear blue/green.

Suspect colonies are subcultured and identified using the conventional biochemical tests employed for the identification of Enterobacteriaceae (see Chapter 3). There are more than 70 serotypes of *V. cholerae* based on the lipopolysaccharide somatic antigen. Only 01 and 0139 have been associated with human disease. Confirmed colonies of *V. cholerae* are therefore serotyped, using a slide agglutination technique employing anti-01 and anti-0139 antisera. Toxin production by the organism is then confirmed, as only toxin-producing strains cause cholera. Non-toxigenic 01 and 0139 strains are not pathogenic, and require no public health action.

Laboratory diagnosis of cholera
1 Comma-shaped bacteria with darting motility in the faeces.
2 Sucrose-fermenting organisms identified on thiosulphate citrate bile sucrose agar.
3 *Vibrio cholerae* confirmed, using biochemical tests.
4 Serotype 01 or 0139 identified by slide agglutination.
5 Toxigenicity confirmed serologically.

For epidemiological purposes, the 01 and 0139 strains can be typed, using agglutination, biochemical or phage reactions, as El Tor or classic types, which also exist in three biotypes (Inaba, Ogawa and Hikojima).

In areas where culture is not possible, serological surveys using techniques to detect antibodies to the 01 lipopolysaccharide antigen can be useful in epidemiological surveys.

Management

Because the mucosal cells are intact in cholera and their absorptive function is undamaged, oral rehydration is successful in over 90% of cases. Intravenous rehydration should be given to exhausted or shocked patients. Very large initial volumes of 4–6 l may be needed, followed by several litres per day while diarrhoea lasts. Spontaneous recovery is usual once hydration is controlled, but the diarrhoea illness may last for 4–5 days. Chemotherapy may be indicated in severe or prolonged disease, or in the elderly and debilitated. Tetracycline is often effective; ciprofloxacin may also be given, and is easier to use if parenteral treatment is required.

While asymptomatic carriage of classic cholera strains is unusual, the El Tor strains may be excreted by asymptomatic carriers and by convalescent patients. Patients and their close contacts should therefore have follow-up stool examination before being released from medical supervision. A 4- or 5-day course of chemotherapy will eradicate excretion in most cases.

Prevention and control

Cholera vaccine is of limited use. The protection afforded is less than 50% and only lasts for about 6 months. The vaccine has no effect on carriage and is therefore of no use in preventing spread. The World Health Organization has now abolished the requirements in the International Health Regulations for a certificate of vaccination against cholera. Nevertheless, evidence of vaccination in travellers from infected areas may occasionally be required.

The most useful measure in preventing the spread of cholera is provision of safe drinking water and sanitary disposal of human faeces. Food likely to be contaminated, especially fish and shellfish, should be thoroughly cooked before eating. Travel and trade restrictions between countries are not effective.

Diseases with arthropod vectors

Dengue fevers

Introduction

Dengue is a common disease in many tropical areas. Although fatalities are rare, the feverish illness is severe and debilitating. Large epidemics can occur and travellers in affected areas are at considerable risk of exposure. Dengue virus is an alphavirus, whose four serotypes are widely distributed in tropical areas. Infection is transmitted by *Aedes* sp. mosquitoes, which bite in the daytime.

Clinical features

The incubation period is 5–7 days. Illness begins abruptly with high fever, often severe arthralgia and frontal headache (this has been called breakbone fever). At this stage the blood count often shows neutropenia and there may be mild hepatocellular disturbance of liver function tests.

Symptoms often abate after 4–6 days but in many cases the disease is biphasic. Fever recommences, there is a generalized lymphadenopathy and a macular rash may appear on the trunk and proximal limbs (Fig. 19.5). The platelet count often falls and the rash can then contain

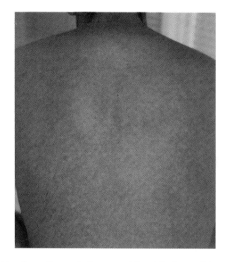

Fig. 19.5 Macular rash seen in the second feverish phase of dengue fever. Courtesy of Dr M.G. Brook.

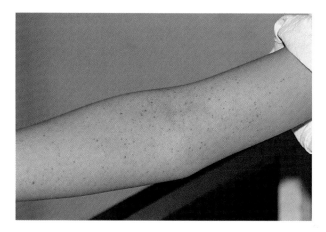

Fig. 19.6 Dengue haemorrhagic fever: positive tourniquet test. Courtesy of Dr D. Lewis.

petechiae (Fig. 19.6), but significant bleeding does not occur and the condition is transient; fever abates in another 5 or 6 days. Convalescence is moderately rapid, taking 2 or 3 weeks.

Diagnosis

This can be suspected in patients who develop typical illness after visiting endemic areas. Virus can be demonstrated in blood during the acute phase. Serological testing of paired samples usually demonstrates a fourfold or greater rise in antibody concentration.

Management

There is no specific treatment. Bed rest is helpful and non-steroidal anti-inflammatory agents significantly reduce discomfort.

Complications

Immunity to dengue fevers is type-specific. Second attacks can occur in individuals partly immunized by previous infection with different serotypes, and the immunopathological features are then enhanced, producing dengue haemorrhagic fever. A typical onset develops into severe disease with profound thrombocytopenia and frank haemorrhage. Pleural effusion and associated secondary pneumonitis may also occur. Shock indicates a poor prognosis. Vigorous supportive treatment is often needed and there is a significant mortality. Children are most often affected, but the disease has been recorded in adults who had a second attack of dengue on revisiting endemic areas.

Other arboviral infections

Introduction

There are many dengue-like viral infections transmitted by sandflies and mosquitoes. They are all characterized by short incubation periods and intense feverish syndromes, some with lymphadenopathy or rash and some without.

Important among these are the zoonotic encephalitides, which cause severe meningoencephalitis with a high risk of long-term sequelae (see Chapter 16). These are mainly carried by rodents or other small mammals and transmitted to larger animals and humans by mosquito bites. In the USA horses are often affected (by eastern and western equine encephalitis), or transmission may be direct from rodents (as in California encephalitis). In Nepal, Korea and other Far Eastern countries pigs and humans are affected by Japanese B encephalitis. Tick-borne encephalitis is endemic in wooded areas of central Europe and eastern Scandinavia.

Prevention and precautions

For many of these diseases the main preventive measure is control of mosquitoes in endemic areas, and avoidance of mosquito bites by humans. Vaccines are available against tick-borne encephalitis and Japanese B encephalitis. They are highly effective and should be offered to travellers who will have rural exposure in endemic areas. They are not necessary unless the traveller remains close to the animals carrying the responsible viruses, as the vectors have a very limited range.

Rickettsioses

Introduction

Rickettsioses are severe systemic diseases, various forms of which are common in many countries. Rocky Mountain spotted fever (caused by *Rickettsia rickettsii*) is tick-borne, and is endemic in the Rocky Mountains and in several rural areas on the eastern seaboard of the USA. Epidemic typhus (*R. prowazekii*) affects many populations infested by lice, which are the reservoir of infection. Both of these diseases are life-threatening if untreated. Less grave but still severe illnesses are tick typhus (*R. conorii*), endemic typhus (*R. mooseri*, transmitted by fleas from mouse to humans) and rickettsialpox (*R. tsutsugamushi*). Similar but rare diseases are trench fever, caused by *Bartonella quintana* and ehrlichosis, caused by *Ehrlichia* spp. The agents of these two diseases are members of the family Rickettsiaceae.

Diseases caused by Rickettsiaceae
1 Rocky Mountain spotted fever (*Rickettsia rickettsii*).
2 Epidemic typhus (*R. prowazekii*).
3 Murine or endemic typhus (*R. mooseri*).
4 Tick typhus (*R. conorii*).
5 Scrub typhus (*R. tsutsugamushi*).
6 Trench fever (*Bartonella quintana*).
7 Ehrlichosis (*Ehrlichia chaffeensis*)

Clinical features

All of these diseases have an incubation period of about 13 days. They begin abruptly with swinging fever and frontal headache. Confusion is common during the peaks of fever and at night. The main pathology of the disease is an endovasculitis, which causes a rash and bleeding diathesis. The rash of Rocky Mountain spotted fever begins as macules on the hands and feet, then spreads over the body, becoming petechial or haemorrhagic. That of epidemic typhus begins in the axillae,

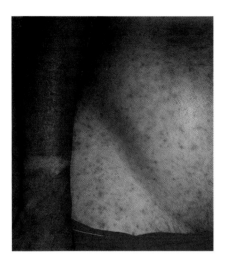

Fig. 19.7 Tick typhus: the patient has a maculopapular rash with a petechial element, conjunctival injection, severe headache and myalgia.

and also becomes purpuric as it spreads. Rashes are also seen in the other rickettsioses and they often have a petechial element (Fig. 19.7). That of rickettsialpox is variegate, having macular, pupuric and pustular elements.

Tick typhus, originating from the Mediterranean countries, the Arabian Gulf or Africa, is the commonest rickettsial disease imported into the UK. The eschar of the originating tick bite may still be visible on admission as a black scab surrounded by inflammation (Fig. 19.8). The rash is generalized and the conjunctivae are suffused. The blood count shows a neutrophilia and transaminases are usually elevated; sometimes clinical jaundice is present. Mild abnormalities of clotting and of renal function are often detectable (a milder version of

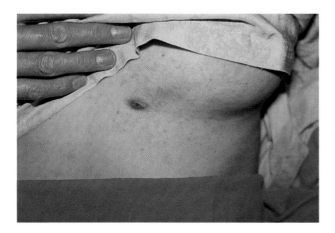

Fig. 19.8 Tick typhus: a black eschar at the site of the infecting tick bite.

the intravascular coagulation, bleeding and systems failure of the more severe rickettsioses).

Untreated tick typhus lasts for about 2 weeks before fever and rash begin to resolve. Although rarely fatal, it is a severe disease followed by debility and prolonged convalescence.

Diagnosis

The travel history and clinical features often suggest the diagnosis. Severe cases with purpura must be distinguished from meningococcal disease. When the rash is absent, a diagnosis of non-A non-B hepatitis may be considered, but the accompanying fever is not typical of jaundice caused by viral hepatitis.

Management

The treatment of choice is tetracycline or chloramphenicol, orally or intravenously. A 10–14-day course is usually required. As in typhoid fever, the temperature may not fall to normal for 3–4 days.

Treatment of rickettsial infections
1 Oxytetracycline orally, 500 mg 6-hourly for 10–14 days.
2 Alternative: chloramphenicol orally or i.v., 500 mg 6-hourly for 10–14 days.

Malaria

Introduction

Malaria is one of the most important imported diseases. The benign malarias are debilitating diseases with a relapsing course. Falciparum (malignant) malaria may be life-threatening and should be treated as a medical emergency. The diagnosis should be actively excluded in every feverish traveller from the tropics, for at least one death occurs almost every year from unsuspected or late-diagnosed falciparum malaria.

Causes of the four types of malaria
1 *Plasmodium falciparum* (malignant tertian malaria).
2 *P. vivax* (benign tertian malaria).
3 *P. ovale* (benign tertian malaria).
4 *P. malariae* (benign quartan malaria).

Clinical features

The only consistent clinical features are fever and rigors. Fever begins abruptly but it rarely assumes a periodic form until synchronous release of parasites is established. Patients therefore present initially with a chaotic, swinging fever; rigors occur when the temperature rises. After 7–14 days fevers begin to occur every third day (tertian fever) in vivax and ovale malaria, or every fourth day (quartan fever) in malariae malaria. In falciparum malaria the fevers are less regular, but approximate to a tertian pattern.

Many non-specific symptoms may be present, including abdominal pain, headache, dysuria and frequency, sore throat and cough. Physical examination may be normal or splenomegaly may be detectable. In chronic or relapsing malaria the spleen can be very large. Hepatomegaly and mild jaundice may also be present.

Malignant malaria is complicated by sludging of parasitized red cells in small blood vessels. The sites predominantly affected determine the range of clinical presentations. Cerebral malaria presents with encephalopathy. It is largely a disease of the non-immune and in endemic areas it mainly affects children below age 4, in whom it must be distinguished from childhood bacterial meningitis. Hypoglycaemia, convulsions and hypoxia readily occur and worsen the prognosis considerably. Blackwater fever results from high parasitaemias causing severe intravascular haemolysis. Profound anaemia, haemoglobinuria and acute renal failure quickly develop in untreated cases. Pulmonary oedema is common in malignant malaria, and frequently coexists with cerebral disease. Jaundice is clinically evident when significant haemolysis occurs; the absence of bile in the urine distinguishes it from the jaundice of viral hepatitis.

Important features of malignant malaria
1 Encephalopathy (cerebral malaria).
2 Pulmonary oedema.
3 Acute renal failure.
4 Severe intravascular haemolysis.
5 Haemoglobinuria (blackwater fever).

Diagnosis

Clinical diagnosis may be possible in established disease with typical periodic fever and splenomegaly, but in early disease the only reliable means of diagnosis is the demonstration of parasites in the red blood cells. This is best done by preparing thick and thin blood films, which are stained with Giemsa or Field's stain respectively. Rapid Romanowsky-type stains are also suitable for thin films. Scanty parasites are easier to detect in thick films, while thin films are often additionally helpful in speciation (Fig. 19.9).

Some automated blood-counting machines can also detect malarial parasites, with an accuracy similar to that of human observers. Speciation is best done by an experienced observer.

A dip-stick test can be used to detect antigens of *P. falciparum* in blood.

Management

Benign malarias

Benign malarias should be treated promptly with chloroquine, to which they are hardly ever resistant. The appropriate regimen is:

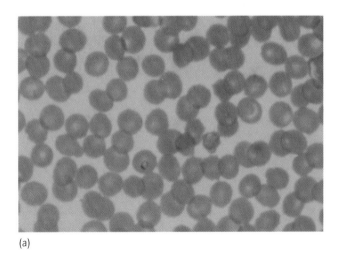

(a)

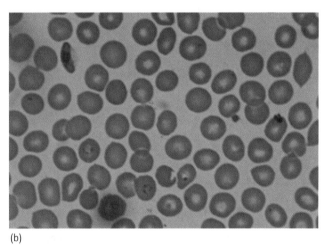

(b)

Fig. 19.9 Malaria: (a) thin blood film, stained with a Romanowsky stain, shows a double chromatin-containing trophozoite of *Plasmodium falciparum*; (b) a gametocyte is also seen, indicating well-established infection in this resident of an endemic area.

1 Chloroquine base 600 mg immediately (four tablets).
2 Next dose 300 mg 6 h later (two tablets).
3 Two more doses 300 mg 24 and 48 h after second dose.

Equivalent doses of chloroquine preparations are chloroquine base 150 mg = chloroquine sulphate 200 mg = chloroquine phosphate 250 mg.

Chloroquine acts quickly and the fever should be abolished within 12–24 h. Nausea or intestinal irritation is rarely severe enough to prevent completion of the treatment. Pruritis can be a difficult problem. It particularly affects dark-skinned people and may make continued treatment intolerable, in which case quinine therapy may be substituted.

Chloroquine exacerbates skin conditions such as psoriasis. Alternative agents such as quinine should be used in this situation.

Eradication of liver parasites

Eradication of liver parasites is necessary after treatment of acute vivax or ovale malaria (hypnozoites are not killed by chloroquine or quinine, which mainly affect developing schizonts).

Liver parasites are eradicated by a 2-week course of primaquine 15 mg daily (250 µg/kg daily for children).

Difficult cases

Chloroquine resistance has been well-documented in a few cases of vivax malaria contracted in Papua New Guinea. Quinine is probably the treatment of choice. In the same area, primaquine tolerance has caused failure of eradication of liver parasites. A further course at twice the dose should be successful.

Falciparum malaria

Falciparum malaria has become resistant to chloroquine in most of its endemic areas. Only a proportion of parasites are chloroquine-resistant, but this is sufficient to make chloroquine an unreliable choice. Uncomplicated cases should be given quinine 600 mg 8-hourly. The dose may be reduced to 400 mg 8-hourly if nausea, tinnitus or deafness occurs. The temperature drops slowly or erratically, often remaining normal only after 2–3 days. Parasitaemia should disappear after 48 h treatment.

For complete eradication of disease 7–10 days' quinine treatment is needed. This can be shortened by giving Fansidar, three tablets, as a single dose on the fourth or fifth day, and discontinuing the quinine thereafter. Fansidar resistance exists in the Far East and some East African countries. If this is suspected, or if a further

episode of malaria occurs after quinine–Fansidar treatment, quinine treatment can be completed with tetracycline 250 mg 6-hourly for 1 week.

Cerebral malaria

Cerebral malaria or other severe forms of malignant malaria must be treated immediately with intravenous quinine. This is not given by bolus injection because of the high risk of cardiac depression, cerebral irritation, nausea and vomiting. The safest procedure is to give an infusion of 10 mg/kg in 5% dextrose over 4 h. This dose can be repeated 8- or 12-hourly until oral therapy is possible. In gravely ill patients or those from the Far East where a degree of quinine tolerance is reported in some *P. falciparum*, the first dose of quinine may be doubled. Quinidine 10–15 mg/kg 8-hourly is an effective substitute if quinine is unavailable.

Other important aspects of treatment include maintenance of adequate blood glucose levels, correction of anaemia by transfusion if necessary, and avoidance of convulsions. Many experts advocate the use of prophylactic phenytoin in patients with coma.

Pulmonary oedema may require vigorous treatment; diuretics and fluid restriction are not highly effective (and in excess could contribute to reduced cerebral blood flow). High inspired oxygen tension and intermittent or continuous positive-pressure ventilation are required in many cases.

Acute renal failure will often respond to conservative management, with a diuresis occurring in 4–7 days. A minority of patients need dialysis.

In spite of severe cerebral disturbance and difficulties with fluid handling, there is little evidence that treatment for cerebral oedema is helpful in cerebral malaria. Indeed, it has been shown that dexamethasone therapy may *prolong* coma without improving the outcome.

Other treatments for malignant malaria

1 Mefloquine — two doses of 10 mg/kg, 6 or 8 h apart; maximum dose 1500 mg. Unfortunately, psychotic side-effects are common at therapeutic doses. Mefloquine may be teratogenic in the first trimester of pregnancy. The drug is contraindicated in epileptics, in severe liver disorder and in pregnancy. Mild ataxia and nausea are common. Rare side-effects include skin rashes and cardiac conduction defects.
2 Halofantrine — recommended only for uncomplicated, chloroquine-resistant falciparum malaria. It must not be given after mefloquine prophylaxis. Give three doses of 500 mg at 6-h intervals. This should be repeated

1 week later. This drug is not recommended for children under 23 kg in weight. Larger children may be given 250 or 375 mg doses, depending on their weight. The adult dose may be given to children over 37 kg.

Halofantrine causes prolongation of the Q-T interval. Sudden cardiac dysrhythmias have occurred in predisposed patients, in those taking other drugs which have the same effect and, rarely, in individuals with no known predisposition. It should not be given to individuals who have been taking mefloquine for this reason. If quinine treatment is unavoidable after halofantrine medication, cardiac monitoring should be considered. Halofantrine is no longer recommended for standby self-treatment of malaria.

3 Artemesin — (extracted from *Artemesia* spp. plants) shows great promise as treatment for malaria, including *P. falciparum*. Preparations for clinical use are being developed.

Proposed treatments also include exchange transfusion to reduce parasitaemia, and prostacyclin therapy to enhance blood flow. These produce a measurable effect in peripheral blood, but it is not known whether they affect occluded small blood vessels in which parasitized red cells are already immobilized.

Prophylaxis of malaria

The risk of malaria is reduced as much by avoidance of mosquito bites as it is by chemoprophylaxis. The anti-mosquito measures already described should always be used by travellers to endemic areas, as they greatly augment the protective effect of chemoprophylaxis.

Two main types of chemoprophylaxis are recommended by British experts:
1 For benign malarias: chloroquine 300 mg weekly *or* proguanil 100 mg daily.
2 For falciparum malaria: chloroquine 300 mg weekly *plus* proguanil 200 mg daily.
3 Mefloquine is available for malarial prophylaxis. The dose is 250 mg (one tablet) weekly. Unfortunately, *P. falciparum* has begun to develop mefloquine resistance in a number of areas, but this is not currently widespread. Mefloquine in therapeutic doses can cause acute psychosis, nightmares or restlessness. At prophylactic doses significant adverse effects occur in about 1 in 10 000 recipients. This drug is contraindicated in epileptics, and those with a history of psychiatric disease. There are no data on its safety in the first trimester of pregnancy. Mefloquine is now the drug of first choice in Central, East and West Africa and in parts of South America where resistant *P. falciparum* occurs.

In all cases medication should be commenced 1 week before entering the endemic area, and continued for 4 weeks after leaving. There is no contraindication to malarial prophylaxis. Falciparum malaria threatens life, and in pregnancy endangers both the mother and the pregnancy itself. Neonates and infants are susceptible to severe disease. Malarial prophylaxis is much less risky than the disease itself and should never be omitted. Both chloroquine and proguanil are safe and well-tolerated by infants and pregnant women. Doses for children under 12 years old are:
1 Up to 6 weeks — one-eighth of adult dose.
2 Up to 1 year — one-quarter of adult dose.
3 Up to 5 years — half of adult dose.
4 6–12 years — three-quarters of adult dose.
Even if prophylaxis has been taken continuously, malaria should be considered and actively sought if the traveller becomes feverish after returning home.

Standby treatment for malaria

Even when prophylaxis is properly used, there is a risk of breakthrough attacks of malaria. Travellers in remote areas, who cannot obtain timely investigation and treatment, may be given a supply of emergency treatment. The only safe drugs for this are quinine (600 mg 8-hourly for 7–10 days) and Fansidar (single dose of three tablets). Medical attention should be sought as soon as possible after their use, so that the blood can be checked for parasites and anaemia, and other investigations performed if indicated.

Leishmaniasis

Introduction

Leishmaniasis is the term given to diseases caused by protozoa of the genus *Leishmania*. Although there are a number of different species, all of which are transmitted by sandflies, there are two main types of clinical disease. Cutaneous leishmaniasis is extremely common in tropical countries, in the Middle East and in many Mediterranean areas. Small rodents, and sometimes dogs, are the reservoir of infection. A severe mucocutaneous disease, called espundia, occurs in tropical Latin America. Systemic leishmaniasis is somewhat less common, affecting tropical areas of the old world. It is a rare disease in the northern and central Mediterranean area, but a common form exists in the eastern Mediterranean area.

Cutaneous leishmaniasis

In the old world this is caused by *L. tropica* (var.) *major* and (var.) *minor*. A typical oriental sore is caused by (var.) *major*, and has an incubation period of 2–6 weeks. The ragged, punched-out ulcer appears usually on the face or extremities, and is accompanied by regional lymphadenopathy. The lesion reaches up to 2.5 cm in diameter and heals slowly over 3–6 months, leaving a depressed, tissue-paper scar.

A more indolent, granulomatous type of lesion follows infection with (var.) *minor*, whose incubation period can be as long as a year. It appears as a purplish nodule, which gradually breaks down and slowly heals over several months. Lymphadenopathy is rare.

Diagnosis is made by demonstrating the protozoa in scrapings from the base of the lesion or in biopsy material. Specific treatment is not often required, but disfiguring facial lesions may be treated with intramuscular sodium stibogluconate for 10 days. Secondary infection may complicate the lesion and should be treated promptly to avoid further scarring.

Espundia causes destructive, scarring lesions of the oropharyngeal mucosa and surrounding structures, including the nasal septum. Secondary infection commonly exacerbates the condition. Vigorous and prolonged treatment with systemic antimonial drugs is necessary, and surgical aftercare may be required.

Systemic leishmaniasis

In most tropical areas the cause is *L. donovani*, which is mostly transmitted from human to human. In the Mediterranean it is caused mainly by a variant, sometimes called *L. infantum*, for which dogs and foxes are an important reservoir. The incubation period is variable but averages about 3 months. Fever is constant for the first few weeks, but then becomes intermittent. The typical features of hepatosplenomegaly, pancytopenia and increased skin pigmentation (which gives the disease the name kala-azar — the black sickness) develop over several weeks. The erythrocyte sedimentation rate is often very high, and is related to a polyclonal elevation of immunoglobulin G (IgG).

The diagnosis may be made by demonstrating protozoa (Leishman–Donovan bodies) packed into the mononuclear phagocytes of the spleen (Fig. 19.10), liver or bone marrow. Splenic aspiration is most likely to give positive results. Serodiagnosis by ELISA test is also possible. Culture is performed in reference laboratories.

The treatment of choice is with organic pentavalent arsenic in the form of sodium stibogluconate 10 mg/kg

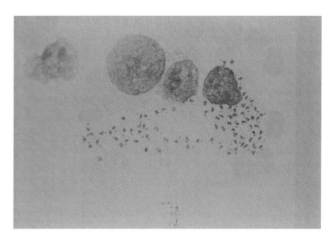

Fig. 19.10 Systemic leishmaniasis: this patient had typical hepatosplenomegaly, pancytopenia and persisting fever. Splenic aspirate revealed Leishman–Donovan bodies — macrophages packed with the protozoan parasites.

daily by intravenous injection. Treatment is made difficult by side-effects such as vomiting, coughing and substernal pain. Injections should be given intramuscularly if coughing and pain occur, but are themselves painful. The duration of treatment varies from 20 to 30 days, and depends on the type of disease and the response to treatment. Failure of response sometimes occurs. The treatment of systemic leishmaniasis is a specialist procedure. Alternative treatments include paromomycin (an aminoglycoside), amphotericin or mixtures of allopurinol and fluconazole.

Filariasis

This is a disease caused by the nematode worms *Wuchereria bancrofti* and *Brugia malayi*. Adult worms live coiled together in the lymphatics of humans. Pregnant female worms release large numbers of microfilariae, which reach the peripheral blood, and must then be ingested by a biting mosquito to complete their life cycle. Several species of mosquito can transmit the disease.

Clinical manifestations usually begin 9–12 months after infection. They are mainly due to inflammation around dead or dying worms in the lymphatics. There is usually a series of episodic fevers, each of which lasts a few hours. The fever is rarely high, but shivering and sweating are common. Lymphangitis may be visible if it is near to the skin surface; common sites are the lower leg or the thigh. Pain and redness of the skin look very like cellulitis or erysipelas. Abdominal pain or scrotal inflammation are rarer manifestations.

The last filariae die within about 5 years of a single infecting episode, and no further symptoms occur. In rare cases with many reinfections, accumulating fibrosis of affected lymphatics can eventually produce lymphoedema (elephantiasis).

Diagnosis is made by demonstrating microfilariae in the peripheral blood. These are most easily found at night, but occasionally have a daytime periodicity; midday and midnight blood films cover both situations. Serodiagnosis by ELISA is also possible.

Treatment is with diethylcarbamazine, which kills both adult worms and microfilariae. The dose is 6 mg/kg daily in divided doses. Febrile allergic reactions are common as worms die at the onset of treatment. It is usual to commence treatment under close medical supervision, starting with 1 mg/kg daily and working up to a therapeutic dose. Full dosage is then continued for 21 days. Antihistamines and/or corticosteroids may be needed until febrile reactions cease.

Treatment of filariasis (excluding onchocerciasis)
Give diethyl carbamazine orally:
1 Day 1: 1 mg/kg as a single dose.
2 Day 2: 3 mg/kg as a single dose.
3 Day 3: 6 mg/kg as a single dose.
4 Next 20 days: 6 mg/kg daily.

Other forms of filariasis

These are caused by *Loa loa* and by *Oncocerca volvulus* (the agent of river blindness). Loiasis is often asymptomatic but may produce localized allergic skin swellings (Calabar swellings), or is visible if an adult worm migrates across the eye. If it requires treatment, diethylcarbamazine is effective.

Onchocerciasis is transmitted by *Simulium* flies which deposit their eggs near fast-flowing water. Adult worms live in the skin, often forming macroscopic nodules. The illness is caused by inflammatory reactions to the millions of microfilariae which invade the skin and eye. Treatment with diethylcarbamazine is dangerous because of severe inflammatory reactions with possible destructive involvement of the eye. Ivermectin 150 mg produces gradual and sustained reduction in microfilariae with little allergic reaction, and the dose can be repeated annually until infection is eradicated. Surgical excision of skin nodules has also been used as a means of reducing microfilarial numbers.

Important zoonoses

Brucellosis (see also Chapter 20)

Introduction

Human infection with *Brucella* spp. is usually acquired from the natural hosts, cattle (*B. abortus*) or goats (*B. melitensis*). Less common forms occur in sheep, pigs and, rarely, dogs. Brucellosis is an important disease worldwide, but is extremely rare in the UK because of successful eradication programmes, particularly for cattle. Imported cases arrive particularly from rural Africa, Mediterranean countries and from the Middle East, where brucellosis is very common (and can also affect camels). The disease affects many body systems, causing severe morbidity and some mortality.

Clinical features

These are variable, ranging from acute illness with swinging fever to chronic symptoms affecting a variety of body systems.

Acute brucellosis

Acute brucellosis has an incubation period of 1–3 weeks. Fever is usually an important finding. It may be continuous, swinging or undulating (rising steadily for 7–10 days and then falling for a day or two). Weakness, shivering and sweating are prominent features and most patients have arthralgia, particularly of large joints. In spite of the severity of the illness, mortality is low and untreated cases tend to recover after anything from 3 or 4 weeks to several months (average 3 or 4 months).

Physical findings are rarely impressive. They include tender splenomegaly in about half of patients, mild cervical and axillary lymphadenopathy, and tenderness of the spine.

Chronic brucellosis

Chronic brucellosis is not common. It may be mistaken for tuberculosis, or for chronic disease of the systems mainly involved. There may well be a considerable element of hypersensitivity in cases of longer duration, but granulomatous inflammation also occurs and may cause arthralgia, uveitis, orchitis, meningoencephalitis and liver abnormalities.

Important complications

Important complications are really local manifestations of a multisystem disease. The commonest is bone and joint disease, in which brucellae can be recovered from inflammatory effusions. Spinal brucellosis is often seen in endemic areas and must be distinguished from tuberculosis and other chronic osteomyelitis.

Less common, but requiring urgent diagnosis and treatment, are neurobrucellosis, with fits, cranial nerve lesions or neuropsychiatric features, and *Brucella* endocarditis, which usually affects previously damaged valves.

Diagnosis

Clinical diagnosis is rarely possible; signs and symptoms are non-specific and the blood count usually shows neutrophilia in acute disease, otherwise neutropenia with a few activated mononuclear cells. Liver granulomata are often present, but are indistinguishable from those of sarcoidosis and non-caseating tuberculosis. The diagnosis must be suspected from the epidemiological circumstances, and appropriate laboratory tests performed.

Diagnosis of brucellosis
1 Blood cultures (maintained for up to 6 weeks).
2 Culture of joint effusions or pus from bone.
3 Antibody detection (usually enzyme-linked immunosorbent assay).

Management

The treatment of choice is tetracycline, which should be given for at least 6 weeks. There may be less likelihood of relapse if demeclocycline is used rather than other formulations. The incidence of relapse is reduced if an aminoglycoside is added for 2–3 weeks of treatment. Although the need for intramuscular injections is inconvenient, the alternative additional drug, rifampicin, is not so effective. Other treatments, such as co-trimoxazole and ciprofloxacin, will achieve defervescence of fever and reduced local inflammation, but recurrence is common after their use. These drugs can be used for treating children.

Treatment of brucellosis
1 Demeclocycline orally 150 mg 6-hourly or 300 mg 12-hourly; *plus*
2 Gentamicin or Netilmicin i.m. or i.v. in standard doses, with blood level monitoring; *or*
3 (Second choice) rifampicin orally 600 mg daily for 14 days during weeks 3 and 4.

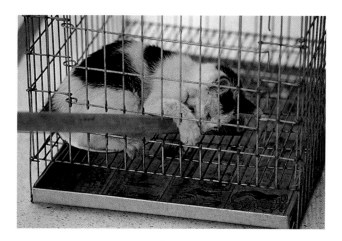

Fig. 19.11 A cat with furious rabies attacks an object which has entered its cage. Courtesy of Dr D. Lewis

Recurrences can occur, even after full tetracycline plus aminoglycoside treatment. They should be treated with a second course of the same therapy.

Rabies (see also Chapter 16)

Rabies is a rhabdovirus infection which can affect many warm-blooded animals including birds, bats, squirrels, skunks, cats, horses and cattle, but is most often transmitted to humans by canines such as dogs, wolves and foxes. The virus causes myeloencephalitis and is excreted in tears and saliva. It is inoculated by bite, scratch or mucosal contamination from animals with rabies, incubating the disease or excreting the virus. Virus enters the peripheral nerves via which it travels to the central nervous system.

The incubation period is short after bites on the head or face — often 10–14 days — but may be over a year for bites in sites such as the lower leg, remote from the central nervous system. Illness often begins with paraesthesiae at the inoculation site. Extreme anxiety is common at this stage. The main clinical features are then either ascending polyneuritis or rapidly developing encephalitis. The patient may be obtunded or speechless (dumb rabies), or excitable and aggressive (furious rabies; Fig. 19.11). In either case, painful spasms of the pharynx often cause the typical, distressing signs of hydrophobia. There is no specific treatment, and survival has not followed even prolonged and intensive supportive care.

Early diagnosis depends on clinical suspicion, and exclusion of more treatable causes of myelitis or encephalitis. Rabies virus can be recovered from saliva, tears and corneal scrapings. Rising titres of antibodies can be demonstrated. Established rabies produces typical appearances in brain biopsy, with Negri bodies in both humans and animals.

Plague (see also Chapter 20)

Plague is the systemic disease caused by *Yersinia pestis*. In nature it is a disease of rats but, as the rats die, the rat fleas are obliged to find alternative hosts and begin to bite humans. The fleas themselves are affected by the infection, for bacteria block their foregut, causing regurgitation of infected material when they attempt to bite.

> Plague is an internationally notifiable disease. Countries in which human plague cases are currently occurring are listed weekly in the World Health Organisation *Weekly Epidemiological Report*.

The incubation period is short, averaging 4 or 5 days, and three-quarters of all cases develop the bubonic form of the disease. After a day or two of fever the bubo appears, usually in an inguinal node, sometimes in the axilla and rarely elsewhere. The degree of swelling is variable. Many patients are bacteraemic. In those who recover untreated the bubo usually discharges offensive pus some time after the fever subsides.

A minority of patients develop pneumonic plague, in which an initially trivial chest infection rapidly evolves into severe pneumonia, often with watery, blood-stained sputum and early respiratory failure. Large numbers of bacteria are excreted and secondary cases may occur.

The diagnosis may be suspected on epidemiological and clinical findings. *Y. pestis* can be recovered from blood, pus or sputum. Tetracycline or chloramphenicol is effective treatment, and the organism is also sensitive to modern agents such as ciprofloxacin. Tetracycline prophylaxis may be offered to those in contact with pneumonic cases.

Anthrax

Introduction and epidemiology

Anthrax is a disease particularly of hoofed animals, caused by *Bacillus anthracis*. *B. anthracis* is an aerobic, spore-bearing, Gram-positive rod, closely related to *B. cereus* and *B. subtilis*, but with a wider range of antibiotic sensitivities than either. In its natural hosts it causes a fatal septicaemic disease in which the animal's blood becomes packed with bacilli. After the host's death, the bacilli form spores which remain viable in the soil for decades. Farm animals are susceptible to anthrax;

an outbreak in the UK in the 1980s affected pigs. Humans become infected by close contact with infected or dead animals, with bones, bonemeal, hides, hooves or meat. Badger-hair shaving brushes occasionally caused infection in the past. The usual route of infection is inoculation into the skin, less often by inhalation or ingestion of large numbers of spores.

Clinical features

Oedematous skin lesion

An oedematous skin lesion (malignant pustule) is the commonest feature. An inflamed site blisters, and forms a black scab, surrounded by a halo of vesicles or pustules. A common site is the neck at the collar, or the arm. Local draining lymph nodes are enlarged and tender. A helpful diagnostic feature is the large extent of oedema. The skin lesion may be 2–4 cm across, but the oedema may extend from the forehead to the costal margin, or involve the whole arm.

Pneumonia

Pneumonia can follow inhalation of massive spore loads, often from hides or dusty bonemeal. It is often fulminant, leading to death in 2 or 3 days. Patients exhale many organisms, and are infectious.

Gastrointestinal anthrax

Gastrointestinal anthrax is probably acquired by ingestion of large spore loads. It causes abdominal pain and severe watery diarrhoea, which contains many sporing organisms.

Septicaemia

Septicaemia is often fatal. It can occur with untreated skin infection, but is common with pneumonitis and gastrointestinal disease. The mode of death is often pulmonary embolism or cerebral vein thrombosis, both of which can occur even after antibiotic treatment has resulted in loss of fever.

Diagnosis

Lesion swabs or vesicle fluid will produce colonies in blood agar, which are composed of tangled chains of square-ended Gram-positive rods. These filamentous colonies are called Medusa head colonies. Spore stains will demonstrate central spores in mature colonies. Blood cultures readily produce a heavy growth; indeed methylene blue-stained blood smears from septicaemic animals and humans will often demonstrate bacilli (without spores, which do not form in the living host).

Treatment

This should be commenced while the diagnosis is confirmed, to minimize the risk of bacteraemia. Intravenous benzylpencillin 2.4–3.0 g 6-hourly is the treatment of choice. Oral ampicillin 500 mg to 1 g 6-hourly should be used for continuation. Ciprofloxacin intravenously 200 mg 12-hourly or orally 500 mg 12-hourly is a good alternative. Treatment should be continued until the lesion is healed, and the oedema completely resolved.

Prevention and control

Anthrax vaccines are available for animal and human use. They cause significant reactions in humans and are nowadays rarely indicated, as personal hygiene and adequate working clothes protect against skin infection with this rare disease. Hides, and hoof and bone products, must be heat- or chemically treated to destroy spores before they are moved between countries or used in manufacturing processes. The tanning process renders hides and leather safe.

Tularaemia (see also Chapter 20)

This is a disease caused by *Francisella tularensis*, an organism of rodents. Hunters and woodsmen can be infected by direct contact or inoculation from live animals, skins or carcasses. The disease may be localized to the skin and local lymph nodes (ulceroglandular form) or behave like a systemic infection with non-specific symptoms, including variable rashes (typhoidal form). Rare cases of ocular, pharyngeal or abdominal infection also occur. Half of patients with the typhoidal form also have a generalized pneumonitis and in these patients there is a significant mortality.

Blood cultures are usually negative, so diagnosis rests on clinical suspicion or recovery of organisms from affected tissue sites. Serological diagnosis can be made by reference laboratories.

Aminoglycosides and tetracycline are effective in treating tularaemia.

Viral haemorrhagic fevers

Introduction

Viral haemorrhagic fevers is a general term describing several groups of severe viral infections in which haemorrhage is part of the clinical picture. These include some diseases already discussed in this and other chapters.

DISEASE LIST

Arboviruses
  Dengue haemorrhagic fever (flavivirus)
  Yellow fever (flavivirus)
  Congo-Crimean haemorrhagic fever (bunyavirus)
  Haemorrhagic fever with renal syndrome (hantavirus)
  Others (Chikungunya, Rift Valley fever).

Arenaviruses
  Lassa fever
  Argentinian haemorrhagic fever (Junin virus)
  Bolivian haemorrhagic fever (Machupo virus)
  Rarer pathogenic arenaviruses occur, also in South America (Guanarito, Sabia).

Filoviruses
  Marburg disease
  Ebola virus haemorrhagic fever.

Yellow fever is an internationally notifiable disease. Countries where human cases are currently occurring are listed in the *Weekly Epidemiological Report*.

These viral infections tend to cause severe systemic diseases with an anonymous insidious onset comprising fever, malaise, variable sore throat and headache, arthralgia and increasing prostration. All severe filovirus infections ultimately give rise to multiorgan damage with evidence of liver dysfunction, bone marrow depression, renal impairment and evidence of widespread tissue damage (falling sodium levels, elevation of non-liver transaminases, falling blood pressure, encephalopathy and extreme lassitude). These problems may be accompanied by specific features such as rash, diarrhoea or renal failure.

Haemorrhagic fevers with renal syndromes

These diseases are caused by viruses of the Hantavirus family. They are natural diseases of rodents, transmitted to humans either by inoculation or by inhalation of body fluids from host animals. Korean haemorrhagic fever is a severe disease, caused by Seoul virus, and is endemic in Korea and many parts of China and the Far East. Milder diseases of the same type occur in eastern Europe and forested parts of Scandinavia. These are often caused by the Puumala virus.

The disease occurs in three main phases: (i) an acute influenza-like syndrome; (ii) an intermediate stage of hypotension or shock, accompanied by haemorrhagic features and thrombocytopenia; and (iii) a late stage of oliguria and renal failure.

Diagnosis is based on demonstrating IgM antibodies, usually by ELISA. The viruses can be recovered in cell cultures of blood or serum.

Management is mainly supportive. Early treatment with tribavirin can abort the hypotensive and nephropathic phases of the disease.

Managing the major viral haemorrhagic fevers

Although these diseases are serious for affected patients, most are not transmitted from person to person. However, some have caused significant nosocomial transmission and are therefore subject to special precautions when diagnosed or suspected in western countries. These are (in approximately increasing order of infectiousness) Lassa fever, Marburg disease, Ebola virus haemorrhagic fever and Congo-Crimean haemorrhagic fever. The maximum incubation period of viral haemorrhagic fevers is 3 weeks. The diagnosis can be excluded if more than 21 days have elapsed between leaving the endemic area and the onset of fever.

Lassa fever

Introduction

Lassa fever is an arenavirus infection whose natural reservoir is the multimammate rat *Mastomys natalensis*, which only carries Lassa virus in West Africa (other arenaviruses less pathogenic to humans exist in other parts of Africa). Transmission is probably by inoculation or mucosal contamination by infectious urine from asymptomatic rats. Small numbers of medical and laboratory staff have been infected when handling cases or specimens.

The disease has an insidious onset with fever, malaise, aches and pains, dry cough, sore throat, moderate gastrointestinal symptoms and increasing prostration. Many cases may be mild or self-limiting, but Lassa fever is a common cause of hospital admission in endemic areas and many patients have severe illnesses of 2–3 weeks' duration. Those who have high transaminases (more than 10 times the upper reference level) usually

have high viraemias (more than four log tissue culture infective dose 50), and suffer a mortality of up to 15%.

Late and fatal cases have haematuria, blood-streaking of sputum and easy bruising, due to poor platelet aggregation. Hypotension can be profound and encephalopathies may occur. Peripheral blood granulocytosis reflects extensive tissue damage. There is often extensive non-pitting oedema of the lower face and neck. Severe haemorrhage is a rare or terminal event.

Diagnosis

Diagnosis depends on clinical and epidemiological suspicion. In the UK *The Management of Viral Haemorrhagic Fevers* (HMSO 1996) sets out the recommendations of the Department of Health for obtaining advice and arranging management for suspected cases. High-security infectious diseases units (HSIDUs) have special clinical and laboratory facilities for handling patient management, and can liaise with the Central Public Health Laboratory: Virus Reference Division* to arrange diagnostic tests.

Laboratory diagnosis is based on demonstrating IgM or IgG antibodies by ELISA, or by recovery of viruses in vero-cell cultures of blood. Urine cultures become positive later than blood cultures and may remain positive for several weeks. Positive blood cultures have also been demonstrated in afebrile patients in early convalescence. Viraemia can nowadays be detected rapidly, using polymerase chain reaction techniques.

Treatment

Treatment is based on intensive support and tribavirin therapy. It is important to exclude immediately life-threatening diseases such as malaria, and no patient should be referred as a case of viral haemorrhagic fever before malaria has been adequately considered and investigated.

Haemorrhagic conditions which should be considered before a diagnosis of viral haemorrhagic fever is assumed
1 Malignant malaria.
2 Meningococcal disease.
3 Severe rickettsial infections.
4 Gram-negative septicaemia with disseminated intravascular coagulation.

*Central Public Health Laboratory: Virus Reference Division, 61 Colindale Avenue, London NW9 5HT.

Supportive measures, with attention to perfusion, fluid balance and fever are important in reducing mortality. Tribavirin is available in HSIDUs, and can reduce mortality in severe disease. Follow-up is necessary to confirm eventual clearance of virus from blood and urine.

Prevention and control

Prevention and control measures are concentrated on close family members and medical contacts with the patient and his or her blood. Casual and social contacts are not at risk. In most cases surveillance of health and temperature during the possible incubation period is sufficient. Tribavirin has been given to high-risk contacts such as sexual partners or persons contaminated with the patient's blood, but there is no firm evidence of its effectiveness.

Argentine haemorrhagic fever

This disease is caused by Junin virus, an arenavirus whose natural hosts are harvest mice. Epidemics occur in northern Argentina, particularly during the corn harvest. The disease is like Lassa fever; petechial rashes and platelet dysfunction are common. Patients with severe disease may have encephalopathies. The mortality is 10–15%.

Convalescent plasma, containing neutralizing antibodies to Junin virus, can reduce mortality to 3%, but a late mild encephalopathy is common in treated patients. An effective vaccine is now available.

Bolivian haemorrhagic fever

This arenavirus infection, caused by Machupo virus, is endemic in rural Bolivia. Several other strains of arenavirus exist in rodent populations in South America, but most are not pathogenic to humans.

Marburg disease and Ebola haemorrhagic fever

Epidemiology

The epidemiology of these filovirus infections is not understood. The original outbreak in Marburg followed the importation of infected vervet monkeys into a scientific laboratory. However, the monkeys also suffer life-threatening disease and no monkeys in the wild have been found to carry these viruses (though some harbour other filoviruses less pathogenic to humans).

Transmission occurred from monkeys and their tissues to laboratory workers, from patients to medical attendants and from one convalescent patient to his wife (the patient's semen was found to contain virus). The main route of transmission is via the blood and body fluids. One patient in a South African outbreak had Marburg virus isolated from the anterior chamber of the eye many weeks after her illness.

Ebola infection has caused large community outbreaks with high mortality. The pattern of the outbreaks was complicated by extensive hospital transmission, perhaps associated with re-use of needles. Countries affected include Zaire, Sudan, Kenya and Northern Uganda.

Clinical features

The clinical picture is similar in both diseases. After 3 or 4 days' insidious onset with high fever and prostration, diarrhoea and a measles-like rash are usually seen. Mild or gross haemorrhagic features may quickly develop, including bloody diarrhoea with abdominal pain. Leukocytosis develops, and transaminases rise as tissue damage proceeds. There is little evidence of intravascular coagulation, as platelet dysfunction is the main cause of haemorrhage.

Diagnosis

Diagnosis may be suspected on clinical and epidemiological grounds. The viruses grow readily in cell cultures and can be demonstrated by immunofluorescence. IgM and IgG antibodies can be demonstrated at appropriate stages of the disease.

No antiviral agent, including interferon, has a significant beneficial effect; vigorous supportive treatment must be given. Removal of the patient from a general hospital setting is more urgent than with Lassa fever, as both the patient and his or her body fluids are more infectious, and there is a small possibility of aerosol infection from either source.

Congo-Crimean haemorrhagic fever

Epidemiology

The natural epidemiology of this nairovirus disease depends on tick-borne transmission between warm-blooded animals. Cattle are important in many African countries but other animals, including small rodents, may be important elsewhere. Congo-Crimean haemorrhagic fever is not restricted to tropical Africa, but is endemic in the Middle East and parts of Bulgaria, former

Yugoslavia and the former southern USSR. It is an infectious condition. Secondary cases are relatively common, particularly among clinical care personnel.

Clinical features

The clinical picture follows an average incubation period of 4–10 days. Abrupt onset of severe viral symptoms is followed in 2 or 3 days by collapse, extensive bruising and purpura, haematemesis and melaena. In these patients there is clear evidence of intravascular coagulation. Cases of intermediate severity can occur, and must be differentiated from meningococcal or rickettsial diseases or from haemorrhagic chickenpox.

Tribavirin may have some action in Congo-Crimean haemorrhagic fever, but treatment is mainly supportive.

Public health measures for viral haemorrhagic fever cases

Viral haemorrhagic fevers are unfamiliar diseases in the UK, where they are extremely rare. There are several important aspects to their safe and expeditious management.

1 Ensure that common severe infections are not missed. The commonest cause of tropical fevers is malaria, and malignant malaria can cause haemorrhagic disease mediated by disseminated intravascular coagulation (see text note, p. 380). This potentially life-threatening disease must not be overlooked because of anxieties about possible viral haemorrhagic fever. Blood films can be examined to exclude malaria before the question of viral haemorrhagic fever is considered in most cases. Seriously ill patients can be commenced on quinine treatment while the differential diagnosis is considered.

2 Obtain advice from a specialist. Regional infectious and tropical disease specialists will have up-to-date information on endemic areas, and will often be able to exclude the diagnosis of viral haemorrhagic fever on telephone enquiry simply on the basis of epidemiological and clinical data.

Cases where the diagnosis cannot readily be excluded fall into two main categories:

(a) Medium-risk cases, whose investigation should be handled in a specialist infectious diseases unit, with the aim of making an alternative diagnosis and treating the patient appropriately.

(b) High-risk cases, when the diagnosis of viral haemorrhagic fever is known, obvious or strongly suspected, or is indicated after investigation as a medium-risk case. Such cases should be managed in an HSIDU, where special control of infection measures are employed during investigation and management. The staff at the HSIDU will accept such cases, and will liaise with regional ambulance services to arrange transfer.

3 Viral haemorrhagic fevers are notifiable diseases. They should be notified by telephone to the appropriate proper officer, with follow-up in writing. The names of face-to-face health care contacts should be recorded for the use of the public health specialists. Contacts of high-risk cases are followed up for 3 weeks after the last contact, or until the diagnosis is disproven.

Local public health specialists will advise on cleaning and disinfection of premises and equipment used by the patient. Standard hospital procedures are usually adequate for this. Special disinfection or fumigation is hardly ever indicated.

Summary of personal health measures recommended for travellers

1 Vaccinations for epidemic diseases. The desirability of these will depend on the current prevalence of epidemics in the destination country. Vaccines available include:

(a) Influenza vaccine.

(b) Meningococcal vaccine.

(Cholera vaccine is no longer required by any country.)

Other vaccines for personal protection will depend on whether a traveller will have other occupational or social exposures:

(a) Tetanus vaccine or booster.

(b) Hepatitis B vaccine.

2 Protection from food- and water-borne diseases is recommended for travellers to tropical countries, particularly where efficient sanitation and safe water supplies cannot be guaranteed. The following measures may be considered:

(a) Typhoid immunization.

(b) Hepatitis A prophylaxis with human normal immunoglobulin or inactivated vaccine.

(c) Polio immunization, or booster if required.

(d) Chemoprophylaxis for diarrhoea (special circumstances only).

(e) Water filter/purification kits (campers and independent travellers).

3 Malaria prophylaxis is essential for everybody who travels to an endemic area. Measures to avoid insect bites should also be emphasized.

4 Yellow fever vaccination is recommended for all travellers who will enter an endemic area. Certificates of vaccination are often required for travellers passing from endemic areas to other countries. Certification is subject to International Health Regulations, and is available only from accredited centres.

5 Immunization against local infections may be advisable for travellers having rural exposure, especially during certain seasons. Diseases to consider include:

(a) Japanese B encephalitis (stays of more than 1 month in rural farming areas of affected countries).

(b) Tick-borne encephalitis (camping, walking or rural work in forested areas of affected countries during late spring and summer).

(c) Rabies (independent travel in remote areas of affected countries; relief work, especially if involving animal contact in those countries; caving in areas where bat rabies occurs).

Assessment of fever in a returning traveller

Different diseases may become evident at different times after a traveller returns from an overseas visit, depending on the incubation periods of the various infections (Table 19.1).

Time after return home	Disease
During first week	Viral gastroenteritis
	Traveller's diarrhoea
	Bacillary dysentery, sexually transmitted diseases, influenza, dengue (and other arboviral infections)
1–2 weeks	Malaria
	Hepatitis A
	Typhoid fever
	Paratyphoid fever
	Rickettsial infections
2–4 weeks	Typhoid fever
	Amoebiasis
	Hepatitis C
	Katayama fever
1–6 months	Hepatitis B
	HIV seroconversion illness
	Hepatitis E
	Amoebiasis
	Rabies
	Cutaneous leishmaniasis
	Systemic leishmaniasis
More than 6 months	Relapses of vivax or ovale malaria
	Reactivation of malariae malaria
	Strongyloidiasis (larva currens)
	Rabies
	Systemic leishmaniasis
	AIDS

AIDS, acquired immunodeficiency syndrome; HIV, human immunodeficiency virus.

Table 19.1 Intervals between a traveller's return home and the presentation of imported diseases

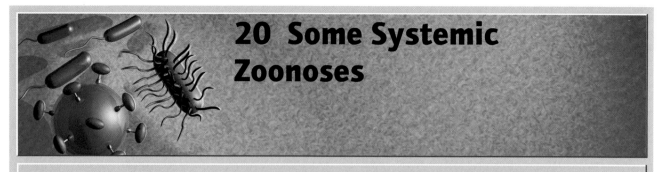

20 Some Systemic Zoonoses

Introduction

A zoonosis is an animal disease which can be accidentally transmitted to humans. Several such diseases, including anthrax, Q-fever, ornithosis, hydatid disease and Lassa fever, have already been mentioned in other chapters of this book. A few diseases, such as *Campylobacter* infections and salmonelloses, are common to animals and humans and are relatively readily transmitted between humans as well as between animals. True zoonoses are not easily transmitted from person to person, save for cases of exceptional pulmonary disease, as in pneumonic plague or anthrax pneumonia.

Most zoonoses are acquired when humans intrude into the animals' daily environment. This occurs during farm work, during the handling of raw animal products such as hides, meat or bones, and during camping or safari expeditions. Consumption of untreated or uncooked products such as milk, soft cheese or preserved but uncooked meat can also be a means of aquiring a zoonosis.

Common activities which predispose to zoonoses
Consuming untreated milk, cream, yoghurt and curd cheese
1 *Salmonella* or *Campylobacter* infections.
2 Brucellosis.
3 Q-fever.
4 Haverhill fever.
5 Tick-borne encephalitis (when the animal is infected).

Hunting, trapping, skinning and butchering wild animals
1 Plague.
2 Tularaemia.
3 Rabies.

Butchering farm animals
1 Q-fever.
2 Streptococcal skin infections.
3 *Erysipelothrix* skin infections.
4 *Streptococcus suis* systemic infections.

Eating undercooked meat
1 Toxoplasmosis.
2 Trichinellosis (from pork).
3 Pork or beef tapeworms.
4 *Salmonella, Escherichia coli* 0157 or *Campylobacter* infections.

Handling dead animals, untanned hides or unpasteurized bonemeal
Anthrax.

Ingestion or inoculation of animal urine
Leptospirosis.

Camping, hiking or forestry working in warm climates
1 Tick-borne encephalitis.
2 Borreliosis.
3 Arboviral encephalitides.
4 Hantavirus (nephropathia epidemica, HFRS or Hantavirus pulmonary syndrome).

Brucellosis

Introduction and epidemiology

Brucella spp. are common pathogens of warm-blooded animals, particularly hoofed animals. When clinically evident in the natural host, they often cause infectious abortion, but inapparent infection and excretion of the organisms also occur. The animal's milk may be contaminated, either by excretion in the milk itself or by contamination during unhygienic milking processes.

Humans aquire infection by consuming unpasteurized dairy products or by contact with infected products of conception, either during delivery or abortion. The earliest description of acute brucellosis was in British soldiers in Malta, who developed severe fever after drinking raw goats' milk. Cases were subsequently recognized associated with cows' milk. Chronic brucellosis or undulant fever was described later, again after consumption of cows' milk.

Occupational exposure is important in the occurrence of brucellosis. Cowhands, veterinary practitioners and goat-keepers are at some risk. However, control programmes have made the infection extremely rare in the UK, as most herds are nowadays *Brucella*-free. The great majority of cases are now imported, and are associated with consumption of untreated milk or dairy products. Brucellosis is still extremely common in the Middle East (where the disease also affects camels) and in rural parts of Africa and Asia; a large outbreak occurred in Malta in 1995. Milk is important for its nutritious value, but is often consumed straight from the cow or goat, and is sometimes preserved by adding the animal's urine.

Clinical features

Brucellosis is an unpredictable disease with a variable clinical picture. The incubation period ranges from 5 days to several weeks, and the onset of the disease may be acute or insidious.

Acute brucellosis

Acute brucellosis has an abrupt onset, with high swinging fever, often rigors and sometimes myalgia and arthralgia. The patient feels severely unwell, but often has few physical signs. About half have enlarged lymph nodes in the cervical chain, and about a quarter have splenomegaly. The white cell count is often, but not always, raised and the liver function tests may be slightly abnormal because of granulomatous hepatitis. Untreated acute brucellosis is rarely fatal, but causes severe morbidity for 5 or 6 weeks.

Chronic brucellosis

Chronic brucellosis is uncommon. It may follow on from an acute attack or commence insidiously. Typically, it causes malaise, depression and a fever which waxes and wanes over periods of 2 or 3 weeks (undulant fever). The white cell count is often low, because of a neutropenia.

Local effects

Local effects of brucellosis are many. Almost any organ or tissue can be involved, although granulomatous inflammation of reticuloendothelial organs is the most constant feature. This causes lymphadenopathy, splenomegaly and abnormalities of the liver function tests.

Bone and joint involvement

Bone and joint involvement can affect the spine or sometimes a large joint. Effusion of a large joint or a chronic osteomyelitis picture in the spine are the usual manifestations. The differential diagnosis from tuberculosis is important in patients from areas where brucellosis is common, and this depends on clinical suspicion and performing the appropriate diagnostic tests (see also Chapter 18).

Orchitis

Orchitis is relatively common. It develops after several days of fever, and may be associated with chills and increased malaise. Physical signs vary from pain in the testicles to acute tenderness and swelling.

Renal involvement

Renal involvement is usually evidenced by proteinuria and 'sterile' pyuria.

Neurobrucellosis

Neurobrucellosis is uncommon, but can be severe. Partly due to an encephalitis or encephalopathy, it can take the form of an acute psychosis. Occasional cases of meningoencephalitis can be life-threatening.

Endocarditis

Endocarditis is a rare manifestation of brucellosis.

Clinical features of brucellosis
1 Fever (undulant in chronic infection).
2 Pyogenic arthritis.
3 Spinal osteomyelitis.
4 Lymphadenopathy.
5 Splenomegaly (especially in acute disease).
6 Abnormal liver function.
7 Orchitis or testicular pain.
8 Endocarditis.
9 Meningoencephalitis.
10 Depression or psychosis.
11 Sterile pyuria.

Diagnosis

Diagnosis depends on suspicion of the disease, eliciting the epidemiological history, and on appropriate laboratory tests.

Blood cultures are often positive, but *Brucella* spp. may be very slow-growing, and cultures must be maintained for up to 6 weeks until they are declared negative. Culture of specimens such as aspirated joint effusions or bony abscesses may also yield positive bacteriological results.

Serological tests are useful, and often give faster results than blood cultures. Traditional agglutination reactions can be carried out; occasionally they are strongly positive in previously immune individuals after new exposure to antigens. This may give rise to an erroneous diagnosis of active disease. Enzyme-linked immunosorbent assay (ELISA) tests are widely performed, and can detect immunoglobulin M (IgM) antibodies in acute disease, or high levels of IgG in chronic infection.

Liver biopsy will often show multiple granulomata, especially in established disease. These are rarely caseating, unless caused by *B. suis*, and must be distinguished from the granulomata of sarcoidosis or miliary tuberculosis.

Treatment

The disease is shortened by treatment with tetracycline, which should be continued for 4–12 weeks. Chlortetracycline or oxytetracycline can be given in divided doses, or demeclocycline or doxycycline in less frequent doses. Some experts believe that demeclocycline has an advantage in producing optimum tissue levels and reducing the risk of relapse (but it is probably also more likely to cause significant photosensitization and/or diabetes insipidus). Relapse can occur, and is less likely if gentamicin 2–5 mg/kg daily or netilmicin 4–6 mg/kg daily (with blood level monitoring) or rifampicin 600 mg daily is given for at least 2 weeks. Aminoglycoside plus tetracycline probably offers the best chance of relapse-free recovery, but is less convenient than rifampicin because of the need for intramuscular injection and blood level monitoring. Positive blood cultures persist after treatment in 10–15% of patients treated with tetracycline for 2 months combined with aminoglycoside for the first month. For endocarditis or neurobrucellosis, tetracycline therapy should be continued for a total of 3 months.

Co-trimoxazole produces early improvement, but is followed by relapse with positive blood cultures in 35–50% of cases. It is not recommended as monotherapy. Quinolones have not been found as effective as tetracycline–aminoglycoside.

Depression or psychotic symptoms do not always respond as readily as other features of the disease. Psychiatric support may be required, and symptoms may need to be treated with psychotropic drugs as well as with antimicrobials.

Treatment in pregnancy is unsatisfactory, as tetracyclines cannot be given. A reasonable compromise is to treat with co-trimoxazole plus rifampicin, and to offer retreatment after delivery if bacteraemia recurs. Children may also be treated with a combination of co-trimoxazole and rifampicin.

Treatment of brucellosis
1 Demeclocycline orally, 300 mg 12-hourly; *or*
Doxycycline orally, 200 mg first doses, then 100–200 mg daily both for 2–3 months; *plus*
Gentamicin i.m., or i.v., 2–5 mg/kg daily in three divided doses (with blood level monitoring); *or*
Netilmicin, single dose i.m. or i.v., 4–6 mg/kg daily (with blood level monitoring); *or*
Rifampicin orally, 600 mg twice daily (or 300 mg 6-hourly), for the first month.
2 In pregnancy co-trimoxazole orally, 960–1440 mg 12-hourly for 2 weeks, then 480 mg 12-hourly for 6 more weeks; *plus*
Rifampicin orally, 300–600 mg twice daily for the first 4 weeks (give first-choice treatment after delivery if indicated).
3 For a child under 12 years tetracycline is contra-indicated; use co-trimoxazole orally; 6 months to 5 years, 240 mg twice daily; 6–12 years, 480 mg twice daily for 8 weeks; *plus*
Rifampicin 10 mg/kg daily for the first 4 weeks.

Lyme disease (borreliosis)

Introduction and epidemiology

Lyme disease has a prolonged natural history and several stages affecting different body systems. It is caused by infection with *Borrelia* spp., which are transmitted from animals to humans by the bite of hard ticks of the genus *Ixodes* (Fig. 20.1). The natural hosts of the *Borrelia* species are small rodents, but human disease is often acquired via deer. Dogs can also be infected. The main organism causing borreliosis is *B. burgdorferi*. However different strains of the organism exist in the USA and in various parts of Europe (where *B. garinii* exists), and they appear to cause diseases with slightly differing clinical characteristics; US strains seem more likely to produce carditis, while European strains may be more likely to produce central nervous system manifestations.

Clinical features

A tick must remain attached for several hours before it has transferred enough borrelias in its saliva to infect a human host. Following this there is an incubation period of 1–3 weeks.

Early Lyme disease — erythema chronicum migrans

About 80% of infected patients develop a characteristic rash surrounding the tick bite. A disc of erythema expands, often clearing in the centre to produce a ring-shaped eruption (Fig. 20.2). This may enlarge sufficiently to encompass a limb before gradually fading. Multiple erythema chronicum migrans (ECM) lesions are occasionally seen. Patients often have fever, aches and pains, and malaise during the eruption, which can last for 2–4 weeks. There may be a mild leukocytosis, and the erythrocyte sedimentation rate is often raised to 40–60 mm/h.

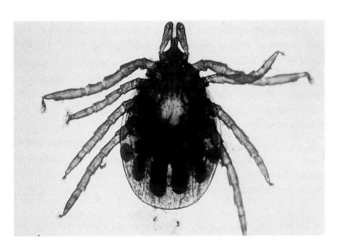

Fig. 20.1 Hard ixodid tick, the vector of borreliosis. Hard ticks are also vectors for tick-borne encephalitis and some rickettsial infections. Courtesy of the Ministry of Defence.

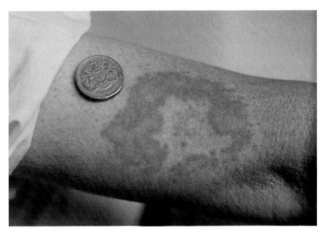

Fig. 20.2 Erythema chronicum migrans. (Courtesy of Dr M.G. Brook.)

Borreliosis is most common following occupational or leisure exposure to open forest or parkland, where ticks inhabit the vegetation. The presence of large animals such as deer seems to increase the likelihood of infection. Transmission has been recorded in the New Forest, the deer parks of London and South-east UK, and in parts of Scotland. Imported cases may originate in European countries such as Germany or Austria, in Scandinavian countries and in eastern and central areas of the USA.

Borrelial lymphocytoma

Borrelial lymphocytoma is a rarer skin manifestation which can occur at the same time as ECM, after it, or occasionally in late Lyme disease. Although it may occur at or near the site of the original tick bite, it has a predilection for the ear (especially in children) or the breast. It is usually a dusky nodule or plaque which may last for several months if untreated, and reaches 1–5 cm diameter. Not all patients have associated constitutional symptoms. Histology is not specific for borreliosis; it shows lymphocytic infiltration with germinal centres, and must be differentiated from other granulomatous disorders and lymphomata.

Later or secondary manifestations

The most common of these are arthritis, neurological disorders and cardiac abnormalities. They can follow the original infection after an interval varying from 2 or 3 weeks to 2 or 3 months.

Lyme arthritis

Lyme arthritis is particularly common in the USA, affecting about half of all patients whose early infection is untreated. Its onset varies from a few days to 2 years after exposure. It is usually an asymmetrical large joint arthritis, but is occasionally palindromic. There is synovitis and often moderate effusion of affected joints. The effusion has a high protein level and contains a polymorph pleiocytosis. This, with an accompanying high erythrocyte sedimentation rate, makes it easy to interpret the illness as seronegative rheumatoid arthritis. Untreated, the arthritis tends to occur in repeated episodes, ocurring progressively less frequently over 2–4 years. Very few patients have permanent or erosive joint disease.

About 1 in 10 untreated patients develop intermittent arthralgias and periarticular pain without objective synovitis or effusion. In some cases these symptoms persist for 5 years or more.

Relapsing lymphocytic meningitis

Relapsing lymphocytic meningitis was recognized long before Lyme disease. It is now known that a significant proportion of these cases are caused by neuroborreliosis.

Peripheral neuropathies

Peripheral neuropathies are common in many types of Lyme disease, and may accompany other manifestations. Facial paralysis is one of the most common neuropathies, but others, including unilateral phrenic nerve palsy, have been described. They tend to resolve spontaneously over a period of weeks.

Polyradiculitis

Polyradiculitis is a disabling and progressive feature of Lyme disease. It appears to be more common in European types of infection. It presents as localized pain in the affected roots, with dysfunction of the associated

nerves. A typical presentation would be low back or sacral pain with a weak knee or foot drop. Paraesthesiae, loss of sensation and absent reflexes are common physical findings.

The radiculitis is often accompanied by meningism and a pleiocytosis in the cerebrospinal fluid (CSF). Although lymphocytes predominate, occasional plasma cells are also seen, and the CSF glucose level may be slightly lowered. The syndrome of relapsing CSF pleiocytosis with nerve root symptoms was described before the aetiology was understood, and was called Bannwarth's syndrome.

Cardiological effects

The cardiological effects are a result of myocarditis. This is often evidenced by conduction defects. Complete heart block is not unusual (Fig. 20.3). Prolonged and progressive cardiomyopathy has been described in occasional cases.

Late chronic Lyme disease

This has been described as a peripheral neuropathy of the glove-and-stocking type, associating with a typical violaceous inflammation of the skin called atrophic acrodermatitis. Histology of affected skin shows a lymphocytic infiltrate, often with many plasma cells. The acrodermatitis is asymmetrical, most commonly affecting a foot or heel, sometimes the elbow or hand. After months or years without treatment the lesions change from oedematous to thin and atrophic. Even though this syndrome may have existed for months or years, together with malaise and mild depression, it is amenable to treatment.

Clinical manifestations of borreliosis
Early
Flu-like illness.
Erythema chronicum migrans.
Borrelial lymphocytoma.

Secondary
Arthritis.
Myocarditis.
Neuropathies.
Relapsing lymphocytic meningitis.
Polyradiculitis.

Late
Peripheral neuropathy.
Atrophic acrodermatitis (acrodermatitis chronica atrophica).

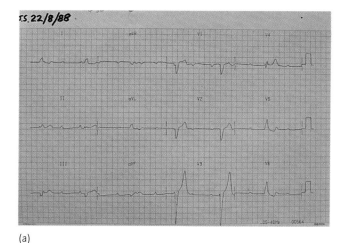

(a)

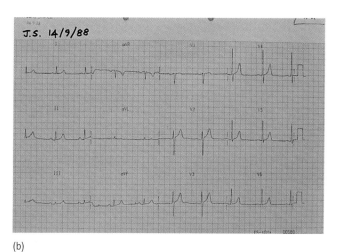

(b)

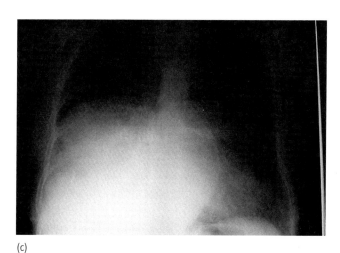

(c)

Fig. 20.3 (a) Electrocardiogram (ECG) showing a complete heart block in a young patient with secondary Lyme disease. (b) The second ECG after treatment shows that conduction is normal. (c) The same patient had a transient phrenic nerve palsy, with raised right diaphragm.

Diagnosis

Many features of Lyme disease are non-specific. Without appropriate suspicion, and unless a history of tick exposure or bite in endemic areas is elicited, the diagnosis may be overlooked.

In specialist laboratories, *B. burgdorferi* can be cultured from active skin lesions. There is also evidence on polymerase chain reaction of *Borrelia* spp. in the synovium and CSF, as well as bacteraemia in the early stages of the infection during the skin rash.

IgM antibodies can be demonstrated by ELISA tests during early infection. These use flagellar antigens to demonstrate the presence of borrelial antibodies. They persist in the blood for a variable time, but have often been replaced by exclusively IgG antibodies by the time secondary features appear.

Although serological tests are evolving as the infecting organism is better understood, and confirmatory Western blot tests are possible, there is a significant prevalence of false-positive IgG antibody tests, probably due to cross-reaction with other spirochaetal antibodies. Isolated positive IgG tests should therefore be interpreted with great caution, unless accompanied by appropriate symptoms and physical signs.

When there are neurological features, locally produced antibodies can be demonstrated in the CSF, and this is useful evidence of infection. Blood antibodies may not become detectable if treatment is given very early.

Treatment

There is still some doubt as to the best approach to treatment.

Early infections

For early infections tetracycline is the most reliable antibiotic, usually given in a 3-week course. This is usually curative if given at the stage of ECM.

Later infections

For later infections more intensive and prolonged treatment is necessary, as relapse commonly follows short courses of tetracycline. Cefotaxime and ceftriaxone have both been used successfully in neuroborreliosis, but in half or more of patients symptoms persist after a 2- or 3-week course. Even longer courses are not always followed by cure, and it is worth giving oral tetracycline, doxycycline, or ampicillin plus probenecid to give a total of 8–12 weeks' antibiotic treatment. Longer continuation courses may have some benefit in late disease.

Penicillin is effective initially, and may be curative in early infections, but carries a risk of recrudescence and relapse if used in secondary or late disease. Erythromycin is less effective than tetracyclines.

Treatment of borreliosis

1 (a) Early: doxycycline orally 200 mg, then 100 mg daily for 20 days more.

(b) Alternative, or for child: ampicillin orally, 500 mg 6-hourly (child under 10 years, 250 mg 6-hourly) *or* amoxycillin orally 500 mg 8-hourly (child under 10 years, 250 mg 8-hourly) for 3 weeks.

(c) Second choice: erythromycin orally, 500 mg 6-hourly (child up to 2 years, 125 mg 6-hourly; 2–8 years, 250 mg 6-hourly) for 3 weeks.

2 Secondary or late: cefotaxime i.v., 1–2 g 8-hourly *or* ceftriaxone i.v., 1–2 g daily, both for 2–4 weeks *followed by* doxycycline orally, 100 mg daily *or* ampicillin 250 mg 6-hourly *plus* probenecid 500 mg twice daily (child under 10 years, half adult dose) for 4–8 weeks.

Toxoplasmosis

Introduction and epidemiology

Toxoplasmosis is the infection caused by *Toxoplasma gondii*. This is a protozoan parasite of the family Sporozoa. It is found in the tissues of almost all warm-blooded creatures, but the only hosts for its definitive life cycle are the cat family. Cats are infected by predation on other infected creatures, or by consumption of oocysts derived from the faeces of recently infected cats.

The oocysts develop in the cat's intestine, and release parasites which enter the blood stream and the tissues. These replicate rapidly by fission, and are called tachyzoites. Parasites within tissues tend to form pseudocysts by replicating to form a mass of many organisms within an expanded cell. The organisms then become quiescent, and are called bradyzoites. Meanwhile some parasites enter the enterocytes and develop into oocysts, which are eventually shed in the faeces. Shedding of oocysts begins about 10 days after infection and persists for 2–3 weeks.

Infection can result from ingestion of tachyzoites, bradyzoites or oocysts. Humans may be infected by contact with cat faeces, particularly those of kittens, who become infected as they begin to predate. However, contact with uncooked or lightly cooked meat is also a major route of infection. Bradyzoites can be demonstrated in many types of butcher's meat, and in meats such as pork, which are preserved and eaten without cooking in many countries. Toxoplasmosis can be transmitted by living tissue, and has occurred when a transplanted heart has contained bradyzoites. Of course, the recipient is immunosuppressed by antirejection medication, and this may modify the presentation of the disease, as will the previous level of immunity against toxoplasmosis.

In the UK the peak age for seroconversion to toxoplasmosis is 15–35 years, and about half of all middle-aged people have evidence of past infection. Very few immunocompetent individuals have a recognizable illness. The importance of the disease lies in its ability to cause transplacental infection with damaging consequences (see Chapter 12). It is also an important opportunistic infection in acquired immunodeficiency syndrome (AIDS) sufferers (see Chapter 21).

Clinical features

Patients who recognize an illness associated with toxoplasmosis (Fig. 20.4) tend to present in one of three ways:

1 A mononucleosis syndrome is common in young adults. The features are fever, malaise, and one or more enlarged lymph nodes. There is an atypical mononucleosis in the peripheral blood but the heterophil antibody test is negative. The illness is self-limiting, with a duration of 2–5 weeks.

2 Patients may present with a single, persistently enlarged lymph node, or occasionally a skin or soft-tissue nodule. The differential diagnosis of lymphadenitis is large, and such lesions often come to excision biopsy because of the need to exclude tuberculosis, sarcoidosis or lymphoma.

3 Acute choroidoretinitis is a feature of late-stage toxoplasmosis. Although there may have been a feverish illness some weeks or months before the onset of eye symptoms, such a history is rarely elicited.

Rare manifestations include myocarditis, encephalitis, encephalomyelitis and pneumonitis. All of these are much more common in the immunosuppressed.

Diagnosis

This is based on serological tests and on histology of the affected tissue.

Several serological tests are useful in the diagnosis of toxoplasmosis. A latex agglutination test is widely used by laboratories for screening sera. Titres rise rapidly during acute disease, and fall slowly over 18–24 months to reach background seropositivity. Titres of 1 : 4000 to 1 : 64 000 are easily reached in the acute stages of disease.

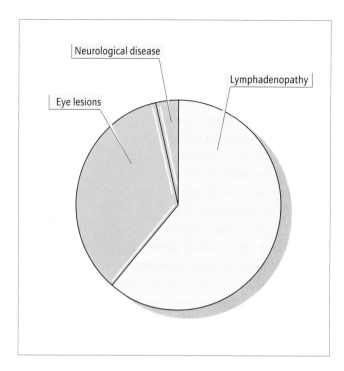

Fig. 20.4 Pie chart of the clinical features reported in cases of toxoplasmosis in England and Wales 1989–1992.

Confirmatory tests carried out in reference laboratories include IgM ELISA tests, the *Toxoplasma* dye test (which uses live trophozoites to measure antibody-mediated inhibition of intravital dye uptake), a complement fixation test and a haemagglutination test. The dye test is the gold standard against which other tests are compared.

The *Toxoplasma* dye test rises and falls in parallel with the latex agglutination test, but is less prone to false-positive results. The complement fixation test has a similar time course. Dye-test antibody titres may reach 1 : 32 000 to 1 : 64 000 in acute disease.

A positive IgM test is evidence of recent infection. IgM antibodies persist for 6 months or more, possibly suggesting that the initial infection subsides only slowly, as bradyzoite cysts form and are maintained inactive by immune reaction. In a few patients IgM antibodies persist for more than 1 year. This is a problem for women who wish to conceive although, if the dye test and latex agglutination titres are falling after 1 year, the risk of parasitaemia and transplacental infection are almost certainly negligible.

Late toxoplasmosis: eye disease

Choroidoretinitis is a late manifestation of toxoplasmosis, and occurs when acute antibody titres have fallen

considerably. Dye test and latex agglutination titres of 1 : 256 to 1 : 512 (dye test) or 1 : 128 (latex agglutination) are not uncommon. The haemagglutination test, however, has a slower response to acute infection, and may show significantly elevated titres at the time that eye disease occurs.

Histological diagnosis

This is the means by which *Toxoplasma* lymphadenitis is often diagnosed. The histological picture is strongly suggestive of toxoplasmosis.

Giemsa-stained tissue smears, myocardial biopsy or brain biopsy preparations can occasionally be shown to contain cysts or typical crescent-shaped trophozoites.

Culture

Culture of CSF may be helpful in acute brain infection. This is a specialist procedure, and must usually be pre-arranged with a reference laboratory. Positive cultures can also be obtained from infected placenta, products of conception, CSF and brain in congenital infection.

Diagnosis of toxoplasmosis
1 Serological tests: immunoglobulin M enzyme-linked immunosorbent assay, latex agglutination, complement fixation testing (and haemagglutination test in later eye disease).
2 Histological appearance of biopsied nodes.
3 Giemsa-stained tissue specimens.
4 Culture of cerebrospinal fluid or affected tissue (rarely performed).

Treatment

Toxoplasmosis is a self-limiting disease in most cases, and is often diagnosed relatively late in the acute stage. The risks of treatment must therefore be balanced against the likely benefit. However, treatment is always justified in myocardial or central nervous system disease.

The treatment of choice is a combination of sulphonamide and pyrimethamine. Sulphadimidine is the best choice of sulphonamide available in the UK. The doses should not be less than 1 g 6-hourly. Sulphadiazine may be superior in penetrating the tissues, if it can be obtained. Pyrimethamine is given in a dose of 50 mg daily. Both of these drugs are folate inhibitors, and in the high dose given can cause a significant fall in the white cell count. The blood count should be closely monitored during treatment, which must often be continued for 4 weeks or more.

Sulphonamides are contraindicated in pregnancy. The treatment of choice is then spiramycin. This is not available in the UK, and must therefore be purchased for the individual patient (see Chapter 12).

Plague

Introduction

Plague, caused by *Yersinia pestis*, is naturally a disease of rodents, and exists in many rural and wooded areas throughout the world. Urban foci of transmission also exist, where feral animals, humans and rats share the environment (Fig. 20.5). Human cases tend to result from close association between humans and rats. Plague is transmitted from rat to rat by the rat flea, whose pharynx becomes blocked by oedema and replicating bacteria. When the diseased flea bites, bacteria are regurgitated through its mouthparts, inoculating a large infective dose into its host. As rats die and the fleas run out of their preferred hosts, humans are increasingly bitten, and sporadic or epidemic human cases of plague occur.

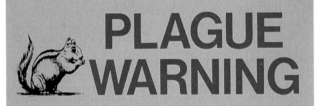

PLAGUE WARNING

Chipmunks, ground squirrels, or other wild rodents in this area may be infected with plague. Plague can be transmitted to humans by the bite of an infected flea or by handling an infected animal.

USE THESE PRECAUTIONS:

1. See a physician if you become ill within 7 days of your visit to this area. Early symptoms include: Malaise (feeling of illness), high fever headache, muscle aches, nausea, and often swollen painful lymph glands. Inform the physician about your travels. THE DISEASE IS CURABLE WHEN DIAGNOSED EARLY.

2. Protect pets with flea powder or flea collars. Keep pets confined or on a leash. It is better to LEAVE PETS HOME.

3. AVOID ANIMAL FLEAS. Do not camp, rest, or sleep near animal burrows. Insect repellent sprayed on socks and trouser cuffs may help.

4. Avoid all contact with chipmunks, squirrels, or other wild animals. DO NOT FEED.

5. DO NOT TOUCH sick or dead animals.
          REPORT THEM to:

Distributed by
California Dept. of Health Services
Vector Biology and Control Section
714 P Street, Sacramento, CA 95814
(916) 445-0498 Rev. 4/80

Fig. 20.5 Plague hazard warning in an urban setting.

Clinical considerations

The incubation period is usually 2–4 days, but can be up to 12 days. The onset of disease is abrupt, with fever, prostration and rigors. Plague is a toxaemic as well as a local disease. Its characteristic clinical features are enlarged, suppurating regional lymph nodes (buboes) and haemorrhagic manifestations.

Buboes

The buboes affect the nodes which drain the flea-bitten area, though the flea bites are rarely apparent. Inguinal nodes are more often affected than others. The mass of enlarged nodes is surrounded by boggy, often haemorrhagic oedema, and in untreated cases will often point and discharge pus after a week or two.

Skin and mucous membranes

The skin and mucous membranes are often affected by petechial and ecchymotic lesions. In bacteraemic plague, an intense haemorrhagic rash may quickly appear.

Pneumonitis

Pneumonitis is a less common feature, but is often rapidly fatal. Extensive lung involvement and respiratory failure can develop in 24–36 h. Patients with pneumonitis are highly infectious, and readily infect numbers of family members and health care workers.

Diagnosis

Diagnosis may be suspected on clinical and epidemiological grounds. Gram-stained smears of lymph-node aspirate, pus or infected sputum often show numerous small, Gram-negative rods with characteristic bipolar staining. The organism grows readily in standard cultures and blood culture media.

Treatment

Treatment with broad-spectrum antibiotics is usually highly effective, though it must be begun promptly, as the disease evolves quickly. Chloramphenicol, tetracycline and aminoglycosides are all effective drugs. Quinolones also have a high level of activity against *Y. pestis*. Doxycycline is effective prophylaxis for those exposed to cases of plague pneumonitis.

Tularaemia

Introduction

This is a disease of rodents and birds caused by *Francisella tularensis*. It is transmitted to humans by inoculation, either by bite or scratch, or by injuries acquired when handling or skinning carcasses. Ticks may also transmit tularemia. It is usually a sporadic disease affecting hunters, trappers and tourists.

Cutaneous-lymphatic presentation

A cutaneous-lymphatic presentation is common. A nodular or suppurative lesion develops at the inoculation site, with extension up the lymphatic channels and enlargement of draining lymph nodes. The lymph-node enlargement is considerable, and often very tender and painful. Occasionally the primary lesion takes the form of a painful conjunctival ulcer.

The lymph-node pathology can exist without a detectable skin lesion.

Typhoidal presentation

A typhoidal presentation is a feature of bacteraemic disease. The patient presents with persisting high fever, but without any local features. The severity of the illness varies from inconvenient fever to prostrating and debilitating disease. Some typhoidal cases develop a widespread pneumonitis which can lead to respiratory failure. Splenomegaly and a transient rash are sometimes seen.

Diagnosis

Diagnosis depends on suspicion, and differentiation from brucellosis and typhoid fever. Blood cultures are rarely positive, but organisms can be cultured from skin lesions and lymph-node aspirate or biopsy specimens. Sputum may also be positive in cases of pneumonitis.

Serological tests are available at reference laboratory level. False-positives and cross-reactions occur, so that interpretation of results must be discriminating.

Treatment

Treatment is always warranted, as there is a mortality of 5–8% in systemic cases. Aminoglycosides are the treatment of choice, producing a rapid response in lung and systemic disease. The skin and lymph-node lesions often continue to evolve, and heal more slowly, even when treated with antibiotics. Tetracycline or chloramphenicol will produce improvement, but relapse often follows treatment with these drugs. Experience with new drugs, such as quinolones, is limited.

Rat bite fever (Haverhill fever)

Introduction

Two organisms may be transmitted by the bites of rats — *Streptobacillus moniliformis*, with an incubation period of 7–10 days, and *Spirillum minus*, with an incubation period of 1–4 weeks. *Streptobacillus moniliformis*, the cause of Haverhill fever, can also be transmitted by contaminated food or milk; indeed quite large milk-borne outbreaks have been described.

Both pathogens cause fever and peripheral rash. The fever tends to be relapsing when caused by *Spirillum minus* and swinging when caused by *Streptobacillus moniliformis*. The rash is variable, sometimes papular, sometimes petechial and occasionally containing small pustules. Arthritis is also common in *S. moniliformis* infections. Both types of infection are rare causes of pyrexia of unknown origin with a rash. They are both usually accompanied by significant neutrophilia. The liver function tests may be slightly abnormal, and prolonged prothrombin times can be demonstrable.

S. moniliformis is a rare cause of endocarditis.

Diagnosis

Diagnosis depends largely on cultures of pus, joint fluid and blood. *S. moniliformis* can be fastidious, but in appropriate culture media produces tangled chains of Gram-negative bacteria. *Spirillum minus* does not grow well in artificial media.

Treatment

Treatment with parenteral benzylpenicillin is effective against both organisms. A course of 1.2 g 6-hourly for 7–10 days is usually sufficient. Streptobacillary endocarditis requires 4–6 weeks' treatment.

Zoonotic streptococcal infections

Introduction

Some animals are colonized and may become infected by pyogenic streptococci which rarely affect humans. Two well-recognized examples of this are *Streptococcus suis*, of pigs, and *S. zooepidemicus*, which can affect horses.

Streptococcus suis

S. suis has an epidemiology in pigs similar to that of the meningococcus in humans. The organism is carried in the nasopharynx, particularly of piglets. When subjected to crowding, or the stress of transport, these young animals may develop clinical meningitis. Humans are infected through close contact, usually with pig carcasses, and tend to develop meningitis with bacteraemia.

Gram-positive cocci may be seen in the CSF of human cases. A beta-haemolytic *Streptococcus* is demonstrated on culture, but is not group A (C or G), as expected. Most *S. suis* are of Lancefield group R or S. Treatment with benzylpenicillin, with or without an aminoglycoside, is appropriate. A course of 10–14 days is usually required.

Streptococcus zooepidemicus

S. zooepidemicus causes bacteraemic or soft-tissue infections, usually in people who have close contact with horses. It appears in culture as a beta-haemolytic *Streptococcus* of Lancefield group C. It may have reduced sensitivity to benzylpenicillin, requiring the addition of an aminoglycoside for optimum therapy.

Herpesvirus simiae infection

Herpesvirus simiae inhabits the mouth and mucocutaneous borders in monkey species, in a similar way to which herpes simplex virus affects humans. It causes cold-sore lesions in a proportion of affected animals. Monkey handlers can become infected if the animal's saliva is inoculated via a bite or scratch.

Human infections may be local, producing herpetic vesicles, but there is a severe risk of potentially fatal viral encephalitis. Treatment with aciclovir is effective in suppressing the skin lesions, but relapse often follows cessation of therapy. Affected individuals therefore often require long-term aciclovir treatment.

The nature of a herpetic lesion in a monkey handler can be confirmed by isolation and characterization of the virus from vesicle or skin scrapings. H. simiae is a dangerous virus for which there is no reliable treatment or prophylaxis. Diagnostic culture is therefore carried out in reference laboratories such as the Virus Reference Division of the Central Public Health Laboratory in London, or the Centers for Disease Control in Atlanta, Georgia, USA, where suitable containment facilities exist.

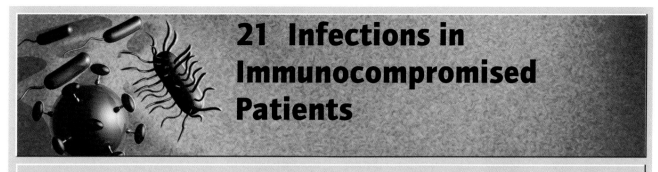

21 Infections in Immunocompromised Patients

Introduction

Earlier chapters have described how organisms can overcome host defences and cause infection. This chapter discusses the infections which occur when host defences are reduced by disease, treatment or inherited disorders.

Each or all of the components of the immune system can be compromised. Various patterns and degrees of immune compromise result in different patterns of infection as different opportunities are opened to invading organisms. Many agents implicated in infections of immunocompromised patients are of low intrinsic virulence. In a normal subject, they might be disregarded as they form part of the bacterial flora, or are incapable of causing primary infection. This makes the interpretation of microbiological culture results more difficult than in non-compromised patients. Nevertheless, pathogens which affect non-compromised patients will also infect the immunocompromised, often causing severe or persisting disease. The lack of immune response may modify the clinical picture, so that typical clinical features are lacking (for instance, the typical rash in varicella or measles). This further increases the difficulty of making a prompt diagnosis.

Classification of infections in immunocompromised patients

Immunodeficiencies are conventionally classified into primary/congenital immunodeficiency (including defects in B cells, T cells, complement and phagocytes) and secondary or acquired immunodeficiency resulting from malignancy or immunosuppressive therapy.

Immune deficiencies can also be conveniently classified into seven groups:
1 Disorders of the innate immune system.
2 Neutropenia and neutrophil dysfunction, e.g. congenital granulomatous disease (CGD).
3 T-cell deficit.
4 Hypogammaglobulinaemia.
5 Complement deficiencies.
6 Splenectomy.
7 Broad-spectrum immunodeficiency related to haematological or other malignancy, intensive chemotherapy or after transplants.

The description here looks at the consequences of deficiency in each of the components of the immune system. This is a simplification, as the patient's immunodeficiency is rarely single and deficiency in one component of the system leads to imbalance and failure of other components (for example, T cells are the main component of cell-mediated immunity, but T-cell help is also essential for the optimal activity of the humoral response).

Disorders of innate immunity are often found in hospital practice, when, for example, treatment breaches the physical barriers to microbial invasion (see Chapter 23). Infections associated with acquired immuno-deficiency syndrome (AIDS) are discussed in Chapter 11. The other immunodeficiencies and the common infections associated with them are summarized in Table 21.1.

With the exception of some congenital abnormalities, immune deficits are rarely single. Patients undergoing chemotherapy for leukaemia or bone marrow transplantation are primarily neutropenic, but also have impaired cell-mediated immunity, predisposing, for example, to cytomegalovirus (CMV) infection. Treatment involves the use of many skin-piercing cannulae, predisposing to *Staphylococcus epidermidis* and other skin-derived infections. Fungal infections are also common in these patients, facilitated by the combination of neutropenia and decreased cell-mediated immunity. Although AIDS primarily causes T-cell dysfunction,

patients show evidence of deficient humoral immunity and susceptibility to pyogenic infection because of a lack of T-cell help for B-cell function.

Neutropenia

This can be an adverse reaction to treatment with a number of drugs, but also accompanies acute leukaemia or its treatment. The risk of infection increases significantly once the neutrophil count falls below $0.5 \times 10^9/l$, and is proportional to the period of neutropenia. More than half of all patients suffering an episode of neutropenia will develop an infection. The mortality from these infections is high if not promptly treated.

Epidemiology

The epidemiology of infection in neutropenic patients is complex. Not only are patients and their underlying diseases diverse, but treatment protocols are constantly evolving and this results in a changing pattern of infec-

Immune deficit	Caused by	Bacterial infections	Other infections
Complement	Congenital	*Neisseria* spp. *Streptococcus pneumoniae*	
Spleen	Surgery, trauma, sickle-cell anaemia (functional)	*S. pneumoniae* *Haemophilus influenzae* (type b)	*Plasmodium* spp *Babesia* spp.
Gamma-globulin	Congenital, multiple myeloma, CLL, AIDS	*S. pneumoniae* *H. influenzae* (non-capsulate)	*Pneumocystis carinii* *Giardia intestinalis* *Cryptosporidium parvum*
Neutrophils	Chemotherapy of leukaemia and bone marrow transplantation dysfunction, e.g. CGD	Enterobacteriaceae Oral streptococci *Pseudomonas aeruginosa* *Enterococcus* spp.	*Candida* spp. *Aspergillus* spp.
T cells	Marrow and other transplantation, AIDS, cancer chemotherapy, lymphoma, steroids	*Listeria monocytogenes* *Mycobacterium tuberculosis* *M. avium-intracellulare* *Salmonella* spp. *Rhodococcus equi*	*P. carinii* *Toxoplasma gondii* *Cryptosporidium parvum* *Leishmania* spp. Herpesvirus spp. CMV Varicella-zoster virus *Cryptococcus neoformans* *Histoplasma* spp. and other systemic yeast infections

AIDS, acquired immunodeficiency syndrome; CGD, congenital granulomatous disease; CLL, chronic lymphocytic leukaemia; CMV, cytomegalovirus.

Table 21.1 Common deficits in immune function and the infections with which they are associated.

tion, both between patients and at different stages of treatment in the same patient.

Bacterial infections

Bacteraemia occurs in 20–30% of neutropenic patients. The principal bacteria implicated in these patients are Gram-negative rods, but Gram-positive cocci are also important. The frequency with which these organisms cause infection changes with developments in treatment and antimicrobial prophylaxis.

Enterobacteriaceae and *Pseudomonas* spp. are the most commonly isolated Gram-negative rods. They are usually derived from the patient's own intestinal flora, gaining access to the circulation when the rapidly multiplying intestinal epithelium is damaged by antineoplastic agents or X-irradiation. The introduction of antimicrobial prophylaxis and improvements in drug treatment of these pathogens have reduced both the incidence and mortality associated with them.

Hospital patients are susceptible to colonization with resistant organisms because of both the administration of antibiotics and the effects of serious underlying disease. Hospital organisms may be transmitted on the hands of medical and nursing attendants or ingested in food, notably washed vegetables.

Although Enterobacteriaceae and *P. aeruginosa* remain the commonest Gram-negative bacilli isolated, the prophylactic use of broad-spectrum 4-fluoroquinolones has diminished the incidence of these infections. A decreasing incidence of *Klebsiella* spp., *Serratia* spp. and *Enterobacter* spp. has been noted in many centres.

In recent years, infections with Gram-positive organisms have become more common in neutropenic patients, rising from around 30% of bacterial infections in the mid-1960s to 60% in the mid-1990s. In most centres, the main organisms reported are *Staphylococcus epidermidis*, the oral streptococci *Streptococcus mitis* and *S. oralis*, *Enterococcus* spp., *Staphylococcus aureus* and *Corynebacterium jeikeium*. The almost universal use of long-term intravascular access devices such as Hickmann and Portacath catheters favours infection with organisms derived from the skin. Infection with oral streptococci may be favoured by severe mucositis secondary to chemotherapy. Although uncommon, enterococcal infection is increasing because of the use of 4-fluoroquinolones for prophylaxis and cephalosporins for treatment of fevers. Methicillin-resistant *S. aureus* (MRSA) strains are an increasing problem in hospitals where these organisms have established themselves.

Bacteria associated with infections in neutropenia
1 Enterobacteriaceae (*Klebsiella*, *Serratia* and *Enterobacter* spp.).
2 Skin-derived organisms: *Staphylococcus epidermidis*, *S. aureus*, including methicillin-resistant *S. aureus* and corynebacteria, including *Corynebacterium jeikeium*.
3 Other streptococci including oral streptococci and enterococci.
4 *Pseudomonas* spp.
5 *Bacillus cereus*.
6 Coagulase-negative staphylococci.

Fungal infections

Patients with prolonged neutropenia are at risk of invasive fungal infection. The frequent use of potent antibacterials encourages colonization by *Candida albicans*, the most commonly isolated organism. More recently, there has been an increase in infection with yeasts such as *C. krusei*, which are naturally resistant to antifungal prophylaxis. Infections with *Torulopsis glabrata* and *C. parapsilosis* have been associated with intravenous cannulae.

Aspergillus spp. are the most common filamentous fungi causing invasive disease, although infections with *Fusarium* spp. and *Pseudoallerchia boydii* have rarely been reported. *Aspergillus fumigatus* is the most commonly isolated species, but *A. flavus* is increasing and *A. niger* is also reported. Infection is aquired by inhalation. *Aspergillus* spores are normally present in the air, and more are released during building work. They pose a grave threat to severely neutropenic patients.

Fungi associated with infections in neutropenia
1 *Candida albicans*.
2 *Candida parapsilosis*.
3 *Candida krusei*.
4 *Torulopsis glabrata*.
5 *Aspergillus fumigatus*.
6 Other *Aspergillus* spp.

Prevention of infection during neutropenia

Protective isolation (see Chapter 23) is intended to reduce the risk of infection in neutropenic patients. The patient is nursed in a side room, and is given sterile water and low-microorganism-content food. Attendant staff should observe hand-washing routines and may use sterile gloves when working with patients. *Aspergillus* infection can be reduced if the air entering the patient's room has been high efficiency particulate air

(HEPA)-filtered. This regimen is designed to prevent the replacement of the normal flora with potential pathogens or resistant organisms.

As the major infecting agents in neutropenic patients come from their own indigenous flora, various suppressive antimicrobial regimens have been used to prevent infection. Non-absorbable antibiotics have been given orally to reduce the numbers of bacteria in the bowel. A combination of framycetin (later replaced with neomycin), colistin and nystatin (fracon), or of gentamicin, vancomycin and nystatin have both been used. The efficacy of these regimens has never been clearly established, but they do appear to select for aminoglycoside-resistant organisms, notably strains of *Klebsiella* spp.

Current antimicrobial prophylaxis is based on the concept of colonization resistance, which suggests that the obligate anaerobic flora prevent colonization by facultative Gram-negative organisms, by competing for intestinal attachment sites and nutrients, and by production of bacteriocins and toxic free fatty acids. Antibiotics should therefore be targeted to facultative organisms, sparing the protective obligate anaerobic flora. Co-trimoxazole prophylaxis had some success, but patients still became colonized with resistant organisms. This has been prevented by the addition of colistin to the regimen. Side-effects such as skin rashes and neutropenia are common.

The introduction of 4-fluoroquinolone prophylaxis has proved to be a major advance. Norfloxacin, ofloxacin and ciprofloxacin have been employed for this purpose. Quinolone prophylaxis is usually combined with agents active against fungi (see below). Such regimens are superior to neomycin–colistin and co-trimoxazole–colistin, both in preventing infection with Gram-negative bacilli and in selection of resistant organisms. Ofloxacin and ciprofloxacin may be more effective than norfloxacin, which is less well-absorbed. This suggests that these agents have a role both in suppressing Gram-negative bacilli in the gut and in inhibiting the early stages of infection. Although effective against Gram-negative bacilli, the quinolones are less active against Gram-positive infections, which are currently increasing.

Antifungal prophylaxis

Oral nystatin alone or in combination with oral amphotericin B is a useful non-absorbed prophylaxis, as it reduces fungal colonization of the mouth and gut. More recently, fluconazole, which is well-absorbed orally, has been successful in preventing yeast infections, but it has no useful activity against *Aspergillus* spp. and some yeasts such as *C. krusei* and *T. glabrata*. Itraconazole has useful activity against *Aspergillus* spp. but its bioavailability is unpredictable in neutropenic patients.

Prevention of infection in neutropenic patients
1 Protective isolation.
2 Ward hygiene, including steam-pressed linen (to kill spores).
3 Filtered air supplies.
4 Suppressive antimicrobial regimens.
5 Antifungal prophylaxis.

Treatment of fever in neutropenic patients

Fever in neutropenic patients is assumed to indicate infection unless proved otherwise. Untreated bacterial infections progress rapidly; more than half of patients with *Pseudomonas* bacteraemia will die within 24 h unless appropriate treatment is prescribed.

Many trials of empirical therapy have been performed in search of a best treatment. Consideration of local organisms and their resistance pattern is important. Aminoglycosides alone are inadequate therapy in neutropenic patients and are therefore usually combined with a beta-lactam antibiotic. The importance of *Pseudomonas* as a pathogen means that the regimen should have optimal activity against this agent. A ureidopenicillin, such as azlocillin or piperacillin, plus amikacin, has obtained response rates above 60% —greater if Gram negative bacteria were isolated. A combination of ceftazidime and amikacin has also been effective in clinical trials, and continuing aminoglycoside therapy for 7 rather than 3 days was shown to be superior.

In this environment of empirical, broad-spectrum treatment, several organisms are major opportunistic pathogens because of their innate resistance to many antimicrobials. These include MRSA, *S. aureus*, *Stenotrophomonas maltophilia* and *Enterococcus faecium*. The emergence of the latter has been favoured by the use of quinolones for prophylaxis, and third-generation cephalosporins for treatment, as both agents have poor activity against enterococci.

Some isolates of enterococci are now resistant to glycopeptide antibiotics (vancomycin and teicoplanin). *Corynebacterium jeikeium* is naturally resistant to many antibiotics, usually excluding vancomycin. This, and the increasing incidence of MRSA, *Staphylococcus epidermidis* and oral streptococci, means that many empirical regimens for febrile neutropenic patients now include vancomycin. When aminoglycosides and glycopeptides must be used in combination, extra care should be given to monitoring renal function and antibiotic serum levels, as their nephrotoxicity can be additive and both are renally excreted.

Treatment of fever in neutropenic patients
1 For *Pseudomonas* and/or enterococcal infection:
azlocillin by i.v. infusion, 2–5 g 8-hourly; *or*
Piperacillin by i.v. infusion 150–300 mg/kg daily; *or*
Cefotaxime i.v. 2–4 g 8-hourly; *or*
Ceftazidime i.v. 2 g 8–12 hourly; *plus*
Amikacin by slow i.v injection or infusion, 7.5 mg/kg
   12-hourly (peak concentrations 1 h after injection
   should be below 30 mg/l, trough below 10 mg/l).
2 For Gram-positive infection, especially aminoglycoside-resistant enterococci and methicillin-resistant
Staphylococcus aureus: vancomycin by slow i.v. infusion
(at least 90 min), 500 mg 6-hourly (peak levels after 1 h
should be below 30 mg/l, trough below 10 mg/l); *or*
Teicoplanin by i.v. injection or infusion, 400 mg
   12-hourly for three doses, then 400 mg daily.

The outcome of therapy is related to the degree and duration of neutropenia. The cytokines GM-CSF (granulocyte–monocyte colony-stimulating factor) and G-CSF can be used to stimulate neutrophil production. This significantly shortens the period of neutropenia, reducing the number of infections and the days of fever.

Patients with chronic granulomatous disease are treated with interferon, which restores the defect in granulocyte function.

T-cell deficiency

T-cell deficiency is increasingly common, with increasing use of corticosteroids, cyclosporin and other immunosuppressive agents in the chemotherapy of malignancies, and in transplantation medicine. The human immunodeficiency virus (HIV) epidemic has also contributed. Congenital T-cell deficiencies are rare and often associated with T-cell dysfunction or combined with a hypogammaglobulinaemia.

Opportunistic pathogens in T-cell deficiencies

These are mainly microorganisms which, in the human host, have an intracellular location.

Bacterial infections

The principal bacteria associated with T-cell deficiency are mycobacteria, including *Mycobacterium tuberculosis*, *M. kansasii*, *M. avium-intracellulare* and *M. chelonei*. *M. tuberculosis* and *M. kansasii* are primarily respiratory pathogens, and often cause typical granulomatous lung disease but in severe T-cell deficiency they can cause dis-

seminated or miliary disease. *M. avium-intracellulare* is acquired by the gastrointestinal or respiratory route, and may cause bowel infection, lung infection or disseminated disease. *M. chelonei* is often acquired by inoculation and then causes local abscesses, but it has also been found to cause bacteraemia and fever of unknown origin. *Listeria monocytogenes* is an important cause of meningitis, and occasionally of peritonitis or bacteraemia. Often the only clue to the listerial aetiology is a history of immunosuppression.

Treatment of mycobacterial infections in T-cell deficiency
1 *Mycobacterium tuberculosis* and *M. kansasii*: treat as routine with triple or quadruple therapy, guided by antibiotic sensitivity testing (see Chapter 18).
2 *M. avium-intercellulare*: useful drugs include rifabutin orally, 450–600 mg/kg daily, ethambutol orally, 15 mg/kg daily, clarithromycin orally, 250–500 mg 12-hourly for 2–4 weeks, then 250 mg 12-hourly, and amikacin i.m. or i.v. 7.5 mg/kg 12-hourly.
3 *M. chelonei*: co-trimoxazole 960 mg 12-hourly, reducing to 480 mg 12-hourly after 2–4 weeks.

Fungal infections

In contrast to neutropenia, superficial fungal infections are uncommon in patients with deficient T-cell function, but deep-seated or disseminated infection can be caused by organisms such as *Histoplasma capsulatum*. Cryptococcal infections, although increasing, are usually found only in patients on high doses of corticosteroids or with HIV infection. Patients with HIV disease often suffer from oropharyngeal candidiasis.

Treatment of systemic yeast infections in the immunosuppressed
1 Amphotericin by i.v. infusion, starting with 250 µg/kg daily and increasing over 3–4 days to 1 mg/kg daily; adjust dose to minimize fever, nausea, hypokalaemia, renal impairment (which may be ameliorated by giving prednisolone before each dose), and rare neurological or haematological effects; some experts stop at a total dose of 1.0 g, others are guided by clinical cure; *or*
Liposomal amphotericin (must be made up in warmed solution) i.v. tolerated in doses of 3–4 mg/kg daily; indicated for severe infections, or when standard preparation is not tolerated.
2 For histoplasmosis or sensitive cryptococcal meningitis: fluconazole orally or i.v. 400 mg daily reducing after response to 200 mg daily; treat until clinical features are abolished (at least 6–8 weeks for cryptococcal meningitis).

Viral infections

Many viral infections occur in the course of leukaemia treatment, or transplantation immunosuppression (see below), often caused by herpes simplex, CMV and varicella-zoster virus. Many of these infections can be prevented by prophylactic aciclovir. Unfortunately, a few herpes simplex and CMV isolates are now resistant to aciclovir and ganciclovir, respectively. Hepatitis B, adenovirus, papillomavirus, polyomavirus and EBV may also cause clinical problems.

In children, measles can be life-threatening, complicated by giant-cell pneumonia and encephalitis. Predisposed children who have been exposed to measles virus should be protected passively with normal immunoglobulin. Live attenuated vaccines are contraindicated in children with immunodeficiencies. Because of the risk of intrafamilial transmission, live oral polio vaccine is also contraindicated in the siblings of immunodeficient children.

Parasitic infection

Pneumocystis carinii pneumonia (PCP) is the commonest infection in AIDS patients (see Chapter 11). Before the HIV epidemic, it was usually reported in patients with leukaemia (particularly lymphoblastic leukaemia), congenital T-cell defects and corticosteroid therapy.

Prophylaxis of PCP

In patients at risk of *P. carinii* infection, prophylaxis initiated before immunosuppression can prevent the development of this condition. It is particularly valuable when immunosuppression is related to bone marrow or organ transplantation but it can also be instituted in patients with AIDS. It has been demonstrated that PCP is uncommon in HIV-positive patients with a T-cell count of greater than 200 lymphocytes/μl, so regular monitoring of CD4 counts can indicate the appropriate time for institution of prophylaxis. Prophylaxis may take the form of oral co-trimoxazole 480–960 mg daily, but unfortunately many patients are unable to tolerate this regimen and alternatives must be sought. Substitution of the sulphamethoxazole with dapsone has been shown to provide equivalent protection with a lower incidence of adverse events. It also has a useful side-effect of decreasing the likelihood of reactivation of toxoplasmosis. Another effective prophylactic is aerosolized pentamidine 150 mg every 2 weeks or 300 mg 4-weekly, although this is less effective in children or in those who have already had an episode of pneumocystis infection.

Treatment of PCP

Co-trimoxazole orally or intravenously, 120 mg/kg per day in divided doses, is indicated. Pentamidine is an alternative to co-trimoxazole and is indicated for patients with a history of adverse reaction to co-trimoxazole. It is potentially very toxic and can cause hypotension during or immediately after intravenous administration. The dose is 4 mg/kg daily for at least 14 days; inhaled pentamidine 600 mg daily may be effective, and avoids severe systemic side-effects. A number of regimens have been developed to treat patients who fail on the primary therapies. These include trimetrexate, an antifolate drug related to methotrexate, which is given with folinic acid. Atovaquone, a ubiquinone which interferes with parasite cytochrome metabolism, has recently been licensed for use in *P. carinii* infections.

Toxoplasma gondii infection

Toxoplasma gondii often presents as a central nervous system infection, with multiple space-occupying lesions. As with PCP, HIV infection is now the commonest predisposition. Hodgkin's disease, cardiac transplantation and acute leukaemia are non-HIV conditions associated with *Toxoplasma* infection. In most cases, disease follows reactivation of previously dormant infection.

Treatment and prophylaxis of toxoplasmosis

Usually toxoplasmosis is an asymptomatic infection. In immunocompromised patients fulminant infection may occur and in others reactivation of cerebral toxoplasmosis may develop, generating space-occupying lesions. Treatment with a combination of pyrimethamine 50 mg daily and sulphadiazine 4 g daily in divided doses is usually required. This is well-absorbed orally and crosses the blood–brain barrier, though sulphadiazine can be given intravenously if necessary. Patients with cerebral toxoplasmosis usually respond by lysis of fever within 48 h of the institution of therapy. Failure to respond should prompt a search for an alternative diagnosis. In patients with persisting immunocompromise, suppressive treatment after successful therapy may be required. Dapsone is usually indicated for this purpose. A number of salvage treatments have been devised for cerebral toxoplasmosis and these include clindamycin and pyrimethamine, trimetrexate and leucovorin.

Cryptosporidiosis

Cryptosporidium parvum infection is one of the most difficult to manage. Acute self-limiting diarrhoea which is profuse and watery develops in immune-competent infected children and adults, but when there is a deficit in T-cell-mediated immunity, resolution does not occur.

C. parvum is naturally resistant to a wide range of disinfectants and antibiotics. A small proportion of patients appear to gain some benefit from spiramycin and others from paromomycin. Recent reports suggest that azithromycin in daily dosage produces a significant benefit. At present, treatment is mainly symptomatic.

Isopora belli infection

Isopora belli is a coccidian parasite which, unlike *Cryptosporidium*, is susceptible to antimicrobial therapy. Patients should be treated with co-trimoxazole. Alternatives include metronidazole, furazolidine, quinacrine, nitrofurantoin and newer macrolide antibiotics. Patients may be maintained on a suppressive dose of co-trimoxazole or a weekly dose of sulphadoxine–pyrimethamine (Fansidar).

Strongyloides stercoralis infection

Strongyloides stercoralis, a nematode infection, is acquired by direct penetration of infective larvae through intact skin followed by invasion of the small bowel by adults which produce further larvae, perpetuating the infection (see Chapter 8). Infection can remain largely asymptomatic for more than 40 years. When cellular immunity is reduced, uncontrolled multiplication of the parasite can develop. This is known as the hyperinfection syndrome, which may be complicated by Gram-negative septicaemia, pneumonia or meningitis, as larvae deposit bacteria in the tissues.

Management of strongyloidiasis

Treatment with albendazole 400 mg daily for 3 days results in eradication in up to 80% of immunocompetent patients, but courses of 400 mg 12-hourly for up to 4 weeks may be needed in the immunosuppressed. Ivermectin is a potentially useful alternative. The complication of Gram-negative septicaemia or meningitis which may arise during uncontrolled hyperinfection syndrome should be treated vigorously with third-generation cephalosporins such as cefotaxime.

Diagnosis of opportunistic infection

Because of the diversity of potential infectious agents and the need for urgent therapy, rapid, accurate diag-nosis is required. All patients should have at least two blood cultures taken from different sites.

If the specimens are taken via an indwelling intravenous cannula, parallel cultures should be taken from a peripheral vein. Blood should also be drawn for mycobacterial culture by conventional liquid medium, or in a radiometric detection system, which gives the advantage of earlier positive results (see Chapter 18). In patients potentially exposed to the systemic mycoses, subcultures should be made to appropriate media in appropriate containment facilities (see Chapter 23).

The diagnosis of pulmonary lesions should be made by bronchoalveolar lavage (see Chapter 7). The washings are examined by Gram, Ziehl–Nielsen and silver methenamine methods for the diagnosis of bacterial, mycobacterial pathogens and PCP. Herpesviruses may be detected by electron microscopy, by rapid CMV culture methods and by polymerase chain reaction (see Chapter 5).

Regular sets of cultures for surveillance or screening are taken in some units, particularly haematology services. The intention is to give early warning of colonization with a potentially dangerous opportunistic pathogen. Sites cultured include mouth swabs, sputum, urine, sites of indwelling cannulae and any area of skin inflammation. Referral to the results of recent surveillance cultures may assist in choosing empirical therapy when fever occurs, but the cause of the fever is not always derived from the superficial sites which can be routinely screened.

Cerebral toxoplasmosis can be suggested by the clinical picture of focal neurological deficit, and appearances seen on computed tomographic scanning. Serology is not diagnostic, as only immunoglobulin G antibodies are detectable, indicating either past infection or reactivation. Definitive diagnosis, however, depends on brain biopsy. In most cases, specific antitoxoplasma therapy is instituted and biopsy undertaken only if there is failure to respond.

The diagnosis of strongyloidiasis should be attempted in all patients exposed to this infection before immuno-compromising therapy is commenced. It can be made by serology and/or jejunal sampling using the Enterotest string test (see Chapter 8).

Diagnosis of opportunistic infection
1 Blood culture.
2 Bone marrow culture.
3 Broncheolar lavage.
4 Cerebrospinal fluid culture.
5 Brain scan.
6 Surveillance cultures: mouth swabs, sputum, urine, sites of indwelling cannulae, areas of skin inflammation.
7 (Tests for strongyloidiasis if indicated.)

Hypogammaglobulinaemia

Congenital hypogammaglobulinaemia

Congenital hypogammaglobulinaemia has two forms: (i) X-linked agammaglobulinaemia, in which patients become susceptible to infection in the first 6 months of life when maternal antibody is lost; and (ii) common variable immunodeficiency, which can occur at any age, most commonly the third decade.

Functional hypogammaglobulinaemia

Functional hypogammaglobulinaemia develops in patients with multiple myeloma, due to arrested B-cell maturation. It also occurs in patients with chronic parasitic infections such as leishmaniasis and trypanosomiasis, due to polyclonal B-cell activation and overproduction of low-affinity, non-specific antibody.

Patients with deficiency in T-cell function are also susceptible to pyogenic, particularly respiratory, infections due to the loss of T-cell help in antibody production.

Opportunistic infections

The main impact of hypo- or agammaglobulinaemia is on the respiratory and gastrointestinal tracts. Patients suffer recurrent and chronic respiratory infections with *Streptococcus pneumoniae* and non-capsulate *Haemophilus influenzae*. *Mycoplasma pneumoniae* and chlamydial pneumonias are also more common and persistent in affected adults. In the intestinal tract, infections with *Giardia*, *Cryptosporidium* and *Campylobacter* may be more persistent than in normal subjects. Rare cases of progressive enteroviral meningoencephalitis occur in agammaglobulinaemic patients.

Recurrent suppurative lung infections lead inevitably to bronchiectasis if immunoglobulin is not replaced regularly. Intravenous immunoglobulin is readily available and effective in preventing this. It is, therefore, indicated in infection-prone patients with congenital agammaglobulinaemia. The role of immunoglobulin in myeloma and other malignant diseases is less clear.

Complement deficiency

Hereditary complement deficiencies are rare but give rise to recurrent pyogenic infections, depending on which component of the complement pathway is deficient. Deficiency in the later components of the complement cascade, C7–C9, results in reduced ability to generate the membrane attack complex and achieve lysis of Gram-negative bacteria. The clinical consequence is recurrent infection with Gram-negative cocci, usually *Neisseria meningitidis*. Kindreds with deficiency of components of the alternative complement pathway suffer more frequent and more serious *S. pneumoniae* infections, including meningitis. This is due to the importance of the alternative complement pathway in opsonizing pneumococcal cell wall components for clearance (see p. 137). Defects in this pathway increase the likelihood, but not the severity, of meningococcal and gonococcal bacteraemias. Rare cases with properdin deficiency can develop devastating meningococcal infection.

Deficiencies of individual complement components have been described affecting each of the components of the cascade. Acquired complement deficiency occurs in immune disorders such as systemic lupus erythematosus.

Splenectomy

Following splenectomy there is a continuing risk of serious sepsis, with an incidence of approximately 0.5–1.0% per year. The risk varies with age and is particularly high in infants and children. Risk also varies with the indication for splenectomy; high mortality is associated with splenectomy for lymphoma and thalassaemia. The risk diminishes with time after splenectomy, but is never eliminated. Patients with sickle-cell disease have functional asplenia and suffer similar susceptibility to sepsis.

The most important infecting organism for splenectomized patients is *S. pneumoniae*, which causes approximately two-thirds of infections in most series. Other important bacteria are *H. influenzae* and *Escherichia coli*. Malaria may follow a fulminant course in patients with splenectomy. Splenectomy is an important predisposition to rare *Capnocytophagia canimorsis* infections, which usually follow a dog bite.

Preventing infections in asplenic patients

Prophylactic vaccination with 23-valent capsular polysaccharide pneumococcal vaccine should be offered 2 weeks before an elective splenectomy. Antibody responses are reduced in magnitude and duration after splenectomy, so vaccination should be repeated 3–6 years later. Local reactions are common on revaccination. Improved responses may be obtained with protein conjugate vaccine, currently under trial. *Haemophilus influenzae* type b (Hib) vaccine should also be given.

Antimicrobial prophylaxis with penicillin V should also be prescribed but its value may decrease as the prevalence of penicillin-resistant pneumococci increases. Patient education is important in encouraging patients to consult their physician quickly at the onset of a fever, or possibly to use an antibiotic regimen prescribed for early treatment without consultation. In reality many patients undergo splenectomy and are lost to effective follow-up, occasionally with disastrous consequences.

Prevention of infection in splenectomized patients
1 Immunization against *Streptococcus pneumoniae* and *Haemophilus influenzae,* preferably before splenectomy.
2 Antimicrobial prophylaxis.
3 Patient education and information.
4 Use of alerting card or bracelet.

Infections in transplant patients

Organ transplant patients

Organ transplant patients have usually received their transplants because of underlying disease of the organ concerned. This may be non-infectious, as in terminal renal failure or ischaemic heart disease. Some transplants, however, are performed for disease caused by severe or persisting infection; examples include liver transplants for acute or chronic liver failure caused by viral hepatitis, and heart transplant for myocarditis of infective origin. Fortunately, the original infection has often been terminated by the same immune and inflammatory response which damaged the affected organ. In a few cases, the infecting agent is not entirely removed with the infected organ, and recrudescence of local or generalized infection can occur. Thus hepatitis B virus can exist in the pancreas, and possibly other tissues, and reinfect a transplanted liver.

Antirejection therapy

Antirejection therapy neccessitates a major suppression of cell-mediated immune responses, to disable the effects of cytotoxic and natural killer cells on the transplanted organ. In the early posttransplant period, aggressive treatment with corticosteroids, azathioprine and cyclosporin is needed. Corticosteroids and azathioprine are broad-spectrum immunosuppressants, which affect both B- and T-cell function, and also depress phagocytes and eosinophils. Cyclosporin has a narrower but strong effect against cell-mediated immune responses. As the transplant stabilizes and the early risk of acute rejection

passes, the degree and spectrum of immunosuppression can be reduced. Many patients take maintenance doses of cyclosporin or azathioprine, sometimes with a small supplement of corticosteroids.

There is therefore an evolution of susceptibility to infection after a transplant.

Evolution of infection risks in transplant patients
1 Risk derived from original disease (e.g. renal failure).
2 Risk of hospital admission and surgery.
3 Risk of disease contracted from transplanted tissue (e.g. toxoplasmosis).
4 Early risk of opportunistic infections during strong immunosuppression.
5 Later risk of opportunistic infections due to chronic suppression of cell-mediated immunity.

The patient will begin with an increased susceptibility to infection simply because of chronic underlying disease. Hepatic cirrhosis causes splenic dysfunction and increased risk of pneumococcal disease. Hypersplenism may cause pancytopenia. Renal failure causes a broad-spectrum susceptibility to infections.

Since the transplant itself is a surgical procedure, the patient will bear the infection risks of hospital admission, anaesthetic and surgery, and sometimes also those of intensive care.

On rare occasions, the transplanted organ contains infective agents. These may be persisting or latent viruses, such as CMV, or dormant organisms such as *Toxoplasma*. Donors from tropical countries may have migrating parasites such as *Strongyloides* in their organs. Infections originating in this way usually become evident soon after the transplant. Efforts are made to eliminate the possibility of transmissible infection in the donor, or to ensure that the recipient has antibodies to agents such as *Toxoplasma* and CMV if the donor is also positive.

The effects of strong immunosuppression are usually important for about 3 months. During this time a wide range of viral, fungal, parasitic and atypical infections may occur. Bacterial infections can occur, and are vigorously investigated and treated. Skin and bowel suppressive treatment may be given with topical disinfectants and non-absorbable antibiotics and antifungal agents. Aciclovir prophylaxis can be given, and protects against herpes simplex infections and also against CMV disease (though the mechanism for the latter is poorly understood). Anti-CMV immune globulin is also used in some cases, and has an additive effect with antivirals.

Importance of cytomegalovirus in posttransplant patients

One of the most difficult infections to treat in the first 3 months after a transplant is CMV infection. Unlike AIDS patients, whose pulmonary CMV infections are rarely clinically important, more than half of transplant patients with CMV pneumonitis in the first 3 months will die. The treatment of CMV pneumonitis depends on the use of the analogue of aciclovir, ganciclovir. This drug can cause neutropenia, thrombocytopenia and oncogenesis. If given with zidovudine, it causes bone marrow depression. Foscarnet, used for CMV retinitis in AIDS, is not recommended for other CMV infections. It is extremely toxic, causing renal impairment in half of those treated and making cyclosporin therapy difficult.

> **Ganciclovir treatment of cytomegalovirus pneumonitis**
> Ganciclovir by i.v. infusion over 1 h, 5 mg/kg 12-hourly for 14–21 days, may be continued at 5 mg/kg daily (or 6 mg/kg daily on 5 days per week), if risk of recurrence exists.

The later risks of reduced cell-mediated immunity are largely related to infections caused by reactivation of latent infections, such as herpes zoster, toxoplasmosis or progressive multifocal leukoencephalopathy (caused by JC virus), or to infection with environmental agents of low pathogenicity, such as *Listeria monocytogenes* or *Nocardia asteroides* (Table 21.2).

Bone marrow transplant patients

Bone marrow transplant patients have slightly different problems because, as well as the immunosuppressive effects of their underlying disease and treatment, their transplant is preceded by ablative chemotherapy and radiotherapy, causing virtually complete suppression of immune responses. The transplanted bone marrow is also often treated to suppress its cytotoxic cell function, in an effort to avoid severe graft-versus-host disease. As the transplanted bone marrow gradually becomes established, many of its functions will recover (Table 21.3).

The need for immunosuppressive maintenance therapy will depend on the source of the transplanted marrow, and its degree of tissue match with the recipient. Autologous transplants (the patient's own bone marrow, harvested during remission of malignancy) rarely need immunosuppressive follow-up. Transplants from close relatives may require little or no antirejection treatment once they are established. Transplants from unrelated donors can require permanent immunosuppression, and may also cause graft-versus-host disease, which itself carries a risk of infection and/or rejection.

Time after transplant	Disease risk
First 2 weeks	Infectious complications of anaesthetic and surgery: *Staphylococcus aureus* or enterobacterial infection of wound, enterobacterial, staphylococcal or candidal infection of organ or deep tissues. Pneumococcal or other chest infection
First 3 months	Chest infections with CMV, *Legionella*, *Aspergillus*, *Mycobacterium*, *Candida* or other fungus. Skin and mucosal infections with herpes simplex, *Candida* or other yeast. Infection of long-term indwelling cannula. Cerebral infections with *Toxoplasma*, *Aspergillus* or *Candida*
After 3 months	Skin infection (herpes zoster). Pneumonia with *Nocardia*, *Aspergillus* or CMV. Cerebral infection with *Listeria*, *Cryptococcus*, *Nocardia*, *Toxoplasma* or JC virus

CMV, cytomegalovirus.

Table 21.2 Range of infection risks following organ transplantation

Duration of effect	Type of defect
First month	Lack of natural killer cells (and other non-CD8 cytotoxic cells)
3–4 months	Total T-cell count deficiency. Decreased interleukin-2 production. Decreased neutrophil chemotaxis
4–6 months	Decreased CD4 (helper/inducer) cells. Decreased CD8 (cytotoxic) cells. Decreased response to polysaccharide antigens and reduced immunoglobulin A responses to antigen
1 year or more	Decreased secondary antibody responses. Decreased alveolar macrophage functions. Reduced proliferative responses by CD4 cells

Table 21.3 Spectrum of immune dysfunction following bone marrow transplant.

As bone marrow transplants are becoming more successful, and will be used to treat metabolic and other non-malignant disease, immunosuppressive therapy is likely to evolve, and possibly become narrower in spectrum. Expertise in long-term follow-up and the treatment of late manifestations of opportunistic infection (possibly including slow infections similar to slow virus diseases) will become increasingly important.

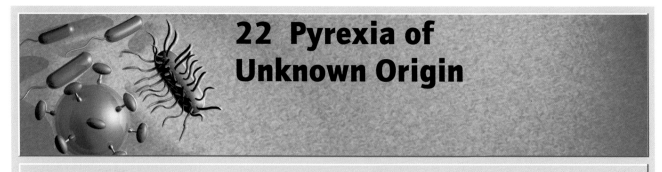

22 Pyrexia of Unknown Origin

Introduction: causes of pyrexia of unknown origin

A pyrexia of unknown origin (PUO) is an elevation of body temperature for which there is no obvious cause. As has been seen in earlier chapters, fever must be defined as a body temperature reaching at least 37.8–38°C. There are many trivial and self-limiting infections which cause short-lasting fevers. Most of these are 'anonymous' viral infections whose formal diagnosis would be tedious and unproductive. They are excluded from the list of conditions to be investigated in PUO by making a more detailed definition: pyrexia of unknown origin is a fever which has continued or frequently recurred for a period of at least 3 weeks, and for which no cause has been found after one or more medical consultations or assessments.

Infection is not the only type of disease which can cause fever. There are several important non-infectious causes of PUO and also a number of rare ones. The causes of fever can be described under six main headings:

1 Infections (45–55% of cases).
2 Malignancies (12–20% of cases).
3 Connective tissue disorders (10–15% of cases).
4 Hypersensitivity disorders.
5 Rare metabolic conditions.
6 Factitious fever (fever induced deliberately by the patient).

Important infectious causes of pyrexia of unknown origin
1 Tuberculosis (usually non-pulmonary, miliary or cryptic).
2 Sepsis (especially in a hollow organ) or abscess.
3 Imported diseases (such as typhoid fever or brucellosis).
4 Subacute endocarditis.
5 Zoonoses with a long time course (such as toxoplasmosis or Q-fever).

Important malignant causes of pyrexia of unknown origin
1 Lymphomata (Hodgkin's and non-Hodgkin's).
2 Leukaemias (especially monocytic or myelomonocytic types).

3 Histiocytoses (usually in small children).
4 Renal adenocarcinoma.
5 Primary hepatic carcinoma.
6 Rare, atrial myxoma.

Connective tissue disorders which may present as pyrexia of unknown origin
1 Sarcoidosis (and rare granulomatous diseases).
2 Polyarteritis nodosa.
3 Systemic lupus erythematosus.
4 Wegener's granulomatosis.
5 Juvenile rheumatoid arthritis.
6 Dermatomyositis.

Common causes of hypersensitivity with fever
Drugs
1 Sulphonamides.
2 Penicillins.
3 Rifampicin.
4 Isoniazid.
5 Streptomycin.
6 Phenytoin.
7 Phenobarbitone.
8 Methyldopa.

Environmental factors
1 Fungus-infected hay (farmer's lung).
2 Bird proteins (pigeon-fancier's lung).

Rare metabolic causes of pyrexia of unknown origin
1 Porphyrias (acute intermittent or mixed types).
2 Familial relapsing polyserositis (familial Mediterranean fever).
3 Some cases of vasoactive intestinal polypeptide-producing tumour (VIPoma) and glucagonoma.

The causes of PUO are not exotic diseases. Most of them are common diseases which have presented without their usual symptoms and physical signs.

Initial assessment

The assessment of a patient with PUO must include a search for both infectious and non-infectious conditions. All screening procedures work more efficiently if the population to be screened is preselected to include a high proportion of likely positives. Collation of an epidemiological and clinical database will allow the physician to choose initial and follow-up investigations in a structured way, and to proceed efficiently to screen for likely causes. Otherwise an almost infinite range of possible tests could be performed, each with a different sensitivity and specificity, presenting the investigator with a hugely complex task when interpreting results.

Epidemiological database

While this applies particularly to infection, it also includes the history of exposure, predisposition and protection for other types of disease. A patient may have been exposed to infection by known contact with other cases, by travel, food, water, occupation, recreation or by association with animals, including farm animals or pets.

Exposure to allergens should also be sought; this could be iatrogenic exposure to agents such as antibiotics or other drugs, or to environmental agents at work, home or play. Such agents might include bird proteins (as in pigeon-fancier's lung), organic dusts such as cotton or contaminated hay (byssinosis and farmer's lung) or to industrial dusts and vapours, including vinyl chloride monomer or beryllium, which can both cause inflammatory or granulomatous lung disease.

Predisposition may be indicated by a family history of an inflammatory condition. This applies not only to rare familial disorders like relapsing serositis, but to Reiter's syndrome and many connective tissue diseases, such as systemic lupus erythematosus and rheumatoid arthritis.

In rare cases the patient will have a history of exposure to carcinogenic agents, such as radiation, including intensive radiotherapy as used to be given for ankylosing spondylosis. A history of sustained immunosuppressive therapy, for instance with cyclosporin, also indicates an increased likelihood of some malignant diseases because of impaired responses to early malignant changes.

Protection or resistance may be the result of natural immunity following previous infection with an agent, or it can be induced by immunization. Temporary resistance can also be obtained by the use of chemoprophylaxis, as commonly used for malaria, or immunoprophylaxis, as for hepatitis A. While none of these confers absolute protection from a condition, they reduce the likelihood of a particular disease to a predictable extent, and allow the investigator to choose priorities in the differential diagnosis of the fever.

Evolution of the feverish condition

Although the current complaint may be fever, this might have been preceded by symptoms either of an earlier stage of the disease or of a recent condition to which the fever is a late sequel.

The severity or behaviour of the fever itself is not often helpful. A truly intermittent fever, such as the tertian fever of malaria, is an exception, but it is not apparent until the disease is well-established. Similarly, the undulant fever of chronic brucellosis, the escalating fever of early typhoid and the relapsing fever of *Borrelia recurrentis* infection can be diagnostically helpful (Fig. 22.1), but they do not always occur in their classic form.

The early stages of viral infections are often marked by prostration, myalgia, arthralgia and shivering attacks. Transient diarrhoea, constipation, sore throat or cough could hint at the systemic site of the problem. Bacterial infections may similarly produce transient localizing symptoms. Abscesses and loculated sepsis are often accompanied by intermittent episodes of bacteraemia. These are marked by rigors — severe shaking chills which make speech and other movement difficult (Fig. 22.2). In postinfectious conditions and connective tissue diseases transient rashes can occur and recur. They may last only minutes or hours, being visible only when the temperature is highest (Fig. 22.3) or when the skin has been warmed by bathing.

If the fever is due to a postinfectious disorder, the precipitating infection probably occurred at least 10–14 days earlier. Typically it would be a sore throat or a viral-type infection with respiratory symptoms or a rash. Next most likely would be a gastrointestinal complaint. Such a history can point to appropriate diagnostic tests at an early stage in the investigation.

Physical examination

By definition, physical signs are few and subtle in this condition. However there are some which can be very helpful in making a diagnosis; they should always be sought, and acted upon when found.

Localized bone or joint pain

Localized bone or joint pain can be extremely mild at the onset of skeletal infections. They may appear as discomfort, stiffness or, particularly in children, reluctance to move the affected part. When they affect the leg or lumbar spine, they are often more obvious when the patient is asked to stand or walk. They are important because such symptoms precede X-ray changes by many

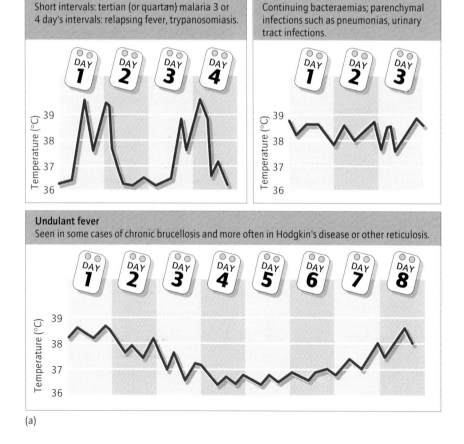

Fig. 22.1 Some classic patterns of fever.
(a) Intermittent, constant and undulant fever.

(a)

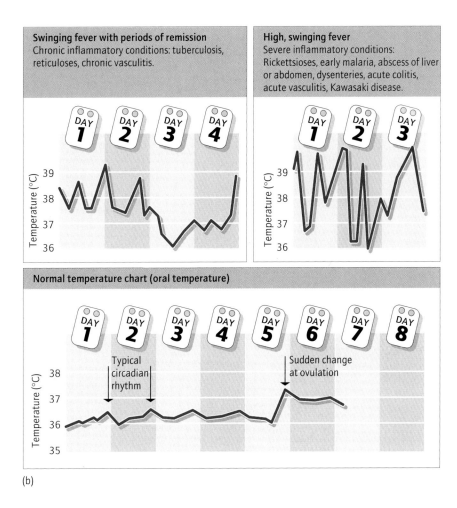

Fig. 22.1 *Continued.* (b) Swinging fever with periods of remission, high swinging fever and a normal temperature chart.

(b)

days or weeks, and should therefore be further investigated by other imaging techniques (see Chapter 17).

Soft systolic murmurs

Soft systolic murmurs may be flow murmurs in feverish patients, but may also be signs of endocarditis, or even pericarditis or myocarditis. They should be reassessed regularly to detect changes, and further investigated at an early stage.

Subtle skin rashes

Subtle skin rashes may be the only sign of embolic or vasculitic phenomena. Showers of petechiae, Osler's nodes or simply small, vasculitic lesions of the digits can be signs of endocarditis or immune vasculitis. Splinter haemorrhages, small retinal haemorrhages and cytoid bodies have a similar significance.

Mild meningism

Mild meningism is easy to pass off as 'difficult' or 'uncooperative' behaviour when such behaviour may really be part of a central nervous system disease. In tuberculous meningitis, as in rarer inflammations of the brain and meninges, it is important to suspect the disease before more definite (and often more irreversible) signs develop. If there is doubt, early investigation is essential.

Mild localized abdominal tenderness

Mild localized abdominal tenderness is also easily dismissed. Certainly the patient may be excessively sensitive, or may be trying to assist the investigation by pointing up every possible sign, but it is difficult to describe the vague sensations of visceral discomfort.

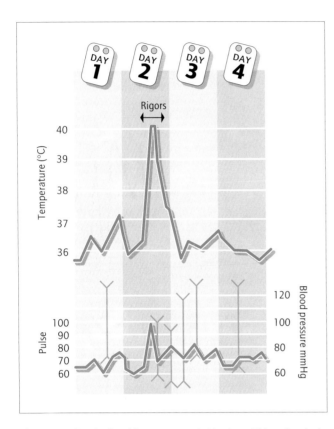

Fig. 22.2 Isolated spike of fever accompanied by rigors. This patient had a *Klebsiella pneumoniae* infection of the obstructed biliary tree, with intermittent bacteraemias.

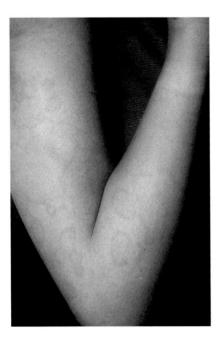

Fig. 22.3 Postinfectious rash: erythema marginatum appearing during an episode of fever.

Trivial abdominal signs may indicate the existence of a peritoneal or subphrenic abscess. If vague signs persist, they should be followed up.

Chest X-ray

The chest X-ray is so important in assessing PUO that initial examination is not complete without it. Extensive pulmonary consolidation or cavitation can exist with few or absent physical signs (Fig. 22.4); granulomatous and other infiltrations and mediastinal swellings are other important abnormalities immediately detectable by X-ray.

Initial laboratory investigations

Full blood count

This is an extremely helpful starting-point. In particular the total and differential white cell count can assist in determining the disease group causing the fever.

A high neutrophil count may indicate bacterial infection. Some infections tend to induce very high neutrophil counts, for instance pneumococcal and *Haemophilus influenzae* infections, in which the white cell count may reach $15–25 \times 10^9/l$. Intermediate elevations of white cell count, around $12–16 \times 10^9/l$, are common in *Streptococcus pyogenes* infections and in the presence of abscesses. While most bacterial infections are accompanied by neutrophilia, there are a few important exceptions. The count is often normal in early *Staphylococcus aureus* infections, even bacteraemias. However, the disease may still

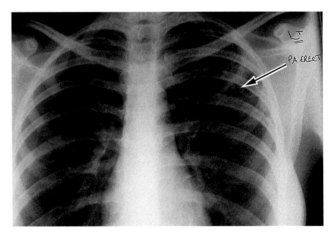

Fig. 22.4 Chest X-ray of a midwife returning from work in Africa with persisting low-grade fever and cough. The chest was clinically clear, but this cavitating opacity (arrow) prompted investigation and treatment for tuberculosis.

be suspected if the differential count is performed, because of the high proportion of neutrophils — often 90–95%. Enteric fevers and brucellosis are said to induce neutropenia, and this is true in established disease. In the early stages, however, there may be a neutrophilia as inflammation begins.

Lymphocyte count

The lymphocyte count is not usually raised in viral infections, with the exception of the mononucleoses. The proportion of lymphocytes may appear raised because of mild neutropenia, possibly caused by the toxic effects of interferon. Small numbers of atypical or activated mononuclear cells are often seen in the blood film of patients with acute viral infections such as hepatitis A or rubella, but these do not approach the numbers seen in the mononucleoses. Pertussis toxin causes marked lymphocytosis ($15–25 \times 10^9/l$), which is an important diagnostic feature of pertussis.

A raised eosinophil count may indicate a tropical parasitic infection. It is a helpful sign in early and late schistosomiasis, strongyloidiasis and liver fluke infection. It is rarely seen in malaria, leishmaniasis or *Toxocara* infections.

Platelet count

The platelet count is rarely altered. Exceptions are severe Gram-negative sepsis in which intravascular coagulation may deplete platelet numbers, and falciparum malaria in which a similar mechanism operates. A high platelet count is usual in established Kawasaki disease and other severe vasculitides, and is a rare finding in disseminated tuberculosis.

Red cells

The red cells may show altered morphology in some infections. Apart from obvious parasitization in malaria, sometimes with distortion and granule formation, there may be abnormalities of red cell production or survival. In parvovirus B19 infection, erythropoiesis is arrested by viral invasion of red cell progenitors. This is detectable as a fall in the reticulocyte count. Conversely, the reticulocyte count will rise if haemolysis occurs, as in *Mycoplasma pneumoniae* infections. The accumulation of larger reticulocytes causes an increase in the mean corpuscular volume.

Stained blood film

The stained blood film can be diagnostic if it contains tropical parasites such as microfilaria or trypanosomes. It may be worth examining films taken in special circum-

stances, e.g. at night or after a dose of filaricide, to increase the likelihood of detecting parasitaemia.

Non-specific tests for inflammation

Plasma viscosity and the erythrocyte sedimentation rate

These are both determined by the complex effects of dissolved proteins in the blood. The erythrocyte sedimentation rate (ESR) is further influenced by the red cell count, but this rarely makes an important difference to its clinical interpretation. The ESR is more commonly used in clinical practice. When inflammation causes changes in the concentrations of acute-reacting proteins, the ESR rises. The rise is not fast; indeed it can take some days for the ESR to reach its height, or to fall to normal after inflammation resolves. This is not always a disadvantage, as it gives an overall indication of the intensity and duration of inflammation.

The ESR is moderately raised (e.g. 35–50 mm/h) in acute infections and other inflammatory conditions. It is often markedly raised (e.g. over 70 mm/h) in the presence of persisting abscesses, in some pneumonias, such as legionnaire's disease and *Mycoplasma* pneumonia, and in severe connective tissue diseases and hypersensitivity reactions.

The plasma viscosity behaves in almost exactly the same way as the ESR.

C-reactive protein

C-reactive protein is often measured because of its rapid response to changing levels of inflammation. It has not proved as helpful as expected in indicating the likely aetiology of the inflammation, being elevated to an unpredictable extent in bacterial infections, viral infections and parasitic disease, as well as in non-infectious conditions. Its best use is in monitoring the response of inflammation to treatment (as in the management of endocarditis) rather than in primary diagnosis.

Blood biochemical tests

Aspartate transaminase and alkaline phosphatase levels

These can be useful in suggesting further investigations in PUO. Slight elevations of transaminases are relatively common in acute viral infections, but this rarely gives levels greater than 55–60 U/l. Higher levels point to local liver inflammation or occasionally to severe and widespread tissue damage. Elevated alkaline phosphatase levels are usually of liver origin. They can indicate space-occupying lesions in the liver, but do not distinguish many small lesions, such as granulomata, from larger lesions, such as abscesses or tumours.

Blood amylase levels

Blood amylase levels may be high in pancreatitis or inflammation of the salivary glands.

Urine examination

Urine microscopy

Urine microscopy can reveal pus cells, red blood cells, casts of various types and occasionally the eggs of *Schistosoma haematobium* (Fig 22.5). Red blood cells or red cell casts should arouse suspicion of renal inflammation, while pus cells usually indicate infection.

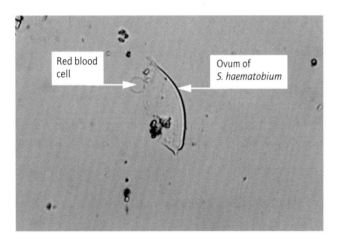

Red blood cell

Ovum of
S. haematobium

Fig. 22.5 Ovum of *Schistosoma haematobium* with red blood cells in the urine of an engineer with episodic haematuria: he had been working on a river estuary in Africa.

Urine biochemical tests

Urine biochemical tests should be combined with microscopy. Protein and blood may indicate infection. Products of haemolysis may be present in severe malaria, and are related to prognosis. Bilirubin is often detectable in urine before clinical jaundice appears in hepatocellular disease.

Initial microbiological investigations

Simple microscopy

This is a rapid diagnostic procedure which is easy to overlook. It has already been mentioned in the context of blood and urine examination, but is also applicable to other specimens.

Stool microscopy

Stool microscopy, either of wet preparations or of concentrated supernatant, can reveal important parasites. These include pathogenic amoebae, the eggs or larvae of invasive helminths, or protozoa such as *Cryptosporidium* sp. which can cause feverish illness in immunosuppressed patients (see Fig. 3.1).

Aspirate

Aspirate from an enlarged spleen or lymph node may contain tropical parasites, such as *Leishmania* (see Fig. 19.10) or trypanosomes.

Pus from abscesses

Pus from abscesses or sinuses can be examined by Gram's stain or acid-fast stains. Fluid from vesicles or bullae may also be useful specimens for microscopy.

Cells

Cells recovered from washings, scrapings or aspirates can be examined with tissue stains to reveal typical inclusion bodies or cytopathic effects; examples include the diagnosis of measles or chickenpox pneumonia by bronchial washings in immunosuppressed children who lack the typical rash. Immunological stains may reveal pathogens such as cytomegalovirus in cell preparations.

Electron microscopy

Electron microscopy can also assist in rapid diagnosis, particularly in examination of vesicle fluid (e.g. to demonstrate herpesvirus particles).

Initial cultures

Blood cultures

Blood cultures are essential, and should be obtained before antimicrobial treatment whenever possible. At least two sets should be taken, at different times and preferably when the temperature is rising or has just risen. This is because temperature rises tend to occur when pathogens are released into the blood. The likelihood of obtaining positive results is not increased by taking more than three sets of blood cultures. The microbiologist should be informed if the illness may be caused by slow-growing organisms, such as brucellae, so that the cultures can be maintained for the appropriate time.

Urine culture

Urine culture is also an important initial investigation. Urinary infections, both acute and chronic, can exist without localizing symptoms or signs. The early morning urine (EMU) can be examined and cultured for mycobacteria.

Stool culture

Stool cultures may be positive in enteric fevers when blood cultures have failed for any reason.

Pus and discharge

Pus, discharge or vesicle fluid must always be collected for culture. It is more helpful to the microbiologist if a significant volume can be obtained, rather than just a smear on a swab.

Cultures for virological investigation

Cultures for virological investigation are equally important, especially in the immunosuppressed. For respiratory viruses, nose and throat swabs, nasopharyngeal aspirate, bronchial aspirate and lavage specimens may be processed. For enteroviruses, throat swabs, stool and (if appropriate) cerebrospinal fluid may be examined. Urine can be cultured for cytomegalovirus and mumps virus. Respiratory specimens, vesicle scrapings and fluid are appropriate for herpesvirus cultures.

Initial serological investigations

These need not be elaborate, unless the clinical situation suggests or compels it. The need for paired sera, taken 10–14 days apart, means that many serological tests must be deferred. The results of initial tests so far described will then be available, and will assist the choice of further investigations. Some immunological tests, however, are useful screening tests and can provide early results.

Heterophile antibodies

Heterophile antibodies, the basis of the Paul–Bunnell test, are detectable in almost all adults with Epstein–Barr virus infection. The monospot test is sensitive and will be positive in most children over the age of about 5; below that age, heterophile antibody tests are less reliable. A positive monospot test is virtually diagnostic of Epstein–Barr virus infection and can solve the diagnosis in patients lacking a significant mononucleosis.

Tuberculin test

The tuberculin test has poor specificity, but is helpful if strongly positive. Tuberculosis is common among PUO patients, so a tuberculin test should be performed as soon as possible. A strongly positive Mantoux test, or Heaf reaction of grade three or more, indicates active tuberculosis unless proved otherwise.

Initial work-up plan for pyrexia of unknown origin
1 Full history.
2 Physical examination.
3 Chest X-ray.
4 Blood count, differential count and morphology.
5 Erythrocyte sedimentation rate (and/or C-reactive protein).
6 Liver and renal function tests.
7 Dipstick urine tests.
8 Microscopy of blood film and urine (cerebrospinal fluid (CSF), stool and lesion fluid if indicated).
9 Culture of blood, urine and respiratory specimens (CSF, stool, pus and lesion fluid if indicated).
10 Acid-fast stain and tuberculosis cultures (sputum, gastric aspirates, EMUs and CSF) if indicated.
11 Heterophil antibody detection test.
12 Tuberculin test.
13 Save baseline serum.

Interpretation of initial findings

The results of initial tests will gradually become available between the first day and about the seventh day of investigation. Many diagnoses will be made from these results alone. Such diagnoses include bacteraemias, culture-positive endocarditis, pneumonias, urinary tract infections, pulmonary tuberculosis, Epstein–Barr virus infection and common parasitic diseases. Some malignancies such as leukaemias will also be revealed.

While results are accumulating, the physical examination should be reviewed a number of times, both to check on doubtful signs and to detect new or changing ones. It is surprising how suddenly a cardiac murmur can become obvious, finger clubbing can develop or lymph nodes enlarge.

Further investigation is indicated if no diagnosis is apparent or if initial assessment suggests a line of investigation. In some cases the patient's condition is poor, and a wider range of tests must be completed without delay. Three main types of investigation are possible:

1 Serological tests for infections.
2 Tests for connective tissue diseases.
3 Tissue diagnosis (imaging and/or biopsy and culture).

Serological tests (and probes) for infections

Demonstration of pathogens in specimens

When pathogens cannot be demonstrated by staining or culture, serological tests can still reveal them in a variety of ways.

Antigen detection

Antigen detection is a reliable diagnostic test for a wide range of pathogens. Examples include latex and other tests on cerebrospinal fluid for cryptococcal antigen, and also the immunological tests for *Chlamydia trachomatis* which can be performed on genital swabs. Detection of hepatitis B antigen in blood is still an important test of active hepatitis B virus disease. Immunological stains can be used to demonstrate whole organisms or antigens in cells or tissues, and these can be made more sensitive by intermediate amplifying steps in which large amounts of antibody are 'stuck' to the antigen and then shown up by fluorescent or enzymic techniques (see Chapter 3).

Genome detection by probes

Genome detection by probes is a relatively recent diagnostic method in which the nucleic acid of an organism is revealed by marking it with a labelled complementary sequence of DNA. Small amounts of nucleic acid in a specimen can be amplified by repeated replication in the polymerase chain reaction. This has proved useful in the examination of cerebrospinal fluid for traces of herpes simplex virus in encephalitis, and of mycobacteria in tuberculous meningitis. Both diagnoses are otherwise extremely difficult because of the very small numbers of organisms present in early disease. Polymerase chain reaction amplification and hybridization to detect viral

RNA is the only means of demonstrating hepatitis C viraemia.

Detection of antibodies to pathogens

There are numerous ways of detecting specific antibodies; these are described and discussed in Chapter 3. Different approaches may be taken to the demonstration of antibodies, depending on the disease concerned.

Diseases with unique antibody responses

Diseases with unique antibody responses are those which are rare in a population, so that few individuals possess antibodies, or those in which an antibody appears quickly and then soon disappears after recovery. Examples of the first alternative are legionellosis, leptospirosis or rickettsial infections, which are rare, even in immigrants to western countries. A diagnosis of one of these diseases can be assumed on a single serum test if the level of antibodies is higher than standard baseline level (e.g. >1:64 for *Legionella pneumophila*). Examples of the second type include systemic amoebiasis in which detectable gel precipitin antibodies correlate closely with active infection. (The heterophile antibody test for Epstein–Barr virus infection is also used in this way.)

Primary infections

Primary infections producing an immunoglobulin M (IgM) response are common causes of fever. In these cases demonstration of IgM antibodies is diagnostic. Examples include hepatitis A, hepatitis B (by IgM anticore antibodies), toxoplasmosis and common diseases such as rubella. Rarities include borreliosis and brucellosis.

Postprimary infections

Infections which may be postprimary require more exacting diagnosis. They include such conditions as *C. pneumoniae* or cytomegalovirus infections. After primary infection many members of a population have background levels of IgG antibodies and produce a secondary response to subsequent infections with the same organism. They do not usually produce a second IgM response. Diagnosis cannot then be made by demonstrating IgM antibodies, but depends on detecting a significant increase in IgG antibody titres. This is impossible if no early serum specimen has been saved; the importance of collecting serum from PUO cases cannot be overemphasized.

Serological and probe tests for infection in pyrexia of unknown origin
1 Antigen detection (blood antigen for hepatitis B or D, cerebrospinal fluid (CSF) antigen for cryptococcosis, tissue antigen for cytomegalovirus, blood probes for hepatitis C RNA, CSF probes for herpes simplex virus DNA and mycobacterial DNA).
2 Single-serum antibody tests (immunoglobulin M for acute viral infections, borreliosis or toxoplamosis, gel precipitin test for amoebiasis, diagnostic titres of *Legionella* antibodies).
3 Paired-serum antibody tests (for atypical pneumonias, leptospirosis, yersiniosis).

Some patients take longer than the traditional 10–14 days to produce diagnostic titres or rises of antibody levels. A serological diagnosis cannot be made before 7–9 weeks in some cases of legionellosis, borreliosis and leptospirosis. Even the anti-streptolysin O titre (ASOT) may take 3 or 4 weeks to reach diagnostic levels. It is always worth taking a late serum specimen if a serological diagnosis has not been evident in the first month of fever.

Tests for connective tissue and granulomatous diseases

Connective tissue and granulomatous diseases are good mimics of infection. Some are particularly like viral infections, presenting with fever and neutropenia, and sometimes rash. A good example of this is systemic lupus erythematosus. Others may cause neutrophilia, for example polyarteritis nodosa and Wegener's granulomatosis. These further mimic bacterial disease by producing focal inflammatory lesions in the respiratory system. The granulomatous disease sarcoidosis must be distinguished from tuberculosis, especially when it presents without its typical pulmonary features.

Elevated ESR

An elevated ESR is a feature of all of these conditions and is usually a prominent finding. While a high ESR is not exclusive to connective tissue diseases, it is unwise to dismiss such a diagnosis unless the finding can be otherwise explained.

Autoantibodies

Autoantibodies are detectable in the blood in many connective tissue diseases, and may be diagnostic.

Sarcoidosis is not associated with autoantibodies but if there is lung involvement the serum angiotensin-converting enzyme level is elevated. This is often detectable even when pulmonary function and chest X-ray appearances are normal.

Serological tests for connective tissue disorders
1 Rheumatoid factor.
2 Antinuclear factor, DS-DNA antibodies.
3 Other specific antibodies (smooth-muscle, mitochondrial, etc.).
4 ANCA (antineutrophil cytoplasmic antibodies).
5 SACE (serum angiotensin-converting enzyme).

Tissue diagnosis (imaging and biopsy)

For many years it has been possible to demonstrate distortion of tissues by X-ray examination, or to perform open or needle biopsies of tissues. The availability of many other imaging techniques has greatly simplified the investigation of PUO. It is now possible to demonstrate the anatomy of tissues and organs, to test their function and to detect inflammation within them. Imaging can suggest whether biopsy may contribute to the diagnosis of PUO, and can also assist in guiding the biopsy needle. It has almost abolished the need for diagnostic laparotomy which was such a feature of PUO investigation in the 1950s and before.

Ultrasound scans

Ultrasound scans are non-invasive and relatively inexpensive. The technique depends on showing differences in the sonic density of tissues and will delineate the anatomy of organs, and lesions within organs, especially if these are outlined by thin fatty planes. It is particularly useful for demonstrating enlargement of the liver, gallbladder, spleen or kidneys and for detecting abscesses, cysts or space-occupying lesions. It can demonstrate soft-tissue swelling and periosteal elevation in early osteomyelitis. It can also define pelvic lesions, particularly in and around the female genital tract. It can be used to guide needles during aspiration and biopsy.

Its limitation is its requirement for expert operation and interpretation, as the anatomical definition is not perfect and the ultrasonic beam makes shadows which can be confused with lesions. Nevertheless, it is justly the first imaging technique used in investigation of PUO cases, and is often diagnostic.

Echocardiography

Echocardiography is ultrasonic imaging of the heart. It is now so sophisticated that it can show a two-dimensional picture of the beating heart and its valves. Doppler echocardiography demonstrates the direction, velocity and turbulence of blood flow. These techniques can show vegetations on heart valves, abscesses of the valve rings and septum, pericardial effusions and even

dilatations of the coronary arteries. The only limitation of echocardiography is its occasional inability to demonstrate small lesions, giving rise to false-negative results.

Computed tomographic scans

Computed tomographic scans are highly refined computed tomograms derived from axial X-rays of the body. They produce high-definition pictures of the anatomy of

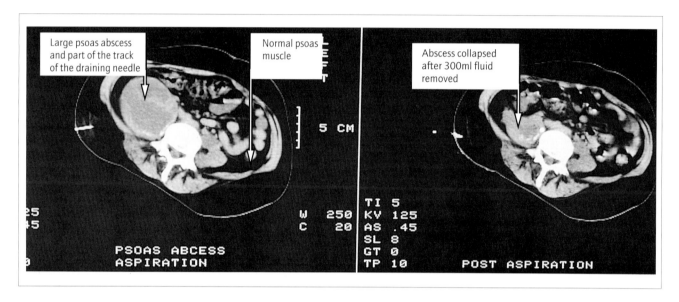

(a)

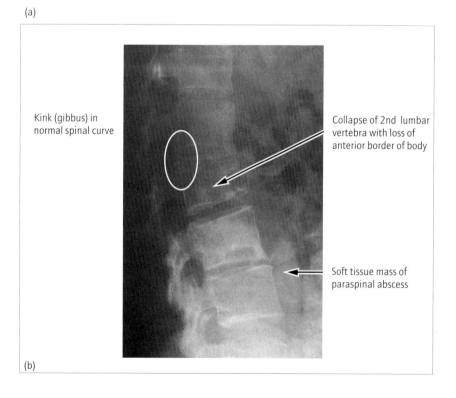

(b)

Fig. 22.6 (a) Computed tomographic-guided aspiration of pus from a large psoas abscess: as well as confirming tuberculosis this was a therapeutic procedure – 300 ml of infected material was removed; (b) X-ray appearance of the same abscess.

organs and can demonstrate lesions of 0.5 cm or less. Contrast media can be used to demonstrate increased blood supply to inflamed lesions; the media cause enhanced radiodensity of affected tissue. Computed tomographic guided biopsy and aspiration can be performed (Fig. 22.6).

Isotope scans

Isotope scans involve the intravenous injection of radioisotopes which will become concentrated in abnormal tissues. Subsequent scanning with an appropriate detection system, usually a gamma camera, will produce a picture demonstrating the affected area. The most commonly used isotopes are technetium, which demonstrates increased blood flow to inflamed tissues, and gallium, which accumulates in areas rich in inflammatory mediators. Technetium is used for bone scans, which can demonstrate inflammatory lesions in bone long before X-rays can show altered bone anatomy. Gallium can reveal abscesses or foci of inflammation in many organs and tissues (Fig. 22.7).

Isotope scans can also be used to demonstrate the relationship between structure and excretory function in the kidneys and liver. Obstruction of urinary or biliary outflow commonly results in infection. Appropriate isotope scans can show whether the isotope is concentrated in the excreted fluid, and can use the concentrated isotope to make an image of the ureter or the bile ducts.

Magnetic resonance scans

Magnetic resonance scans make images of the concentrations of magnetic atoms in the tissues. The most abundant magnetic atom in the body is hydrogen, present in the tissues as various concentrations of water. Magnetic resonance scans are therefore good for showing vascularity of tissues, but can also demonstrate subtle variations of the water content. Oedema is easily seen, so inflammation is detectable by magnetic resonance imaging, even before there is a change in radiodensity (i.e. in X-ray or computed tomographic appearance). It is possible to enhance magnetic resonance images with media containing magnetic atoms, some of which are radioisotopes, but radioisotopes are potentially damaging to some tissues, while magnetic fields are not. The disadvantage of magnetic resonance scans is that they cannot be performed on patients who contain magnetically active metal structures such as steel joint prostheses or haemostatic clips. These ferrous objects would be disastrously attracted to the scanners' enormously powerful magnets.

X-ray techniques

X-ray techniques are still important in the investigation of PUO. This is particularly true in bowel disease, where scanning images may not be able to distinguish between the fluid-filled lumen of the bowel and an abscess in the folds of the peritoneum. Contrast studies can demonstrate mucosal disease (Fig. 22.8) perforations and fistulae of the bowel, and indeed of many other hollow organs.

Laparoscopy

Laparoscopy allows direct examination of organs in the abdomen or pelvis. It is useful for detecting abnor-

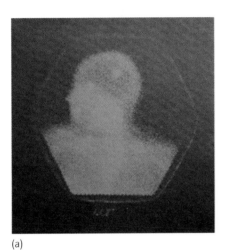

(a)

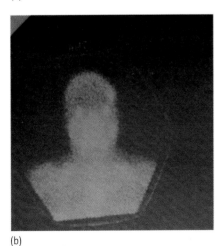

(b)

Fig. 22.7 (a and b) Gallium scan showing concentration of activity in the left parietal bone: this teenager with fever, anaemia and weight loss had a lymphoma.

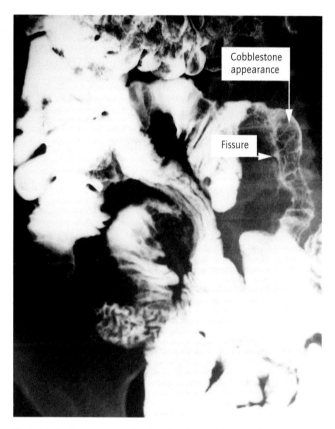

Fig. 22.8 Barium meal examination showing cobblestone change and fissuring in the terminal ileum: this Indian patient had ileal tuberculosis.

malities of the abdominal lymph nodes, the liver and the genital tract. Biopsies can be obtained under laparoscopic control. Other procedures for examining tissue planes or the lumen of the organs include mediastinoscopy, bronchoscopy and endoscopy of the bowel, biliary tract and urinary system.

Laparotomy

Laparotomy is hardly ever necessary in the investigation of PUO. It can, however, be helpful on rare occasions when lesions are demonstrable by imaging of the liver or lymph nodes but biopsy has proved impossible or unproductive. A minilaparotomy can then be performed, which really amounts to no more than an open biopsy. This permits distinction between, for instance, tuberculosis, sarcoidosis and reticulosis.

Making the most of biopsy material

This means more than simply performing histological examination. It is usual to fix biopsy material in formalin, but portions should also be retained in sterile water or saline, for bacteriological and virological examination. Different tissues may be handled in a number of ways.

Bone marrow or aspirates from abscesses and cysts can be cultured like blood cultures, or directly inoculated on to culture media. Solid tissues must be treated in the laboratory before inoculation. Smears may be prepared for later virological or bacteriological study. Specimens for viral culture may be refrigerated, but should not be frozen. Although cultures cannot be performed on fixed specimens and serology is rarely possible, DNA can survive fixation and may still be detectable by hybridization techniques.

Imaging and biopsy procedures in the diagnosis of pyrexia of unknown origin

1 Ultrasound scans (especially abdominal and pelvic; B, C).
2 Computed tomographic scan of the head or body (B, C).
3 Magnetic resonance scan of the head or body.
4 Gallium scan (whole-body).
5 Technetium bone scan.
6 Laparoscopy (B, C).
7 Bronchoscopy (B, C).
8 Minilaparotomy (B, C).
9 Liver biopsy (C).
10 Lymph-node biopsy (C).
11 Bone marrow biopsy (C).
12 Temporal artery biopsy .
13 Skin lesion biopsy (C).
B indicates that biopsy may be performed; C indicates that standard and tuberculosis culture should be performed.

Trials of therapy

Risks of trials of therapy

As a general rule, trials of therapy should be done late or not at all in the investigation of PUO. This is because the drugs usually trialled can make further investigation difficult or impossible. Many antimicrobial agents can also cause hypersensitivity reactions, which can exacerbate fever or cause problems such as rash, blood disorder or organ failure.

Broad-spectrum antimicrobial therapy may prevent recovery of organisms by culture while failing to treat the disease adequately. This is common in enteric fevers, brucellosis and *Streptococcus pyogenes* infections. Antimicrobial therapy alone may fail to resolve abscesses or loculated infections, which must still be identified and drained before fever will resolve. Standard multiple therapy for tuberculosis includes broad-spectrum agents such as rifampicin or streptomycin, which will also interfere with culture of pyogenic organisms. Tetracycline and co-trimoxazole may partly inhibit malarial parasites or other protozoa, masking parasitic infections.

Finally, corticosteroids can inhibit the immune responses which make serodiagnosis possible, and can make the difference between a useful or an unproductive tuberculin test response. By inhibiting protective inflammatory responses and producing 'false' improvement in fever, corticosteroids can allow untreated infection to advance, leading to complications such as perforation of hollow organs or dissemination of infection.

Risks of trials of therapy
1 Reduced usefulness of diagnostic cultures.
2 Modification of infection without cure.
3 Adverse reaction to therapy complicating the illness.
4 Corticosteroids may reduce the usefulness of immunological tests.
5 Corticosteroids may permit progressive infection with reduced signs of inflammation.

Uses of trials of therapy

In spite of the risks, there are situations where trials of therapy are unavoidable, and indeed indicated. The most important of these are cases in which a diagnosis is strongly suspected after investigation, but cannot be proved. If the suspected diagnosis is a specific infection, treatment may be attempted, using the narrowest possible antimicrobial spectrum which includes the relevant pathogen. Obtaining the expected response is then indicative of the presumed diagnosis.

Care must be taken not to treat another condition inadvertently; for instance, trial of antituberculosis treatment should be performed using isoniazid (INAH), pyrazinamide, ethambutol, etc., rather than drugs also active against pyogenic organisms. Patients undergoing a trial of corticosteroids should be examined frequently, and X-rays or imaging results should be reviewed, in case infection is potentiated by immunosuppression. Inability to stabilize the condition on reducing doses should cause review of the presumed diagnosis.

When the patient's condition is critical a 'blind' trial of therapy may be unavoidable. All possible specimens should first be obtained for culture. The physician must then make a best-guess decision on the treatment or treatments to try. If possible, treatments should be introduced sequentially but this is not always feasible in an emergency. Once started, treatment should not be stopped before it has had a chance to produce results; while many pyogenic infections improve promptly, enteric fevers may take up to a week and tuberculosis as much as a month to respond by improvement of fever.

Reasons to attempt trials of therapy
1 To gain further evidence for a suspected diagnosis by obtaining the expected response to therapy.
2 In an emergency when the patient's condition is unsatisfactory.

When treatment is apparently effective the difficult decision must be made as to how long it should be continued. This will depend on the type of condition suspected and on any laboratory data available. The temperature chart gives the earliest indication of success. Other helpful data include the C-reactive protein, which is a good indicator of response in endocarditis, and the ESR in tuberculosis. Successful treatment of tuberculosis may remove inhibition of cell-mediated immunity, causing the tuberculin test to become strongly positive and confirming the diagnosis. Treatment can then be continued for the appropriate 6 or 9 months. In connective tissue disorders the ESR or autoantibody levels are often useful guides to response. Non-specific indicators of response include the restoring of serum albumin levels and regaining lost body weight.

When no improvement can be obtained in PUO

This situation prevails in about 5% of most published series. It is not an indication for despair, for it is most common in cases with mild or subacute fevers. About half of these cases eventually recover and most of the others remain feverish but do not deteriorate. The commonest cause of prolonged high fever, defying diagnosis is lymphoma.

Investigation of PUO is therefore well worthwhile, usually leading to diagnosis and cure, and rarely ending in failure.

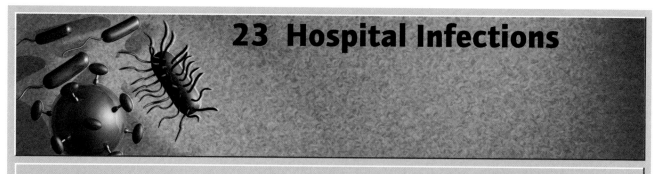

23 Hospital Infections

Introduction

The hospital is an ideal environment for the transmission of pathogens, because patients with similar diseases and susceptibilities are housed in an enclosed community. Patients share contact with many health care workers each day. In this setting, the ward, patients and workers become colonized by organisms adapted to the special environment. New susceptibles are frequently added to the population, and are at risk of colonization and infection. Approximately 10% of patients admitted to hospital develop a hospital-acquired infection at some point during their hospital stay.

Most hospital infections are wound, urinary and respiratory tract infections. In addition, immunocompromised patients readily develop infection with organisms of low virulence. Patients in the intensive therapy unit, where many antibiotics are used, can be colonized with naturally resistant organisms, which may invade, often causing pneumonia or bacteraemia.

Organisms with multiple antibiotic resistances can also cause problems on general wards. So-called methicillin-resistant *Staphylococcus aureus* (MRSA) strains are an example. Many are not only resistant to antistaphylococcal penicillins, but also to a range of other antistaphylococcal agents. If they cause infections, prolonged treatment may be necessary, using expensive or toxic drugs, such as teicoplanin or vancomycin.

Hospital infection not only imposes a burden of illness and prolonged admission on the patient; it also imposes the cost of investigation and treatment on the hospital, as well as preventing the use of the bed for other patients. It carries the risk of spread, particularly to other patients, and demands time-consuming and expensive control measures.

The concepts of host, organism and environment have already been discussed (see Chapter 1). The same approach can be applied to the behaviour of hospital infection. In this chapter the main hospital pathogens will be described. We will also review the special susceptibilities of patient populations to organisms which often have low pathogenicity in the community, and discuss features of the hospital environment which influence the transmission of these pathogens.

Patient susceptibilities to hospital infection

Although it seems glib to say that patients are in hospital because they are sick, the need for admission implies an alteration in host defences. This is obvious in patients immunocompromised by an illness such as leukaemia, or by treatment such as cytotoxic chemotherapy or high-dose corticosteroids. It is less obvious in fit patients admitted for routine surgery. However, the effects of anaesthesia and postoperative pain may inhibit coughing, leading to postoperative hypostatic pneumonia, or they may make micturition difficult, leading to urinary infection. It is essential therefore to assess each patient carefully for such factors.

Patient predispositions to hospital infection
1 Pre-existing condition (chronic chest disease, obstructed urinary outflow or previous immuno-suppression).
2 Need for invasive devices (intravenous cannulae, urinary catheters, etc.).
3 Effect of surgery (skin wound, tissue trauma, opening colonized viscus, anaesthetic, immobilization, introduction of foreign material such as joint prosthesis or arterial graft).
4 Effect of antibiotic treatment (antibiotic-associated diarrhoea, colonization by resistant organisms, predisposition to superficial fungal infections).
5 Effect of immunosuppressive treatment (corticosteroids, cancer chemotherapy or transplant immuno-suppression).
6 Exposure to health care workers and other patients who may transmit pathogens.
7 Exposure to pathogens in the environment, especially bedding and food.

Infection due to intravenous cannulae

Intravenous devices of many kinds can be placed in the vascular system for varying periods. The time for which they can be maintained depends partly on the likelihood of infection in each site. Peripheral venous catheters are readily colonized by organisms of the skin flora. Trivial infection, with mild inflammation, is common but more invasive disease with organisms such as *S. aureus* can cause significant morbidity and mortality (Fig. 23.1).

Many patients now have venous catheters which enter the right atrium. These may be used for intravascular monitoring, as with Swan–Ganz catheters, or to give intravenous feeding or drugs which are irritant to peripheral veins. When long-term intravenous therapy is required, long lines, such as Hickman or Portacath catheters, can be inserted via a subcutaneous track or tunnel. Infection in these devices is serious as, besides the infectious complications, the line must be replaced using a new tunnel. This is costly in terms of time and resources, and also requires a second operative procedure.

The common pathogens of intravenous catheters are flora from the skin of the host, particularly *S. epidermidis* and *S. aureus*. More rarely, corynebacteria may be implicated, especially the naturally multidrug-resistant species *Corynebacterium jeikeium*, which may cause line-related sepsis in leukaemic patients.

Clinical features

These are usually mild unless septicaemia supervenes. Vigilance is important in detecting this early stage, when treatment is likely to be successful, and complications few. There may be signs of inflammation at the site of the skin entry, with tenderness, cellulitis or slight purulent exudate. As in infective endocarditis, bacteraemia is usually continuous. Fever is often present but is usually mild — around 37.5–38.5 °C. When line-related sepsis is likely, the patient should also be examined for signs of metastatic infection or endocarditis.

Prevention and control

The control of line-related sepsis must start in the medical and nursing schools. A strict protocol of skin disinfection and sterile technique must always be used when inserting intravenous access devices. The choice of device is also important. Those with side ports are prone to colonization at the site where no flow occurs. Giving sets may also provide a nidus for colonization. This is especially true if multiple access points are available, each with a dead space where fluids can become static. Contamination can be introduced into intravenous fluids and giving sets by repeated addition of drugs to the intravenous system. Ideally additive drugs should be incorporated into intravenous fluids in the manufacturing pharmacy, under sterile and controlled conditions.

The most important factor in preventing line-related sepsis is the regular review of inserted lines. To facilitate this the date when lines were inserted must be documented in the patient's case record. Peripheral intravenous lines should ideally be resited every 48 h. Central lines should be changed at least weekly. The life of tunnelled lines is much longer, but clinicians must be aware of the risks of infection, and intervene to remove the line whenever it occurs. Special situations, such as intravenous feeding, encourage infection by providing a rich supply of nutrients within the lumen. They are best managed by a specialist team which includes clinicians, pharmacists and microbiologists.

Measures to prevent line-related sepsis
1 Choice of device (excluding side ports and dead spaces).
2 Aseptic and atraumatic insertion.
3 Additive drugs and parenteral feeds prepared in the pharmacy.
4 Maintaining adequate hygiene and dressing of insertion site.
5 Regular review of insertion site.

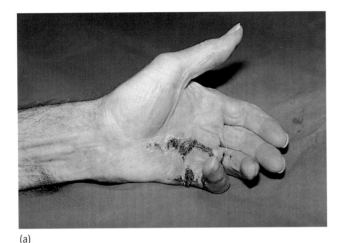

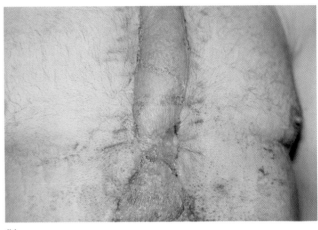

(a)   (b)

Fig. 23.1 (a) An infected minor operation wound on the hand. Methicillin-resistant *Staphylococcus auraus* (MRSA) was recovered from swabs. (b) A patient in the same ward required skin grafting after MRSA infection of a sternotomy wound.

6 Replacing giving set (and cannula when indicated) at appropriate intervals.
7 Removing cannula from inflamed site.
8 Removing or changing cannula in a bacteraemic patient.

Treatment

When bacteraemia is associated with an intravenous access device the device should be removed. The skin insertion site and the cannula tip should both be cultured, and blood culture should be obtained, both through the infected device and via a separate, peripheral site. When the infecting organism is of low virulence such as *S. epidermidis*, this should be sufficient but if the infection is severe a glycopeptide antibiotic can be given for 48 h. When *S. aureus* is the infecting organism, 2 weeks' intravenous antistaphylococcal therapy is needed to minimize mortality and complications. After completion of treatment, physical review should be performed to exclude persisting focal infection, such as endocarditis or osteomyelitis. When *S. epidermidis* colonizes a 'precious' cannula, an attempt to eradicate the organisms by intracannular treatment with a glycopeptide is sometimes made. Even if successful, this should be followed by vigilant review to detect recrudescence.

Management of line-related sepsis
1 Removal of the affected device.
2 Culture of site, cannula and blood.
3 Short course of glycopeptide antibiotic (active against staphylococci and corynebacteria).
4 Full treatment if *Staphylococcus aureus* is isolated.
5 Review need for insertion of new device.

Infection associated with urinary catheters

Indwelling urinary catheters provide an easy route for ascending infection of the urinary tract. After a number of days organisms will reach the bladder, often by ascending between the catheter and the urethral wall. Permanent bladder catheterization is always associated with bacterial colonization of the urine.

Gram-negative organisms are the commonest colonizers of the catheterized bladder. *Escherichia coli*, *Klebsiella pneumoniae* and *Pseudomonas* spp. are often seen. *Proteus* spp. are also seen in chronically stagnant urine; their ability to metabolize urea and produce alkaline ammonia predisposes to the deposition of calcium as stones or 'sand'. In turn, these deposits can act as a reservoir of infection.

After transurethral prostatectomy, *S. aureus* or coagulase-negative staphylococci can cause urinary colonization, occasionally complicated by epididymitis.

Catheter-related urinary colonization is often asymptomatic, but there is a risk of ascending infection or bacteraemia if the catheter becomes blocked or is vigorously manipulated. Colonization is inevitable and is not treated, in case a more aggressive and resistant organism should replace the existing one. If fever, urinary tract symptoms or rigors occur, appropriate antibiotic therapy should be given. The catheter should usually be replaced before chemotherapy is discontinued, to ensure adequate drainage of the bladder and to remove a possible nidus of infection.

Closed drainage systems, in which the catheter is never opened directly to the environment, delay the entry and ascent of organisms, and afford a barrier to the introduction of hospital pathogens from attendants' hands. The risks can also be minimized by careful attention to aseptic technique when the catheter is inserted, and to the personal hygiene of the catheterized patient.

> **Avoiding urinary catheter-related sepsis**
> 1 Sterile, atraumatic insertion.
> 2 Appropriate choice of catheter type and size.
> 3 Use of closed drainage systems.
> 4 Maintenance of good patient hygiene.
> 5 Replacing catheter at appropriate intervals.
> 6 Removing calcific deposits from the bladder (if they form).
> 7 Avoiding excessive catheter manipulation or unneccessary bladder washouts.
> 8 Treating bacteriuria only when symptomatic.

Susceptibilities of intensive therapy patients

Patients in the intensive therapy unit (ITU) are susceptible to infection for several reasons. Immune responses are often diminished by the stress and metabolic effects of existing disease. Many patients in intensive care have recently undergone anaesthetic and surgical risks. Additionally, many of the barriers to infection provided by innate immunity (see Chapter 1) are breached because of the need for complex intravenous therapy, invasive monitoring, artificial ventilation and the need for extracorporeal procedures such as dialysis or haemofiltration.

Tracheal intubation and artificial ventilation

The endotracheal tube provides a route for organisms in the pharynx to overcome the mucociliary blanket defence and gain access to the lower respiratory tract. As the patient has been in hospital for some time and may have received several courses of antibiotics it is not unusual for the normal upper respiratory flora to have been replaced with Gram-negative organisms or enterococci, which may be resistant to many first-line antibiotics. Artificial ventilation usually imposes the need for muscular paralysis; this inhibits the normal sighing and coughing reflexes, further reducing the ability of patients to resist bacterial invasion of the lungs.

The patient in the ITU has a multiplicity of intravenous and intra-arterial cannulae. To reduce the risk of cannula-related sepsis, regular changes of cannulae, giving sets, three-way taps and other associated equipment are required.

In addition to the special risks of intensive care, many patients will have reduced innate and specific immunity because of organ failure, underlying malignancy, previous or pre-existing infection or chronic airways disease.

> **Common causes of lung infections in hospital settings**
> 1 *Streptococcus pneumoniae* (often local strains, may be penicillin-tolerant).
> 2 Methicillin-resistant *Staphylococcus aureus* (usually needs glycopeptide treatment).
> 3 *Moraxella catarrhalis* (usually produces beta-lactamase).
> 4 *Klebsiella pneumoniae* (always resistant to ampicillin).
> 5 *Escherichia coli*.
> 6 Enterococci (need beta-lactam/aminoglycoside, alternatively aminoglycoside–glycopeptide combination, meropenem or imipenem; a few are aminoglycoside- or glycopeptide-resistant).
> 7 *Pseudomonas* or related organisms (need aminoglycoside, ureidopenicillin or antipseudomonal cephalosporin).
> 8 *Candida* (needs fluconazole as itraconazole is unpredictably distributed in critically ill patients).
> 9 Other yeasts (may need amphotericin treatment).

Most patients in the ITU also have an indwelling urinary catheter, and this may also act as a source of sepsis and secondary septicaemia.

The types of organisms causing local and bacteraemic infections in the ITU depend on local environmental factors and antibiotic usage. Common pathogens causing problems of treatment include *Klebsiella*, other antibiotic-resistant Gram-negative rods and enterococci. MRSA can cause intermittent outbreaks of colonizations and infections.

Surgery and its contribution to infection

Very extensive and complex surgery is possible, using modern techniques and anaesthetics, but the impact of infection on the outcome should not be forgotten. Lister, the pioneer of antiseptic surgery, said that each operation was an experiment in bacteriology. This remains true today, though more control can be exerted over the experiment and its adverse effects. Patients must often be admitted to the ITU after a complex operation. This adds to the range of infections to which they are susceptible.

A number of factors influence the occurrence of infection in surgical patients: the patient, the operation, the antimicrobial prophylaxis, the surgical team and the postoperative care.

The patient

Patients often come to surgery with pre-existing health problems. Minimizing the time between admission and the surgical procedure will limit the opportunity to acquire resistant hospital pathogens. Wherever possible, existing infection should be treated before surgery is undertaken. Patients with respiratory infections should receive appropriate antibiotics and physiotherapy. Antimicrobials should not be prescribed for trivial reasons in advance of surgery, as these may allow the replacement of sensitive normal flora with multidrug-resistant hospital strains.

Prophylaxis of surgical infections

The introduction of antimicrobial prophylaxis has done much to reduce the incidence of surgical infection. There are a number of basic principles which guide its use. The agents used should be bactericidal and active against the organisms likely to be implicated in infection. To ensure that they are available at the susceptible site at the time of operation, the first dose is often given as part of pre-medication if intramuscular, or at induction if intravenous. There is no evidence that additional benefit is gained by continuing prophylaxis for more than 1–3 days.

Choosing appropriate surgical prophylaxis

For this purpose, operations can be classified into three categories: clean, contaminated and infected.

Clean operations

In clean operations only the skin, or a site such as a joint which is normally bacteriologically sterile, is breached. In this case, the common organisms implicated in postoperative infection are staphylococci from the skin. Postoperative infection after clean operations is almost always mild wound infection, and affects less than 2% of patients. Antimicrobial prophylaxis is not usually indicated.

The exception is when a prosthetic device, such as a vascular graft or hip prosthesis, is to be inserted. In these circumstances the consequences of infection are catastrophic and prophylaxis is indicated.

Systems designed to minimize the transmission of skin bacteria into the operation site include filtered air supplies to the operating theatre and impermeable, ventilated suits for surgeons.

Attempts to eradicate those bacteria which enter the wound include the use of antibiotic-impregnated orthopaedic cement, and even antibiotic-impregnated intravascular prostheses. Nevertheless, the most common organisms infecting implanted devices remain staphylococci from the patient's own skin.

Neurosurgical operations in which the meninges are opened carry a risk of postsurgical meningitis. This is rare, but when it occurs it is often with *S. aureus* or Gram-negative organisms, including *Pseudomonas* spp. and *Acinetobacter* spp.

Contaminated operations

In these operations the surgeon opens an organ, such as the large bowel, which possesses a normal flora. Without prophylaxis the risk of infection varies between 10 and 40%. When the bowel is opened, a mixture of facultative and obligate anaerobes are released, and prophylaxis active against these organisms should include metronidazole and a broad-spectrum antibiotic such as a second-generation cephalosporin. In the upper gastrointestinal tract obligate anaerobes are uncommon and prophylaxis with a second-generation cephalosporin alone is adequate. After gastric and duodenal surgery, candidal infections occasionally occur. When obstruction is present, obligate anaerobes may accumulate, for example in the biliary tree or stomach, and the prophylaxis must be adjusted accordingly.

Instrumentation through a colonized or infected hollow organ is similar to a contaminated operation. Examples are cystoscopy or ureteroscopy of the infected urinary tract and endoscopic retrograde cholangiopancreatography, when the endoscope must enter the sterile biliary tree after passing through the colonized duodenum. Prophylaxis must be given in these circumstances, as the risk of infection approaches 100%, and bacteraemia is common.

Infected operations

Infected operations are those in which infection already exists, and contamination with pathogens is inevitable. Drainage of an intraperitoneal abscess and excision of perforated bowel are good examples. Appropriate antimicrobial therapy, rather than prophylaxis, should be prescribed in this situation.

> **Examples of prophylactic regimens for surgical procedures**
> 1 For upper gastrointestinal tract, endoscopic retrograde cholangiopancreatography or infected biliary tree: single dose of gentamicin *or* broad-spectrum cephalosporin 2 h before surgery.

2 For colonic and rectal surgery: single dose of gentamicin *or* cefuroxime *plus* metronidazole 2 h before surgery.
3 For hysterectomy: single dose of metronidazole, rectally or i.v. 1–2 h before surgery.
4 For high amputations of the leg: benzylpenicillin i.v. or i.m. 300–600 mg 6-hourly for 5 days *or* metronidazole rectally 1 g or i.v. 500 mg 8-hourly for 5 days.
5 For joint replacement: cefuroxime or co-amoxiclav in standard parenteral doses for not more than 3 days (bone cement also contains aminoglycoside to inhibit skin-derived staphylococci).

The surgical team

The surgical team, or scrubbed team, is intimately involved with the operation. If one of the team has an infected or colonized skin or respiratory site, the pathogen involved, often a streptococcus or staphylococcus, may be shed into the patient's wound. The number of bacteria released into the operating theatre air depends on the number of persons in the theatre and their movement. The surgical team should therefore be as small as possible, and movements should be limited as much as possible.

The number of organisms shed can also be related to the design of surgical gowns and the type of material used. A direct relationship between this and postoperative infection is less clear. Impervious materials reduce shedding to a minimum but are very uncomfortable to wear. In the Charnley system, where the surgical team wear impervious 'space suits', these have individual air supplies and are cooled.

Surgical infections in immunocompromised patients

Modern medical practice means that there are now many patients with severe immunocompromise (see Chapter 21). These patients, however, do not form a homogeneous group. In addition to their underlying condition which imposes differing infection risks, the nature of the immunocompromise will alter the range of infections to which they are subject. Renal and liver transplant patients require less immunosuppression to prevent rejection and are therefore subject to fewer opportunist infections than cardiac or bone marrow transplant patients, in whom infection is a more important determinant of outcome. In understanding the nature of the infection risks to which patients are exposed it is convenient to discuss these under treatment and immune factors.

Treatment considerations

In many patients the transplantation or other therapeutic intervention imposes particular surgical risks. In cardiac transplantation the chest wall wound is a common site of infection, as is the urinary tract in renal transplant patients. For patients given radiotherapy, radiation damage to the intestinal epithelium makes bacterial escape across the gut wall more likely. After liver transplantation, postoperative infections such as cholangitis and biliary peritonitis are related to the surgery on the biliary tract.

Immune considerations

Different diseases have a differing impact on the various components of the immune system. In some, such as human immunodeficiency virus (HIV) infection, the major effect falls on T-cell function. Cyclosporin treatment also has a major immunosuppressive effect on T cells. In multiple myelomatosis the main effect is on humoral immunity. Neutrophils are principally affected in patients undergoing induction chemotherapy for leukaemia. Other conditions such as splenectomy can cause poor clearance of blood-borne parasites, and a defect in control of capsulate organisms. Immunodeficiency is seldom purely cellular or humoral: for instance, T-cell disorder also leads to humoral deficiency, because of the lack of T-helper function.

Environmental factors in hospital infection

The hospital environment is very different from the general environment, and poses particular dangers to patients least equipped to resist infection. Hospitals provide many opportunities for person-to-person transmission by contact. Hospital food may transmit food-borne disease if kitchen hygiene or food handling is unsatisfactory. Food is often a reservoir of local *Pseudomonas* strains. The air supply in the hospital environment is controlled and may allow for the transmission of aerosol-borne organisms such as legionellae if systems are not properly maintained. Similarly, air-borne organisms such as varicella-zoster virus can spread rapidly in the hospital environment if the appropriate control measures are not taken. *Aspergillus* spores always exist in unfiltered air, and can infect neutropenic patients.

Water supply

The water supply of a hospital is complex. Unlike a domestic building or an office system there are great demands for water which must be delivered to a very large number of sites and often with different requirements. In addition to supplying wash-hand basins and showers, there is a need for central heating and air-conditioning. Several departments also require the delivery of steam for heating or disinfection.

In the life of a hospital, water use will evolve with changing demands, and changes of use of ward and laboratory areas. This affords many opportunities for lengths of pipework to be extended, or to go out of use. Cold water may become stagnant in these areas, or hot water may lose its heat. A great danger is that *Legionella* spp. will colonize the warm water, especially when stagnant water has given up its protective chlorine. Sporadic cases or outbreaks of legionellosis may then occur. Inadequately cleaned and disinfected air-conditioning systems or cooling towers are also common sources of legionellosis (see p. 141). *Legionella pneumophila* serogroup 1 tends to cause classic legionnaire's disease, while other strains have reduced virulence, usually only causing disease in immunocompromised patients.

Any area where fast-running water may cause aerosols is a potential source of infection. Shower heads and spray-type taps may harbour legionellae in rubber washers, and disperse large numbers.

Frequent use, adequate maintenance and cleaning are all important in minimizing risk. Legionellae cannot survive at temperatures above 55°C, or replicate below 20°C. The risk of scalding by adequately hot water can be reduced by installing mixer taps. Redundant or overlong stretches of pipework, where legionellae could multiply in stagnant water at suitable temperature, must be avoided. Pasteurizing the hot water system, by applying extra heat, may help to clear legionellae from the system. In addition it may be necessary to add additional chlorine to the cold water system. These measures may be necessary after pipework has been decommissioned for repair or alteration.

Control of legionellae in hospitals

1 Minimize long or redundant runs of pipework.
2 Ensure adequate chlorination of cold water.
3 Ensure adequate temperature of hot water.
4 Avoid spray taps and rubber washers.
5 Maintain taps, shower heads and cooling systems meticulously.
6 Consider pasteurization of colonized hot water systems.

Air supply

The piping and trunking of hospital air-conditioning may accumulate much dust and building debris over a period of years. Sporing organisms and fungi such as *Aspergillus* spp. may thrive in these conditions. They can be discharged into the air and cause respiratory or systemic disease in susceptible individuals. Operating theatres, laboratories and individual patient isolation rooms are sites of particular risk.

Operating theatres

The construction and maintenance of operating theatres is a specialist subject. The emphasis is on easy-to-clean, impermeable surfaces, including those of movable equipment. Design is intended to minimize the need for movement of staff, and to direct the movement of patient, staff and theatre waste away from the operating or clean areas, rather than towards or through them.

There are guidelines which set out the maximum number of organisms tolerable in the air of an operating theatre. Air is supplied to the theatre through filters. Before the theatres may be used, and following repairs to the filters or other decommissioning, air quality should be tested. A special air sampler (e.g. Casella slit sampler) is used, which draws a known volume of air through a slit and deposits particles on solid bacteriological medium. Colonies of organisms can be counted after the medium is incubated, and speciation performed if indicated.

Hospital equipment and the spread of infection

Disposable hospital equipment such as syringes, needles, blood lancets, scalpels, intravenous cannulae and urinary catheters makes the introduction of infection by often-repeated invasive procedures very rare. Blood-borne infections can still be transmitted, however, by inoculation accidents with used sharp instruments. Most hospitals have strict protocols for the handling and disposal of sharps.

Some equipment is too complex and expensive for single use. Examples include endoscopes and associated biopsy equipment, complex surgical instruments, positive-pressure ventilators and high air-loss beds. These all have internal channels which can come into contact with body fluids, wound exudates or infected tissues. All have been involved in hospital outbreaks of infection. Automated cleaning systems, in which a sequence of cleaning solutions and disinfectants are pumped through the equipment for a fixed time, have reduced mishaps in decontamination after use. Such systems are expensive, and can only be used properly if the hospital possesses enough equipment to allow a satisfactory cleaning cycle before the next use.

Even such apparently simple equipment as mattresses, linen and beds can contribute to infection. The impermeable covers of mattresses can develop holes, allowing moisture and bacteria to enter. Linen which is washed at too low a temperature, or not pressed, can be contaminated by spore-bearing organisms. Low skin-pressure beds may be made of foam components, plastic beads or air-filled rubber bubbles, all of which can accumulate fluid and pathogens if not properly maintained and cleaned. All of these have caused outbreaks of skin infection, sometimes with systemic extension, often in patients with burns, skin grafts or immunosuppressive conditions.

Isolation facilities in hospitals

There are two main types of patient isolation, designed for different purposes. In source isolation the aim is to ensure that the organisms infecting or colonizing the patient are not transmitted to other patients or staff. In protective isolation the aim is to prevent organisms being transmitted to patients with special susceptibility to infection.

Source isolation

There are several types of source isolation depending on the infection that is being controlled. It is traditional to divide these into groups depending on the routes of transmission. These include blood, wound and enteric, and respiratory isolation. It is simpler, and mistakes are less likely, if a universal type of isolation is practised for all infected patients, and this is now becoming common practice in many western hospital settings.

More stringent, high-security isolation is occasionally indicated for dangerous infections, whose treatment is difficult and which may be transmitted to medical carers. Only a few viral haemorrhagic fevers, rare bacterial pneumonias such as plague and anthrax, and some fungal pneumonias fall into this category.

Blood, wound and enteric isolation

The purpose of blood, wound and enteric isolation is to prevent the transmission of organisms normally spread by contact or ingestion. Patients are nursed in a side room which contains a wash-hand basin and preferably a separate toilet facility. Nursing and medical staff remove white coats before entering the room and put on an apron or gown. The apron is discarded and hands are washed before leaving the room. Gloves are worn when handling the patient's body fluids or excreta.

Infections which can be contained by blood, wound and enteric precautions
1 Most bacteraemias.
2 Localized infections and wounds of the skin.
3 Infections with methicillin-resistant *Staphyloccus aureus*.
4 Viral hepatitides.
5 Infectious diarrhoeas.

Respiratory isolation

The precautions taken here are similar to blood, wound and enteric precautions, but the patient's room should be ventilated by a system that extracts the air to the exterior, and does not permit air flow into other ward areas. If the patient is transferred to another department of the hospital for further treatment or investigations, such as the radiology department, the patient may wear a face mask. The mask does not prevent contact with organisms suspended in droplet nuclei, but it does provide a barrier against gross contamination by fragments or large droplets of sputum which may be produced during coughing. Nurses or physiotherapists having close facial contact with a patient may wear face masks for similar reasons.

Contamination of the air outside the patient's room can be minimized by keeping the door closed. This will also ensure that the ventilation system is not overloaded by extraneous air flows.

Infections which can be contained by respiratory isolation
1 Pulmonary tuberculosis (sensitive organisms; for first two weeks of treatment: resistant organisms; until sputum smear is negative).
2 Varicella and herpes zoster.
3 Measles.
4 Pertussis.
5 Diphtheria.
6 Skin infections in patients with exfoliative conditions.
7 Chest infections caused by unusually resistant organisms.

Control of drug-resistant pulmonary tuberculosis in hospitals

Patients should be managed in single-room isolation until two or three successive sputum smears are negative for acid–alcohol bacilli. The patient's room should be at negative pressure relative to the adjacent hospital areas. To reduce the bacterial load in the room, air should be extracted to the exterior to be replaced by clean air which will dilute organisms in the room (the US Centers for Disease Control recommend six complete air changes per hour).

Susceptible visitors to the room should wear close-fitting filter masks which cover nose and mouth. Care attendants who have received BCG immunization, or who are tuberculin text reactors may not require routine respiratory protection, but should use it for such procedures as obtaining induced sputum specimens or performing bronchial lavage, bronchoscopy or upper GI endoscopy.

High-security isolation

Highly secure isolation is provided by rooms in which the air flow is strictly controlled, and all air leaving the room is filtered to remove droplet or viral particles. Attendant staff wear protective clothing, including face protection, gloves, trousers and boots which provide a barrier to personal contamination. In exceptional cases, filtered respiratory protection is indicated, or the patient may be cared for in a filtered environment such as a bed isolator. All infectious waste from such units is decontaminated by heat or chemical methods before leaving the area. These facilities are only available in specialist units. Small-scale, negative-pressure filtered isolators are available for the laboratory handling of specimens containing dangerous pathogens (Fig. 23.2).

Strict isolation methods have recently been applied to the control of multidrug-resistant tuberculosis, after the occurrence of outbreaks in patients and care workers. Patients have been nursed in negative-pressure single rooms and this has assisted in the control of epidemics. In the UK, bacillus Calmette–Guérin (BCG) vaccine is offered to all individuals, and this may have helped to prevent outbreaks among health workers (see Chapter 18).

Protective isolation

Protective isolation is used for patients who are highly susceptible to infection (see Chapter 21). Patients with severe neutropenia are nursed in protective isolation when their neutrophil count falls below $0.5 \times 10^9/l$. Protection is not only physical, in the form of single-room isolation and filtered air to reduce the risk of *Aspergillus* infection, but must also include arrangements to control the risk of infection from such sources as Gram-negative organisms in food or *Listeria* in soft cheeses.

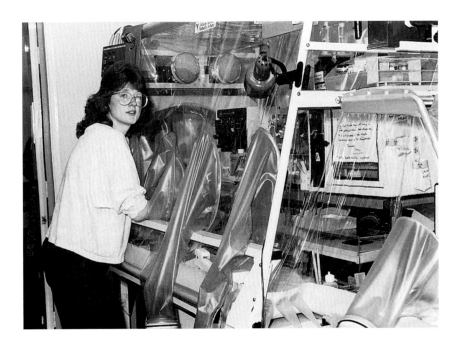

Fig. 23.2 Negative-pressure filter isolator for high-security laboratory work. This laboratory contains an incubator, an automated blood count machine, a cassette-based biochemistry analyser, a coagulometer, a plain patometer, a microscope and a centrifuge in a bench area of 2 m².

Often the most difficult aspect of all these forms of isolation is ensuring that staff adhere to the effective policies. Large ward rounds, many ancillary staff, numbers of untrained voluntary workers and crowds of visitors all contribute to transmission of infection, and busy staff may often neglect the simple precautions of hand-washing when work pressures become intense.

Prevention of infection in laboratories

In European legislation, pathogens come under the heading of biological agents and are classified into categories depending on the hazard that they present to the people who work with them. Where they are handled in the workplace, an assessment of the resulting risk must be made, and protocols to minimize this designed in accordance with the provisions of the Control of Substances Hazardous to Health (COSHH) regulations.

Definition of a biological agent
Any microorganism, cell culture or human endoparasite, including any which have been genetically modified, which may cause any infection, allergy, toxicity or otherwise create a hazard to human health.

In the UK the Advisory Committee on Dangerous Pathogens (ACDP) is a committee of the Health and Safety Executive, which advises on the design and operation of laboratories and other workplaces, depending on the type of organisms handled. Pathogens may be classified according to the recommendations of the ACDP and other countries have similar systems. They give four hazard groups:

Category 1: An organism that is most unlikely to cause human disease.

Category 2: An organism that may cause human disease and that might be a hazard to laboratory workers but is unlikely to spread in the community. Laboratory exposure rarely produces infection and effective prophylaxis or treatment is usually available.

Category 3: An organism that may cause severe human disease and presents a serious hazard to laboratory workers. It may present a risk of spread to the community, but there is usually effective prophylaxis or effective treatment available.

Category 4: An organism that causes severe human disease and is a serious hazard to laboratory workers. It may present a high risk of spread to the community and there is usually no effective prophylaxis or treatment (Table 23.1).

Pathogen	Laboratory procedures
Category 2	
Staphylococcus aureus	Open, easily cleanable bench with
Streptococcus pyogenes	adequate workspace; dedicated working
Escherichia coli	overall; separate rest area; no eating,
Cytomegalovirus	drinking, smoking, etc. in the laboratory;
	hand-washing facilities available in the
	laboratory
Category 3	
Salmonella typhi	As above, plus: separate room dedicated
Shigella dysenteriae	to this category; manipulations must be
Brucella spp.	performed in class 1 safety cabinets;
Mycobacterium tuberculosis	dedicated overalls; hand-washing
Hepatitis B virus	facilities in room; ventilation by
	air extraction to exterior
Category 4	
Rabies virus	As above, but separate unit away
Lassa virus	from general circulation; HEPA-filtered,
Marburg virus	negative-pressure ventilation; all work
Ebola virus	in class 3 cabinets or laboratory isolator;
	all laboratory waste and effluent
	disinfected before leaving unit

Table 23.1 Examples of the categorization of pathogens and their laboratory handling. HEPA, high efficiency particulate air.

Laboratory safety requires a well-designed laboratory suite. Attention must be paid to the materials employed in floors, walls and benching, and to the provision of services, including water supply and ventilation.

High containment facilities (level 3) must be provided for any laboratory likely to isolate organisms in hazard group 3 or which examines specimens which might contain such organisms (e.g. sputum). A laboratory suite may contain many laboratories and facilities, such as media preparation rooms, autoclave facilities, an incubator room and a cold room. Each of the individual laboratories within the clinical microbiology suite should conform to containment level 2 or containment level 3 (COSHH regulations).

A containment level 3 laboratory should be sited away from the main work of the department and access limited to authorized personnel who are trained in the use of the room and in the manipulation of hazard group 3 organisms. The doors should be locked when not in use. A continuous air flow through the laboratory must be maintained when work is in progress. A system must operate to prevent positive pressurization of the room if the extraction fans fail. Reversed air flows into the ventilation system must also be prevented. A microbiological safety cabinet of class 1 or class 2 conforming to British Standard (BS) 5726 or its equivalent must be available and all procedures where cultures or specimens are manipulated must be performed in this cabinet. It should be exhausted through a HEPA filter to the outside air. The laboratory should be sealable so that it can be fumigated.

Safety cabinets

Class 1 cabinets

Class 1 cabinets or exhaust-protective cabinets (BS 5726) are simple in design, with air being drawn through the face of the cabinet and out through the HEPA filter to the outside air.

Class 2 cabinets

Air is drawn into the cabinet through a HEPA filter and directed downwards on to the work surface. A portion of the filtered air is extracted. Class 2 microbiological safety cabinets provide protection to the operator and also to the work. They are, therefore, suitable for tissue culture, where contamination of cell-lines is minimized.

Class 3 cabinets

These are similar in clinical design to class 1 cabinets. However, air is drawn into the cabinet and exhausted through a HEPA filter. It is fully enclosed and the operator works through glove ports (Fig. 23.3). This type of cabinet provides maximum protection to the worker from aerosol hazard. Some argue that the need to manipulate all materials and equipment with gloved hands increases the risk of accidental self-inoculation when needles and other sharp implements must be used.

Containment level 4

Containment level 4 laboratories are rare and usually localized at national reference or research laboratories. They are operated on the basis of complete security of the material used in the laboratory. Laboratory workers change fully before entering the laboratory via an air-lock while work is contained in class 3 cabinets and there is a negative pressure between the laboratory, the air-lock and the outside. Air enters through HEPA filters and is extracted through a pair of HEPA filters. A double-sided interlocked autoclave ensures that all material leaving the laboratory is rendered safe. The worker

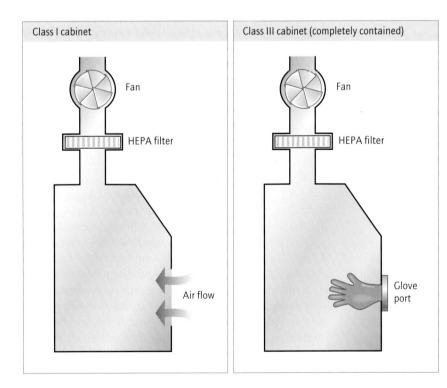

Fig. 23.3 Class 1 and class 3 exhaust-ventilated cabinets. HEPA, high efficiency particulate air.

should be visible within the laboratory through glass panels and an intercom or telephone system provided with an additional competent person available to assist in emergencies. Respirators must be available for this contingency.

Control of infection in hospitals

Appropriate organization and effective management protocols are essential to the control of hospital infection. These arrangements promote good clinical practice to minimize the occurrence of infection, and allow co-ordinated response to outbreaks when they arise. The control of infection organization has two main strands: the control of infection committee and the control of infection team.

Control of infection committee

The control of infection committee is generally a subcommittee of the senior medical committee of the hospital, and is empowered to develop and implement infection control policies and procedures. The chairperson of the committee is usually the consultant microbiologist or a consultant of equivalent expertise, such as the consultant in infectious diseases or communicable disease control. Other key staff include a hospital manager, and senior representatives from hospital services involved in infection control procedures (operating theatres, sterile supplies, nursing staff, cleaning and catering services, maintenance services and medical and surgical departments). The committee should be able to co-opt those professionals whose expertise or co-operation are required.

When an outbreak occurs, the control of infection committee may meet to coordinate a response, although in general a smaller group is often more practical, and clinicians and nursing staff from the affected area can be co-opted.

Control of infection team

The control of infection team is the core group whose role is to implement the control of infection policy, and to monitor its effectiveness. This team usually consists of the control of infection officer who is also the chairperson of the control of infection committee, and the control of infection nursing staff, often including ward-based control of infection 'link' nurses. They work together to manage the control of infection policy on a day-to-day basis, to collect statistics on infection rates

and to identify any problems. The team will monitor compliance with the policy at ward level and will implement emergency control measures when indicated. It will undertake specific surveillance of particular organisms, such as MRSA in surgical units, *Klebsiella* endemicity in ITUs and antibiotic-resistant urinary pathogens, and will screen suspected carriers. It will also provide assistance and advice to hospital staff on current policy, and on developments made necessary by changes of activity or procedures in various hospital departments.

The remit of the control of infection team and committee is necessarily wide and impact closely on the activity of many clinical and other departments. This is because apparently trivial factors can have a profound effect on transmission of microorganisms in the hospital environment.

Control of infection standards

Examples of these have been drawn up by the Association of Medical Microbiologists, the Hospital Infection Society and the Infection Control Association in the Public Health Laboratory Service. The Department of Health has recently issued guidelines developed by a broad-based advisory group. It sets out criteria for management structure and responsibilities related to control of infection. It recommends policies and procedures for appropriate microbiological services, surveillance for the control of infection, and relevant education policies.

It suggests that an infection control structure with sufficient resources and clear lines of responsibility should be set out. This responsibility should lie directly with the senior management of the hospital. A control of infection committee and effective control of infection team should be present. The plans for controlling outbreaks of infection should be laid down by the control of infection committee. The remit is very wide, involving all aspects of the hospital, including the mortuary services, sterile supply services, the hotel services, engineering, disposal of waste products and purchase of all equipment. None of these ideals can be serviced without an adequate microbiological laboratory and standards related to this are laid down. Regular surveillance for infections should be in place. Education is the main method of preventing transmission of infection and the infection control team should be central to the education of medical, nursing and paramedical staff. Adequate resources and staffing should be provided by the hospital management to ensure that this important task can be carried out.

Control of an outbreak

With effective control of infection procedures in place, outbreaks ideally should be the exception. They are inevitable however because of the nature of the hospital environment, admitting patients from the community who may be incubating diseases such as *Salmonella* infections or chickenpox. Each department must have a plan for responding to outbreaks which can be foreseen, such as *Salmonella* infections, MRSA, legionnaire's disease and multidrug-resistant Gram-negative organisms.

There are three main strands to controlling outbreaks within the hospital. Once a true outbreak has been confirmed they are: (i) to identify the source or reservoir; (ii) to halt the transmission; and (iii) to modify the host risk.

Identifying sources and reservoirs

The reservoirs are identified by screening patients within the hospital environment or before admission to hospital. Patients coming from hospitals with known epidemics, e.g. MRSA, may be screened for the presence of this organism and isolated until shown to be negative. Where the environment is the reservoir of infection, for example in legionnaire's disease, it may be necessary to sample the water supply at various points. Outbreaks such as MRSA infections may continue by person-to-person spread. Testing other patients and staff then becomes important in identifying the source of the problem.

Halting transmission

This is the most difficult aspect of infection control as it involves improving routine procedures such as hand-washing and asepsis, isolating colonized and infected patients, and modifying the way in which patients are nursed. Cohort nursing or targeted nursing may allow individual groups of infected patients to be nursed by a team not involved with caring for other, non-infected patients. It may be necessary to stop admitting new patients until the situation is controlled.

Modifying host factors

It is more difficult to modify the host risks. Some of these remit naturally as patients recover from operations or can cease immunosuppressive drugs. Where epidemics of multidrug-resistant organisms are the problem, it may be possible to modify the host risk by controlling antibiotic usage. This will require liaison between the prescribing clinicians and the microbiology and infection control teams.

Hospital cleaning and disinfection

These are two important aspects of the control of infection committee's work. If the hospital is clean and its equipment and special areas adequately disinfected, staff can work safely and the risk of spreading infection is minimised.

Disinfection

Disinfection is the removal of sufficient microbial contamination from equipment to allow its safe use. This may range from the cleaning and disinfection of a vacated bed to the removal of all microbial contamination from a reusable surgical instrument.

Disinfection by cleaning

This is an extremely effective way of cleaning floors, furniture and ordinary work surfaces. It entails the removal of dust and organic matter by wiping or washing with detergent solution, and then wiping dry with a clean cloth. Machine-washing cutlery and crockery at an adequate heat (above 80°C) is a good method of decontamination, as is washing linen at an adequate temperature (above 75°C). Steam-pressing bed sheets and towels is sufficient to remove many bacterial spores.

In some circumstances additional treatment with disinfectants (various types of antibacterial agents) is necessary to reduce bacterial contamination further. Different types of disinfectants are used for different purposes:

1 Chloros (sodium hypochlorite or bleach) is an oxidizing agent which kills most vegetative bacteria and many viruses. A 1% solution is used for cleaning surfaces, and for disinfecting spillages, a 10% solution is poured over, before they are wiped up, or absorbed into granules and swept up. It is toxic to humans and corrodes many metals.

2 Halogen disinfectants (chlorides and iodides) have low toxicity to human skin. They kill many bacteria, and iodine can kill spores. They are used as skin washes, scrubs and disinfectants, for example chlorhexidine and Betadine, which are extensively used in intensive care units and operating theatres.

3 Alcohols act rapidly to kill vegetative bacteria, many viruses and fungi. They may be used as sprays to disinfect surfaces, such as trolley tops, and also as rubs for rapid hand disinfection. Halogen disinfectants can be dispensed as alcoholic solutions, for additional bactericidal effect. Alcohols are easily diluted to below effective concentrations by evaporation, and penetrate

organic matter poorly. Their flammability makes them too dangerous to use near diathermy units and other operating theatre equipment.

4 Aldehydes are non-corrosive and kill a wide range of organisms. Glutaraldehyde (Cidex) solution is widely used in automated decontamination systems. Sealed rooms and large equipment are occasionally decontaminated by fumigation with humid formaldehyde vapour.

5 Phenol-based disinfectants such as Hycolin are noncorrosive, and highly toxic to microorganisms but are not very active against viruses. They are used to disinfect contaminated surfaces such as the floors of ambulances, bed frames and bathroom equipment. Suspensions of tarry phenolics, such as Sudol, are used for cleaning highly contaminated stone and ceramic floors, such as mortuary areas. They are highly microbicidal, but leave a residue which is hard to remove from instruments and equipment.

6 Ethylene oxide is a gas which kills bacteria, viruses, fungi and bacterial spores. It can penetrate complex instruments, and is used for cleaning laparoscopes, arthroscopes, reusable cardiac catheters and delicate surgical instruments. It is applied at low pressure, usually mixed with carbon dioxide to avoid risk of explosion, and at a temperature of 55°C. Instruments must be aired after treatment to remove the irritant gas.

Disinfectants do not work adequately in the presence of organic matter, which may degrade them. Debris can also prevent the disinfectant from reaching its target surface. All equipment should be cleaned or washed before being disinfected.

Physical methods of disinfection

Heat is the most commonly used physical disinfection method in hospitals. Superheated and pressurized steam is used in autoclaving. Porous material such as operating gowns and drapes are prepared for use by this method. Stainless steel and some plastic and rubber equipment can also be autoclaved.

Adequate sterilization is a function of temperature and time of exposure. In an autoclave, air is drawn out of the load by creating a vacuum, and is replaced by pressurized steam. This process is repeated in five to eight cycles. The temperature in the vessel is then held, usually at 134°C, for 3–20 min. An extended cycle is used for potentially contaminated material from patients with Creutzfeldt–Jakob disease.

The effectiveness of the cycle can be tested by including heat-stable bacterial spores in the load, and showing that they do not germinate after treatment. The attainment of adequate temperatures can be shown by using autoclavable tape to wrap the load; the tape shows a colour change at the correct temperature–time combination. Equipment can be prepacked in semipermeable paper or plastic wrappers, and the whole package autoclaved. The equipment is then sterile until the pack is broken.

Closed jars and bottles would rupture in the waves of heat and pressure produced by standard autoclaves. Special autoclaves with balanced pressure and heat cycles must be used for these.

Gamma radiation is widely used in industry to remove microbial contamination after manufacture from plastic, silicon and rubber equipment, usually after packaging. As the gamma rays penetrate deeply, the method can be used to sterilize fragile and complex equipment such as cardiac catheters, pacemaker controllers and complex interventional radiology equipment.

Hospital waste disposal

A hospital produces a huge amount of waste. This includes:

1 Domestic-type waste from kitchens, washrooms, dining facilities and public areas.

2 Clinical waste such as used dressings, wound drainage, used disposable equipment and even organs and limbs from the surgical department.

3 Discarded, used sharps.

Domestic waste can be removed by local authority services and disposed of in various ways without hazard to disposal workers or the public. Clinical waste must be safely packed and clearly identified. In the UK it is put into strong, yellow plastic sacks at the site where it is generated. These sacks are stored in strong bins or skips until they are removed intact for incineration locally, or by a licensed disposal firm. Used sharps are disposed of directly into strong, leak-proof bins at the site where they are generated. These bins are sealed when full, and are removed intact for storage and incineration.

Laboratory waste contains high concentrations of pathogens. All used containers, media and disposable equipment are autoclaved before they are either disposed of in the hospital waste system or recycled for laboratory use. Laboratories use the same sharps disposal system as the other hospital areas.

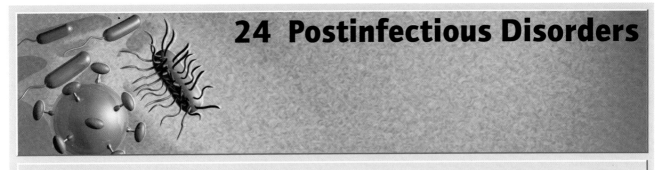

24 Postinfectious Disorders

Introduction

Most people who have suffered an infectious disease expect to make a steady improvement when the infection is controlled. This process of convalescence is very complex, and depends on a number of more or less simultaneous events.

Normal features of convalescence

Suppression of active infection

In many cases, as in the cure of influenza, meningitis or endocarditis, this is probably achieved by complete eradication of the causative pathogen. Sometimes the pathogen is destroyed by the action of antibiotic, antibody, phagocytosis or cytotoxic immune reaction. In other cases the infected cells are shed, as in influenza, or destroyed, as in hepatitis A.

In some diseases it has long been known that the pathogen is suppressed rather than destroyed. Toxoplasmosis is such a case, in which tissue cysts are maintained inactive and the egress of parasites is prevented by an immune reaction. Viruses of the herpes group remain latent unless the immune system is impaired sufficiently for recrudescent or secondary infections to occur. It is now suspected that some viral pathogens are suppressed by selecting inactive mutants from the range of mutations which occur during rapid replication. Hepatitis e antigenaemia may cease when an e-antigen-negative mutant is selected, while e-antigen-positive viral products are destroyed by anti-e antibodies.

Methods of terminating active infection

1 Destruction of pathogens and their antigens.
2 Shedding or destruction of virus-infected cells.
3 Making pathogens inaccessible to the immune system (e.g. in pseudocysts).
4 Selecting antigenically inert mutants of the pathogen.
5 Establishment of latency.

Return of immune responses to resting states

As the amount of microbial antigen falls with suppression of infection, antigen presentation will lessen and the stimulus to further activation of immune responses will subside. However, many activated lymphocytes will remain, including helper T cells, cytotoxic

T cells and clonally proliferating B and T cells, as well as suppressor T cells. It is now known that many T cells are inactivated by a process of enzymic self-destruction (called apoptosis) that limits their activated lifetime. The presence of increased levels of interleukin-2 while infection persists tends to delay this destruction and maintain immune activation.

As antigen levels decline, the production of immune complexes slows down, slowing the activation of the classical complement pathway and the coagulation cascade.

The reduction in the intensity of immune responses permits the reduction of inflammatory reactions in the tissues.

Events favouring reduced immune activity and inflammation
1 Falling levels of antigen and immune complexes.
2 Reduced antigen presentation.
3 Reduced cytokine production.
4 Reduced immune complex-mediated complement activation.
5 Apoptosis.

Repair of tissue damage

The catabolic state usually found in acute infection must be reversed to allow protein construction and repair of destroyed or damaged tissue. This in turn permits the restoration of normal bodily functions, for instance, absorption of nutrients after bowel infection or glucose metabolism after severe liver infection. The time needed to complete this process can be surprisingly long; for instance, there is mild but measurable hypoxaemia for several weeks after acute bronchiolitis in infants. During this period the metabolic rate is often increased, with concurrent tachycardia and often a feeling of easy fatiguability.

Features of postinfectious disorders

In postinfectious disorders the process of convalescence is prolonged, sometimes for a considerable time. This is often because of an inflammatory condition which arises in different tissue from that affected by the original infection. In some cases the postinfectious condition overlaps the acute infection in time; this is the case when erythema nodosum complicates primary tuberculosis. In other instances it follows the acute infection with little or no interval; erythema multiforme complicating episodes of herpes simplex tends to do this. Finally the postinfectious condition can follow an interval of 2 weeks or more after apparent cure of the acute infection; this is seen in poststreptococcal nephritis and postmeasles encephalitis (Table 24.1).

Persisting low-grade infection

Persisting low-grade infection has been considered as a pathogenic mechanism, especially in postinfectious encephalitis, which may be histologically indistinguishable from acute infectious encephalitis. Early evidence for persistence of infection came when measles virus was recovered from the brain tissue of cases of subacute sclerosing panencephalitis (SSPE). Immunoglobulin M antibodies can persist for weeks or months in some infections such as hepatitis A, infectious mononucleosis and toxoplasmosis, which can all be followed by a debilitating and prolonged convalescence. More recent work on erythema multiforme associated with herpes simplex has used polymerase chain amplification to demonstrate herpes simplex virus DNA in epidermal lesions.

Molecular mimicry

Molecular mimicry also offers a good explanation for some conditions. In the Guillain–Barré syndrome there is evidence of immunological attack against components of myelin. Experimental demyelination of nerve roots very similar to that seen in Guillain–Barré syndrome can be produced in animals by antimyelin antibodies.

Nephritogenic strains of *Streptococcus pyogenes* produce a unique antigen which cross-reacts with glomerular structures.

Immune complex disease

Immune complex disease has been postulated as a cause particularly of postinfectious arthritis. In the synovitis which often follows meningococcal disease, meningococcal antigen has been demonstrated in biopsies of affected synovium. Similarly, in Reiter's syndrome, chlamydial antigen has been found in synovium.

Possible pathogenesis of postinfectious conditions

There are several mechanisms by which postinfectious conditions may arise. However, although theoretical considerations can offer a number of explanations, the true pathogenesis of most conditions is poorly understood.

Disorder	Common associations	Rare associations
Aplastic anaemia		Non-A /non-B hepatitis
Arthritis	Rubella Meningococcus *Yersinia*	*Salmonella* *Shigella* *Campylobacter* Mumps
Encephalitis	Varicella Measles Influenza Mumps	Rubella Yellow fever vaccine
Erythema multiforme	Herpes simplex	*Mycoplasma pneumoniae*
Erythema nodosum	Tuberculosis Leprosy	*Yersinia*
Glomerulonephritis	*Streptococcus pyrogenes*	Hepatitis B Mumps
Guillain–Barré	Cytomegalovirus *Campylobacter*	Hepatitis A or B Respiratory viruses
Haemolysis	*Mycoplasma pneumoniae*	Epstein–Barr virus Syphilis
Haemolytic–uraemic syndrome	*Escherichia coli* 0157	
Haemophagocytic syndrome		Epstein–Barr virus Cytomegalovirus
Reiter's syndrome	Chlamydial genital infections	*Shigella*
Reye's syndrome	Varicella Influenza	Aspirin as a cofactor
Rheumatic fever	*Streptococcus pyogenes*	
Serositis	Meningococcus	
Thrombocytopenia	Rubella Mumps Varicella	Epstein–Barr virus Tuberculosis

Table 24.1 Some postinfectious disorders and associated pathogens

Persisting inappropriate immune reaction

Persisting inappropriate immune reaction is probably a mechanism in some of the cytopenias. It is known that haemolysis in *Mycoplasma* pneumonia and Epstein–Barr infections is related to the inappropriate production of anti-I and anti-i anti-red-cell antibodies respectively. Thrombocytopenia is likely to be caused by a similar mechanism; indeed, antiplatelet antibodies can be demonstrated in some cases.

A condition like systemic lupus erythematosus occasionally occurs after infectious mononucleosis. This is associated with positive anti-DNA antibodies, joint pains and raised erythrocyte sedimentation rate (ESR), but has a limited duration of several months.

Failure of termination of immune response

Failure of termination of the normal acute immune response may be responsible for severe conditions such as the haemophagocytic syndrome. Apparently uncontrolled proliferation and activity of macrophages and other immune cells produces infiltration of the liver, spleen and bone marrow which is hard to distinguish from a malignant histiocytosis. Immunosuppression predisposes to this condition.

Susceptibility of the patient

Special susceptibility of the patient may also influence the occurrence of postinfectious conditions. It has long been recognized that non-secretors of blood group sub-stances are more likely than others to develop rheumatic fever. Reiter's syndrome is almost exclusive to patients with the human leukocyte antigen (HLA) B27 tissue type, but in non-Reiter's arthropathies they are not over-represented. A total of 88% of patients who have recur-rent erythema multiforme after herpes simplex episodes have tissue type DQw3, and 71% have DRw53.

Possible mechanisms of postinfectious disease
1 Persistent low-grade infection.
2 Molecular mimicry.
3 Immune complex disease.
4 Persisting inappropriate immune activity.
5 Failure to terminate the normal acute immune response.
6 Special immunological susceptibility of the patient.

Erythema multiforme

Epidemiology

This skin disorder affects mainly teenagers and young adults. It has been described after streptococcal infec-tions, *Mycoplasma pneumoniae* infections and after exposure to drugs such as sulphonamides and long-acting penicillins. The authors have seen it as an accom-paniment of Epstein–Barr virus infection in toddlers. Rarer causes include barbiturates, diphenoxylate and traumas such as radiotherapy.

Repeated episodes of erythema multiforme occur in some patients who have cold sores. The skin rash often follows 2 or 3 days after the onset of the mucocutaneous lesions, and lasts up to a week. The severity of the rash is related to the extent of the herpetic lesions on each occasion.

Pathology

The skin lesions are associated with oedema and necro-sis of epidermis with dilatation and inflammatory infiltration of the subepidermal blood vessels. The oede-matous epidermis may become raised, forming bullae. In herpes simplex-associated disease, viral antigen and viral genome can both be demonstrated in the keratino-cytes of the affected skin, but are not present in normal skin.

Clinical features

Illness begins abruptly, with fever and developing rash. Typically, many of the lesions are target or iris-shaped

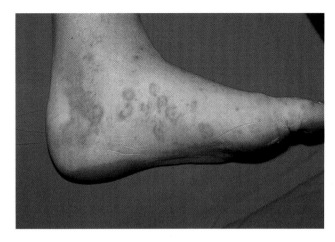

Fig. 24.1 Target lesions of erythema multiforme.

with an erythematous halo surrounding an oedematous or dusky centre (Fig. 24.1). The rash is densest on the extremities, including the palms and soles (Fig. 24.2), but is also exaggerated in areas exposed to sunlight or trauma. Untreated, the lesions last for 2–6 weeks, some of them coming and going all the time. There may be arthralgia, especially of the ankles. There is no charac-teristic change in the white cell count. The ESR is usually high — 70 mm/h or more.

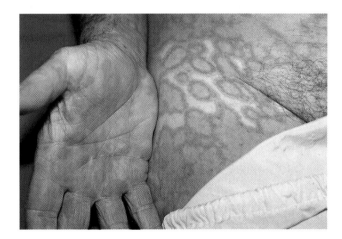

Fig. 24.2 Erythema multiforme: lesions on the palms.

Stevens–Johnson syndrome

Stevens–Johnson syndrome is the term used when ery-thema multiforme affects mucosae as well as skin. The disease is usually severe, with many skin bullae and severe, sometimes haemorrhagic inflammation of the oral, conjunctival and genital mucosae. There is danger of widespread epidermal necrolysis, in which the surface of the epidermis shears off the lower layers (Fig. 24.3).

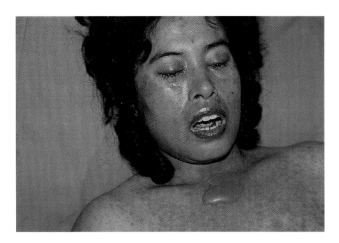

Fig. 24.3 Stevens–Johnson syndrome: severe involvement of the oral and conjunctival mucosae and epidermal necrolysis.

The keratinized layer becomes loose, and can be moved over the lower epidermis, or rubbed off it (Nikolsky's sign).

Management

The rash will often resolve progressively if the cause can be identified and removed. Severe cases, however, and all cases of Stevens–Johnson syndrome are often treated with corticosteroids, though there is little firm evidence of benefit. The ESR can be used as an objective measure of improvement.

Patients with epidermal necrolysis should be nursed in a warm room and kept well-hydrated, as heat and moisture are rapidly lost from the exposed lower epidermis. There is risk of secondary infection, particularly with *Staphylococcus aureus*, which may cause bacteraemia. If a patient develops fever, tachycardia or shock, blood cultures should be obtained and early treatment commenced.

Complications

These are few, once the patient has passed the severe part of the illness. The inflammation is very superficial, and the epidermal layers are replaced with only an occasional atrophic scar. After particularly severe mucosal ulceration, adhesions may develop, for instance between the lip and gum, or in the conjunctival sac. These may require division and split-skin grafting.

Guillain–Barré syndrome (ascending polyneuritis)

Epidemiology

This is a condition in which there is demyelination of the nerve roots. It often follows a viral-type respiratory infection or a gastrointestinal illness, with an interval of 1–3 weeks. Specific conditions in which it can occur include cytomegalovirus infections, infectious mononucleosis, *Campylobacter* infection of the bowel and legionnaire's disease.

The disease affects all age groups, but tends to be more prolonged in middle-aged individuals and the elderly.

Pathology

There is inflammation and demyelination of nerve fibres in the spinal and cranial nerve roots. This can be demonstrated electrophysiologically by special electromyographic studies, but in practice this is rarely done as the diagnosis is often clear, and management does not depend on test results. If inflammation is sufficiently severe, degeneration of some nerve fibres in nerve trunks may follow.

Clinical features

The first symptoms are usually paraesthesiae followed by weakness in the feet and lower legs. At this stage there may be no objective signs, and the patient may be thought hysterical. The disease progresses up the spinal levels, with weakness of the trunk and arms, and finally facial paralysis. Some patients describe prodromal aching or pain in the muscles. As the paralysis intensifies, tendon reflexes are lost and the patient becomes immobile. There may be respiratory failure because of intercostal and diaphragmatic paralysis. Early facial paralysis warns of sudden respiratory failure. There is little involvement of sphincters, and this is transient if it occurs.

Sensory features include loss of light touch and joint position sense. There are no upper motor neuron signs; the plantar responses, when they can be elicited, are downgoing.

Abnormal laboratory findings are confined to the cerebrospinal fluid (CSF). Early in the course of the illness there is an excess of lymphocytes, related to the inflammation of the nerve roots. The CSF protein level gradually rises, and may reach levels of some grams per litre.

Paralysis may cease to progress at any stage, but rarely takes longer than 2 or 3 weeks to stabilize. Some cases progress to complete paralysis within 2–3 days. After stabilization there is progressive recovery. This may be rapid, taking 2 or 3 weeks until the patient can walk independently. In very elderly patients, or when significant nerve fibre degeneration has occurred, it can take 3–12 months or more, and the recovery of muscle strength may be compromised by atrophy due to disuse and a degree of denervation.

There is a 10–20% mortality, largely from the side-effects of respiratory intensive care. Of those who recover, 90% return to full motor activity; the remainder have variable residual weakness.

Management

Patients should be carefully observed as paralysis develops, as ventilation is often required for those with respiratory paralysis. The paralysed patient also needs skin care and attention to pressure areas. Monitoring of the vital capacity and the arterial oxygen saturation are helpful.

Plasmapheresis has resulted in remission in prolonged paralysis, but may require supplementation with immunosuppressive therapy for a variable time to prevent relapse. Intravenous immunoglobulin is a safer and more convenient means of obtaining remission, and is probably as effective as plasmapheresis.

Henoch–Schönlein disease

Epidemiology

This is a vasculitic condition which presents with fever, purpuric rash, arthralgia and synovitis, abdominal pain and a characteristic type of glomerulonephritis. There is no unique precipitating condition, but there has often been a preceding respiratory infection and some sufferers have evidence of recent streptococcal disease. Children and young adults are most often affected, though cases occasionally occur in the middle-aged.

Clinical features

Rash

The rash affects mainly the extensor surfaces of the feet, ankles and legs, and commonly affects the buttocks. The lesions are raised and of variable size. Not all are purpuric, but a proportion usually are, and those on the feet often take the form of haemorrhagic vesicles (Fig. 24.4).

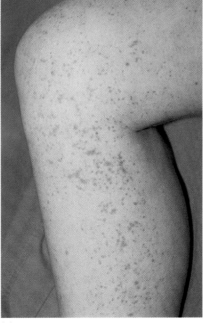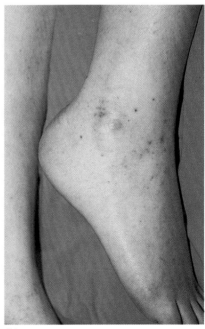

Fig. 24.4 (a and b) Henoch–Schönlein disease: characteristic rash with raised and haemorrhagic elements.

(a)   (b)

Synovitis

The synovitis most often affects the ankles and knees, but any joint can be involved. Tendon sheaths around the ankle, and sometimes the wrist, are often swollen and painful.

Abdominal pain

The abdominal pain is caused by swelling and haemorrhagic lesions of the bowel. Severe cases may have vomiting and abdominal rigidity. Nodular swelling occasionally predisposes to intussusception. Blood is sometimes seen in the stools.

Nephritis

The nephritis is a focal glomerulitis. Haematuria and proteinuria are common. Renal failure can occur, with hypertension and oedema.

> **Main features of Henoch–Schönlein disease**
> 1 Rash on the legs and/or buttocks.
> 2 Joint pain.
> 3 Abdominal pain.
> 4 Proteinuria (and often microscopic haematuria).
> 5 Reduced renal function.

Management

Management is usually symptomatic, as the disorder is self-limiting and usually benign. Non-steroidal anti-inflammatory agents often help pain, especially of the joints. Corticosteroids do not alter the course of the disease. Most children who develop nephritis will recover, but about a quarter are at risk of deteriorating renal function later in life.

Problems in the course of the disease may be due to bowel haemorrhage or intracerebral haemorrhage. A minority of patients require dialysis for renal failure and a few do not recover. Adults are thought to be more at risk of persisting renal impairment.

Poststreptococcal glomerulonephritis

Epidemiology

This disorder affects children of age 1–5 years, and is rare in other age groups. It can follow *Streptococcus pyogenes* infection of the skin or throat. It usually occurs 10–14 days after the initiating infection, but can appear after as long as 4 weeks.

Clinical features

The onset is abrupt, with fever, malaise and often loin pain. There is puffiness of the child's feet and face. Haematuria and oliguria are often noticed by the mother.

Physical findings are of mild loin tenderness and hypertension. There is mild to moderate haematuria and proteinuria; significant protein loss is rare. Urine microscopy shows epithelial casts which contain red blood cells, confirming the glomerular origin of the problem.

> **Main features of poststreptococcal nephritis**
> 1 Fever and loin pain.
> 2 Facial and dependent oedema.
> 3 Haematuria and oliguria.
> 4 Impaired renal function.
> 5 It follows 10–21 days after streptococcal infection.

Diagnosis

Transient haematuria is common at the onset of acute streptococcal infections and does not indicate the presence of glomerulonephritis. Glomerulonephritis can occur in a variety of other infections, including viral hepatitis, infectious mononucleosis, atypical pneumonias and childhood viral infections. Drugs, including penicillins and cephalosporins, occasionally cause idiosyncratic nephritis. Care should be taken to show that the glomerulonephritis is truly associated with streptococcal infection, especially if it is severe or prolonged.

Evidence of recent streptococcal infection is provided either by persisting positive culture from throat or skin, or by significantly elevated anti-streptolysin O titre (ASOT) or other antibody titres (see Chapter 6).

Renal biopsy is rarely carried out as the natural course of the disease is short; diuresis and improvement in creatinine levels occur within 7–10 days. Histology shows swollen glomeruli with endothelial proliferation and neutrophil infiltration. Irregular deposits of immune complexes can be demonstrated on the glomerular basement membrane.

Management

The throat or skin infection should be treated with penicillin or a suitable alternative (see Chapter 6). The glomerulonephritis almost always resolves without specific treatment. Diuretics may be indicated to reduce oedema; a few patients require protein and potassium restriction. It is rare for dialysis to be indicated. Once the kidneys have recovered, renal function should be expected to remain normal.

Reye's syndrome

Introduction and epidemiology

This is a rare childhood disease consisting of encephalopathy, cerebral oedema and fatty infiltration of the liver, with a characteristic picture of liver dysfunction. It is associated with transient but severe damage to mitochondrial structure and function. Disrupted and necrotic mitochondria are demonstrable on liver biopsy in affected cases.

In the USA the syndrome more often follows infection with varicella or influenza B than other infections. In the UK it has followed these diseases, but also echovirus infections, atypical pneumonias and adenovirus infections.

A number of epidemiological studies have suggested that Reye's syndrome is more likely to occur in children who have received aspirin treatment for the preceding feverish illness. Aspirin is therefore no longer recommended as an antipyretic for children below the age of 12.

Clinical features

Typical clinical features begin a few days after the onset of a viral-type infection. There is increasing drowsiness, vomiting and often convulsions. Hepatomegaly is common, but jaundice is not often seen.

There is biochemical evidence of liver dysfunction, with a raised blood ammonia and low blood urea. The blood glucose may also fall, leading to hypoglycaemic convulsions. There is sometimes significant impairment of blood clotting.

The most important aspect of the disease is the raised intracranial pressure and reduction of cerebral perfusion, which can cause permanent cerebral damage.

Main features of Reye's syndrome
1 Drowsiness and vomiting.
2 Raised intracranial pressure.
3 Hepatomegaly.
4 Biochemical signs of liver failure.
5 It occurs within 1 week of respiratory or gastro-intestinal illness.

Diagnosis

Diagnosis is not always easy, as there is a clinical overlap with the effects of several inborn errors of fatty acid

oxidation and urea synthesis. These possibilities should be investigated, particularly in children below the age of 15 months. Expert clinical advice is helpful in this respect.

Management

Management is directed at maintaining adequate cerebral perfusion pressure, with the aid of intracerebral pressure monitoring and paediatric intensive care facilities. Admission to such facilities is a matter of urgency. The disease is self-limiting; recovery occurs slowly as the mitochondria recover from the temporary insult. If cerebral damage can be prevented, full recovery can be achieved.

Rheumatic fever

Introduction and epidemiology

Rheumatic fever is a multisystem inflammatory disease which follows throat infection with *S. pyogenes*. It does not occur after streptococcal skin infections.

It has been a rare condition in western countries for some decades, but in the 1980s large epidemics occurred in North America. This may be because of the reappearance of certain epidemic types of *S. pyogenes* with an antigenic structure related to that of cardiac and other tissues, leading to the development of rheumatic fever. The streptococci recovered from North American cases produced mucoid colonies, and most were of M-type 18.

The throat infection preceding the development of rheumatic fever is variable in severity. Only half of the recent North American cases had throat symptoms sufficient to warrant a medical consultation, and only a quarter of all cases had received antibiotic treatment. Most affected individuals are between the ages of 5 and 16 years, though a few may be up to age 25 or 30. After this age, the susceptibility to rheumatic fever seems to be lost.

Clinical features

There is an interval of 2–3 weeks between the acute infection and the onset of rheumatic fever. The various manifestations of the disease have been classified into major and minor features, or criteria, to aid clinical diagnosis (Table 24.2).

The commonest presentation is with fever and flitting or migratory polyarthritis.

Major manifestations	Minor manifestations
Arthritis (70%)	Fever
Carditis (50%)	Previous episode(s)
Chorea (20%)	Raised ESR or CRP
Rash (12%)	ECG abnormalities
Nodules (5%)	Arthralgia

The percentages shown are for recent North American cases. CRP, C-reactive protein; ECG, electrocardiogram; ESR, erythrocyte sedimentation rate.

Table 24.2 Major and minor manifestations of rheumatic fever

Arthritis

The arthritis is acute and painful, with synovitis and often effusion. It affects large joints, particularly the knees and ankles, but the joints of the arm can also be involved. Typically, one joint is affected for a few days, but then improves rapidly while another becomes inflamed.

Carditis

The carditis is a pancarditis. The combined pericardial, myocardial and endocardial disease can cause heart failure. About 10% of cases have evidence of this at presentation.

There is acute inflammation of the pericardium, often with a degree of purulent exudate.

The myocardium is inflamed, and may contain typical Aschoff bodies. These are inflammatory bodies consisting of somewhat degenerative epithelioid central areas surrounded by haloes of inflammatory cells. As a postmortem finding these are pathognomonic of rheumatic fever. The myocardial inflammation is often reflected by cardiographic changes, such as prolongation of the P-R interval, axis changes or other conduction changes.

Endocarditis

The endocarditis is usually macroscopic, with verrucous vegetations on the affected valves. The mitral valve is most often affected, the aortic valve less so (boys are more likely than girls to have aortic disease). The right heart valves, especially the pulmonary, are rarely affected. The most common valve lesion is mitral regurgitation, but vegetations can cause stenotic features. When heart failure occurs, it is often related to severe valvular disease, but exacerbated by myocardial inflammation.

Chorea

Chorea is often seen in older children and girls, and on occasions it is the sole major manifestation of the disease. The abnormal movements may be mild and partly disguised, making the patient appear restless, or they may be more gross and obtrusive. They can develop late in the illness, when other manifestations are subsiding, and can last for several weeks or even months.

Rash

The rash is classically erythema marginatum (see Fig. 22.3), a rash of raised, serpiginous lesions which comes and goes rapidly, waxing and waning with the fever from hour to hour. More often there is an urticarial, multiform or even erythema nodosum-like rash, which is similarly changeable.

Nodules

Nodules are usually less than 1 cm in diameter. They are subcutaneous and often found over tendons on the extensor surfaces of the arms. They are most often seen in patients with severe carditis.

Diagnosis

This is based on clinical assessment using the major and minor criteria, and on demonstrating evidence of recent streptococcal infection (see Chapter 6).

The commonest findings on examination of the heart are a soft first heart sound, a third heart sound or a short systolic or diastolic (Carey Coombs) murmur. Echocardiography is useful to demonstrate the valvular lesions.

The presence of Aschoff bodies in biopsy material such as skin nodules may be helpful, but the inflammatory changes in tissue other than myocardium are rarely specific.

Management

The treatment of choice is aspirin, but other non-steroidal anti-inflammatory agents may be used, and are preferred in younger children, if they are sufficiently effective. Corticosteroids are said not to influence the inflammation significantly.

Bed rest and/or diuretic treatment may be indicated if there is heart failure. Fatalities from acute rheumatic fever are rare, but severe congestive heart failure can sometimes be life-threatening.

Prevention

This is important, as a first attack is often followed by recurrences each time a streptococcus invades the throat. With each succeeding attack there is fibrosis of the valve rings, shortening of the chordae tendinae and increasing deformity of heart valves, leading to the risk of valve failure and of subacute endocarditis.

Phenoxymethyl penicillin is very effective prophylaxis. It is given in a dose of 250 mg twice daily. An oral sulphonamide, erythromycin or co-trimoxazole may be given to penicillin-allergic patients. Prophylaxis is usually continued until the individual leaves school. For those working in schools or hospitals it may be continued for longer, but the risk of rheumatic fever becomes very small after the age of 30.

Reiter's syndrome

Introduction and epidemiology

Reiter's syndrome is a multisystem disorder which affects almost exclusively individuals with tissue type HLA B27. In its commonest form it follows non-specific genital infection (usually chlamydial) in men. It can also affect patients of either sex after an attack of bacillary dysentery.

Clinical features

Illness begins 10–14 days after the acute precipitating condition. The syndrome consists of synovitis, sacroileitis, conjunctivitis, mucocutaneous rashes and aortitis.

Synovitis with associated conjunctivitis

This is the commonest presentation. The synovitis typically affects tendon sheaths, especially of the hand and foot, but also of the elbow and shoulder. There is also arthritis of both large and small joints (Fig. 24.5). The knee, ankle and shoulder are often affected. Sacroileitis is prominent, causing low back pain, local tenderness and discomfort on 'springing' the pelvis. The patient usually has a fever.

Circinate balanitis

Circinate balanitis is the typical mucocutaneous rash. This is often a red, roughly circular slightly weeping lesion with scaly margins, affecting the periurethral part of the glans penis. Non-specific papular or scaly rashes

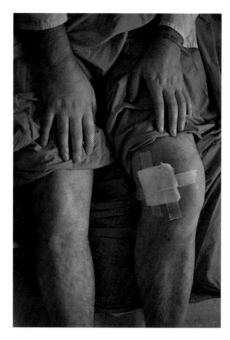

Fig. 24.5 Reiter's syndrome: synovitis of the left knee and tendinitis of the dorsum of the right hand.

may also occur on the glans and at the angles of the mouth.

Aortitis

Aortitis is not always clinically evident. Sometimes a soft systolic murmur is audible, but in rare, severe cases aortic incompetence may occur and lead to sudden heart failure.

There may be a polymorph leukocytosis in the peripheral blood. The ESR is usually raised to 70 mm/h or more and the C-reactive protein is also very high. Chlamydial antigens have been demonstrated in the affected synovium, but this and tissue typing are expensive and not necessary for an adequate diagnosis in most cases. Sacroileitis is often radiographically demonstrable, showing as soft-tissue swelling and perisacral sclerosis. As it does not occur in rheumatic fever, this helps to differentiate between that condition and Reiter's syndrome with aortic valve involvement.

Keratoderma blennorrhagica

Keratoderma blennorrhagica is a thickened, scaling rash of the palms and soles, in which flat vesicles are often seen. It is characteristic of late Reiter's syndrome. It often presents after the earlier features have responded somewhat to treatment.

Uveitis and cardiac dysrhythmias

Uveitis and cardiac dysrhythmias are rarer manifestations.

> **Main features of Reiter's syndrome**
> 1 Synovitis.
> 2 Sacroileitis.
> 3 Conjunctivitis.
> 4 Aortitis.
> 5 Circinate balanitis.
> 6 Late keratoderma blennorrhagica.

Management

This is symptomatic. The initiating illness should be treated if it is still active, but the Reiter's syndrome is probably related more to antigen already fixed in the affected tissues than to continuing active disease.

Non-steroidal anti-inflammatory drugs are the mainstay of treatment. Systemic corticosteroid treatment is avoided, if possible, but corticosteroid eye drops may be necessary to control uveitis. Rare cases of aortic valve disruption may need to be treated surgically, but control of inflammation is important to provide a good basis for any implanted valve structure.

The disease has prolonged and relapsing course, often requiring several weeks or months of treatment with anti-inflammatory agents.

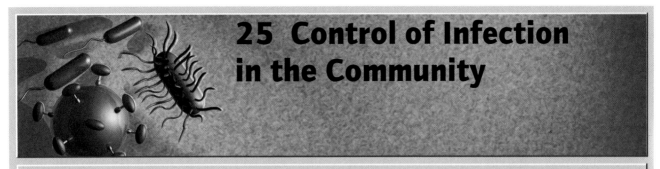

25 Control of Infection in the Community

Communicable disease and the law

The legal framework for control of infection in the community has developed over the past 150 years. In the UK, much of the old legislation was brought together under the Public Health (Control of Disease) Act 1984 and the Public Health (Infectious Diseases) Regulations 1988. These acts do not apply in Scotland, which has similar legislation, however.

Responsibility for the control of communicable disease was vested in local authorities during the 19th century, when the post of medical officer of health (MOH) was established. When the National Health Service was created, the MOH, who was employed by the local authority, retained responsibilities for control of infection and related activities such as immunization. The post of MOH was abolished in 1974; however, some residual functions including communicable disease control were retained by local authorities.

Each local authority has a designated proper officer (in Scotland, medical officer) with statutory powers for prevention and control of infection. These statutory powers relate to the notifiable diseases (see p. 455) and to certain other diseases, usually defined. The proper officer is usually (but not always) a consultant in communicable disease control (CCDC) who is a health authority employee acting on behalf of the local authority. The post of CCDC is sometimes referred to as MOEH (medical officer for environmental health). In Scotland, the equivalent post is the consultant in public health (communicable disease and environmental health).

In addition to the CCDC in the community, hospitals have a control of infection officer who is often the local microbiologist. Air and sea ports have a medical officer who liaises with the local CCDC.

Functions of the consultant in communicable disease control
1 Surveillance of communicable diseases.
2 Development of policies for control of communicable disease.
3 Investigation and control of outbreaks.
4 Coordination of immunization and acquired immuno-deficiency syndrome prevention programmes.
5 Provision of advice on prevention and control.

Role of national agencies

In England and Wales, the Communicable Disease Surveillance Centre (CDSC) was established in 1979 as part of the Public Health Laboratory Service (PHLS). The laboratory network of the PHLS had existed for many years, and the government inquiries that followed two incidents of laboratory-acquired smallpox infection in the 1970s recommended the creation of an epidemiological unit within the PHLS that could coordinate the management of major incidents. The functions of the CDSC are:
1 Surveillance of communicable diseases and of immunization programmes.
2 Investigation of outbreaks.
3 Epidemiological research.
4 Training in the epidemiology and control of communicable disease.

In Scotland, the equivalent agency is the Communicable Diseases (Scotland) Unit (CD(S)U). Most countries have similar organizations, for example the Centers for Disease Control in the USA. In some countries the functions are performed by the Ministry of Health.

The Office of Populations Censuses and Surveys (OPCS) collects vital statistics (births, marriages and deaths), provides population estimates and projections and administers the notification system (see p. 455). The equivalent organization in Scotland is the General Register Office (Scotland).

The Ministry of Agriculture, Fisheries and Food (MAFF; Department of Agriculture and Fisheries in Scotland) is responsible for the control of infection in animals. Close collaboration between MAFF, CDSC/ CD(S)U and CCDCs is important in relation to control of zoonotic infections.

Communicable disease surveillance

Principles and practice of surveillance

Surveillance of disease is the continuous systematic collection and analysis of relevant morbidity and mortality data. The primary aim of surveillance is to identify trends or clusters of disease which require preventive action; thus surveillance is *information for action*. Surveillance is also used to evaluate control measures such as vaccination programmes, to plan resource allocation and to provide baseline epidemiological information for research workers.

The process of surveillance involves four basic steps:
1 Collection of data.
2 Analysis of data to provide statistics.
3 Interpretation of statistics to provide meaningful information.
4 Dissemination of narrative reports to those who need to know.

An ideal surveillance system should meet the following criteria:
1 The disease under surveillance must be of sufficient importance to justify the resources required to undertake effective monitoring.
2 The surveillance should be timely — the data should be collected and interpreted sufficiently quickly to enable effective control measures to be taken. This is particularly important for communicable diseases, where large outbreaks can occur very suddenly and cause considerable morbidity.
3 The data collected should be representative of the total population. In practice this is difficult to achieve as surveillance systems usually build on routine data sources from atypical populations such as hospital inpatients. The role of the epidemiologist is to understand and take account of the biases inherent in surveillance systems when interpreting the data.

4 It should be consistent over time and between geographical areas. If the proportion of cases detected by a surveillance system is not constant, it becomes difficult to interpret any changes in reported disease incidence. During periods of increased disease incidence the efficiency of reporting tends also to increase. A change in the criteria for reporting a disease can have a large effect on reported incidence. For example, the inclusion of patients with a CD4 count of less than $200/\mu l$ in the case definition for acquired immunodeficiency syndrome (AIDS) resulted in a 200% increase in the cumulative total of cases reported in the USA.
5 Reporting should be complete wherever possible.
6 It should be simple, in both structure and ease of operation.
7 It should be flexible, thus capable of adapting to changing information needs (for example, emergence of a new disease).

> **Criteria for an effective surveillance system**
> 1 Disease under surveillance is of sufficient public health importance.
> 2 Timeliness.
> 3 Representative of the total population.
> 4 Consistency over time and between geographical areas.
> 5 Completeness of reporting.
> 6 Simplicity.
> 7 Flexibility.

A surveillance system may be active, passive or stimulated-passive. A passive system relies on routinely collected data, e.g. notifications of infectious disease, where cases are reported without any specific encouragement or inducement. When special efforts are made to improve reporting to a passive surveillance scheme, e.g. by written reminders or following up non-reporting centres, the scheme becomes stimulated-passive. An active surveillance system is where all potential reporting units are contacted at regular intervals and specifically asked to report the condition under surveillance; in addition, if no cases have been seen, a 'negative' report is requested. The British Paediatric Association Surveillance Unit (BPASU; see p. 456) is a good example of an active surveillance system.

In general, passive surveillance systems are used for common or less severe diseases such as food poisoning where it is not essential (or possible) to ascertain every case. Active-passive or active reporting is usually only necessary for rare or serious conditions, or those where a public health programme of elimination is planned, for example poliomyelitis.

Sources of data

Reports of outbreaks and other infectious disease incidents are often provided on an *ad hoc* basis. There are however many sources of data, routine and non-routine, that constitute the formal communicable disease surveillance network.

Routine sources of data on infectious disease in the UK
1 Statutory notifications to the consultant in communicable disease control.
2 Laboratory reports.
3 General practitioner reporting schemes.
4 Hospital inpatient and outpatient statistics.
5 Returns from sexually transmitted disease clinics.
6 Death certificates.
7 School medical officers.
8 Occupational health departments.

Routine data sources

There are several routine sources of data on infectious disease in the UK. The most important are notifications, laboratory reports, general practitioner surveillance schemes, hospital data, clinic returns and death certificates.

Notification

Notification is a statutory requirement. All doctors are required to notify any cases of specified infections seen by them to the designated proper officer for the relevant local authority. Notification is based on clinical suspicion and does not require laboratory confirmation, although if the diagnosis is altered as a result of laboratory investigations, the notification can be corrected by the notifying doctor. A small fee is payable for each notification.

Notifiable diseases in the UK (differs in Scotland)
1 Acute encephalitis.
2 Acute poliomyelitis.
3 Anthrax.
4 Cholera.
5 Diphtheria.
6 Dysentery (amoebic or bacillary).
7 Leprosy.
8 Leptospirosis.
9 Malaria.
10 Measles.
11 Meningitis.
12 Meningococcal septicaemia (without meningitis).
13 Mumps.
14 Ophthalmia neonatorum.
15 Paratyphoid fever.
16 Plague.
17 Rabies.
18 Relapsing fever.
19 Rubella.
20 Scarlet fever.
21 Smallpox.
22 Tetanus.
23 Tuberculosis.
24 Typhoid fever.
25 Typhus.
26 Viral haemorrhagic fever.
27 Viral hepatitis.
28 Whooping cough.
29 Yellow fever.

Weekly summaries of notifications are forwarded from local authorities to the OPCS where they are collated into weekly, quarterly and annual reports. These reports are transmitted to the national agencies for communicable disease surveillance (CDSC and CD(S)U).

The notification system has developed over more than 100 years. Many of the conditions are of historical interest only, whereas others, e.g. legionellosis, are noticeable by their absence. A local authority has the discretion to add conditions to the list that occur in that authority; addition of a disease to the national list requires approval by the Secretary of State.

Laboratory reports

Laboratory reports provide reliable information on many infections. These are provided on a voluntary basis by National Health Service, public health and private laboratories to the CDSC and CD(S)U. The main limitation of laboratory data is that they are biased towards patients with severe infections or where laboratory confirmation is likely to influence management. For some conditions, especially many viral infections, laboratory reports do not therefore provide a representative picture of infection in the community.

General practitioner surveillance schemes

The Royal College of General Practitioners (RCGP) operates a national network of 'spotter' practices, serving a population of approximately 750 000, who provide weekly reports of first-time consultations on a variety of infectious and non-infectious conditions. It provides a particularly sensitive index of influenza activity.

In addition to the RCGP scheme, local general practitioner surveillance networks operate in several parts of the country, including Wales, Oxford and Surrey.

Hospital data

Hospital data provide useful information on infections that usually require admission, such as meningococcal meningitis. They tend however to be incomplete and out of date.

Clinic data

Clinic data are useful for certain conditions, particularly sexually transmitted diseases. Annual returns of numbers of diagnoses from sexually transmitted disease clinics are collected by the Department of Health.

Death certificates

Death certificates have a limited contribution to surveillance, as deaths from infection are rare. However, the ratio of deaths to cases (the case fatality ratio) can provide useful information on the changing severity of some diseases and the effectiveness of new treatment measures.

Other useful routine sources of data include the Medical Officers of Schools Association (MOSA) which reports incidents in boarding schools, the Emergency Bed Service and some occupational health departments.

Special surveillance schemes

For some infections, routine data are not available and special surveillance systems have been established. Examples in the UK include the confidential reporting of AIDS and human immunodeficiency virus (HIV)-related disease to the CDSC and CD(S)U, the National Congenital Rubella Registry at the Institute of Child Health, and the BPASU. Under the BPASU scheme, all consultant paediatricians are sent a monthly card with a menu of about 12 reportable conditions. Any cases seen are then followed up by the lead investigator for that condition. Conditions may be added to or deleted from the menu on application to the BPASU. The BPASU scheme has been particularly useful for ascertaining cases of rare infectious disorders such as subacute sclerosing panencephalitis.

Dissemination of information

Notification data are published in the Registrar General's *Weekly Return*, the quarterly OPCS *Infectious Disease Monitors* and an annual volume, *Communicable Disease Statistics*. The weekly *Communicable Disease Report* (CDR) is published by the CDSC and contains both laboratory and notification data. The CDR is distributed to CCDCs, microbiologists, infectious disease physicians and others with an interest in communicable disease control. Similar bulletins are published in other countries, for example the *Morbidity and Mortality Weekly Report* (MMWR) in the USA.

Surveillance in other countries

Most countries operate a notification system for communicable diseases, although the list of reportable conditions varies widely from one country to another. In North America, the use of standardized case definitions has been widely adopted. In some countries, telephone reporting is used. In France, general practitioners report through minicomputer terminals linked via the national telephone network. Pan-European surveillance is now being developed for a number of infections including AIDS, travel-associated legionellosis, meningococcal infection and influenza.

Prevention and control of communicable disease

Prevention may be primary, secondary or tertiary. Primary prevention aims to prevent or reduce exposure to the infectious agent. This is the most effective method, but also the most difficult to achieve. The purpose of secondary prevention is to detect infection at an early stage, so that control measures to prevent further spread can be taken. Much of the day-to-day work of a CCDC is secondary prevention. In tertiary prevention, the aim is to minimize the disability arising from infection.

There is a wide range of measures that may be taken to prevent or control infection in the community and in hospitals (Table 25.1). Some of these measures may be used for more than one type of prevention. Control procedures that relate mainly to the control of infection in the community are discussed in this chapter; for the control of infection in hospitals see Chapter 23.

Social and environmental factors

Although infection is still an important clinical problem in developed societies, many of the more serious diseases that were common in the past have largely been brought under control. In contrast, infectious disease remains a major cause of morbidity and mortality in developing countries.

Primary prevention	Secondary prevention	Tertiary prevention
Immunization (pre-exposure)	Immunization (postexposure)	Effective treatment of acute infection*
Improved housing and sanitation	Contact tracing	Management of postinfectious disorders†
Provision of safe food, pasteurization of milk	Screening of food handlers, health workers, etc.	Physiotherapy, speech therapy
Vector control	Chemoprophylaxis	
Behaviour modification (sexual, hygiene, etc.)	Effective surveillance	
Isolation, barrier nursing‡	Outbreak investigation and management	
Disinfection, sterilization‡		
Laboratory safety‡		

*See Chapter 4.
†See Chapter 24.
‡See Chapter 23.

Table 25.1 Prevention and control of infection

The main factors in reducing the burden of infectious disease in western society were the improvements in social and environmental conditions that took place in the late 19th and early 20th century. Public health legislation forced industry and local government to spend money on sanitation and better housing. The average family size shrank rapidly during the early part of the 20th century, resulting in less crowding. Better nutrition meant that the population was less susceptible to disease.

The most important environmental measures are provision of adequately treated drinking water and safe disposal of faeces. Water-borne infection accounts for more deaths in developing countries than any other disease (Fig. 25.1). The recent spread of cholera throughout South America illustrates the vital importance of basic sanitation. Even in the UK, water-borne outbreaks, for example of cryptosporidiosis, are relatively common, due to treatment failures and posttreatment contamination of water supplies.

Better housing conditions have made a major contribution to controlling respiratory infections such as tuberculosis that are spread by close person-to-person contact. The reduction in tuberculosis illustrates the relative importance of environmental conditions compared to more high-tech prevention methods. Cases of respiratory tuberculosis have markedly declined since reliable records began last century. The introduction of mass radiography, chemotherapy and

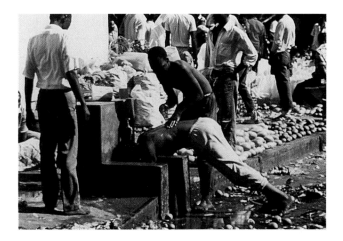

Fig. 25.1 Consumption of untreated water in a developing country: a major source of infection. Courtesy of SmithKline Beecham.

bacillus Calmette–Guérin (BCG) vaccination in the second half of this century has made virtually no difference to the rate of decline (Fig. 25.2).

Paradoxically, the burden of some infectious diseases actually rises as living conditions improve. This applies to conditions where the rate of complications is greater in adults than in children. The epidemics of paralytic poliomyelitis that occurred in the 1940s and 1950s are attributed to improved sanitation with a consequent reduction of wild virus circulation in young children

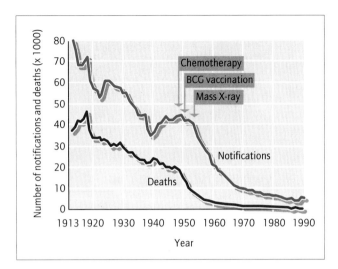

Fig. 25.2 Respiratory tuberculosis in England and Wales from 1913 to 1990. The disease started to decline long before chemotherapy and other medical interventions became available, due to improvements in living conditions.

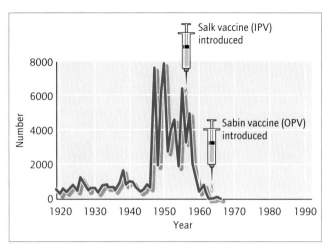

Fig. 25.3 Paralytic poliomyelitis in England and Wales from 1914 to 1992. The outbreaks in the 1940s and 1950s were associated with an increasing age at infection, with a corresponding increase in the ratio of paralytic to non-paralytic cases. IPV, inactivated poliovaccine; OPV, oral poliovaccine.

(Fig. 25.3). This led to an increase in the average age at which infection occurred. As the ratio of paralytic to non-paralytic cases rises with age, the number of paralytic cases actually increased. A similar phenomenon has recently been observed for hepatitis A in some countries, where the number of cases with jaundice is rising as the average age at infection increases.

Another infection to emerge as result of modern living is legionnaire's disease. The causal agent, *Legionella pneumophila*, thrives in microenvironments such as showerheads, cooling towers and air-conditioning units. Outbreaks of legionnaire's disease occur when bacterially contaminated aerosols are generated from these water systems, particularly when the systems are not properly maintained (Fig. 25.4).

Health education

Many health education programmes have been conducted at local and national levels with the aim of reducing exposure to infectious diseases. These include safe sex campaigns, needle exchange schemes, advice to pregnant women, guidance on food hygiene and advice to travellers. These campaigns have been conducted by government bodies such as the Health Education Authority, voluntary agencies and industry (especially in relation to food hygiene). At the local level many individuals and agencies may be involved, including CCDCs, general practitioners, health promotion departments, health visitors and voluntary groups.

With a few notable exceptions, health education has met with limited success in preventing exposure to communicable disease. Research has shown that campaigns often succeed in raising public awareness, but seldom result in behaviour modification. Where behaviour modification does occur, it is often short-lived. Many infectious diseases are considered by the public to be relatively unimportant. The smaller the perceived risk of infection, the less likely that an education programme will succeed. The advent of AIDS, together with the high media profile for diseases such as food poisoning, legionellosis and meningococcal meningitis, has however shifted the public perception of infectious disease in recent years.

In general, the education programmes most likely to succeed are those that involve the local community in their design and implementation, and are ongoing rather than one-off events.

Food safety

Salmonellosis and other bacterial causes of food poisoning have increased considerably in recent years (see Chapter 8). This has attracted considerable public attention and led to a major review of the legislation governing food safety, culminating in the Food Safety Act 1990. Food law has now been harmonized across the European Community since the introduction of the single European market.

Much of the responsibilty for enforcement of food safety legislation lies with environmental health officers

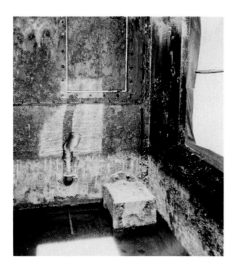

Fig. 25.4 Inside view of a cooling tower — a potential source for *Legionella pneumophila*. This badly maintained tower was the source of a large outbreak of legionnaire's disease.

Arthropod	Diseases
Mosquito	Malaria, dengue fever, filiariasis, yellow fever
Sandfly	Leishmaniasis, sandfly fever
Fly	Trypanosomiasis
Flea	Plague, rickettsial fevers, tungiasis
Tick	Relapsing fever
Mite	Scabies, typhus
Maggot	Myiasis
Louse	Pediculosis, relapsing fever, typhus

Table 25.3 Arthropods of medical importance

(EHOs) who are employed by local authorities to inspect food premises. MAFF officers carry out enforcement duties on dairy farms. This includes the extensive legislation which has recently been introduced to control *Salmonella* infection.

Pasteurization of milk greatly reduces the risk of exposure to many pathogens such as *Mycobacterium bovis* and *Campylobacter* sp. In Scotland it is illegal to produce or sell unpasteurized milk, whereas in England and Wales it is not. The ban in Scotland has led to a substantial reduction in the number of milk-associated outbreaks compared to England (Table 25.2).

	England and Wales		Scotland	
Time period	No. of outbreaks	No. of cases	No. of outbreaks	No. of cases
1980–1982	40	540	21	1090
1983–1984	22	518	8	46

Table 25.2 Milk-borne outbreaks of salmonellosis in England, Wales and Scotland, from 1980 to 1984, showing the impact of compulsory pasteurization in Scotland in 1983

Vector control

This is particularly important in tropical countries where arthropods play an important role in many infections,

both as vectors and as primary causal agents (Table 25.3).

Travellers to the tropics can reduce the risk of infection by taking measures to avoid insect bites using, for example, repellents such as diethyl toluamide, mosquito nets and protective clothing. Attempts to control insect populations by the use of pesticides have usually been unsuccessful due to the emergence of resistance.

Immunization

The introduction of effective immunization programmes has been one of the most significant public health achievements this century. The control of smallpox, polio and diphtheria would not have been possible without the development of immunizing agents against these diseases.

Vaccines and immunoglobulins

Immunization may be achieved passively by administration of an immunoglobulin preparation, or actively by use of a live or non-replicating vaccine.

Immunoglobulins

Immunoglobulins are prepared from plasma treated by ethanol fractionation. They provide short-term protection against certain infections and are also used in the treatment of immune disorders and to supplement antiviral therapy, especially in the immunocompromised (see Chapter 21). The most commonly used preparation is human immunoglobulin (HIG) which is prepared from pooled plasma and therefore contains antibodies to viruses that are prevalent in the general population. HIG is mainly used for postexposure prophylaxis of acute hepatitis A. It is also given to travellers to countries where hepatitis A is endemic; however as protection is relatively short-lived and active immunization is now available, its role in pre-exposure prophylaxis is diminishing. The other main indication for HIG is for postexposure prophylaxis against measles in immuno-suppressed contacts.

Other immunoglobulins are available for post-exposure management of specific infections. These are prepared from hyperimmune donors. Hepatitis B immunoglobulin, in combination with active immun-ization, is used for postexposure prophylaxis following accidental exposure to infected blood, and for babies born to acutely or chronically infected mothers. Varicella-zoster immunoglobulin is indicated for sus-ceptible immunosuppressed and pregnant contacts of chickenpox or herpes zoster, for neonates whose mothers develop chickenpox in the period 7 days before to 7 days after delivery and for susceptible neonates in contact with chickenpox or zoster. Tetanus immuno-globulin is used in the management of tetanus-prone wounds in patients who have not been immunized or in whom the last dose of vaccine was given more than 10 years previously. Tick-borne encephalitis immuno-globulin is available in countries where the disease is endemic, notably Austria, for prophylaxis following tick bites. Rabies immunoglobulin is indicated for prophy-laxis following warm-blooded animal bites in countries where the disease is endemic in the animal population.

Immunoglobulins and their use for prophylaxis of infection

1 Human immunoglobulin: pre-exposure prophylaxis of hepatitis A for short-term travel abroad (2 months or less), adult 250 mg; child under 10 years 125 mg; longer-term travel (3–5 months) and for postexposure pro-phylaxis of hepatitis A 500 mg; child under 10 years 250 mg.
Postexposure prophylaxis of measles: child under 1 year 250 mg, 1–2 years 500 mg, 3 years and over 750 mg; to allow an attenuated attack, child under 1 year 100 mg, 1 year and over 250 mg.
2 Hepatitis B immunoglobulin: for postexposure prophy-laxis, adult 500 U, child under 4 years 200 U, 5–9 years 300 U, neonate 200 U as soon as possible after birth.
3 Human rabies immunoglobulin: for postexposure pro-phylaxis, 20 U/kg, half by i.m. infection and half by filtration around the wound.
4 Tetanus immunoglobulin: for postexposure pro-phylaxis, 250 U, increased to 500 U if more than 24 h have elapsed or if there is risk of heavy contamination.
5 Varicella-zoster immunoglobulin: for postexposure prophylaxis (as soon as possible and not later than 10 days after exposure), child up to 5 years 250 mg, 6–10 years 500 mg, 11–14 years 750 mg, over 15 years 1 g;

---

second dose required if further exposure occurs after 3 weeks.
6 Tick-borne encephalitis immunoglobulin: this is avail-able for postexposure prophylaxis after a tick bite in an endemic area.
All of the above preparations should be given intra-muscularly.

Vaccines

Vaccines are derived from whole viruses and bacteria, or their antigenic components. Live vaccines are prepared from attenuated strains that have minimal pathogenicity but are capable of inducing a protective immune response. They multiply in the human host and provide antigenic stimulation over a period of time. This results in durable immunity, usually after a single dose. Vaccine failures are uncommon, and are usually the result of inadequate handling or administration. The main dis-advantage of live vaccines is that they occasionally cause a full-blown infection in the recipient. This is most likely to occur in the immunosuppressed patient; live vaccines are usually contraindicated for this group. Their use in pregnancy should also be avoided because of the potential risk of fetal infection.

Non-replicating vaccines contain either inactivated whole organisms or antigenic components. Increasingly sophisticated methods are being used to produce these vaccines, such as protein–polysaccharide conjugation (*Haemophilus influenzae*) and genetic expression of pro-tective antigens (hepatitis B). Because replication does not take place in the human host, non-replicating vaccines are safe for use in pregnancy and in the immunosuppressed. Their disadvantage is that more than one dose is usually required for protection. Local reactions are relatively com-mon with non-replicating vaccines; this is related to the quantity of antigen they contain.

Types of vaccines, their modes of action and contraindications

Live: examples — bacillus Calmette–Guérin (BCG), measles, mumps, rubella, oral polio, yellow fever
1 Multiply inside the human host and provide con-tinuous antigenic stimulation over a period of time.
2 Provide durable immunity, usually after a single dose.
3 Contraindicated in pregnancy and the immuno-suppressed.

Killed: examples — pertussis, influenza, Haemophilus influenzae type b, rabies, typhoid
1 Do not multiply inside the human host.
2 Antibody response is related to the antigen content and potency.

3 Multiple doses are often required, with subsequent booster doses.
4 No general contraindications.

Strategic aspects of immunization programmes

The aim of an immunization programme may be eradication, elimination or containment.

Eradication is total absence of the organism in humans, animals and the environment. Once a disease has been eradicated, the immunization programme can be discontinued. The only disease that has been eradicated by immunization is smallpox. Smallpox had many features that favoured eradication — an easily recognizable illness with no subclinical or latent infection, no long-term carriers, visible evidence of immunity (a characteristic scar), absence of non-human hosts, low infectivity and a long incubation period. Poliomyelitis shares many of these characteristics, and the World Health Organization now intends to eradicate polio globally by the year 2000. Elimination is where the disease has disappeared, but the organism remains in animal hosts, the environment or causing subclinical infection in humans. Unlike eradication, it is not possible to discontinue immunization. Containment is the point at which a disease, although not eliminated, is no longer considered to be a significant public health problem.

Possible aims for an immunization programme, with examples of diseases for which these have been achieved
1 Eradication: removal of the causal agent (e.g. smallpox).
2 Elimination: absence of disease, although the causal agent remains (e.g. polio).
3 Control: reduction of disease to the point at which it is no longer a public health problem (e.g. *Haemophilus influenzae* type b).

There are two basic approaches to immunization programmes: universal or selective. Universal immunization has been adopted for most of the childhood vaccines. A selective programme aims to protect only those at risk from disease. This is less expensive than universal immunization, and tends to be used for the more costly vaccines such as hepatitis B. In practice it is often difficult to identify and immunize those who are genuinely at risk.

Immunization schedules

The ages at which vaccines are given, and the preparations used, vary considerably from one country to

Age	Vaccines
2 months	Diphtheria/tetanus/pertussis (DTP)
	Haemophilus influenzae type b (Hib)
	Oral poliovaccine (OPV)
3 months	DTP
	Hib
	OPV
4 months	DTP
	Hib
	OPV
12–15 months	Measles/mumps/rubella (MMR)
4–5 years	Diphtheria/tetanus (DT)
	OPV
10–14 years*	Bacillus Calmette–Guérin (BCG)
15–18 years	Tetanus/low-dose diphtheria (Td)
	OPV

* In some parts of the country BCG is given in the neonatal period.

Table 25.4 British childhood immunization schedule (mid-1990s)

another. The approach in the UK has been to minimize the number of clinic visits and to secure protection as early in life as possible, without compromising efficacy. The currently recommended schedule is shown in Table 25.4. The British schedule is similar to that used in many European countries and in the USA.

Surveillance of immunization programmes

The ingredients for a successful immunization programme are a safe, effective vaccine and high coverage (uptake) in the target population. The safety and efficacy of vaccines are established in clinical trials before they are licensed. After licensing, batches of all vaccines are regularly tested for potency and toxicity at the National Institute for Biological Standards and Control (NIBSC) before release. Any severe or unusual reactions to vaccines should be reported on a yellow card to the Committee on Safety of Medicines. Additional surveillance schemes have been established to monitor the efficacy and safety of some vaccines, e.g. BCG. Annual serological surveys of age-specific antibody prevalence to measles, mumps and rubella (MMR) are undertaken by the CDSC to monitor the impact of the MMR vaccine. Coverage of vaccines is assessed from annual returns to the health departments and the COVER (cover of vaccination evaluated rapidly) scheme, which is run by the CDSC.

The target coverage for childhood vaccines is 95% at 2 years of age. Most immunizations are given by general practitioners, who are paid according to whether they achieve targets. Each health district has a designated immunization coordinator, who is usually either a community paediatrician or the CCDC, with local re-

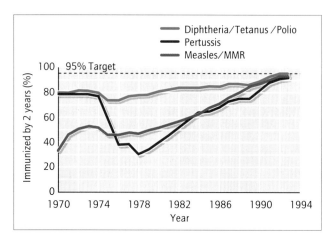

Fig. 25.5 Vaccine coverage in England and Wales from 1970 to 1993.

sponsibility for management of the programme. Vaccine coverage has improved considerably in recent years (Fig. 25.5).

Contact tracing

The principle of contact tracing is to identify those who have been in contact with an infectious disease in order that preventive measures can be taken. These measures may include screening for evidence of infection and subsequent treatment, active or passive immunization and chemoprophylaxis (see below).

For contact tracing to be successful, speed of notification of the index case and follow-up of contacts are of the essence. This poses particular difficulties for sexually transmitted diseases, where patients may be unwilling to notify their partners. Contact tracing is most likely to be effective for infections with longer incubation periods and where adequate chemotherapy is available.

Chemoprophylaxis

This is used for control of more serious infections such as diphtheria and meningococcal disease. It is also sometimes used during influenza outbreaks among high-risk patients, such as elderly nursing-home residents. The aim of chemoprophylaxis may be either to eliminate carriage of pathogenic organisms, reducing the risk of

infection in those not yet exposed, or to treat newly acquired infection in contacts who are non-immune and may be incubating the disease. The former requires prophylaxis of a large contact network, whereas the latter can be achieved by treating only those who have been in close contact with the index case. Both strategies can be difficult to implement as they require healthy individuals to take antibiotics which may produce side-effects. Single-dose regimens are the most effective. It is important to determine the antibiotic sensitivity of the strain from the index case, as this may influence the agent selected for chemoprophylaxis.

Example of a chemoprophylaxis regimen, in this case for meningococcal disease
Rifampicin 600 mg orally every 12 h for 2 days; child 10 mg/kg (3 months–1 year, 5 mg/kg) every 12 h for 2 days; contraindicated in pregnancy, liver disease and alcoholism.
Alternative: ciprofloxacin 500 mg single oral dose (adults and children over 10 years only); contraindicated in pregnancy.

Screening

A screening programme should fulfil the following criteria. First, the disease should be an important public health problem. Second, there should be a recognizable latent or early symptomatic stage. Third, the screening test should be harmless, sensitive and specific. Finally, effective treatment should be available for the condition in question with general agreement on who should be treated.

It is rare that these criteria can be met. Screening for infectious disease is often adopted in response to public and political pressure or for medicolegal reasons rather than on the basis of sound public health. For example, it is commonplace to exclude food-handlers with recent *Salmonella* infection until three consecutive negative stool samples are obtained. This results in unnecessary time off work and contributes little to the control of food poisoning. Screening for tuberculosis by mass radiography has been discontinued, although tuberculin testing is still widely used for screening of health care workers and teachers. The most effective screening programmes have been those aimed at preventing congenital rubella and syphilis (see Chapter 12).

Outbreak investigation

Although there is no legal requirement for CCDCs to investigate outbreaks, there is no doubt that prompt

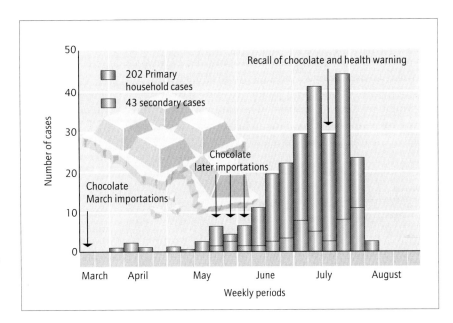

Fig. 25.6 The epidemic curve for an outbreak of *Salmonella napoli* caused by contaminated chocolate, showing the impact of rapid identification and removal of the source.

identification and control of incidents can prevent substantial morbidity. For example, it was estimated that 30 000 cases of salmonellosis were averted following the investigation of a single outbreak which was caused by contaminated imported chocolate (Fig. 25.6).

Methods

Prompt recognition of the outbreak is a prerequisite. For this, adequate surveillance must be in place. When apparent clusters are identified, it is important to distinguish between true outbreaks and those caused by reporting artefacts. A knowledge of the expected incidence for the time of year and place is necessary. Factors that may cause a pseudo-outbreak include the availability of a new or more sensitive laboratory test, the appointment of a physician with a particular disease interest and undue media involvement.

The next step is to confirm the diagnosis. This may seem obvious, but is often overlooked. In 1985, a large outbreak of legionnellosis associated with a hospital outpatient department was initially labelled as epidemic influenza until appropriate laboratory investigations were undertaken. Once the diagnosis has been confirmed, a case definition should be developed. Initially this should be non-specific so that all suspected cases can be identified and investigated; later on in the investigation a more rigorous definition, often with laboratory confirmation, will be required. This case definition should then be the basis for collecting and counting cases. Collection of cases will often involve active case finding, for example, by phoning general practitioners, laboratories and hospitals.

At this stage of the investigation, the aim is to formulate a hypothesis that explains the source of the outbreak, the mode of transmission and the duration. The basic epidemiological information to be collected on all cases must include date of onset of symptoms, age/sex and place of residence (time, person, place). This information should be tabulated and an epidemic curve drawn. Additional information required will depend on the nature of the outbreak. For example, a salmonella incident will involve obtaining food consumption histories, whereas in an outbreak of legionnaire's disease details of likely exposures should be sought, such as foreign travel. These preliminary enquiries should be carefully conducted as face-to-face interviews, ideally with cases affected early in the outbreak.

The hypothesis generated should then be tested by a formal analytical study. This may either be a case-control or cohort study. In a case-control study, exposure histories are sought from cases and healthy controls. The relative risk of exposure to the postulated source of the outbreak is then calculated for cases and controls. The controls must be drawn from the same population as the cases, so that they have had the same opportunity for exposure to the source. Case-control studies are suited to investigation of uncommon infections such as botulism. Their main disadvantage is the potential for bias arising from selection of controls.

In a cohort study, the disease outcome is compared between those exposed and not exposed to the source.

Cohort studies are often used for the investigation of outbreaks with high attack rates such as food-poisoning incidents. They are more time-consuming and expensive than case-control studies, but less prone to bias.

In both case-control and cohort studies a structured questionnaire should be used. The interviews are conducted by phone or face to face; in larger investigations a postal questionnaire may be used.

> **Steps in the investigation of an outbreak of infectious disease**
> 1 Establish that an outbreak exists.
> 2 Confirm the diagnosis.
> 3 Define the population at risk.
> 4 Define, collect and count cases.
> 5 Describe the cases according to time (onset), person (age/sex) and place.
> 6 Formulate a hypothesis to explain the source, mode of transmission and duration of outbreak.
> 7 Test the hypothesis by an analytical study (case-control or cohort).
> 8 Plan and implement control measures.
> 9 Evaluate effectiveness of control measures.

A major difficulty with outbreak investigations is recall bias. The interviews may be conducted several days or even weeks after the event. Patients may not remember their exposures or bias their responses towards their perception of the source of the outbreak. For example, patients affected by food poisoning frequently ascribe their symptoms to the meal consumed immediately before the onset of illness, rather than in the period 24–48 h previously; their recall for the earlier meals may therefore be less accurate. This can be overcome by giving prompts, such as asking patients to consult their diary during the interview. It is also important to conceal the exposure variable in the questionnaire by including questions about other exposures that are not under investigation.

Organization and management

The CCDC should, at an early stage, convene an action committee which should meet frequently to review progress and plan control measures. This group may include the local microbiologist, chief environmental health officer, director of public health, public health laboratory director, hospital control of infection officer, a representative of the suspected source (e.g. a water company) and, where appropriate, representatives of CDSC and MAFF. It is important that all communication with the press is through a single source; the action committee should agree the contents of all press statements.

All stages of the outbreak investigation should be carefully documented. This is particularly important where legal action is likely to ensue. A preliminary report should be prepared within 48 h of the investigation, and interim reports at regular intervals thereafter. These should be approved by the action committee. The final report should be a comprehensive account of the investigation and include an evaluation of the control measures that were implemented as well as recommendations for the prevention and management of future incidents.

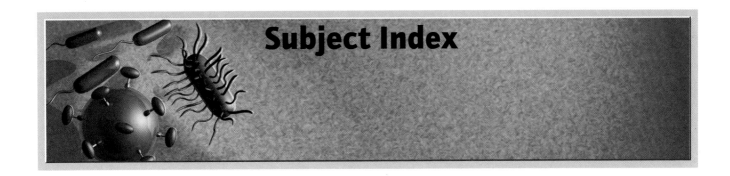

Subject Index

Page numbers in *italics* refer to figures and tables

465

tuberculous peritonitis, 349
tularaemia, 287, 387, 392, 401
  cutaneous-lymphatic, 401
  diagnosis, 401
  treatment, 401
  typhoidal, 401
tumour necrosis factor, 10
  body temperature effects, 17
  inhibition, 295
  meningococcal meningitis, 316
  mycobacterial infection, 345
  production, 16
typhoid, 371–4
  antibiotic treatment, 374
  antigen detection, 373
  clinical features, 371–3
  complications, 372
  diagnosis, 373
  enteric fever, 371
  immunization, 374, 390
  management, 374
  prevention, 374
  relapse, 372–3
typhoid fever, encephalopathy, 324
typhus fever
  encephalopathy, 324
  types, 378
typing microorganisms, 41–4
  auxotyping, 42
  bacteriocin, 43
  biotyping, 42
  molecular methods, 43–4
  nucleic acid, 43
  protein, 43
  serological, 42
  simple laboratory, 41–2

ulcer, tropical, 344
ultraviolet radiation, 369
umbilical infection, 253
upper respiratory tract flora, 103
upper respiratory tract infections, 103
  acute otitis media, 106–7
  conjunctivitis, 103–6
  meningococcal meningitis, 316
  paranasal sinusitis, 107
Ureaplasma urealyticum non-specific genital
  infection, 222
ureteric reflux, 214
ureteric stricture, 287
  Gram-negative septicaemia, 300
urethra
  normal human flora, 3
  symptoms of infection, 208
urethral caruncle, 212, 213
urethral obstruction, 215
urethral strictures, 225
urethral syndrome, 211–13
urethritis, 211–13, 222
  clinical features, 212
  diagnosis, 212
  management, 212–13
urinary bladder, symptoms of infection, 208
urinary catheters, 430–1
  closed drainage systems, 430–1
  colonization, 430
urinary tract
  abnormalities, 215
  mucosa, 8
urinary tract infection, 207

ascending, 213–14
automated identification methods, 211
children, 214–15
culture, 210–11
diagnosis, 208–11
identification, 211
laboratory diagnosis, 210–11
men, 215
microbiological diagnosis, 209–11
microscopy, 210
pathogenesis, 207–8
predisposition, 207
pregnancy, 215
prophylaxis, 214
screening techniques, 208–9
sensitivity tests, 211
specimens, 209–10
symptoms, 208
three glass test, 208, *209*
urethral syndrome, 211–13
urethritis, 211–13
white cells, 209
urine, suprapubic aspiration, 209
uveitis, Reiter's syndrome, 452

V-beta receptors, 14
vaccines, 460–1
  coverage, 461–2
  failure, 460
  killed, 460–1
  live, 460
  non-replicating, 460
vaccinia autoinoculation lesions, *86*
vagina, normal human flora, 3
vaginal intraepithelial neoplasia, 219
vaginosis, bacterial, 228
valaciclovir, 221
  herpes zoster, 83
valproate, 18
vancomycin, 52, 69, 428
  endocarditis, 280, 281
variable surface glycoprotein (VSG), 15
varicella
  embryopathy, 245–6
  vaccine, 270
varicella infection
  intrauterine, 239
  maternal, 246
  neonatal, 246
  Reye's syndrome, 449
  see also chickenpox
varicella zoster
  immunoglobulin, 270, 460
  pneumonitis, 50
vasculitis, 77
vasodilators, 293
vectors, 5
  arthropod, 30, 377–86, 459
  helminths, 33
  protozoa, 31
ventriculitis, *Streptococcus milleri*, 323
verocytotoxin-producing *E. coli*, 159, 160
  laboratory diagnosis, 162
  management, 162
verrucae, 78–9
vertebral body collapse, 359
vidarabine, 86
Vincent's angina, 37, 124–5
viral antigens, 14
  capsid, 110, 112

viral culture, 44
viral encephalitides, 31
viral haemorrhagic fevers, 387–90
  management, 388
  public health measures, 390
  with renal syndromes, 387–8
viral infections
  gastrointestinal tract, 154, 156–8
  liver, 183–95
  lower respiratory tract, 127–35
  mouth, 107–13
  skin/mucosae, 78–86
  T-cell deficiency, 408
  throat, 107–13
virulence, 2
virus, 22
  attachment, 25
  capsid symmetry, 25, *26*
  classification, 22, 24
  envelope, 25
  genomic structure, 24
  nucleic acid, 24
  structure, 22, *23*, 24–5, *26*
Volkmann's canal, 334
Volkmann's system, 331
vomiting, treatment, 153–4
vomitus, 152

warts
  common, 78
  genital, 78, 218
  plantar, 78–9
water
  drinking, 371, 374, 377, 390
    infection spread, 457
  purification, 390
  supply and hospital infections, 433
  systems, *142*, 143
    legionnaire's disease, 458, *459*
watercress, wild, 205, 206
Waterhouse–Friderichson syndrome, 121
Wegener's granulomatosis, 423
Weil's disease, 196
Western blotting, 49–50
whipworms, 179
whooping cough *see* pertussis
Widal agglutination test, 373
winter vomiting disease, 157–8
wound isolation, 435

yellow fever, 194–5, 387
  clinical features, 195
  epidemiology, 194–5
  prevention, 195
  sylvan, 194
  vaccination, 195, 390–1
Yersinia infections, 170–1

zalcitabine, 236
zidovudine, 73, 236
  HIV 1 vertical transmission, 246
Ziehl–Nielsen stain, 37, 38
zoonoses, 5, 6, 392
  hydatid disease, 33
  pregnancy, 255
  streptococcal infections, 401–2
zoster immune globulin (ZIG), 245–6
zymodemes, 44

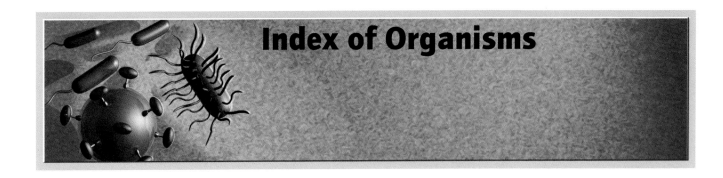

Index of Organisms

Page numbers in **bold** refer to main entries; those in *italics* refer to figures and tables